5,14,15,38

Diseases of the ear

Diseases of the ear

Sixth edition

Edited by

Harold Ludman MA MB(Cantab) FRCS(Eng)

Consultant Otolaryngologist and Surgeon in Neuro-otology, National Hospital for Neurology and Neurosurgery, Queen Square, London; Emeritus Consultant Otolaryngologist, King's College Hospital, London, UK

and

Tony Wright LLM DM FRCS Tech RMS

Head of Department and Professor of Otorhinolaryngology, Institute of Laryngology and Otology, University College London; Honorary Consultant, Royal National Throat Nose and Ear Hospital, London, UK

A member of the Hodder Headline Group
LONDON • SYDNEY • AUCKLAND
Co-published in the USA by Oxford University Press, Inc., New York

First published in Great Britain 1998
Arnold, a member of the Hodder Headline Group,
338 Euston Road, London NW1 3BH

http:\\www.arnoldpublishers.com

Co-published in the United States of America by
Oxford University Press, Inc.,
198 Madison Avenue, New York, NY10016
Oxford is a registered trademark of Oxford University Press

Whilst the advice and information in this book is believed to be true and
accurate at the date of going to press, neither the authors nor the publisher
can accept any legal responsibility or liability for any errors or omissions that
may be made. In particular (but without limiting the generality of the
preceding disclaimer) every effort has been made to check drug dosages;
however it is still possible that errors have been missed. Furthermore,
dosage schedules are constantly being revised and new side-effects
recognized. For these reasons the reader is strongly urged to consult the
drug companies' printed instructions before administering any of the drugs
recommended in this book.

Publisher: Georgina Bentloff
Project editor: Sophie Oliver
Production editor: Julie Delf
Project manager: Alison Creedy
Production controller: Rose James
Cover designer: Terry Griffiths

British Library Cataloguing in Publication Data
A catalogue record for this book is available from the British Library

Library of Congress Cataloging-in-Publication Data
A catalog record for this book is available from the Library of Congress

ISBN 0340 56441 5

Composition by Scribe Design, Gillingham, Kent
Printed and bound by The Bath Press, Bath

Contents

III Congenital ear disease

IV Acquired external ear disease

V Acquired middle ear disease

VI Acquired inner ear disease

Contributors

Peter W Alberti MB PhD FRCS(C)
Professor of Otolaryngology, Department of Otolaryngology, Faculty of Medicine, University of Toronto, Toronto, Canada

Amos Ar PhD
Professor of Physiology, Department of Zoology, George S. Wise Faculty of Life Sciences, Tel-Aviv University, Israel

Derald E Brackmann MD
Clinical Professor of Otolaryngology – Head and Neck Surgery, University of Southern California; President and Associate, House Ear Clinic, House Ear Institute, Los Angeles, California, USA

Paul B Van Cauwenberge MD PhD
Professor and Chairman, Department of Otolaryngology, University of Ghent, B-9000 Ghent, Belgium

Graeme M Clark AO
Professor of Otolaryngology, Special Research Centre for Human Communication Research, Department of Otolaryngology, The University of Melbourne; The Co-operative Research Centre for Cochlear Implant Speech and Hearing Research and the Bionic Ear Institute, Melbourne, Australia

Adrian Davis MSc PhD
Professor of the Department of Surgery (ENT), Head of Epidemiology, Public Health and Clinical Sections, MRC Institute of Hearing Research, University Park, University of Nottingham, Nottingham, UK

Rosalyn A Davies MRCP PhD
Consultant Audiological Physician in Neuro-otology, National Hospital for Neurology and Neurosurgery, Queen Square, London, UK

Ingeborg Dhooge MD PhD
Assistant Professor, Department of Otolaryngology, University of Ghent, B-9000 Ghent, Belgium

Michael E Glasscock III MD
Clinical Professor of Surgery (Otology-Neurotology), Associate Clinical Professor of Neurosurgery, Vanderbilt University School of Medicine, Nashville, Tennessee, USA

Jonathan WP Hazell FRCS
Unit Head and Consultant Neuro-Otologist, The Royal National Institute for Deaf People, Medical Research Unit, Royal National Throat Nose and Ear Hospital, London, UK

Anthony F Jahn MD PA FACS FRCS(C)
Professor of Clinical Otolaryngology, Columbia University College of Physicians and Surgeons; Director of Otology/Neurotology, St Luke's/Roosevelt Hospital Center, New York, New York, USA

P Jani BDS MBBS FRCS
Senior Registrar in Otolaryngology, Addenbrooke's Hospital, Cambridge, UK

Nick Jones BDS MBBS FRCS
Consultant ENT Surgeon, Department of Otolaryngology, Queen's Medical Centre, Nottingham, UK

David T Kemp PhD
Professor of Auditory Biophysics, Institute of Laryngology and Otology, University College London, UK

Harold Ludman MA MB(Cantab) FRCS(Eng)
Consultant Otolaryngologist and Surgeon in Neuro-otology, National Hospital for Neurology and Neurosurgery, Queen Square, London; Emeritus Consultant Otolaryngologist, King's College Hospital, London, UK

Linda M Luxon BSc FRCP
Professor of Audiological Medicine, Institute of Laryngology and Otology, University College London; Honorary Consultant Audiological Physician at the Royal National Throat Nose and Ear Hospital, London; Consultant Audiological Physician, The National Hospital for Neurology and Neurosurgery, Queen Square, London, UK

Henri AM Marres MD PhD
Consultant Ear, Nose and Throat Surgeon, Department of Oto-Rhino-Laryngology, University Hospital Nijmegen, Nijmegen, The Netherlands

A Richard Maw MS FRCS
Consultant Otolaryngologist, Royal Hospital for Sick Children, Bristol; Senior Clinical Lecturer, Department of Otolaryngology, University of Bristol, UK

Mark May MD FACS
Professor, Department of Otolaryngology, University of Pittsburgh Medical School, and the Facial Paralysis/Sinus Surgery Center, Shadyside Medical Center, Pittsburgh, Pennsylvania, USA

David A Moffat BSc MA FRCS
Consultant Otolaryngologist and Clinical Director, Department of Otoneurological and Skull Base Surgery, Addenbrooke's University Hospital Trust, Cambridge; Associate Lecturer, University of Cambridge, UK

Stefan EG De Moor MD
Attending Otolaryngologist, Department of Otolaryngology, University of Ghent, B-9000 Ghent, Belgium

Alec Fitzgerald O'Connor FRCS
Consultant Otolaryngologist and Clinical Director, Department of Otolaryngology, St Thomas' Hospital, London; Consultant Neurotologist, The Royal London Hospital NHS Trust, London, UK

Cliodna F OMahoney MRCGP MRCP(I) MSc
Consultant Audiological Physician, Department of Audiology, Great Ormond Street Hospital for Sick Children (NHS Trust), London, UK

Peter D Phelps MD FRCS FRCR
Consultant Radiologist, Royal National Throat Nose and Ear Hospital, London, and the Walsgrave Hospital NHS Trust, Coventry, UK

James Robinson FRCS
Consultant Otologist, ENT Department, Gloucester Royal Hospital, Gloucester, UK

Jacob Sadé MD
Professor of Otolaryngology, Ear Research Laboratory, Sara & Felix Dumont Chair of Hearing Research, Sackler School of Medicine and Bioengineering Program, Tel-Aviv University, Israel

Barry Schaitkin MD
Associate Professor of Otolaryngology, University of Pittsburgh Medical School, and the Facial Paralysis/Sinus Surgery Center, Shadyside Medical Center, Pittsburgh, Pennsylvania, USA

Susan Snashall MBBS MD
Consultant Audiological Physician, St George's Healthcare NHS Trust, St George's Hospital, London, UK

Dafydd Stephens FRCP
Consultant in Audiological Medicine, Welsh Hearing Institute, University Hospital of Wales, Heath Park, Cardiff, UK

Ian S Storper MD
Assistant Professor, Department Otolaryngology, Head and Neck Surgery, University of Michigan School of Medicine, Ann Arbor, Michigan, USA

Charles A Syms III MD
Assistant Professor of Surgery, Uniformed Services University of the Health Sciences, Staff Otologist/Neurotologist, Wilford Hall USAF Medical Center, San Antonio, TX; previously Clinical Fellow, House Ear Clinic, House Ear Institute, Los Angeles, California, USA

Tony Wright LLM DM FRCS Tech RMS
Head of Department and Professor of Otorhinolaryngology, Institute of Laryngology and Otology, University College London; Honorary Consultant, Royal National Throat Nose and Ear Hospital, London, UK

Robin Youngs MD FRCS
Consultant Otolaryngologist, Department of Otolaryngology, West Suffolk Hospital, Bury St Edmunds, Suffolk, UK

Preface

The first edition of 'Diseases of the Ear' was written in its entirety by Stuart Mawson – every single word from preface to index – and was published in 1963. His aim was to create a book, for candidates for the FRCS examination in Otolaryngology, that would provide all the information needed by trainees, as perceived and presented by a particularly distinguished otologist. That awesome achievement entailed several hard years of lucubration – working at night, early in the mornings and at weekends – while, at the same time, conducting a daunting clinical work load, and meeting the needs of other prestigious roles in the specialty. His personal and elegant writing style, and his renowned otological expertise, marked the work with the qualities that have formed the basis for its persisting success. As his Registrar at King's College Hospital at the time, I had the pleasure of producing all the line drawings for that edition, on the grounds that otolaryngological knowledge would be more valuable than professional artistic accomplishment. During the next 11 years Stuart Mawson undertook the whole single-handed authorship of the next two editions, updating and improving each time, with my new and revised drawings. The fourth edition was written jointly by Stuart Mawson and myself; then, after his retirement, I took on the task of partially rewriting, updating and illustrating the fifth edition. This incorporated a marked change from the previous 'inhouse' King's authorship, with chapters by a handful of additional contributors, to accommodate the needs of increasing supraspecialization.

Supraspecialization has burgeoned apace, and now, for this sixth edition, a large number of contributors have been assembled from all parts of the world. Furthermore editorship has been shared. I have had the incomparable good fortune of per-

suading Tony Wright, Professor of Otolaryngology at the Institute of Laryngology and Otology, Gray's Inn Road, London, to be my co-editor. This has been a collaboration that has proved enjoyable, helpful and enormously valuable. It is no exaggeration to say that, without his participation, it is doubtful whether this sixth edition would have appeared.

The many invited contributors are all acknowledged experts in their individual fields and have introduced strength and authority, but at the inevitable price of some difficulties and risks. The most obvious, which affect all multiauthor publications, are inconsistencies – even contradictions – and repetition. It has been our task as editors to try to strike a sensible balance to maintain consistency throughout. This has meant that many contributions have been radically edited to fit our overall plan, but we have deliberately retained some repetition intending that most contributions shall be self-sufficient without too much cross-reference, and also because we believe that some difficult concepts are better grasped after reading more than one description. We have exercised a certain amount of editorial presumption, some might say arrogance, in choosing and using our own preferred terminology and abbreviations for the many instances where there is no international uniform agreement, and where writers tend to favour their own idiosyncratic preferences. Since this is not a multivolume reference work, we have, occasionally, chosen to be didactic and have avoided polemic.

The overall principle, however, remains unchanged. Here, as with previous editions, we have created, between one set of covers, a book small enough to read comfortably. We hope it presents all the essential otological information for otologists in training, at a stage when, in the UK,

Australia, New Zealand, Canada, India and elsewhere, they would be sitting the relevant FRCS or MS examination in ORL; and in the USA the Boards in Otolaryngology.

The pattern of Specialist examinations in the UK has recently changed. Trainees will start specialist training after a relatively short time, usually with little or no previous ORL experience, and they will not be examined in any aspect of otology until they appear for the so-called 'Intercollegiate examination' towards the end of training. This book, we hope, will be the ideal companion for them throughout those years of otological training, and should contain enough factual material to equip a properly trained candidate to pass the Intercollegiate examination. Of course trainees must expect to consult large reference works and read original literature, but this book should meet the need for a 'vade mecum', – a basic guide – and will, we trust, become a valued friend, as have its predecessors for several generations of otologists. Despite increased specialization, the unique niche for this work, which made previous editions so successful, is still there to accommodate this new one.

The choice of references and extra reading material needs explanation. This is not a book written at a level where every statement throughout needs verification from a source in the literature. There are some chapters where the material is relatively new and specialized, or where it is presented by a world authority who wishes to support the contribution in the traditional scholarly way. There are others treating a large subject, some of which is now part of the accepted knowledge of the specialty. For these a full list of cited references would be excessive, and the need is to direct the reader to sources of more detailed information, and to original seminal contributions. So, some chapters have references cited in the text, whereas others offer lists for further reading. This apparent lack of uniformity is deliberate, and planned to meet the intentions of the editors in the most expeditious way.

Here for the first time, and with some personal regrets, the drawings are not mine, but their production has been rigorously supervised to ensure that the price of artistic professionalism has not been bought at the unforgiveable and base cost of otological inaccuracy.

We are immensely grateful to the librarians at the Institute of Laryngology and Otology, Peter Zwarts and Paul Pearson, for their dedicated help in checking references, and to Andrew Gardner in the photographic department there for his expert photographic illustrations for Chapter 3.

Our wives have suffered and borne the trials of supporting us during the arduous and lengthy production of this book. They deserve our admiration and they have our sincere thanks, and so do Nicola and Elizabeth Wright, who have lost a little of their childhood along the way.

HAROLD LUDMAN 1997

PART I

Introduction

CHAPTER 1

Anatomy and development of the ear and hearing

TONY WRIGHT

Introduction

The ear is conventionally and conveniently divided into three separate but linked, anatomical groupings called the outer, middle and inner ears. The outer and middle ears can be thought of as developing from a common origin during embryonic and fetal life whereas the inner ear has a separate derivation. Congenital abnormalities and some inherited defects frequently involve either the outer or the middle ears but it is less common for both to be involved. Many of these defects will be described in later chapters; however, to have a fuller appreciation of adult anatomy and some of its variations understanding how development occurs is often helpful.

Development of the human ear

THE OUTER AND MIDDLE EARS

The 9 months from implantation of the fertilized and dividing egg – the blastocyst – to birth is divided into three periods namely pre-embryonic, embryonic and fetal (Table 1.1).

During the embryonic phase there is rapid growth and differentiation of the ectoderm, mesoderm and endoderm, so that by the end of this period all the major organ systems have been formed and the late embryo has an external shape that is obviously human. In the fetal period there

Table 1.1 Phases in human development

Phase	Duration (days)
Pre-embryonic, pre-somite stage	21
Embryonic	35
Fetal	210

are changes in the shape, size and orientation of the various structures, as well as rapid overall growth, but no new tissues develop.

During growth from the fertilized egg into the fully formed fetus, animals pass through phases that represent, to a certain degree at least, their evolutionary precursors. The phrase: 'ontogeny recapitulates phylogeny' has been used to express this reflection of earlier forms. In mammals a phase is reached during early embryonic life when the mesenchyme surrounding the primitive foregut and pharynx differentiates into a maxillary and mandibular swelling on each side of the midline just above and below the buccopharyngeal membrane (Fig 1.1). This membrane then breaks down and a space that will later become both nasal and buccal cavities is formed. Further down the embryo and in the mesenchyme surrounding the pharynx, five or six parallel thickenings develop as bands that surround the pharynx. These are the branchial arches, which are numbered 1 to 5 from head to tail. They are formed anterior to the 40–43 paired somites, which subsequently give rise to the trunk and limbs. On the external surface a groove develops between each branchial arch and this is matched by a cleft

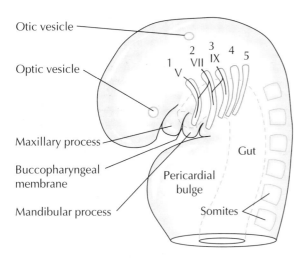

Fig 1.1 Schematic diagram of an early, 16–28 somite embryo with a representation of the mandibular and maxillary processes and the branchial arches. This representation does not exactly relate to any particular time of embryogenesis but is intended to give an impression of development. The branchial arches are numbered in Arabic numerals whereas the the nerves of those arches are given Roman numerals. This simplified diagram illustrates the innervation of these branchial arches.

or pouch on the inner pharyngeal surface. In each branchial arch develops a bar of cartilage, a group of muscles, an associated artery and a cranial nerve, which supplies these structures and their derivatives. This nerve is called the post-trematic nerve. In addition, a nerve from the arch lower down supplies the inner endodermal surface of the arch above and is called the pre-trematic nerve.

The first arch has the trigeminal nerve (V), the second arch has the facial (VII) and the third arch

the glossopharyngeal (IX). These are the post-trematic nerves. The pre-trematic nerves are the chorda tympani (from VII) running to the first arch (V) and Jacobson's nerve (the tympanic branch of IX) running to the second arch (VII) (Table 1.2).

The innervation of the lower arches and indeed their derivation are much less clear. In fish the layers between the arches break down to form the gill clefts, but in mammals this does not occur although grooves on the external surface of the embryo do develop and for a very short time come into contact with the endoderm lining the equivalent pharyngeal pouch. However, mesoderm rapidly intervenes and develops into the normal adult structures. Occasionally there is failure of this system when the various branchial arch defects can occur as sinuses (blind-ended tracts opening onto an epithelial surface), when a cleft or groove fails to regress, or less commonly as fistulae (a tract running from one epithelial surface to another) when the ectodermal endodermal junction breaks down.

The first pharyngeal pouch (on the inside) expands due to the rapid growth of the surrounding mesenchyme and, after dragging in some of the second pouch endoderm, results in the formation of the Eustachian tube, middle ear and mastoid antrum. In creating these large spaces the neural structures are forced to take a convoluted path to stay within mesenchyme and yet remain bound to their original arch structures and the derivatives. The facial nerve is a good example as it turns posteriorly from the geniculate ganglion, then inferiorly and then anteriorly in order to leave the skull. (The adult anatomy of the facial nerve is described in detail in Chapter 16.)

The endoderm of the slit-like sac that is the precursor of the middle ear lies against the ectoderm of the first pharyngeal groove by the fourth week. Mesenchyme grows in between these two layers to

Table 1.2 Derivatives of the first and second branchial arches

	Cartilage	Post-trematic nerve	Pre-trematic nerve	Artery
First arch Derivatives	Meckel's Malleus Incus 'Mandible' Anterior malleolar ligament Sphenomandibular ligament	Mandibular V	Chorda tympani VII	Maxillary
Second arch Derivatives	Reichert's Stapes superstructure Styloid process Lesser cornu of hyoid Stylohoid ligament	Facial VII	Tympanic branch IX	Stapedial

form the middle layer of the future tympanic membrane. The underlying sac expands and as it reaches the developing ossicles and labyrinth, the epithelium is draped over these structures and their associated muscles, tendons and ligaments, so that a complex series of mucosal folds is formed.

The future Eustachian tube lumen and middle ear spaces are formed by 8 months gestation and the epitympanum and mastoid antrum are developed by birth. A few mastoid 'air cells' may be present at birth, albeit filled with amniotic fluid. However, development of the mastoid air cell system does not occur until after birth, with about 90 per cent of air cell formation being completed by the age of 6 years with the remaining 10 per cent occurring up to the age of 18 years.

The ossicles develop from the outer ends of the first arch (Meckel's) and second arch (Reichert's) cartilages, which lie above and below the first pharyngeal pouch (see Table 1.2). The process begins at 4 weeks and adult shape, size and ossification is present by 25 weeks. The muscles attached to an ossicle arise from the arch that contributed to the development of that particular ossicle. Thus the tensor tympani is attached to the upper part of the handle of the malleus, which is derived from the first arch and is, therefore, supplied by a branch of the Vth (mandibular) nerve. By the same argument the stapedius muscle is supplied by the VIIth (facial) nerve. The chorda tympani, which is the pre-trematic nerve of the second arch that supplies endodermal structures of the first arch (i.e. taste to the anterior two-thirds of the tongue and submandibular gland secretomotor fibres) has to run through mesoderm as it cannot run through air. This mesoderm subsequently becomes the middle layer of the tympanic membrane.

The external ear canal develops from the first pharyngeal groove in a complex fashion and a complete description is beyond the scope of this book (see Michaels and Soucek, 1989). It is sufficient to say that the meatus deepens by proliferation of its ectoderm and that an anteriorly placed bud of epithelial cells expands vertically to form the skin that will cover the future tympanic membrane. This clump of cells then opens up as a slit to form the canal lumen and produce the pars tensa and deep external canal epithelium. These two types of skin both have migratory properties so that the ear canal becomes self-cleansing.

The external auricle or pinna develops from a series of small cartilaginous tubercles that surround the first pharyngeal groove. These enlarge and coalesce, although it seems that the majority of the auricle is derived from the second arch cartilages and that the tragus is the only contribution from the first arch. The rudimentary pinna has formed by 60

days although it apparently continues to grow throughout life.

Failure of formation of the first and second branchial arch structures gives rise to problems that range from failure of adequate skin migration with 'ear canal cholesteatoma' (which is very rare) through bat ears, accessory auricles and pre-auricular sinuses, to complete failure of formation of the external ear canal and middle ear. There are also the rare first arch fistulae (col-aural fistulae), which comprise a tract between the external ear canal and the skin of the cheek, with the fistula path passing through the parotid gland and frequently between branches of the facial nerve.

THE INNER EAR (LABYRINTH)

The inner ear initially develops quite independently of the middle and outer ears, although the two become interconnected by the stapes superstructure becoming attached to the stapes footplate thereby giving continuity to the auditory pathway.

The development of the labyrinth can be thought of as the initial development of the generalized structure of the membranous labyrinth, followed by a period of encasement by the bony labyrinth and the production of a further series of spaces within

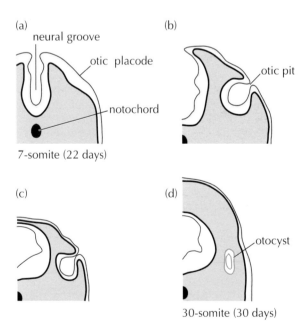

Fig 1.2 (a)–(d) The development of the otocyst. The otocyst develops as a thickening called the otic placode on the surface of the embryo just cranial to the first somite. This thickening sinks into the mesoderm and eventually the otic pit closes off to leave the isolated otocyst, which subsequently becomes the membranous labyrinth.

(a)

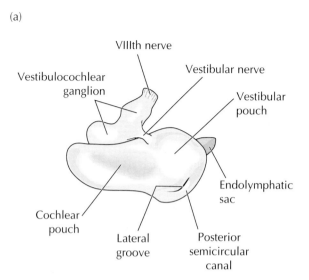

Fig 1.3 The development of the membranous labyrinth. (a) The initial stage of differentiation of the otocyst into recognizable cochlear and vestibular portions. This stage occurs at about 35–36 days and teratogenic agents acting at this time result in severe malformations of the inner ear. (b)–(d) Further growth stages: the fully developed membranous labyrinth is present at the end of the first 10 weeks of pregnancy.

(b)

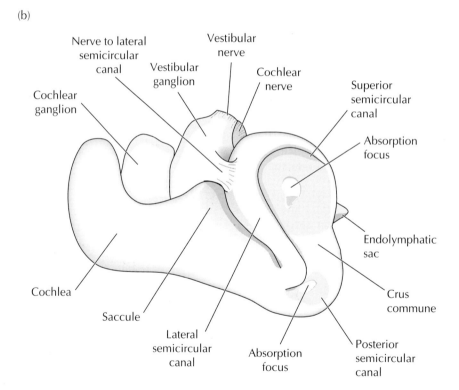

this bony shell, which in turn become the perilymphatic spaces of the complete structure. These different activities are happening at different times in different parts of the labyrinth so that damage or derangements at specific times give rise to many peculiar and varied abnormalities as will be seen in the chapter on the radiology of the inner ear.

Within the first few days of embryonic life (i.e. at about day 22–23) ectodermal thickening forms on the side of the head end of the embryo close to the part of the developing neural tube and neural crest cells that will later become the brain and brainstem and the cranial nerves, respectively. The ectodermal thickening is the otic placode, which deepens and then sinks below the surface as the sides close in to form an otic pit, which eventually loses connection with the surface and forms the otocyst (Fig 1.2).

(c)

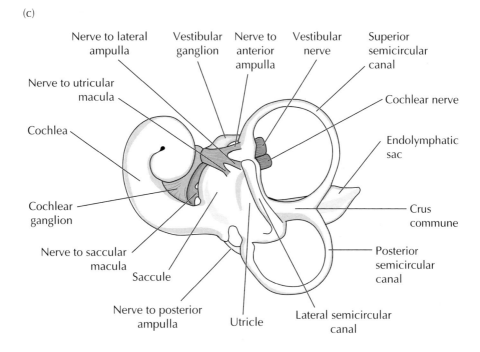

(d)

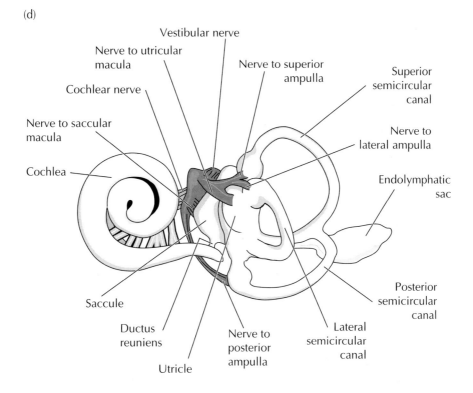

Associated with the otocyst is the cluster of neural crest cells that later become the separate facial (geniculate), auditory (spiral) and vestibular (Scarpa's) ganglion cell bodies. The otocyst then undergoes a series of spectacular changes that result in the full-sized outline of the adult membranous labyrinth by 25 weeks gestation.

The semicircular canals start to develop at around 35 days as three flattened pouches that grow out at right angles from each other from the utricle

(Fig 1.3). At the centre of each semicircular ridge the opposing epithelial surfaces meet, fuse and then coalesce to be replaced by mesoderm. The superior canal is the first to be fully formed by 6 weeks.

As these developments are taking place the cochlea starts to be formed. The saccule, which has separated from the utricle, starts to put out a single pouch-like process that grows and then begins to coil from base to apex to reach its full two and a half coils by 25 weeks.

Within the membranous labyrinth the sensory cells of the three cristae, two maculae and the organ of Corti are beginning to develop from areas of ectodermal specialization. Either this is encouraged by the ingrowth of nerve endings from the cochleovestibular ganglion, which was originally outside the otocyst, or the development of the sensory cells encourages neural ingrowth.

The organ of Corti starts developing as a single block of heaped up ectodermal cells at about 11 weeks. Within this mass develop inner and outer hair cells and then specialized supporting cells. The tunnel of Corti appears between inner and outer pillar cells as clusters of stereocilia and a single kinocilium develops on each hair cell. The cochlear kinocilium regresses to leave the adult configuration of stereocilia, and the spaces between the outer hair cells open up as the supporting cells (Deiter's cells) change shape. Differentiation progresses from base to apex so that at any one time various stages of development can be seen in appropriately prepared material.

Epithelium close to the sensory regions develops into the specialized cell groups that maintain the ionic and electrical stability of the endolymph.

These regions are the stria vascularis of the cochlear duct and the 'dark cell' regions of the vestibular sensory epithelium.

THE BONY LABYRINTH

The mesenchyme enclosing the otocyst becomes chondrified to form the otic capsule. As the membranous labyrinth expands, the otic capsule remodels and in places undergoes dedifferentiation to form fluid-filled spaces that eventually become the perilymphatic spaces. This dedifferentiation does not occur where nerves enter the sensory cell regions. Elsewhere, the perilymphatic spaces become continuous and a communication with the cerebrospinal fluid is formed by the development of the cochlear aqueduct, which runs to the posterior cranial fossa from the base of the cochlea.

Ossification of the cartilaginous otic capsule begins in or around the sixteenth week from a variable number of centres that finally fuse without leaving tell-tale suture lines. This dense bony mass is the petrous bone (Greek *petra* 'rock') and is frequently the last part of a whale to decompose and is sometimes the only remains of those unfortunate enough to be eaten by sharks.

There are certain channels that remain within the otic capsule; one of the most important of these is the oval window in which part of the otic capsule becomes the stapes footplate and the annular ligament, thereby allowing sound from the middle ear to enter the labyrinthine fluids (Table 1.3).

Table 1.3 Development of communication channels passing through the bony labyrinth

Internal auditory meatus	Persisting channel in cartilage model around VII and VIII nerves
Subarcuate fossa	Persisting vascular channel
Vestibular aqueduct	Fifth and sixth ossification centres fuse around the endolymphatic duct
Cochlear aqueduct	Resorption of precartilage
Fossula ante fenestram	Resorption of precartilage
Fossula post fenestram (inconstant)	Resorption of cartilage
Oval window	Otic capsule becomes footplate of stapes and annular ligament
Round window	Persisting cartilage becomes round window niche and membrane

THE TEMPORAL BONE

Four separate elements eventually fuse to form the temporal bone, which is one of the most complex and interesting parts of the bony anatomy of the body (Fig 1.4 and Plate section). These four parts are

- petromastoid
- squamous
- tympanic
- styloid process

The petromastoid is derived from petrous bone described above and the continuing growth of its outer layers, which form the roof of the middle ear; the lateral wall of the Eustachian tube; the floor of the middle ear; the canal of the facial nerve; and the petrous apex.

The squamous bone develops in mesenchyme and starts to ossify from a single centre close to the roof of the zygoma as early as 8 weeks. The posteroinferior portion grows down behind the tympanic ring to form the lateral wall of the fetal mastoid antrum.

The tympanic bone also forms in mesenchyme, but from several centres around the external meatus. These form the major part of a ring with a groove on the inner aspect that becomes the sulcus for the tympanic membrane. Even by late fetal life the bony ear canal is unformed and only after birth do anterior and posterior protuberances grow to form the floor of the canal. These crescentic swellings eventually fuse laterally leaving a gap in the middle of the floor. This is the foramen of Huschke, which is usually closed by adolescence. The tympanic bone fuses with the mastoid process of the petromastoid and with parts of the squamous and petrous bones as the tympanomastoid, tympanosquamous and petrotympanic sutures. The petrotympanic suture has a canal for the chorda tympani nerve.

The styloid develops from two centres at the cranial end of the second arch (Reichert's) cartilage. The part close to the base of the skull starts to ossify before birth, but the styloid process itself does not start to ossify until after birth and fusion of the two parts may not occur until after puberty.

Much of the growth of temporal bone occurs after birth with enlargement of the whole structure and major growth of the mastoid process so that the stylomastoid foramen, which was initially close to the surface, becomes buried by the development of the mastoid tip. At the same time there is generalized downwards rotation of the petrous bone so that the tympanic membrane moves from being almost horizontal in the neonate to an angle of about 55° with the horizontal in the adult. With these changes the floor of the middle cranial fossa flattens and the positions of the geniculate ganglion, the semicircular canals and the internal auditory meatus change in relation to each other, so that middle cranial fossa surgery in the baby is anatomically a different experience from that in the adolescent.

Adult anatomy

THE AURICLE (PINNA)

The body of the auricle (Fig 1.5) is formed from elastic fibrocartilage and is a continuous sheet except for a narrow gap between the tragus and the anterior crus of the helix, where it is replaced by a dense fibrous tissue band. This gap is a site for an endaural incision which, properly performed, should not damage cartilage or its perichondrium and which by splitting the soft-tissue ring surrounding the bony ear canal allows wide exposure of the deeper parts.

The innervation of the auricle and its surrounding regions is shown in Figure 1.6 and described in Table 1.4.

Table 1.4 Sensory innervation of the auricle

Nerve	Derivation	Region supplied
Greater auricular	Cervical plexus C2, 3	Medial surface and posterior portion of lateral surface
Lesser occipital	Cervical plexus C2, 3	Superior portion of medial surface
Auricular	Vagus X	Concha and antihelix, and some supply to medial surface (eminetia concha)
Auriculotemporal	Vc Mandibular	Tragus, crus of helix and adjacent helix
Facial VII		Probably supplies small region in the root of concha

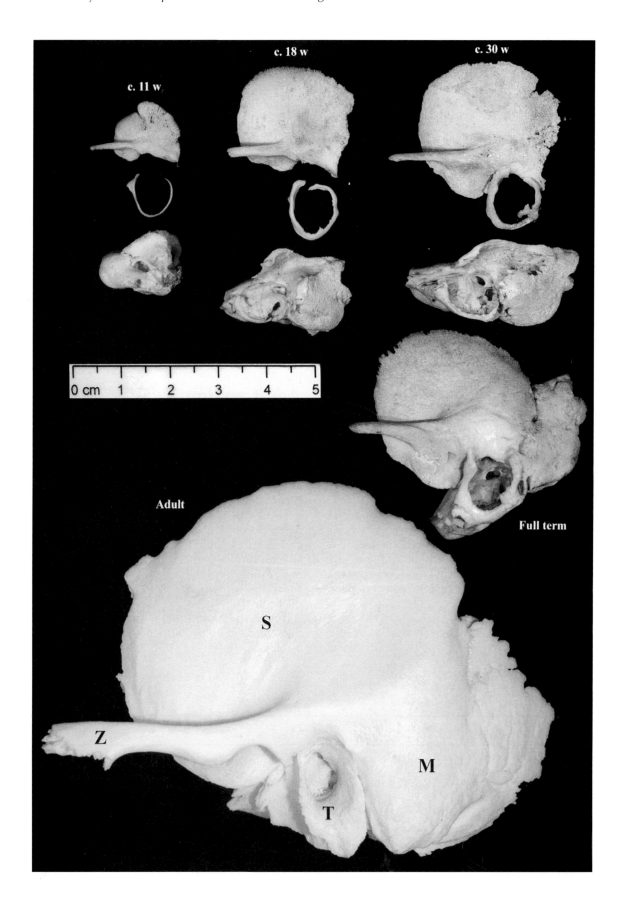

Fig 1.4 Stages in the development of the temporal bone. The illustrations are of lateral views of the temporal bone and the first three are of ancient Roman fetal remains. The very early stages have the separate elements of the developing bone clearly displayed as the flattened squamous portion, the tympanic ring and the petrous segment. At birth the three elements are fused although still very underdeveloped. The oval window for the stapes can be identified and it should be noted that the facial nerve canal is absent in the early bones. The fourth bone is from a term infant. The facial nerve is covered by a bony canal at birth but the stylomastoid foramen is very superficial. It is not until the growth of the mastoid process that the foramen becomes 'buried' in the base of the skull. The full-grown adult temporal bone is shown to illustrate the remarkable growth that occurs postnatally. S, squamous portion; M, petromastoid; T, tympanic ring; Z, zygomatic arch. The styloid process is missing in this specimen. (I am very grateful to Dr Louise Scheuer PhD, Senior Lecturer in Anatomy and Developmental Biology at the Royal Free Hospital School of Medicine, for permission to image these Roman bones digitally and to use the images. These and other images are available for study on the web at www.vml.ucl.ac.uk).

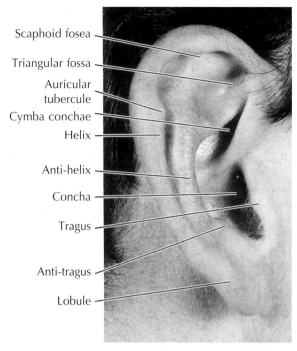

Fig 1.5 A view of the right auricle with the various anatomical parts named.

Scaphoid fosea
Triangular fossa
Auricular tubercule
Cymba conchae
Helix
Anti-helix
Concha
Tragus
Anti-tragus
Lobule

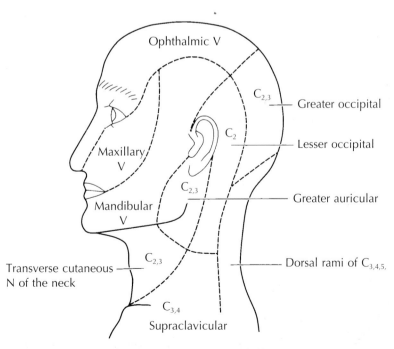

Ophthalmic V

Maxillary V

Mandibular V

$C_{2,3}$

C_2

$C_{2,3}$

$C_{2,3}$

$C_{3,4}$

Transverse cutaneous N of the neck

Supraclavicular

Greater occipital

Lesser occipital

Greater auricular

Dorsal rami of $C_{3,4,5,}$

Fig 1.6 The sensory innervation of the skin around the external ear.

The cartilage extends about 8 mm down the ear canal to form its lateral two-thirds. The cartilage of the auricle is covered with perichondrium from which it derives its supply of nutrients as cartilage itself is avascular. Stripping the perichondrium from the cartilage, as occurs after injuries that cause haematoma, can lead to cartilage necrosis with crumpled up, 'boxer's ears'. The skin of the pinna is thin and closely attached to the perichondrium on the lateral surface. On the medial surface, that is between the mastoid process and the auricle, there is a definite subdermal layer that allows dissection during surgery for bat ears. The skin of the auricle is covered with fine hairs and, most noticeably in the concha and the scaphoid fossa, there are sebaceous glands opening into the root canals of these hairs. The cartilage of the auricle is connected to the skull by ligaments and muscles, which are supplied by the temporal branches (auricularis anterior and superior muscles) and posterior auricular branches (auricularis posterior muscle) of the facial nerve.

The innervation of the auricle derives from first and second branchial arch nerves, as might be expected, but also from the cervical nerves that supply the scalp.

EXTERNAL EAR CANAL

The external ear canal in adults is approximately 2.5 cm long with the lateral one-third having cartilaginous walls and the medial two-thirds bony walls. The diameter of the canal varies greatly between individuals and between different races. Starting from the outside the canal curves forwards and slightly downwards so that a direct view of the tympanic membrane usually requires the auricle to be gently pulled upwards and backwards to straighten out the cartilaginous canal.

The continuing curve of the deep bony canal results in the tympanic membrane lying at a slant across the bony canal with an acute angle between the drum and the anterior canal wall. This anterior recess is a difficult spot for access either in the clinic or at surgery.

The external canal is lined with skin. Skin normally grows directly from the basal layers towards the surface, where it is shed into the surroundings. Excess proliferation of the scalp skin when trapped by the hair is dandruff. If this pattern of direct upward growth were to occur in the external ear canal then the canal would soon become filled with desquamated skin. Instead of maturation taking place directly towards the surface, there is outward, oblique growth of the epidermis of the canal skin and pars flaccida so that the surface layers effec-

tively migrate towards the external opening of the canal. The normal of rate of migration is about 0.05 mm/day, although this range is hugely variable and in some conditions there is complete failure of migration with a consequent build-up of shed keratin in the ear canal.

The skin of the pars tensa has a different derivation from that of the deep canal, and cell divisions occur randomly within the layer of basal cells. The effect of this in a circular sheet with the handle of the malleus forming a central boundary extending halfway down the membrane is to create outward, mass migration of the skin of the pars tensa. Ink dots applied to the surface have an outward pattern of movement. However, if a hole is made in the tympanic membrane and a graft laid underneath the membrane (an underlay graft) then migration of the skin from the outer edge of the perforation is directed centrally to cover the graft. This occurs because the boundary conditions have altered and fortunately provides the basis for the healing of grafts and for the re-epithelization of mastoid cavities. Even a small piece of pars tensa skin has this ability and so is a precious material and needs to be preserved during ear surgery if a bare area needs covering. The property of canal skin to migrate, however, can also bring problems with the formation of cholesteatoma if the skin becomes displaced into the middle ear cleft.

At the outer limits of the ear canal are some short hairs that project towards the opening of the canal. In this region are clusters of ceruminous and sebaceous glands. The ceruminous glands are modified apocrine sweat glands that open into the root canal of the hair follicles and produce a watery, white secretion that slowly darkens turning semi-solid and sticky as it dries. Because these glands are apocrine sweat glands they respond to many stimuli such adrenergic drugs, fever and emotion which, along with direct mechanical stimulation, can all produce increased or altered secretion.

The sebaceous glands produce an oily material (sebum) from the breakdown of their fat-containing cells, which is usually excreted into the root canals of the hair follicles. The mixture of desquamated cells, cerumen and sebum forms wax. This is a good agent for inhibiting the growth of many fungi and bacteria and is strongly bactericidal for certain bacterial species.

Wax is not usually found in the deep ear canal and a lump of 'wax' overlying the upper portion of the tympanic membrane (pars flaccida or attic region) is rarely true wax, but is nearly always associated with an underlying cholesteatoma as it is, in fact, dried-up, oxidized keratin. The sense of the old adage 'beware the attic wax' is still just as true today as it was then.

THE TYMPANIC MEMBRANE AND MIDDLE EAR CLEFT

The tympanic membrane and middle ear constitute a remarkable system that has evolved as an adaptation to living on land. The middle ears of reptiles, birds and mammals all comprise the same basic elements, namely a mobile tympanic membrane, an air-filled middle ear space and a bony connection between the tympanic membrane and the opening into the labyrinth.

The tympanic membrane

The tympanic membrane is slightly oval in shape and is approximately 9–10 mm in its maximum diameter from posterosuperior to anteroinferior. The tympanic membrane not only lies obliquely across the long axis of the ear canal but also is not vertical, forming an acute angle of about 55° with the floor of the canal. Overall the membrane is concave towards the ear canal but each segment is slightly convex between the lateral attachment of the annulus and the centre of the membrane where the tip of the malleus handle is attached at the umbo (Fig 1.7).

The tympanic membrane is divided into two portions, with the pars tensa, the lower of the two forming the majority. The pars flaccida is a rather flat triangular region above this.

The circumference of the pars tensa is thickened to form the annulus, which inserts into a sulcus in the tympanic bone. The sulcus does not, however, extend to the roof of the deep bony canal, and the annulus, which lies in the upper part of the sulcus both anteriorly and posteriorly, then runs centrally to form the anterior and posterior malleolar folds, which attach to the rather prominent lateral process at the top of the malleus handle. The membrane above the malleolar folds is called the pars flaccida.

Above the pars flaccida is the bony deep canal wall. Because the canal is turning gently downwards and because there is an air-filled space housing the head of the malleus and the body of the incus deep to this bony wall, then it is rather wedge-shaped with a sharp inferior edge. This crescent of bone is called the outer attic wall (outer epitympanic wall) or scutum (Latin *scutum* 'shield') and it is easily eroded by cholesteatoma leaving a tell-tale sign on the appropriate coronal CT scan.

The tympanic membrane itself comprises three layers. There is an outer layer of skin, a middle layer of mainly fibrous tissue – the lamina propria – and an inner mucosal layer continuous with the lining of the middle ear cavity.

The lamina propria of the pars tensa has radially oriented fibres in the outer layers and circular, parabolic and transverse fibres in the deeper layer. This arrangement probably accounts for the complex pattern of tympanic membrane displacement during sound stimulation. The pars flaccida has a fibrous layer, although it is less marked, and the orientation of the fibres seems random.

The middle ear space is notionally divided into three compartments: the epitympanic, mesotympanic and hypotympanic spaces, upper, middle and lower, respectively. The epitympanum or attic, lies above the level of the malleolar folds and is separated from the mesotympanic and hypotympanic spaces by a series of mucosal membranes and folds. The hypotympanum lies below the level of the inferior part of the tympanic sulcus and is continuous with the mesotympanum above. These three spaces contain air, the ossicles, their associated tendons and their associated ligaments. The walls of the cavity have nerves running across them and openings into surrounding structures.

Air

The gas filling a normal middle ear is not air but is nitrogen rich; middle ear ventilation is described in Chapter 24. The Eustachian tube, which delivers gas from the nasopharynx and allows the clearance of mucus, is described later in this chapter.

The ossicles

The malleus, incus and stapes form a semi-rigid bony chain for conducting sound (Fig 1.8).

The handle of the malleus lies between the middle and the mucosal layers of the tympanic membrane. It runs downwards, medially and slightly backwards and although it is very closely attached to the membrane at its lower end there is a fine web of mucosa separating the membrane from the handle in the upper portion before it becomes densely adherent again at the lateral process. This slit-like space can be opened surgically without perforating the membrane and allows the wire of a prosthesis to be wrapped around the malleus handle in certain types of ossicular reconstruction.

The lateral process of the malleus is a prominent landmark on the tympanic membrane; deep to this on the medial surface the chorda tympani crosses the upper part of the malleus handle above the insertion of the tendon of tensor tympani but below the neck of the malleus itself. The neck of the malleus connects the handle with the head and amputation of the head by cutting through the neck leaves chorda tympani and tensor tympani intact.

(a)

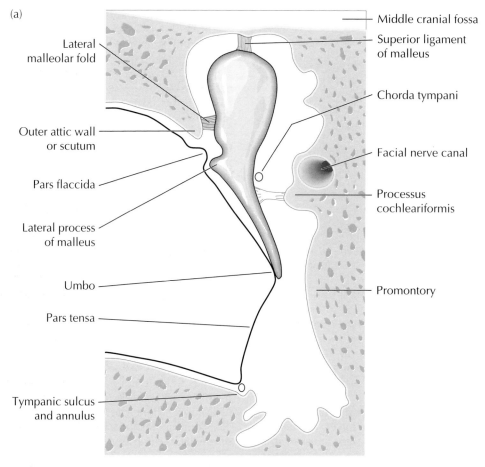

Lateral malleolar fold

Outer attic wall or scutum

Pars flaccida

Lateral process of malleus

Umbo

Pars tensa

Tympanic sulcus and annulus

Middle cranial fossa

Superior ligament of malleus

Chorda tympani

Facial nerve canal

Processus cochleariformis

Promontory

(b)

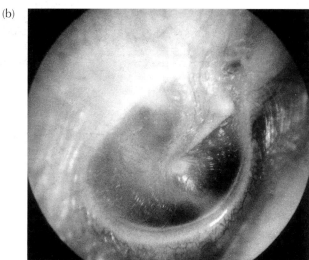

Fig 1.7 (a) A section through the long axis of the external ear canal showing the relationships of the tympanic membrane. (b) An endoscopic photograph of the right tympanic membrane. The malleus handle runs from the middle of the membrane upwards and forwards to the lateral process, which is usually a good landmark.

The head of the malleus lies in the attic and is, in part, suspended by the superior ligament, which runs upward to the roof of the attic – the tegmen tympani.

The head of the malleus articulates with the body of the incus by way of a synovial joint. The surface of the joint is not flat, but on the malleus is rather like an elongated saddle with the lower and rather

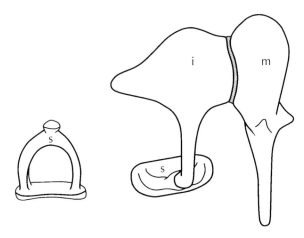

Fig 1.8 The right malleus (m), incus (i) and stapes (s).

The orientation of the articular process of the incus with the malleus means that, fortunately, it is possible to disarticulate the malleoincudal joint and remove the incus from the middle ear after the incudostapedial joint has been divided. The tip of a short hook placed medial to the long process of the incus can be moved laterally so that the incus rotates about its short ligament and the joint conveniently breaks open. Medial pressure on the long process locks the malleoincudal joint against the spur on the malleus, which is a blessing for those learning how to place the prosthesis during a stapedectomy.

The stapes itself has a head and neck, two limbs (crura) and a footplate. The joint between the head of the stapes and the lenticular process of the incus is lined by cartilage and provides an easy plane of cleavage between the two. The stapedius tendon inserts into the posterior part of the neck, and of the two crura the anterior is thinner and generally the lesser curved. The crura are hollowed out on their concave surfaces, which gives an optimum combination of strength and lightness. The footplate is on average 3 mm long and 1.4 mm wide and usually has a convex superior margin and flattish inferior margin. From these descriptions it should be possible to decide from which side an ossicle originates if you have the good fortune to be handed one during an examination (Table 1.5).

The stapes footplate sits in the oval window and is attached to the bony margins of the window by an annular ligament. It can be seen from Figure 1.9 that the oval window is at the bottom of a niche surrounded by the facial nerve above, the processus cochleariformis in front, the promontory below and the pyramid of the stapedius muscle and the second

smaller part projecting posteriorly like a spur or cog. The body of the incus also lies in the attic and has two processes projecting from it. The short process runs posteriorly and is cradled by a depression in the posterior wall of the middle ear – the fossa incudis – where a short ligament holds it firmly in place. The long process descends from the attic into the mesotympanum, posterior to the handle of the malleus, and at the tip of the incus has a small medially projecting mass called the lenticular process. This has sometimes been called the fourth ossicle because of its incomplete fusion with the tip of the long process, thereby giving the appearance of a separate bone or at least a sesamoid bone. The lenticular process articulates with the head of the stapes.

Table 1.5 How to decide from which side an ossicle originates

Malleus
Hold the bone with its head above, handle below. Have the lateral process facing you.
Then if the joint surface is to your left it is the right malleus; if to your right it is the left malleus.

Incus
Hold with the body above, long process below. Hold with the short process in your left hand.
If the lenticular process then faces away from you it is the right incus; if towards you it is the left incus.

Stapes
This bone is now getting rather small. Therefore request a lens. This will probably not be available and if the examiner asks whether your eyesight is sufficient reply that it is perfect, but you want to be certain of your decision. This is a constructive waste of time.
Stand the stapes on its footplate with its long axis pointing away from you. Have the more curved arch towards you.
If the convex surface of the footplate is to the left it is the right stapes; if to the right it is the left stapes.

If after all this you cannot decide from which side the ossicle originates then drop it as the first law of temporal bone dissection is 'An ossicle gone to ground is never found'.

turn of the facial nerve behind. The facial nerve and promontory can be especially prominent, making access to the footplate rather difficult on occasions.

The malleus and stapes have muscles attached to them. The tensor tympani arises mainly from the walls of a long narrow bony canal lying in the roof of the Eustachian tube. Small elements derive from the cartilaginous portions of the tube and from the greater wing of the sphenoid. The muscle runs backwards into the tympanic cavity on its medial wall just below the level of the facial nerve. At about the level of the geniculate ganglion the muscle gives way to a tendon, which is held in a bony spoon-shaped prominence – the processus cochleariformis – by a transverse tendon. The tendon of the tensa tympani then turns through a right angle to pass laterally to the neck of the malleus below the chorda tympani.

The processus partly overlies the facial nerve just posterior to the geniculate ganglion and is a robust landmark that is rarely eroded by disease. The tensor tympani muscle, from its first arch origins, is supplied from the mandibular nerve by a branch from the medial pterygoid nerve by way of the otic ganglion.

The stapedius muscle also arises from the walls of a bony tube that curves downwards and backwards from the pyramid to run anterior and then deep to the facial nerve in its descending (mastoid) portion. Several slender branches from the nerve supply the muscle directly. The tendon emerges from the tip of the pyramid and inserts into the back of the neck of the stapes.

The stapedius muscle sometimes gets confused with the facial nerve during temporal bone dissection, but the level of the muscle and its colour should be definitive. Not only does the stapedius contract in response to loud sound, but if you look carefully with a microscope at the stapes in a patient with a posterior perforation and a deficient long process of the incus and then ask them to count slowly to 10, the stapedius tendon can be seen to pull on the stapes just before each number is spoken. I do not have a reasonable explanation for the function of this action.

The walls of the tympanic cavity

The medial wall of the tympanic cavity

The medial wall of the tympanic cavity is very important for the surgeon. It has many important structures in close proximity and it is vital to have the 'feel' of the quality of the bone, the colour, the shape and the relationships of the various structures before major ear surgery is performed. This means plenty of supervised temporal bone work.

The facial nerve runs across the medial wall separating the epitympanic region above from the mesotympanic below (Fig 1.9). At the geniculate ganglion the facial nerve canal is marked by the processus cochleariformis. In the horizontal segment, the bony canal (the Fallopian canal) often has micro-dehiscences and when the bone is thin or the nerve exposed by disease there are two or three straight blood vessels clearly visible along this line of nerve. These are the only straight blood vessels in the middle ear and indicate quite clearly that the facial nerve is very close by. There are some straight blood vessels in the mastoid itself and these will be described later. Slightly more posteriorly the facial nerve is related to the lateral semicircular canal, which lies above the line of the nerve (Fig 1.10). During a cortical mastoidectomy the triangular relationship of the lateral semicircular canal, the short process of the incus and the facial (VIIth) nerve is often quite helpful.

The course and relationships of the facial nerve are described in more detail in Chapter 16.

Below the facial nerve is the oval window niche at the bottom of which is the oval window itself. The niche is approximately 3.25 mm long and 1.75 mm wide.

Below the oval window is the round window niche lying a little posteriorly. This curved bony overhang obscures the round window membrane, which is roughly oval, about 2.3 by 1.9 mm in dimension and the plane of which lies at right angles to the plane of the stapes footplate.

Deep to the stapes footplate is perilymph filling the vestibule whereas deep to the oval window is the perilymph of the scala tympani of the basal turn of the cochlea. The round window membrane is not at the end of the scala tympani, but forms part of its floor.

Posterior to the two windows is the posterior extension of the mesotympanum medial to the facial nerve. This space is the sinus tympani, probably the most inaccessible site in the middle ear and mastoid. The sinus tympani is of varying extent and on rare occasions communicates with the mastoid air cells. Its importance is that disease, especially cholesteatoma that has extended into the sinus tympani, is extremely difficult to eradicate. The worst region for access is above the pyramid, posterior to an intact stapes and medial to the facial nerve. An approach to this region via the mastoid, that is, a retrofacial approach, is not possible because the posterior semicircular canal blocks access.

The lateral wall of the tympanic cavity

The lateral wall comprises mainly the tympanic membrane, and most of the structures in this wall

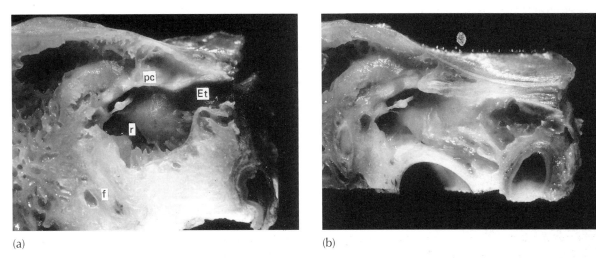

(a)   (b)

Fig 1.9 (a) The medial wall of the middle ear cavity. The cut is rather lateral and shows the facial nerve running across the medial wall backwards from the processus cochleariformis (pc) and above the stapes before it turns down into the descending or mastoid portion (f). Beneath the stapes is the round window (r) and anteriorly can be seen the opening of the Eustachian tube (Et). (b) In a different bone, a slightly more medial cut has been made to show the dome of the jugular bulb posteriorly and the carotid artery as it turns forwards to pass medial to the Eustachian tube. The tensor tympani muscle can be seen in the roof of the Eustachian tube as it passes backwards to the processus cochleariformis.

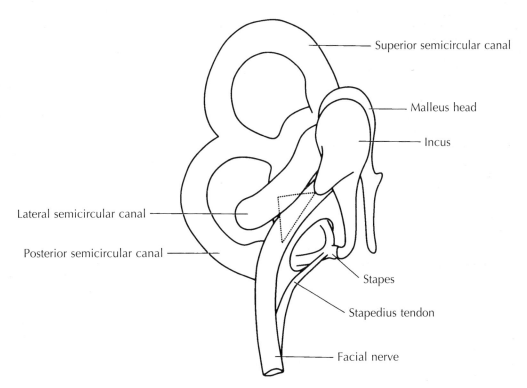

Fig 1.10 The relationship in the right ear between the short process of the incus, the facial (VIIth) nerve and the lateral semicircular canal. The two short sides of the triangle are approximately 1.5 mm in length.

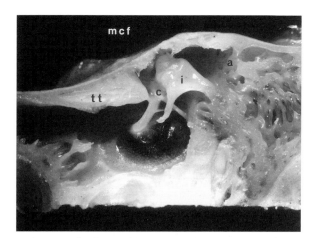

Fig 1.11 The lateral wall of the tympanic cavity. The heads of the ossicles lie in the epitympanum or attic, which extends back to the aditus to the mastoid antrum (a). The chorda tympani (c) passes across the upper part of the handle and the neck of the malleus above the insertion of the tensor tympani before it runs lateral to the long process of the incus.

have already been described and depicted. The chorda tympani nerve, which carries taste sensation from the anterior two-thirds of the same side of the tongue and secretomotor fibres to the submandibular gland, enters the middle ear anteriorly from its canal in the petrotympanic fissure above the opening of the Eustachian tube (Fig 1.11). From these it runs posteriorly between the fibrous and mucosal layers of the tympanic membrane, across the upper part of the handle of the malleus and then continues within the membrane, but below the level of the posterior malleolar fold. The nerve reaches the posterior bony canal wall just medial to the tympanic sulcus, enters its small canal and then runs obliquely downwards and medially until it reaches the facial nerve. The points of entry of the chorda tympani into both the bony canal wall and the facial nerve bundle are quite variable and on occasions the chorda leaves the skull base by a separate foramen before it joins the facial nerve. During cortical mastoidectomy and temporal bone dissection, the fibrous strands of the tympanomastoid suture line can often be confused with the chorda tympani although the angle of the white strands of the suture line is different from the angle of the chorda. Sometimes, however, this difference is not much. I do not feel that the chorda is a good guide to the facial nerve.

The anterior wall of the tympanic cavity

The anterior wall is rather narrow and comprises mainly the opening into the Eustachian tube.

Above this is the canal for the tensor tympani tendon and medial to both of these runs the carotid artery as it turns from the middle ear segment forward into the carotid sinus before entering the skull in the cavernous sinus.

The Eustachian tube

The Eustachian tube is an intriguing part of the middle ear mechanism as it links the middle ear with the nasopharynx. Its function is discussed more fully in Chapter 24, but the anatomical details are described here. The tube is, in the adult, about 36 mm long with the lateral, that is the bony middle ear segment, being approximately 12 mm long. It narrows down from its wide middle ear portion to a narrow part called the isthmus, which has an internal diameter of approximately 1 mm and a length of about 2 mm. A thin plate of bone forms the roof of the Eustachian tube and above this is the tensor tympani muscle. The carotid artery, which lies medially, is separated from the Eustachian tube also by a thin plate of bone.

The medial, cartilaginous portion of the tube is 24 mm long and the bulk of the walls of the tube is formed by a cartilaginous plate. This plate forms the posteromedial wall and the roof, with the anterolateral wall being formed by a mucosal and muscle sheet. The Eustachian tube opens in the nasopharynx behind and below the posterior end of the inferior turbinate. The tensor palati muscle arises from the scaphoid bone and from along the whole length of the upper rim of cartilage that forms the roof of the cartilaginous Eustachian tube (Fig 1.12). From these two origins the muscle converges into a short tendon that turns medially around the hook of the hamulus and then spreads

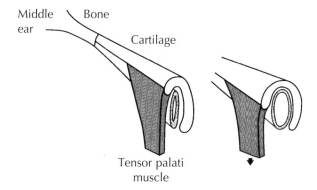

Fig 1.12 Diagrammatic representation of the Eustachian tube with the attachment of the tensor palati muscle. The levator palati runs along the floor of the tube and has some fibres that originate from the cartilaginous border of the tube itself.

out within the soft-palate to join the equivalent muscle from the other side of the skull base. The levator palati muscle contains some fibres that originate from the undersurface of the cartilaginous portion of the Eustachian tube. The tensor palati muscle is supplied by a branch of the mandibular nerve, whereas the levator is supplied from the pharyngeal plexus. In general, it is thought that on swallowing the tensor palati muscle contributes to the opening of the cartilaginous portion of the Eustachian tube, whereas the levator palati muscle, which has a slower response, may contribute to middle ear ventilation (see Chapter 24).

The posterior wall of the tympanic cavity

The posterior wall has at its upper end an opening into the mastoid antrum. This opening is called the aditus and leads back from the posterior epitympanum (attic) into the antrum of the mastoid. Below this opening is a small depression in the posterior wall of the middle ear which houses the short process of the incus and its suspensory ligament. This depression, which is called the fossa incudis, lies above a small outgrowth of bone from the posterior wall called the pyramid. This houses the stapedius muscle and tendon, which inserts into the posterior aspect of the head of the stapes. The stapedius muscle itself curves downwards and posteriorly to run into, or just below, the facial nerve canal. The facial recess is a groove that lies between the pyramid and facial nerve and the annulus of the

tympanic membrane. The sinus tympani lies deep to the pyramid and facial nerve and runs into the medial wall of the middle ear (Fig 1.13).

The roof of the tympanic cavity

The roof of the epitympanum is called the tegmen tympani and is a thin bony roof that separates the middle ear space from the middle cranial fossa. In children, this bony plate is unformed and provides a relatively easy route of access for infection into the extradural spaces.

The floor of the tympanic cavity

The floor of the tympanic cavity comprises the roof of the dome of the jugular bulb and, anterior and medial to this, the bony plate covering the internal carotid artery as it turns forwards from the artery in the neck to run medial to the Eustachian tube before it turns into the cavernous sinus.

The mastoid air-cell system

The mastoid antrum and its related air cells lie within the petrous portion of the temporal bone. The air-filled spaces communicate with the middle ear by way of the attic and some small spaces between the suspensory ligaments of the ossicles. The roof of the mastoid antrum and mastoid air-cell space form the floor of the middle cranial fossa, whereas the medial wall relates to the posterior

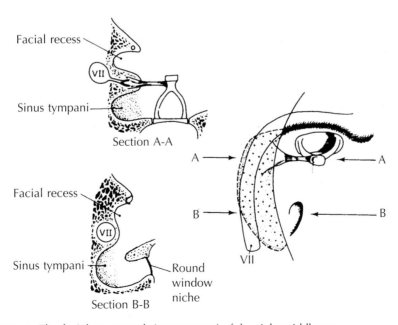

Fig 1.13 The facial recess and sinus tympani of the right middle ear.

cranial fossa. Just deep to the dural plate of the posterior cranial fossa is the saccus endolymphaticus, which derives from the endolymphatic duct, which, in turn, has passed through the vestibular aqueduct of the temporal bone. There are several straight blood vessels running along the length of the sac on its mastoid surface. Posterior to the endolymphatic system is the sigmoid sinus, which curves downwards only to turn sharply upwards to pass medial to the facial nerve and then become the dome of the jugular bulb in the middle ear space. The posterior belly of the digastric muscle forms a groove in the base of the mastoid bone. The corresponding ridge inside the mastoid lies lateral not only to the sigmoid sinus, but also to the facial nerve and is a useful landmark for finding the nerve itself. The periosteum of the digastric groove on the undersurface of the mastoid bone continues anteriorly and part of it becomes the endosteum of the stylomastoid foramen and, subsequently, of the facial nerve canal.

The outer wall of the mastoid lies just below the skin and is easily palpable behind the pinna. MacEwen's triangle is a direct lateral relation to the mastoid antrum and is formed by a posterior prolongation of the line of the zygomatic arch and a tangent to this that passes through the posterior border of the external auditory meatus.

The mastoid air-cell system is, in most of the population, fairly extensive, with air cells extending into the mastoid tip, the retrofacial region, the sinodural angle and anteriorly into the petrous apex and arch of the zygoma. It seems that in individuals with

chronic ear disease the mastoid is not well aerated, although it is still a matter of debate as to whether this is cause or effect (see Chapter 24 for more a more detailed discussion). The lining of the mastoid is, in normal ears, a flattened, non-ciliated epithelium without goblet cells or mucus glands.

The anteromedial apex of the petrous bone is shaped like a foreshortened pyramid and points anteriorly and medially. The posteromedial surface of the petrous apex is part of the posterior cranial fossa, whereas the superior aspect of the bone forms the floor of the middle cranial fossa. Running through the bony petrous apex are the carotid artery and the internal auditory meatus. At the apex of the petrous bone is the trigeminal nerve running into Meckel's cave with the VIth (abducent) nerve passing close to its roof. Gradenigo's syndrome is the result of infection at the petrous apex and comprises a lateral rectus palsy, pain in the face and discharging ear.

The internal auditory meatus

The internal auditory meatus is a short canal running into the petrous apex and carrying both the auditory and vestibular nerves and the facial nerve (Fig 1.14). The apex of this canal is traversed by a crest (the crista falciformis) that separates the nerves into upper and lower groups. The upper group consists of the facial nerve (VIIth), which runs anteriorly, with the superior vestibular nerve (VIIIth) lying in the posterior portion of this superior compartment. Inferiorly and anteriorly, in the

SUPERIOR

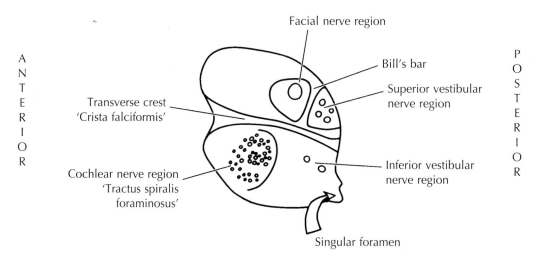

Fig 1.14 The apex of the right internal auditory meatus as seen from the posterior cranial fossa.

lower compartment, is the cochlear nerve (VIIIth), whereas inferiorly and posteriorly are the inferior vestibular nerve and the singular nerve. The superior vestibular nerve supplies the ampulla of the superior and lateral semicircular canals and part of the utricle; the inferior vestibular nerve supplies the rest of the utricle and the saccule whereas the singular nerve supplies the ampulla of the posterior semicircular canal.

THE INNER EAR

The bony labyrinth is derived from the inner periosteal layer of the otic capsule and in the adult comprises a thin but very dense shell. The space within this shell is filled with perilymph and can be divided into three anatomical and functional portions: the semicircular canals, the vestibule and the cochlea. Within the bony labyrinth lies the membranous labyrinth, which is filled with endolymph and which contains the sensory cells of hearing and balance (Fig 1.15).

The three semicircular canals are the most posterior element of the labyrinth. The lateral canal is nearly horizontal and has a small swelling at its anterior end. This is called the ampulla and it contains vestibular sensory cells. The ampulla of the lateral canal lies next to the ampulla of the superior canal, the plane of which lies nearly at right angles to the plane of the lateral canal and in turn to that of the posterior canal. The superior and posterior canals join at their non-ampullated ends as the crus commune, which is the most medial part of the semicircular canal system. The ampulla of the posterior canal is situated inferiorly. Within the fluid-filled spaces of the three bony canals lies a replica in the form of the membranous labyrinth, with the membranous ampullae corresponding to the bony enlargements.

The vestibule lies between the semicircular canals and the cochlear portion of the labyrinth. Within the vestibule are two collections of sensory cells located within membranous compartments called the saccule and utricle. The utricle is the more posterior and the saccule lies underneath the footplate of the stapes. The two interconnect by way of the utricular and saccular ducts. These join and in turn give rise to the endolymphatic duct, which passes posteriorly and medially through the temporal bone in a channel called the vestibular aqueduct to enter the posterior cranial fossa between the bone and the dura. As the endolymphatic duct enters the posterior fossa just medial to the posterior semicircular canal it expands into the flattened endolymphatic sac. The five openings of the ends of the three membranous semicircular

canals open into the utricle. Arising from the anterior part of the saccule is the very narrow ductus reuniens, which joins the cochlear duct

The cochlea

The bony cochlea has a coiled shell-like appearance and houses a spiral structure, part bone, part membrane, called the cochlear duct or scala media. This contains endolymph and the sensory cells of hearing. The ductus reuniens passes backwards from the base of the cochlear duct into the saccule. The saccular and utricular ducts connect the utricle and semicircular canals to the endolymphatic duct and sac. This is not to say that the endolymph, filling the membranous labyrinth, flows from one place to another. Indeed, it seems as if the ductus reuniens, which has only a microscopic lumen, is probably incapable of transmitting fluid from the cochlear duct posteriorly into the saccule and utricle.

The cochlear duct is triangular in section and spirals through approximately two and a half turns from base to apex. The human cochlear duct has a length of approximately 35 mm although there is a wide range of lengths from 29 to 40 mm. The duct has a flat floor called the spiral lamina, a side wall, which is mainly the stria vascularis, and a sloping, diagonal roof called Reissner's membrane. The spiral lamina of the cochlea runs around a central bony core called the modiolus like the thread of a screw. At the apex of the modiolus the thread-like spiral lamina takes off into the fluid-filled spaces of the apex of the cochlea. As this apical crescent is not attached to the modiolus, there is a gap between the space above (scala vestibuli) and the space below (scala tympani), which is called the helicotrema.

The spiral lamina has a bony portion – the bony spiral lamina attached to the modiolus – and a membranous portion or basilar membrane, which extends from the edge of the bony spiral lamina to the outer wall of the labyrinth.

The organ of Corti is a band-like structure situated on the basilar membrane and contains the auditory sensory cells (Fig 1.16). These sensory cells have hair-like stereocilia projecting from their upper, endolymphatic surfaces and have therefore become called hair cells. There are two types of auditory hair cells, the inner hair cells (IHCs) and the outer hair cells (OHCs). The IHC lies closer to the modiolus than the OHC and has a rounded flask-like shape. It is surrounded by supporting cells and has about 10 separate afferent auditory nerve fibres that make synaptic connection with its basal end. There are approximately 3500 IHCs in a healthy human cochlea.

(a)

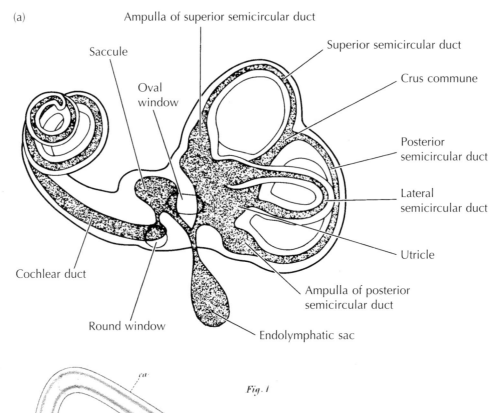

Ampulla of superior semicircular duct

Saccule

Superior semicircular duct

Oval window

Crus commune

Posterior semicircular duct

Lateral semicircular duct

Utricle

Cochlear duct

Ampulla of posterior semicircular duct

Round window

Endolymphatic sac

(b)

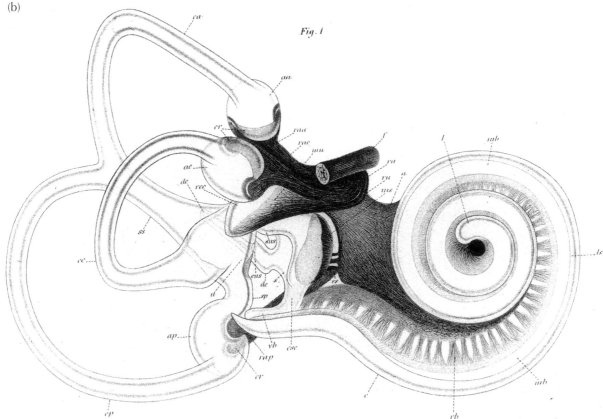

Fig. 1

Fig 1.15 (a) The left bony labyrinth viewed from a lateral aspect with the membranous labyrinth shown stippled. (b) A drawing of the right membranous labyrinth exquisitely executed by Gustav Retzius in compendious works that illustrated the inner ears of a whole range of animals. The work from which this illustration is taken was published in 1882 and I have no idea how he managed to achieve the accuracy shown here and in Figure 1.16(e).

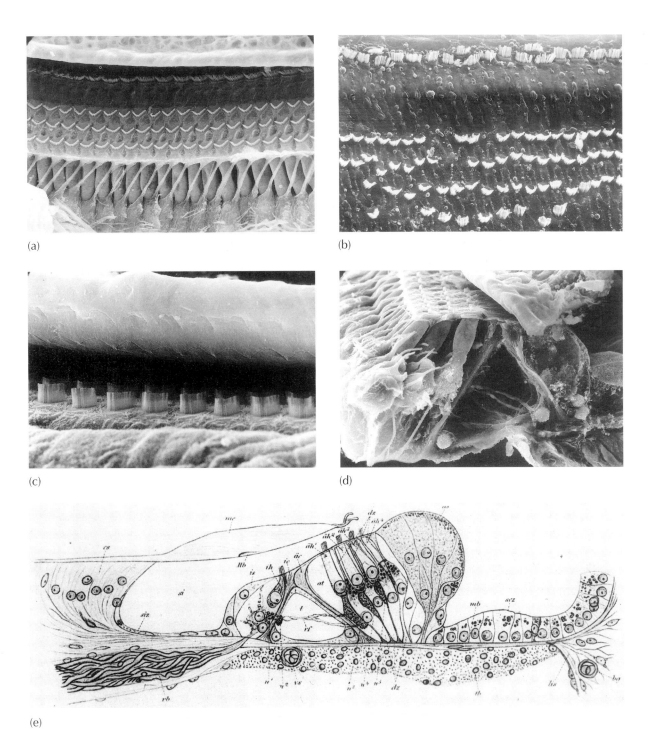

(a)

(b)

(c)

(d)

(e)

Fig 1.16 (a) The surface of the gerbil organ of Corti. The outer supporting cells have been removed to reveal the cylindrical bodies of the outer hair cells and the finger-like processes of the Deiters' cells as they extend up to the surface of the organ of Corti to form a reticular (net-like) pattern. The inner hair cells can be seen as a single row of cells with a straight array of stereocilia. (b) The surface of the human organ of Corti showing a rather disorganized arrangement with missing OHCs and extra IHCs. (c) A different angle of view of the gerbil organ of Corti showing the hair cell bundles and the marks of the insertion of the longest stereocilia into the underside of the tectorial membrane, which has rolled up during preparation. (d) The cut end of the organ of Corti showing the triangular tunnel of Corti bounded by the pillar cells and with the tunnel-crossing fibres on their way to the OHCs. (e) A diagram by Retzius of a section of the organ of Corti showing the beautiful detail that has not been improved upon with modern technology 100 years later.

Between the IHCs and the OHCs is a triangular space called the tunnel of Corti. The roof of this is formed by an arch of the processes of the inner and outer pillar cells. These processes are formed mainly by microtubular elements and seem to give a rigidity to the overall structure. Further out are the OHCs, which are arranged in parallel rows, although in the human this arrangement is rather haphazard and irregular compared with the rodent ear. Each OHC is cylindrical in shape and is supported at its lower pole by the cup-like processes of Deiters' cells. Finger-like projections from the Deiters' cells (the phalangeal processes) extend to the upper, endolymphatic surface of the organ of Corti, where they broaden out to form the supporting network (the reticular network) that surrounds the upper ends of the OHCs. The body of the OHC is therefore surrounded by a space that is filled with a fluid called Cortilymph, which probably has the same composition as perilymph. The OHCs only contribute a little to the afferent inner-vation arising from the cochlea, but they have a good efferent supply coming from the various tunnel-crossing fibres that in turn derive from the olivocochlear bundle (see below). There are approximately 12 000 OHCs in each organ of Corti.

The apical surfaces of the OHCs and the IHCs have stereocilia projecting from them into the endolymph. The stereocilia are not, however, true cilia with a '9 + 2' internal structure of microtubules, but rather have a core of actin molecules packed in a paracrystalline array that gives the stereocilia a rigid and rather fragile structure. The cilia do not bend when displaced, but pivot about their insertions into the thickened upper surface of the hair cell. Each of the stereocilia of a bundle on one hair cell is linked by very fine bands to the adjacent stereocilia (Fig 1.17). The tips of the shorter stereocilia also have links to adjacent taller stereocilia and it is these links that are thought to be responsible for the opening of ion channels during auditory stimulation (see Chapter 2).

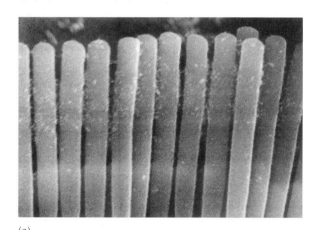

(a)

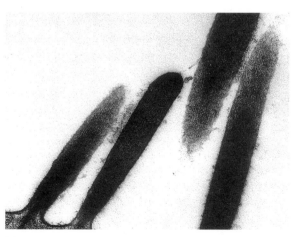

(c)

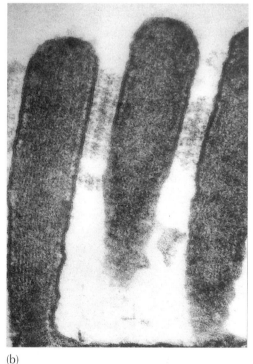

(b)

Fig 1.17 (a) A scanning electron micrograph (SEM) of the stereocilia of an IHC showing the links between adjacent stereocilia. (b) A transmission electron micrograph (TEM) of a similar area showing these links in more detail. (c) A TEM of a cluster of OHC stereocilia showing both a cross link and a tip link between the central stereocilium and the adjacent larger one.

The tectorial membrane arises from a lip or limbus on the edge of the bony spiral lamina. The membrane, which is a fibrogelatinous structure, spreads outwards across the organ of Corti and, in life, attaches to the supporting cells (the Hensen's and Claudius' cells), which lie on the outer side of the OHCs. The tips of the longest stereocilia of the OHCs insert a little way into the tectorial membrane, but in the mature organ of Corti the tips of the stereocilia of the IHCs do not.

Stria vascularis

The lateral wall of the cochlear duct constitutes, in the main, the stria vascularis (Fig 1.18). As the name suggests this strip is highly vascular and consists of a single marginal, endolymphatic layer of cells, an intermediate cell layer and a basal cell layer.

The intermediate and basal cell layers have many capillaries passing through them, although there do not seem to be any nerve fibres attached to the walls of these vessels. The marginal cells are covered with microvilli on their endolymphatic surface and have 'tight junctions' between neighbouring cells. These cells seem to be metabolically very active, being rich in mitochondria and containing a very extensive Golgi apparatus and endoplasmic reticulum. It is generally thought that the stria vascularis maintains the composition of the endolymph with its high concentration of potassium (approximately 140 mM) and high positive endocochlear potential (+80 mV) by its activity. Cell groups very similar to the stria vascularis surround the sensory cell regions of the saccule and utricle (the maculae) and the ampullae of the semicircular canal. These collections of strial-like tissue are called the 'dark cell' regions. It is thought that these areas locally maintain the composition of the endolymph in the vestibular portion of the labyrinth.

The perilymph

The perilymph strongly resembles extracellular fluid and cerebrospinal fluid. Indeed, there is a communication between the cerebrospinal fluid space and the scala tympani of the basal turn of the cochlear. This channel is called the cochlear aqueduct and could be the route of transfer of organisms from the cerebrospinal fluid to the labyrinth during an attack of meningitis. However, whereas the bony cochlear aqueduct may sometimes appear wide on conventional CT scanning the lumen of the duct is filled with a fibrous mesh, which probably limits the free passage of fluid between the two chambers.

The vestibular labyrinth

The sensory cells of the vestibular labyrinth detect acceleration and deceleration of the head in ways that are described in Chapter 2. The sensory cells are found in the maculae of the saccule and utricle and in the crista of the ampullae of the three semicircular canals. The saccule lies within the vestibule opposite the stapes footplate. It is almost globular in shape, but is prolonged posteriorly. The macula lies on the anterior wall of the saccule. The utricle is larger than the saccule and lies in the posterior superior part of the vestibule. The lower part of the lateral wall of the utricle contains the macula, the plane of which lies at right angles to that of the macula of the saccule. Both the maculae contain sensory cells and supporting cells. The sensory cells are of two types – I and II. The type-I cells are flask-shaped (rather like the IHCs) and each cell body is surrounded by a large goblet-shaped nerve terminal or chalice that may enclose many type-I hair cells. From the upper, endolymphatic surface of each type-I hair cell arises a cluster of stereocilia – much as in the cochlea – but in addition there is a single kinocilium, which is a true cilium with an associated basal body (Fig 1.19).

The type-II cells also have an array of stereocilia and a single kinocilium, but have a cylindrical cell

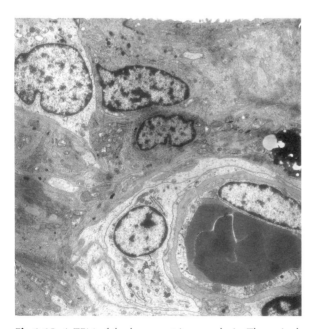

Fig 1.18 A TEM of the human stria vascularis. The apical, endolymphatic surface is at the top of the micrograph and the highly convoluted pattern of attachment between the marginal and intermediate cells can be seen. A capillary is present between the intermediate and basal cell layers.

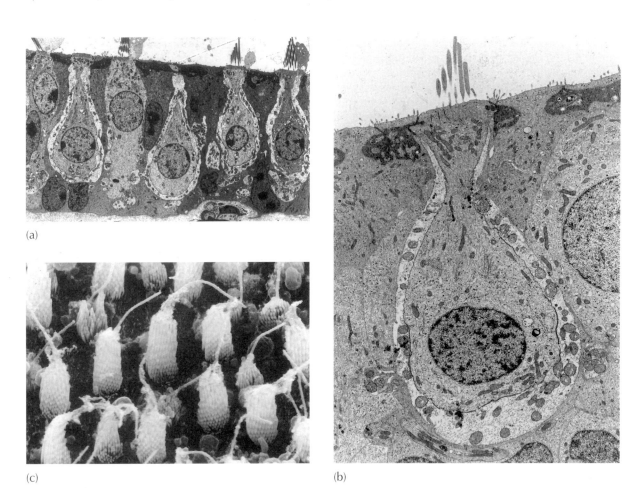

(a)

(b)

(c)

Fig 1.19 (a) A low power TEM view of the macula of the utricle showing the flask-shaped type-I cells and a single cylindrical type-II cell with a cluster of button-like nerve teminals around the base and side walls. (b) A single type-I cell with a nerve chalice. (c) The surface of the macule of the utricle showing the clusters of stereocilia with the single long kinocilium arising from each bundle.

body and a cluster of button-like nerve terminals that make synaptic contact with the basal regions.

The afferent nerve fibres that arise from type-II cells are slightly smaller than those arising from type-I cells. The efferent fibres that supply the type-II cells have granulated button-type nerve endings making direct contact with the cell bodies, whereas the efferent fibres to the type-I cells appear to end on the afferent nerve chalice, rather than the cell body itself.

The sensory cells as well as being able to detect acceleration have a 'direction sense' built in to their physiology by having 'polarity'. That is to say, deflection of the hair cell bundle in the direction of the kinocilium results in stimulation of the hair cell and an increased neural output, whereas deflection in the opposite direction results in inhibition. This is also true for the cochlear hair cells although the kinocilium that was located on the outer edge of the

array of stereocilia regresses as the hair cell matures.

The ampulla of each semicircular canal has a saddle-shaped ridge running across its long axis (Fig 1.20). This ridge is the crista and is located on the wall of the ampulla so that its surface faces the centre of the semicircular canal to which it belongs. Each crista contains type-I and type-II sensory cells and supporting cells. The sensory cells appear to be evenly mixed across the crista but on any one crista the polarity of the sensory cells is always the same. In the lateral (horizontal) semicircular canal the kinocilium is on the utricular side of each hair cell so that deflection of the stereocilia towards the utricle (utriculopetal or ampullopetal) results in an increased neural output.

In the posterior and superior canals (the vertical canals) the reverse holds and the kinocilium is on the semicircular canal side of each sensory cell.

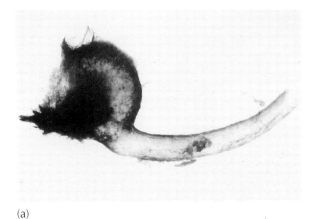

(a)

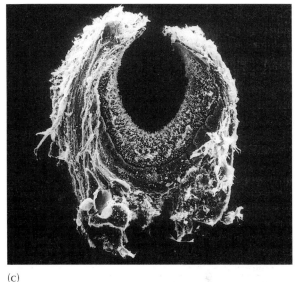

(c)

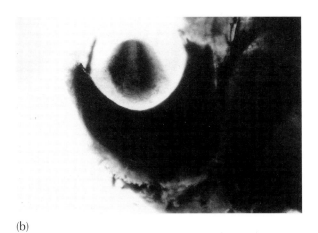

(b)

Fig 1.20 (a) A portion of a human semicircular canal and its associated ampulla. (b) An end-on view of the ampulla showing the saddle-shaped crista and the cupula, which has shrunk considerably during processing. (c) An SEM of the crista of a young woman showing the carpet of stereocilia over the crest of the crista, which has curled up a little with preparation.

Deflection of the stereociliary bundles away from the utricle (utriculofugal or ampullofugal) is therefore needed for stimulation.

The orientation of the hair cells in the maculae is quite different and much more complex (Fig 1.21). In the saccule, which is approximately comma-shaped, and the utricle, which is rather wider, there is a region running approximately along the axis of each macula, in which the polarity of the sensory cells changes abruptly through 180°. This region is the striola. The mechanisms defining the creation of such a level of complexity of hair cell orientation by differential growth from a collection of hair cell precursors are only just being considered.

The otoconial membrane and the cupula

The stereocilia of the vestibular cells extend into the endolymph and are partly embedded in a highly specialized fibrogelatinous structure rather like the tectorial membrane in the cochlea.

In the saccule and utricle this structure is named the otoconial membrane as it contains the otoconia, which are calcium-based 'crystals' (Fig 1.22). In humans these crystals have a consistent shape, but vary in size and can be up to 30 µm long. In the region of the striola they are rather smaller than elsewhere and are usually heaped up in a snowdrift pattern.

The otoconia probably form by the condensation of calcium in the sulphated mucopolysaccharides of the otoconial membrane. The calcium appears to be derived from the unimaginatively named 'globular bodies', which are produced by the supporting cells and are very calcium rich. The otoconia, once formed, are not static bodies and appear to have a slow turnover, with old otoconia possibly being resorbed by the dark cell regions that are adjacent to the maculae. It seems very likely that new otoconia are formed during life although this has not been unequivocally demonstrated.

In the ampullae of the semicircular canals a fibrogelatinous cupula sits on the crista and in life extends to fill the membranous ampullae. There is a narrow endolymph-filled, subcupular space between the crista and the cupula and into this space project the cilia of the sensory cells. During routine histological preservation, the cupula shrinks

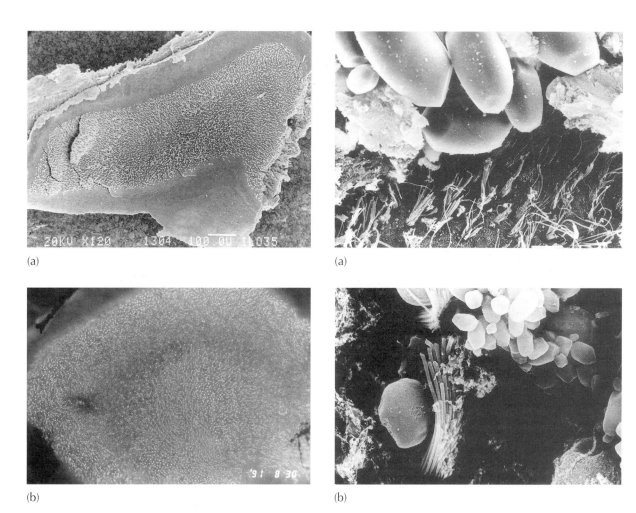

(a)

(b)

(a)

(b)

Fig 1.21 (a) An SEM of the macule of the saccule showing the comma shape and striolar region running along its centre and marked by an apparent lessening of hair cell density. (b) A fluorescence light micrograph of the macule of the utricle stained with phalloidin, which shows stereocilia and which again indicates the striolar region by the reduced staining.

Fig 1.22 (a) An SEM of the surface of the human macula showing the large otoconia embedded in the dried otoconial membrane dwarfing the underlying bundles of stereocilia. (b) A view close to the striolar region showing the cluster of small, possibly newly formed otoconia and a 'globular body' close to the bundle of stereocilia.

dramatically (as does the tectorial membrane and the otoconial membrane) and this anatomical artefact may have resulted in some of the earlier, misleading theories of function (Fig 1.23).

THE INNERVATION OF THE INNER EAR

The afferent innervation

The cochlea

The afferent nerve fibres, which are about 30 000 in number in humans and which arise mainly from the IHCs, pass into the bony spiral lamina and modiolus. The sensory body of each nerve fibre is found in this region and is of interest as it is bipolar and usually unmyelinated unlike most other sensory ganglion cell bodies, which are unipolar and myelinated. The acoustic nerve fibre loses its myelin sheath shortly before it enters the cell body, but soon regains it as it passes further into the modiolus. Subsequently the fibres pass into the acoustic nerve bundle within the internal auditory meatus. The fibres from the apex (low tones) lie in the centre of the bundle, whereas those from the base (high tones) form the outer layer. The nerve can be said to have a tonotopic arrangement with different areas representing different frequencies.

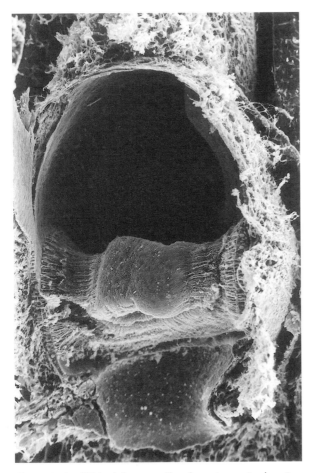

Fig 1.23 An SEM of the ampulla of a guinea pig showing how the cupula has shrunk down to a small mass on the crista.

The nerve bundle now passes into the internal auditory meatus and is joined by the superior and inferior vestibular nerves and subsequently by the singular nerve to form the complete acousti-covestibular bundle. The acoustic nerve is not intertwined with the vestibular nerve and can be surgically separated. There is often a groove between the two divisions with a small blood vessel on its surface to help decide the plane of separation during vestibular neurectomy. When viewed from the brainstem the facial and acousticovestibular nerve bundles make a 90° clockwise rotation about themselves as they pass from the meatus and across the cerebellopontine angle (see Chapter 16).

The efferent fibres to the cochlea leave the brainstem in the superior vestibular nerve and travel with this into the meatus where they cross to the acoustic division by way of Oort's anastomosis, which is a rather small bundle of fibres.

The vestibular system

Large myelinated fibres from the type-I and type-II sensory cells pass into their respective parts of the vestibular nerve. The utricle and the cristae of the lateral and superior semicircular canals provide fibres to the superior division, the saccule to the inferior division and the ampulla of the posterior canal to the singular (posterior) nerve. These three divisions all join within the internal auditory meatus and at a variable distance along the canal can be found the vestibular ganglion (Scarpa's ganglion). This structure comprises primitive bipolar cell bodies like those in the spiral (cochlear) ganglion.

The central auditory pathways

The acoustic nerve enters the brainstem in the groove between the pons and the medulla oblongata. The ascending, afferent fibres first enter the cochlear nucleus, which itself is subdivided into several distinct groupings. The ventral nucleus is the first point of entry and from here fibres pass to the anteroventral, posteroventral and the dorsal nuclei. The tonotopicity of the cochlea and the acoustic nerve is strictly maintained at this level.

From the cochlear nucleus fibres pass to the superior olive on the same side and a large bundle passes to the contralateral superior olive via the trapezoid body so that from very early on in the ascending pathway a binaural representation for auditory processing is established (Fig 1.24). The auditory tract then ascends by the lateral lemniscus to the inferior colliculus and thence to the medial geniculate body by way of the auditory radiation. From the medial geniculate body there are connections with the auditory cortex, which is hidden in the lateral or Sylvian fissure in the superior temporal gyrus (Brodmann area 41 in humans). There are probably several acoustic areas in humans, but this region is termed the 'first acoustic area (A1)'.

The efferent supply

The efferent pathways appear to run from the auditory cortex parallel to the afferent tracts down to the level of the cochlear nuclei. Here there are additional contributions from the superior olive both crossed and uncrossed, which may synapse in the cochlear nuclei or pass directly through to leave the brainstem in the superior division of the vestibular nerve (Fig 1.25). The efferent fibres terminate almost exclusively on the bodies of the OHCs, but the way in which they control cochlear function is unknown.

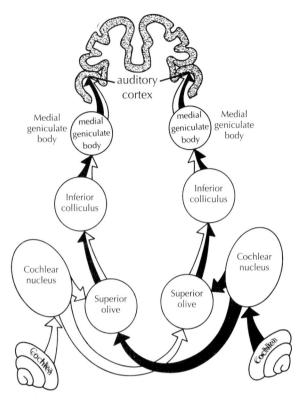

Fig 1.24 A diagram of the ascending auditory pathways.

The central vestibular pathways

The vestibular nerve enters the brainstem at the lower border of the pons and is separated from the facial nerve by the acoustic nerve, the intermediate nerve (sensory – taste and secretomotor – salivary and lacrimal division of VII) and usually by the anterior inferior cerebellar artery.

The vast majority of the vestibular nerve fibres bifurcate into an ascending and descending branch, both of which enter the vestibular nuclei. Further branching of the ascending division allows fibres to enter the cerebellum directly.

In the vestibular nuclear complex there have conventionally been described four main nuclei, although other lesser nuclei also exist.

- superior (Bechterew)
- lateral (Deiters')
- medial (triangular or Schwalbe)
- descending (inferior or spinal)

This vestibular nuclear complex occupies a large area just below the floor of the fourth ventricle. The organization of the vestibular nuclei and their connections with the nuclei that subserve eye-movements (III, IV, VI), the spinal cord, the cerebral cortex and other parts of the brainstem is stunningly complex. Furthermore, there are efferent

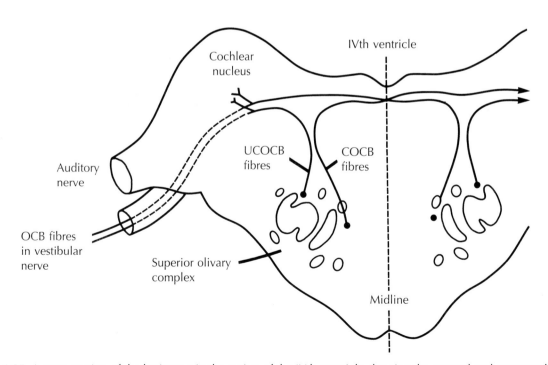

Fig 1.25 A cross-section of the brainstem in the region of the IVth ventricle showing the crossed and uncrossed fibres from the olivary nuclei leaving the brainstem by way of the vestibular nerve roots as the crossed and uncrossed olivocochlear bundle (COCB and UCOCB). (Reproduced with permission of Dr James Pickles.)

fibres, albeit few in number, that leave the vestibular nuclei to act on the type-I and type-II hair cells.

THE BLOOD SUPPLY TO THE LABYRINTH

The labyrinthine artery, which is usually a branch of the anterior inferior cerebellar artery, passes along the internal auditory meatus, usually between the facial and the acousticovestibular nerves. The artery divides subsequently into an anterior vestibular and a common cochlear artery. Further division of the common cochlear artery into a cochlear division and a vestibulocochlear division is seen, although there is great variability. The arterial supply to the labyrinth is of the form of a single feeding artery with no collateral circulation. The supply is also fairly well distributed by its branches to either the cochlear or the labyrinthine segment with little overlap between the two.

Acknowledgement

I am greatly indebted to Dr Andrew Forge, Reader in Auditory Cell Biology at the Institute of Laryngology and Otology for his continuing support and for supplying Figures 1.16 (a), (b) and (c), 1.17 (a), (b) and (c), 1.19 (a), (b) and (c), 1.21 (a) and (b) and 1.23.

Suggested reading

Axelsson A. The vascular anatomy of the cochlea in the guinea pig and man. *Acta Otolaryngologica* 1968; **suppl 243**:6–134.

Brodal A. *Neurological anatomy in relation to clinical medicine, 3rd ed.* New York: Oxford University Press, 1981.

Donaldson JA, Lambert PM, Duckert LG, Rubel EW. *Surgical anatomy of the temporal bone, 4th ed.* New York: Raven Press, 1992.

Michaels L, Soucek S. Development of the stratified squamous epithelium of the human lympanic membrane and external ear canal. *American Journal of Anatomy* 1989; **184**:334–44.

Spoendlin H. Primary neurons and synapses. In: Friedman I, Ballantyne J eds. *Ultrastructural atlas of the inner ear.* London: Butterworths, 1984:133–64.

Stone M, Fulghum RS. Bactericidal activity of wet cerumen. *Annals of Otology, Rhinology and Laryngology* 1984; **93**:183–6.

Webster DB, Fay RR, Popper AN. *The evolutionary biology of hearing.* New York: Springer-Verlag, 1992.

Wright A, Davis A, Bredberg G, Ulehlova L, Spencer H. Hair cell distributions in the normal human cochlea. *Acta Otolaryngologica* 1987; **suppl 444**:1–48.

CHAPTER 2

Applied anatomy and physiology of the ear

TONY WRIGHT

The pinna and external ear canal

In humans the pinna has only a small role to play in the collection of sound although it is common experience that sound collection can be enhanced by 'cupping' the ear with the curved palm of the hand. Indeed, the early acoustic hearing trumpets relied on this principle and were sometimes enough

to overcome a slight hearing loss. Loss of the pinna worsens the hearing level by about 5 dB over the speech frequencies.

The ear canal has a much more important role in hearing. As well as protecting the tympanic membrane from direct damage by its curvature, the physical characteristics of the canal act to enhance the sound pressure levels at the eardrum over a range of frequencies.

It is a property of any tube that is open at one end and closed at the other that sound introduced

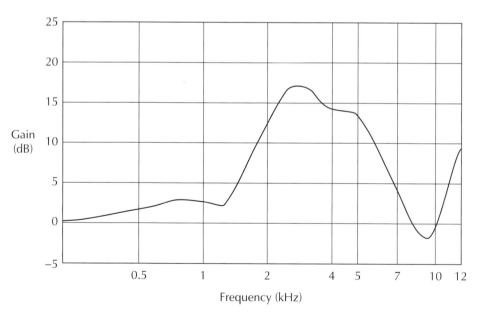

Fig 2.1 Sound pressure levels at the tympanic membrane. The average pressure gain of the external ear canal in humans as measured at the tympanic membrane. The gain in pressure at the tympanic membrane over that in the free field is plotted against frequency for a source at the side of the head.

at the open end will show a distribution of sound pressures along the tube depending on the frequency of the sound and the length and diameter of the tube. There is no 'amplification' of sound because no energy is put into the system. There is merely a redistribution of the energy in the form of resonant peaks. In the ear canal the sound pressures at the eardrum show an enhancement over a 'useful' range of frequencies. This is depicted in Figure 2.1, which indicates a gain of up to 15 dB on the original sound level at the tympanic membrane although elsewhere in the ear canal there will be an overall 15 dB loss in the sound pressure levels at this particular frequency.

Loss of the normal ear canal anatomy as in a modified radical mastoid cavity does affect the resonance properties of the ear canal, but not as much as might be thought.

The middle ear

One of the many problems facing animals changing from an aquatic or marine life to a terrestrial existence was adaptation to an environment in which sound was airborne, rather than transmitted through fluid. Some remedies to this problem have been 'modelled' in certain fishes in which an extension of an air sac or swim-bladder is interposed between the outside water and the inner ear. Among the modern bony fishes only the more primitive species have developed connections between the outside, the swim-bladder and the inner ear, either directly or by way of a chain of ossicles. The great majority of the modern bony fishes have no connection whatsoever between their swim-bladder and the inner ear. Nevertheless, the transition from an 'aquatic' to a 'terrestrial' life has raised the question as to whether the tympanic cavity evolved only once or three times, that is, independently in reptiles, birds and mammals. Whatever the precise mechanism of evolution, there has been a convergence of function in that the stapes has lost its primary role as a support for the lower jaw in the primitive fishes and the hyoid bone has been incorporated into the middle ear. The insertion of a mobile but rigid structure into the ear capsule must have been a crucial event in the evolution of terrestrial hearing. In simple terms the problem has been to overcome the widely different impedances of air and perilymph. Transfer of sound between two media of very different impedances is accompanied by a major loss of energy as sound is reflected from the interface rather than being absorbed by the second medium. Echoes are best heard in rocky caverns containing a lake as at least

99 per cent of sound is reflected from the surface of a large body of water and from the surrounding hard rock.

The impedance of air is 430 N·s/m³ (Newton seconds per cubic metre). The impedance of the cochlea is not the same as that of a large body of water and has been measured experimentally and calculated as approximately 1.5×10^5 N·s/m³ at 1 kHz. Attempting to get sound from air directly into the cochlear fluids results in a reduction of energy transfer that approximates to a 60 dB loss.

This problem has been partly overcome by the development of the middle ear mechanism, which comprises a mobile tympanic membrane, an air-filled middle ear and a system of bones linking the tympanic membrane to the perilymph (Fig 2.2). In birds there is a single bony strut called the columella. In mammals, which are morphologically

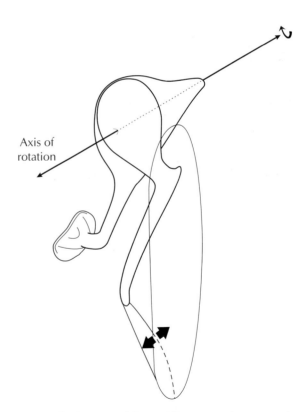

Fig 2.2 The features of the middle ear transformer mechanism. First and most importantly, there is the large area of the tympanic membrane compared with the area of the stapes footplate. Then there is then lever ratio of the effective length of the malleus handle compared with that of the long process of the incus and finally there is the relatively small buckling effect of the tympanic membrane. The areal ratio of the membrane to the stapes footplate has by far the most significant effect.

Axis of rotation

unique, the three ossicles connect the tympanic membrane to the oval window. This arrangement goes a long way to matching the impedance of air to that of the labyrinthine fluids by three different but additive factors.

THE RATIO OF THE AREAS OF THE TYMPANIC MEMBRANE TO THE OVAL WINDOW

The sound pressure collected over the large area of the tympanic membrane is transferred to the small area of the stapes footplate so that the sound pressure at the oval window is enhanced, although this gain is balanced by a loss of displacement. The ratio of the areas of the two structures in different species varies quite considerably, but in the cat the tympanic membrane has an area of 0.42 cm^2 and a stapes footplate about 0.012 cm^2. The pressure on the stapes footplate is, therefore, increased by 0.42/0.012, that is 35 times. In other words, rather large amplitude but relatively low pressure airborne sound is converted to high pressure rather low amplitude movement – albeit of the same frequency – at the oval window.

THE TYMPANIC MEMBRANE'S FLEXIBILITY

The middle layer of the tympanic membrane has a complex arrangement of radial and circular fibres and its shape, although concave towards the external canal, rather like a loudspeaker cone, is convex in each segment from annulus to malleus handle. This results in the membrane having a degree of flexibility so that complex patterns of vibration occur at different frequencies and intensities across its surface. The membrane does not act like a stiff loudspeaker cone, but buckles in response to incoming sound. It is felt by some authors that this buckling factor helps in impedance matching as the sound energy absorbed by the fibres of the middle layer of the drum is, in turn, transferred to the malleus handle. This increases the forces transferred to the labyrinthine fluids although it is relatively a small factor and has been assessed as improving the impedance value by a factor of 4.

THE OSSICULAR CHAIN

The ossicles are surrounded by air, which provides them with a very low friction environment. The ossicular chain, in mammals, also has a small con-

tributory effect in the direct reduction of the impedance mismatch. The malleus and incus are suspended by a series of ligaments that, in effect, reduces their mass and inertia. The two bones, however, also provide a lever effect. The long process of the incus is shorter than the malleus handle and overall this produces a lever action that converts low pressure with a long lever action at the malleus handle to higher pressure, albeit with a short lever action, at the tip of the long process of the incus and subsequently at the stapes footplate. The lever action improves the impedance ratio by a factor of approximately 1.3.

The combination of these three factors reduces the impedance of the inner ear fluids by a theoretical factor of approximately 185 (i.e. 35 × 4 × 1.3). This would effectively reduce the impedance of the inner ear by the same factor to give a figure of 810 N·s/m^3 (i.e. 1.5 × 10^5/185). This figure is still higher than the impedance of air, but nevertheless the mismatch has been greatly reduced and the efficiency of the system improved.

Actual measurements of the impedance of the middle ear system give values of approximately 1680 N·s/m^3 at 1 kHz. This is about twice the expected value and in reality it seems that approximately 50 per cent of the energy arriving at the eardrum is transferred to the cochlea.

Of the 50 per cent energy lost in the middle ear, some is wasted in overcoming the inertia of the ossicular mass and some frictional resistance. A major element of loss is, however, reflection of sound from the tympanic membrane. It is this reflected sound that is measured in impedance tympanometry. Increases in the amount of sound reflected when the tympanic membrane is stretched or distorted indicate a loss of efficiency of the impedance matching and a change in the measured impedance.

The middle ear mechanism is not an amplifier, in that it does not increase the sound energy at the oval window compared with that at the tympanic membrane. However, it does allow airborne sound to enter the perilymph with a relatively high degree of efficiency.

The inner ear

The conversion of sound energy into impulses in the acoustic nerve, or of acceleration of the head into impulses in the vestibular nerves is brought about by the sensory cells of the labyrinth. The basic cell type is similar in both the cochlear and vestibular portions of the labyrinth and, indeed, the

Table 2.1 The relative ionic concentrations and voltages inside the hair cells and in the cochlear fluids of the rat

	Intracellular	Perilymph	Endolymph
Na$^+$	20–40 mM	138 mM	1 mM
K$^+$	120–130 mM	7 mM	154 mM
Voltage	–45 mV	0 mV	+92 mV

stimulus to depolarize the cell is the same, namely the deflection of the stereocilia that project from the apical, endolymphatic surface of these cells. It is the way that this mechanical deformation occurs that differs between hearing and balance, and within balance between linear and angular accelerations. These different mechanisms will be explained after a description of the sensory hair cell itself.

The sensory cell comprises a cell body with a nucleus that is placed towards the lower pole. The apical, endolymphatic surface is thickened to form a cuticular plate and from this project the stereocilia. These are rigid structures comprising a core of actin molecules packed in a para-crystalline array, which makes the stereocilia stiff bundles rather than the floppy structures that they appear to be in some micrographs. The shafts of the stereocilia are covered by a unit membrane that merges with the cell membrane at the cuticular plate. In any bundle of stereocilia there seem to be lateral links joining adjacent stereocilia, and where there are shorter and longer stereocilia, 'tip links' joining the tips of the shorter stereocilia to the shafts of the longer.

The inside of the cell has the normal environment of any non-neural cell with an intracellular potassium level of about 120–130 mM, a low sodium and an intracellular potential of some –45 mV (Fig 2.3). The endolymph also has a high potassium level of around 150 mM which is unusual for body fluid. There is a low sodium of around 40 mM and overall a strongly positive potential of around +80 mV. The endolymph is therefore a rather special fluid, the composition of which is maintained by the stria vascularis in the cochlear duct and by the dark cell regions that surround the cristae of the ampullae and the maculae of the utricle and saccule.

There is thus a large potential difference of some 130 mV across the apical hair cell membrane and it is this potential that drives the positive potassium ions towards the negatively charged cell interior when the cell membrane becomes 'leaky'. The stimulus to convert the stable membrane at rest to a leaky state is the deflection of the stereocilia, although the precise mechanism or the site of initial

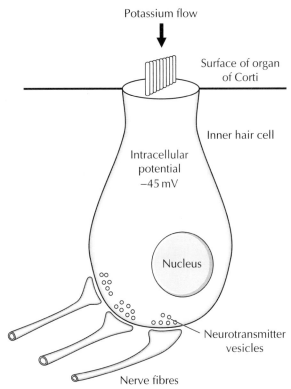

Endolymph — High Potassium
+80 mV

Potassium flow

Surface of organ of Corti

Inner hair cell

Intracellular potential –45 mV

Nucleus

Neurotransmitter vesicles

Nerve fibres

Fig 2.3 Diagram of inner hair cell with ion levels and voltages. A typical cochlear inner hair cell or vestibular sensory cell with its large negative intracellular potential and high potassium levels is shown. The endolymph above its apical surface also has a high potassium level but there is a highly positive endolymphatic potential, which is the driving force to power potassium into the hair cell and thereby depolarize it.

ion transfer is unknown. It may be that as the stereocilia are deflected, the tip links 'drag' on the membrane of the longer stereocilia to which they are attached and the 'ion gate' is deformed thus opening up a channel through which ions can pass. An 'ion gate' can be thought of as a small hole in the cell membrane that is not quite big enough to allow a K$^+$ ion through. A small increase in the diameter of the channel to something slightly more than 2×10^{-10} m will permit the K$^+$ ion to pass.

The potassium floods through these channels down an electrical gradient, and if enough positive charge reaches the inside of the sensory cell, the negative charge is reduced to such an extent that the cell can be said to have depolarized. This alters the membrane properties of the cell and nerve transmitter substances are thereby released at synapses with the afferent nerve endings, which are clustered at the base of the cell.

At 'threshold' the deflection of the stereocilia to allow enough potassium flow for depolarization is extremely small and of the order of the diameter of a few hydrogen ions. It is impossible to imagine this sort of movement, but the remarkable sensitivity is brought about by the combination of the special characteristics of the endolymph and the mechanical structure of the stereociliary bundles.

It is apparent that depolarization should be caused by deflection of the stereociliary bundle in one direction but not in the other if this mechanical opening of the 'ion gates' is to be believed. This does indeed seem to occur. The sensory cells of the vestibular apparatus have a kinocilium, which is a true cilium in the accepted sense of the word with the familiar internal '9 + 2' structure of microtubules. The kinocilium is a feature of the sensory cells of the cochlea during development, but regresses at maturity. When present the kinocilium was sited on the outer, peripheral portion of the cuticular plate of the auditory sensory cells.

In the vestibular labyrinth, deflection of the stereociliary bundle in the direction of the kinocilium results in an increased firing of the associated nerve fibres. Deflection away from the kinocilium causes a reduction of the background firing rate (Fig 2.4). The loss of any minor potassium influx through a few open gates allows the cell to hyperpolarize as the normal homeostatic mechanisms continue unchallenged by potassium influx. This occurs as the reduction of traction on the cell membrane by the tip links makes the ion channels smaller and therefore less likely to allow K$^+$ ions through so that the balance between influx and efflux tilts in favour of efflux and hyperpolarization.

To maintain the sensitivity of the system requires considerable energy consumption. Neither the organ of Corti nor the vestibular sensory regions has a closely associated blood supply and the provision of nutrients and the removal of metabolites has to be by diffusion, often over a considerable distance. The distance factor is presumably to reduce the 'noise' of the vascular system with the non-laminar flow disturbances found at capillary levels.

The sensitivity of the system can, therefore, be changed by several factors without actual mechanical damage occurring to the sensory cells themselves.

CHANGES IN THE ENDOLYMPH

The normal homeostasis of the endolymph is maintained by the highly vascular and metaboli-

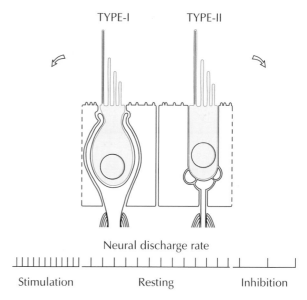

Fig 2.4 Diagram of vestibular hair cells with excitation and inhibition. The typical appearance of type-I and type-II vestibular sensory cells with the cluster of kinocilia arising from the cuticular plate of the hair-cell body is shown. Deviation of the stereociliary bundle towards the kinocilium results in an increased neural output from the cell. The opposite deflection results in inhibition. The cells can, therefore, not only detect acceleration but also detect its direction, in other words, they have polarity.

cally very active cells of the stria vascularis and dark cell regions. Alterations in the blood supply to these structures or drug effects (i.e. the loop diuretics) can probably alter the composition and electrical potential of the endolymph and may even alter its osmotic pressure. Subtle changes bring symptoms that may be out of proportion to the degree of change because of the sensitivity of the system.

MECHANICAL CHANGES TO THE STEREOCILIA

Experimentally, minute pressure changes within the cochlear duct have been shown to disrupt the 'fine tuning' of the cochlea (see below). Presumably distortion of the normal anatomy of the stereocilia alters their response to sound. It is possible to imagine that very small changes in endolymphatic pressure induced by alterations in the strial or dark cell function could account for many of the symptoms that arise from the inner ear when the cause is otherwise unknown (i.e. Menière's disease).

LOSS OF A SUSTAINABLE SUPPLY OF NUTRIENTS

Failure to sustain the metabolic activities of the sensory cells, either by over stimulation or from a poor blood supply, could account for changes at least in the cochlea, whose activity seems to be more energy dependent for normal function than does that of the vestibular regions. Although there is good evidence, as witnessed by the changes in transient evoked otoacoustic emissions and the temporary threshold shift that occurs after prolonged noise exposure, that something is happening, there is no good evidence that ischaemia brings about fluctuations in function by directly challenging the sensory cells rather than the stria or dark cell regions themselves.

Cochlear mechanics

By a series of elegant experiments Georg von Békésy laid the foundation to a modern theory of how the cochlea functions; he was awarded the Nobel Prize in 1961.

Using temporal bones from different species he opened the cochlear duct, sprinkled carbon or silver particles onto Reissner's membrane and stimulated the cochlea by a pure-tone vibrator that was inserted in place of the stapes. He observed the movement of the particles in response to pure tones with a microscope and often had a stroboscope coupled to the vibrator to 'freeze' the movement of Reissner's membrane. He was able to measure the frequency and intensity of the stimulating sound and the displacement of Reissner's membrane from its rest position. He argued that as the whole system was in an incompressible fluid, then the movement of Reissner's membrane mimicked the movement of the basilar membrane and therefore the organ of Corti relative to the tectorial membrane.

Békésy discovered that a 'wave' travelled along the basilar membrane from base to apex, reached a peak and then decayed rapidly (Fig 2.5). This travelling wave took time to reach its maximum displacement and thereby introduced a phase delay between the stimulus entering the cochlea and the peak of basilar membrane displacement. The stroboscope was used to freeze the movement of the basilar membrane at different instances within a sine wave, and thus the wave envelope was seen to comprise the sum of the instantaneous displacements through one cycle of the wave.

Changing the pitch of the incoming pure tone led to a shift in the maximal displacement of the

(a)
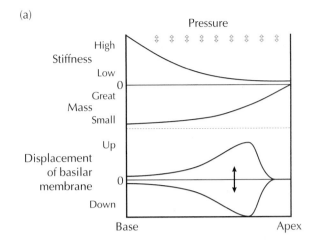
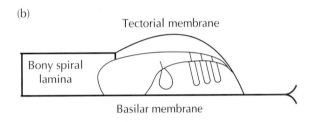

(b)
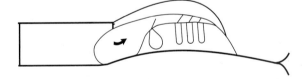

Fig 2.5 Békésy's wave envelope. (a) The composite diagram shows not only the change in stiffness and mass of segments of the basilar membrane from base to apex, but also the displacement of the membrane in relation to distance along the cochlea in response to pure tone stimulation. This is Békésy's travelling wave. (b) This diagram, which is redrawn from Békésy's original work, shows the organ of Corti at rest in the neutral position in the upper illustration. As there is basilar membrane movement with the growth of the travelling wave, there is movement of the organ of Corti relative to the tectorial membrane, which is attached to the immobile bony spiral lamina. This relative movement results not only in shearing forces across the mass of outer hair cell stereocilia but also in fluid movement under the tectorial membrane in the inner sulcus and it is this movement that deflects and consequently depolarizes the inner hair cells, which carry the bulk of the afferent innervation.

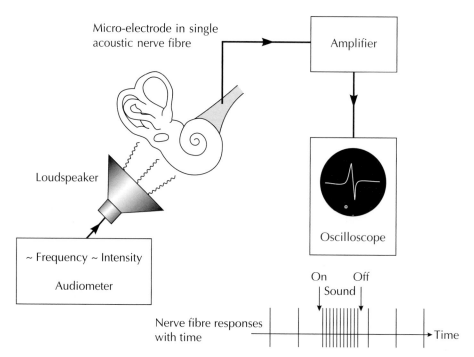

Fig 2.6 Acoustic nerve tuning curves. This is the typical experimental set-up for the detection of individual cochlear nerve fibre tuning curves. A single fine glass electrode is passed into the acoustic nerve bundle until it enters a single nerve fibre as witnessed by a significant potential voltage change. Once stabilized the stimulating source is swept across a single low intensity from low pitch to high. A neural response is recorded when there is a significantly increased output from the individual nerve fibre.

travelling wave. Higher pitches had their maxima close to the base of the cochlea whereas lower pitched sounds had maximal displacement near the apex.

The cochlea was thus tonotopically (pitch-place) organized and Békésy's discovery went a long way to explaining how the cochlea was mechanically tuned to discriminate different frequencies. However, the peak of the travelling wave did not shift until there were quite major shifts in frequency. These changes were much greater than the smallest shifts in frequency that could be detected by the human ear in the speech frequency range. The difference limen, that is the smallest detectable difference, for frequency is in the region of 1 Hz in the speech frequency range. Békésy thought that, whereas the cochlea provided a good but coarse first filter for frequency discrimination, the finer tuning was performed centrally.

However, as electrode technology improved in the 1950s and 1960s, other researchers, most notably Katsuki, Evans and Kiang, were each able to study individual fibres of the acoustic nerve. An individual fibre has a background firing rate that increases dramatically when sound above threshold is presented to the test ear. A block diagram of the experimental set-up is shown in Figure 2.6.

With such an arrangement it is possible to perform an 'audiogram' on an individual nerve fibre. What is found is that at very low intensities a single fibre responds to a single frequency only – the critical frequency (cf) for that fibre. As the intensity is increased, the band of frequencies to which the fibre responds widens until at very high intensities it will respond to most frequencies. The curve separating the area of 'response' from 'non-response' is called the tuning curve, and for virtually all of the fibres in the acoustic nerve this curve is sharply tuned. This means that near the threshold a small shift in frequency away from the critical frequency results in that fibre becoming non-responsive (Fig 2.7).

It was found that there were whole families of overlapping tuning curves and that, starting with a single narrow band of frequencies near threshold, only a small group of fibres would be firing; as the intensity increased, there would be a progressive increase in the numbers of fibres responding. This corresponded with the normal smooth growth of perceived loudness as sound intensity increased.

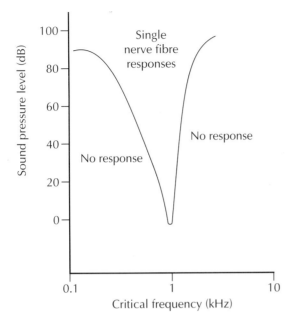

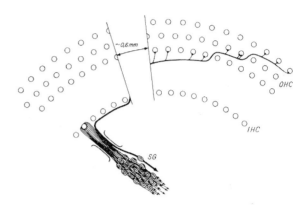

Fig 2.7 Neural frequency tuning curve (ftc). If one follows a stimulus paradigm (or protocol) that involves starting at low sound intensities and sweeping across the frequencies from low to high, a response is detected at a certain critical frequency for that particular fibre. As the intensity is increased, the fibre responds to a very narrow band of frequencies until, at last, the response range suddenly widens and many frequencies can be detected. This pattern of responses is called 'fine tuning' and distinguishes the response from that of the basilar membrane travelling wave, which is coarsely tuned.

Fig 2.8 Afferent innervation of the organ of Corti reproduced with permission of the late and greatly missed Heinrich Spoendlin, one of the great investigators of our times. This diagram represents a surface view of the organ of Corti in the cat and shows the afferent innervation from the inner hair cells (IHCs) and outer hair cells (OHCs). One IHC has about 10 afferent nerve fibres synapsing with the base of the cell body. These fibres pass inwards through the habenula perforata (shown by the tunnel), lose their myelin sheaths and then enter the bipolar cell body of the spiral ganglion (SG). Only about 5 per cent of the afferent fibres arise from the OHCs. From the spiral ganglion a single afferent fibre crosses the tunnel of Corti and then turns basalwards to supply about 10 OHCs.

From threshold to maximum stimulation there was what is called a 'wide dynamic range'.

If the experimental animals were made hypoxic or were given metabolic poison, or lost their outer hair cells through prior treatment with aminoglycoside antibiotics, then the sharp tips of the tuning curves were lost. The rather blunt curves had thresholds elevated some 40–50 dB and the dynamic range from threshold to saturation was dramatically narrowed. Once again, starting with a narrow band of sound and increasing its intensity, there would be no response at low intensities, an elevated threshold when a few fibres would 'switch on' and then, within a narrow range of intensities the fibre response would become saturated. This phenomenon was the beginning of the explanation of auditory recruitment, that is, an unusually rapid growth of loudness with increasing intensity, which is common with cochlear damage.

The finding of sharply tuned responses from the acoustic nerve fibres did not, however, fit in very well with Békésy's travelling wave, which was rather coarsely tuned. It was argued that, if the motion of the basilar membrane was a broad, first filter, then there must be a fine, second filter hidden somewhere within the cochlea in order that the output could be so finely tuned. The hunt was on for some form of second filter mechanism and theories became more and more complex invoking many mechanisms known from other systems, such as lateral inhibition as occurs in the retina, to account for the remarkable properties of the cochlea.

In the 1970s Heinrich Spoendlin began a painstaking and meticulous series of experiments to map out the innervation of the organ of Corti. The inner ear of the cat has about 3000 inner hair cells (IHCs), 10 000 outer hair cells (OHCs) and about 30 000 fibres in the acoustic nerve. Spoendlin found that about 95 per cent of the afferent fibres of the acoustic nerve arose from the IHCs in a one-to-one arrangement and that each IHC had approximately 10 afferent fibres synapsing with it. The remaining afferents arose from the OHCs, but one fibre made contact with many OHCs spread along several millimetres of the organ of Corti (Fig 2.8).

The efferent fibres from the crossed olivocochlear bundle supplied the OHCs. There did not appear to be any fibres linking IHCs together, so that lateral inhibition was an unlikely mechanism for sharpening the tuning.

In the 1970s it became possible to insert electrodes into individual IHCs. As the recording electrode entered a cell, a negative potential could be recorded and loss of this potential, that is, depolarization of the cell, when sound was applied to the ear could be recorded. Russell and Sellick were the first to find that the depolarization of the IHC was also finely tuned, which indicated that the stimulus reaching the IHC must also be finely tuned. As with the experiments relating to nerve fibres, the animals had to be well oxygenated and have intact OHCs for this IHC fine tuning to be intact.

Békésy's original experiment had been performed with dead specimens and he was having to use sound intensities equivalent to 140 dB and more in order to see movement with the light-microscope. New techniques of anaesthesia have permitted living models to be used and advances in measuring techniques allowed more physiological sound pressures of the order of 70 dB to be used as a stimulus.

The capacitance probe technique involved advancing a small plate through the scala tympani until it was close to the basilar membrane and then fixing it rigidly. The basilar membrane, with the 80 mV positive charge of the endolymph above it and the plate, forms a capacitor whose capacitance can be measured extremely accurately. The capacitance of parallel plates is related to the distance between them, and as the basilar membrane moved relative to the plate so the capacitance changed proportionally. An alternative technique – the Mossbauer technique – was to use a speck of radioactive cobalt placed on the basilar membrane, again through an approach by way of the scala tympani. Radioactive cobalt emits gamma radiation of a specific wave length as it decays, which can be detected by an appropriately placed spectrometer. When the basilar membrane vibrates, the wavelength of the emitted radiation undergoes a Doppler shift. As the membrane moves towards the detector, the wavelength shortens and the frequency increases whereas when it retreats from the detector the reverse happens.

With the use of these techniques Békésy's experiments were repeated and confirmed, although when living specimens under optimal conditions were used a peak of enhanced movement of the basilar membrane was found at the leading edge of the travelling wave. This peak of enhanced movement was 'finely tuned' in that it only appeared at one small area in response to a specific frequency. A move away from that frequency results in that region of the basilar membrane not responding with enhanced movement although another region close by did (Fig 2.9).

Once again, this finding required not only a perfectly oxygenated and metabolically active cochlea, but also an intact compliment of OHCs and, furthermore, no pressure deviations within the cochlea.

Thus, on top of Békésy's travelling wave, which was a passive phenomenon relating to the intrinsic mechanical properties of all the elements of the cochlea duct, there was an active region of basilar membrane movement that was energy dependent and required healthy OHCs for its existence. This became called the cochlear amplifier.

In the late 1970s after earlier work with celestial sound waves, Kemp pursued a suggestion first made by Gold that there should be echoes from the cochlea. The system to detect these comprised a plug that sealed the ear canal, with a small sound generator and microphone enclosed within the plug. Clicks were introduced into the ear canal and the resultant sounds detected by the microphone. With repeated clicks the output, which was time locked to the stimulus, was added together to enhance the response; furthermore, it reduced the random background noise, which, with enough time-locked repetitions, tended to cancel itself out. The responses are shown in Chapter 4 Figure 4.24 onwards.

A series of experiments was needed to exclude the middle ear structures as the source of this sound, but it was eventually accepted that the

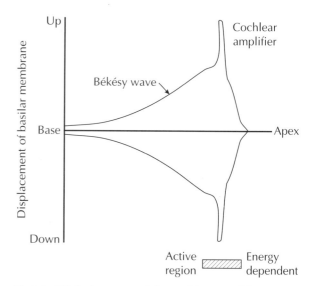

Fig 2.9 Békésy's wave and the cochlear amplifier. Experiments using a capacitance probe or, more recently, the Mossbauer technique, have suggested that on the crest of Békésy's travelling wave there is a small area that, in response to its 'own' frequency, undergoes an enhanced vibration that is 'finely tuned'. This active region of mechanical movement is energy dependent and requires the presence of healthy OHCs for it to be detected. Loss of the OHCs, damage to them from the administration of the ototoxic aminoglycoside, anoxia or metabolic poisons result in the loss of this response.

sounds arose from the cochlea. As before, the inner ear needed to be healthy and to have a functioning set of OHCs. The response was lost or significantly reduced after aminoglycoside toxicity or prolonged noise exposure, both of which damage the OHCs.

Analysis of the echo showed that under appropriate conditions the energy contained within the echo was greater than the energy that reached the cochlea. Thus, there appeared to be a mechanically active, energy-dependent amplifier within the organ of Corti that required the active functioning of the OHCs to be effective. The cochlear echoes became more properly called otoacoustic emissions (OAEs) and it was apparent that at least some of the mechanical activity of the cochlear amplifier used to enhance basilar membrane movement spilled back out of the cochlea and could be detected as an OAE in the external ear canal.

During early noise exposure the OAEs are lost before definite audiometric changes and to have a normal OAE response, the cochlea itself has to be normal. The system, therefore, has great potential as a screening device and, indeed, is becoming increasingly used as such.

The OHCs despite their paucity of innervation have, it seems, a major role to play in the sensitivity and frequency discrimination capabilities of the inner ear. The OHC possesses all the attributes of a sensory hair cell, but there are considerable differences between it and the IHC. Perhaps the most significant is that the cell body is not surrounded by supporting cells. Instead, from its attachment at the endolymphatic surface of the organ of Corti to the base where it is cupped by the bodies of Deiters' cells, it is surrounded elsewhere by fluid that is very similar to perilymph and has been called Cortilymph. OHCs can be dissected out of the organ of Corti and in an appropriate medium are able to expand and contract along their length in response to and in time with stimuli such as applied electric fields.

Whether the OHCs are capable of actual contraction within the organ of Corti remains to be seen, as the organ of Corti appears to be a moderately rigid structure with the triangular tunnel of Corti being bounded by the pillars of Corti and with the phalangeal processes of Deiters' cell apparently buttressing this structure. As the tips of the longest stereocilia of the OHCs are embedded within the tectorial membrane, some slight contraction of a narrow group of OHCs located close to the maximum of the travelling wave could give rise to the extra distortion of the basilar membrane–organ of Corti–tectorial membrane complex. This might induce just enough extra fluid movement within the inner sulcus to create that stimulus needed to deflect the stereocilia of the IHC to result in depolarization. The precise mechanism of the cochlear amplifier and the role of the OHCs in the cochlea's remarkable frequency selectivity and sensitivity should be better understood by the next edition of this book.

Hearing is primarily a warning system, with the receptive part of communication by sound having a secondary role. Anything that can enhance the sensitivity of the IHCs, which are but passive transducers of sound-induced fluid movement, will bring survival advantage to the organism. The OHCs appear to do this by adding about 40–50 dB of gain to the system, which thus becomes very sensitive. However, the price to pay for this specialization is a fragility of the OHCs to all sorts of stimuli, including noise itself. Furthermore, the OHCs in mammals have a spatial arrangement in the organ of Corti without the close contact of supporting cells, which almost certainly precludes natural regeneration after damage (see Chapter 37 on ototoxicity).

The vestibular labyrinth

The vestibular sensory cells detect acceleration or deceleration of the head. They can detect linear and angular changes and any complex interaction of the two. The vestibular system is a very 'old' system and in land-living vertebrates is probably a derivation of the lateral line organ of primitive fishes, which became specialized at the head end and eventually became incorporated into the skull (see Chapter 1 on the embryology of the otocyst). The lateral line contains sensory hair cells that detect fluid movement either in response to the movement of the fish's body in still water or in response to the movement of the water itself, or a combination of the two. The somatosensory or proprioceptive system was, therefore, an integral part of the mechanism to assess the contribution of self-induced and external movements. The visual pathways are also involved, and in the human vision is perhaps the predominant sensory input to the balance system. The vestibular labyrinth is remarkably sensitive and very rapidly reacts to small, non-sustained accelerations, such as turning the head, and quickly and appropriately redirects the eyes to maintain fixation on whatever was the object of interest despite head movement. This response is called the vestibular–ocular reflex (VOR).

The vestibular sensory cells have already been described, as far as their responses are concerned, earlier in this chapter. In short, the cells not only respond to deflection of their stereocilia, but also have polarity. Deflection towards the kinocilium

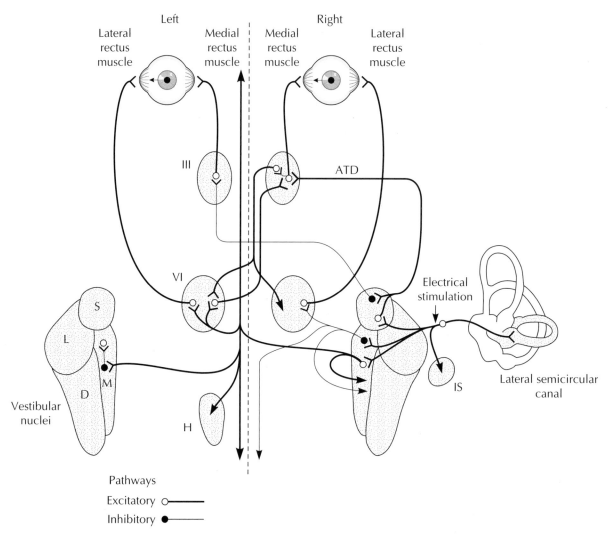

Fig 2.10 Lateral semicircular canal stimulation pattern; direct neuronal connections of the lateral semicircular canals. The small arrows in each eye indicate the direction of eye movement in response to head movement in what is, in effect, the opposite direction. IS, interstitial nucleus of the vestibular nerve; S, superior (Bechterew); L, lateral (Deiters'); D, descending (inferior or spinal); M, medial (triangular or Schwalbe) vestibular nuclei; H, hypoglossal nucleus; III, oculomotor nucleus; IV, abducent nucleus; ATD, ascending tract of Deiter. Stimulation (excitatory) pathways are shown with solid, heavy lines whereas inhibitory pathways are light lines.

results in stimulation and an increased output in the vestibular nerve attached to that particular cell, whereas the opposite deflection results in inhibition. The mechanism of stimulation in the three cristae of each labyrinth is, however, different from that of the two maculae.

THE SEMICIRCULAR CANALS

The ampulla at one end of each semicircular canal houses the crista, which contains the sensory cells.

The polarity of the cells in each crista is always the same so that deflection in one particular direction produces either stimulation or inhibition of the bundle of fibres arising from that particular crista depending on which canal is involved. The lateral (horizontal) semicircular canals have their sensory cells aligned so that relative flow of endolymph around the semicircular canal towards the ampulla and the utricle (ampullopetal: Latin *peto* 'I seek') results in deflection of the stereocilia towards the kinocilium (which lies on the utricular side of each bundle) and stimulation of the afferent nerve fibres

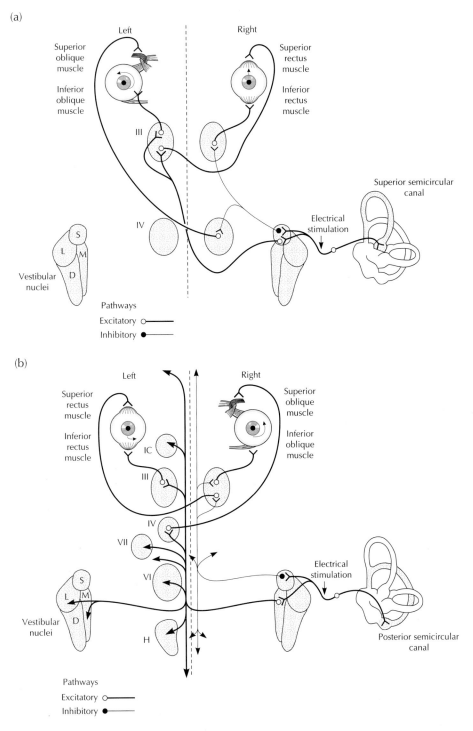

Fig 2.11 Superior and posterior semicircular stimulation pattern. (a) Superior semicircular canal connections. The abbreviations are as used in Figure 2.10. In essence the superior semicircular canal plays onto the superior vestibular nucleus and this results in stimulation of the ipsilateral superior rectus and of the contralateral inferior oblique. At the same time, the ipsilateral inferior rectus and contralateral superior oblique are inhibited thus resulting in an overall movement of the eyes that is opposite to the movement of the head. (b) Posterior semicircular canal connections. The abbreviations are as used in Figure 2.10 but, in addition, IV, trochlear nucleus; VII, facial nerve nucleus; IC, interstitial nucleus of Cajal. The result of activity in the posterior semicircular canal is to stimulate the ipsilateral superior oblique and the contralateral inferior rectus and to inhibit the ipsilateral inferior oblique and the contralateral superior rectus.

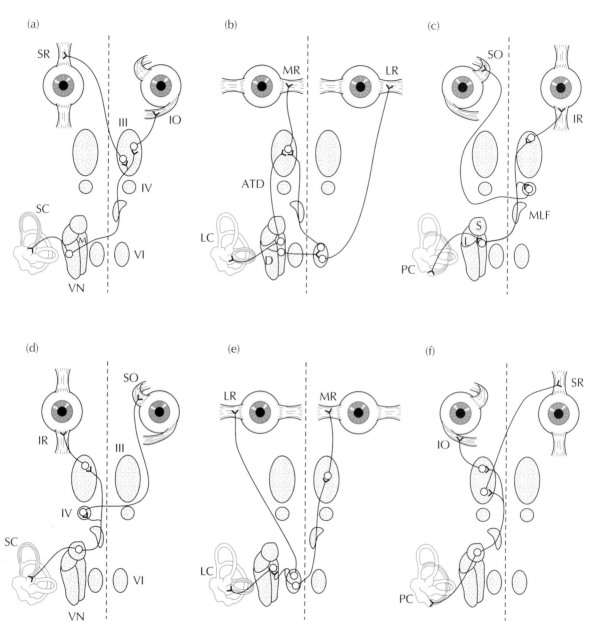

Fig 2.12 Connections of the semicircular canals. (a)–(c) Excitatory pathways and (d)–(f) inhibitory pathways existing between each semicircular canal and the respective extra-ocular muscles. MR, medial rectus; LR, lateral rectus; SR, superior rectus; IR, inferior rectus; IO, inferior oblique; SO, superior oblique; SC, superior semicircular canal; LC, lateral semicircular canal; PC, posterior semicircular canal; VN, vestibular nuclei; MLF, medial longitudinal fasciculus; ATD, ascending tract of Deiter. The remaining abbreviations are as described in Figures 2.10 and 2.11.

(Fig 2.10). The reverse flow (ampullofugal: Latin *fugo* 'I flee') brings inhibition; see Figures 1.20 and 2.13.

The superior and posterior semicircular canals have the reverse arrangement of sensory cells, with the kinocilium being on the canal side of the crista. Flow of endolymph away from the ampulla and the

utricle (ampullofugal) results in stimulation whereas ampullopetal flow causes a reduction of the static output (Fig 2.11).

Thus rotation of the head to the right results in stimulation of the right semicircular canal and inhibition of the left as the endolymph is effectively flowing towards the utricle on the right and away from the utricle on the left. Try it yourself by slowly turning your head from side to side and imagining the anatomy of the lateral semicircular canals with their ampullae at their anterior ends. As the head turns to the right the endolymph tends to remain static because of its inertia. The cristae, however, move with the head as they are attached to the bony labyrinth. There is therefore relative movement between the endolymph and the cristae. On the right the endolymph, in effect, moves towards the crista and, in the lateral canals, ampullopetal flow results in stimulation. On the left side the reverse occurs and the resting output from the crista is reduced.

The cristae are functionally paired as shown in Table 2.2 and the central pathways and the interconnections with the nuclei of the nerves that supply the muscles that move the eyes are such that stimulation of each canal results in movements of the eyes approximately in the plane of the canal in order to maintain visual fixation. These relationships are shown in Table 2.3. Stimulation of one canal not only activates one set of muscles to bring about the desired movement – in our example of turning to the right, the right medial rectus and the left lateral rectus – but also inhibits the antagonists. The increased output from the right canal is also accompanied by a decreased output from the left lateral semicircular canal. The effect of this is to enhance the effect of the stimulus from the right canal by reducing any tonic stimulating influence on the antagonists and by reducing any inhibition of the agonists. There is, in effect, a four-way 'push–pull' mechanism that enhances the sensitivity of the system and yet still allows it to function should one labyrinth stop working. The central connections of the canals and their subsequent paths are shown in Figures 2.10, 2.11 and 2.12.

The oblique rotations are specifically detected by the left posterior and right superior canals together and the left superior and right posterior canals together. The situation is not, of course as simple as

Table 2.2 The functional pairing of the semicircular canals

Right and left lateral (horizontal)
Right posterior and left superior
Right superior and left posterior

this because it is probably uncommon for there to be pure stimulation of a single pair of semicircular canals. These complex patterns are likely to be added to by the changing pattern of the image on the retina when the central response to this is to try to maintain position by way of the optokinetic reflex (OKN) which will be discussed further in Chapter 5. To make matters even more complicated there are likely to be proprioceptive impulses from the neck muscles and the numerous synovial joints in the cervical spine that will also send in relevant information to oculomotor centres by way of the spinovestibular tracts. In spite of this seeming complexity, the VOR is very fast and accurately maintains visual fixation despite rapid head movement. This presumably has a major survival advantage for prey and predator.

Generation of the stimulus to the hair cell

The early experiments involving the semicircular canals and their mechanism of stimulation tended to use supramaximal, non-physiological forces to detect change within the system. Pressures were used that caused actual movement of the cupula and it was this movement that was thought to be the direct stimulus to the hair cells of the crista. This belief was encouraged by the histological studies, which showed the cupula to be a small paddle or flap attached to either the crista or the dome of the ampulla. These earlier histological findings were artefact as the cupula is a fibrogelatinous structure that shrinks considerably during

Table 2.3 The effect of increased afferent output from the semicircular canals

Semicircular canal	Stimulates		Inhibits	
Lateral	ipsi:	medial rectus	contra:	medial rectus
	contra:	lateral rectus	ipsi:	lateral rectus
Superior	ipsi:	superior rectus	ipsi:	inferior rectus
	contra:	inferior oblique	contra:	superior oblique
Posterior	ipsi:	superior oblique	ipsi:	inferior oblique
	contra:	inferior rectus	contra:	superior rectus

standard histological preparation, much as the tectorial membrane shrinks and loses its lateral attachment to the organ of Corti in the cochlea.

Nevertheless, most modern theories of semicircular canal stimulation envisage some form of deflection of the cupula as the link between flow of endolymph along the semicircular canal and the deflection of the stereocilia, which in turn results in stimulation or inhibition of the sensory cell.

In reality the cupula fills the ampulla and is loosely attached at its lateral margins. Much of the rest of the dome of the ampulla is filled with a loose-knit fibrogelatinous matrix. Dohlman, who had been researching the vestibular system for over 50 years, finally came to the conclusion that much of his earlier work was misguided because the vestibular system is trying to maximize sensitivity and any system that had to move the large masses of the cupula in order to stimulate the hair cells was inefficient. Furthermore, if cupular deflection were the method of stimulation, then the semicircular canals should enter the dome of the ampulla rather than the base for maximal effect. He, therefore, postulated that fluid was channelled by the angle of approach of the semicircular canals and by the loose packing of the ampulla with fibrogelatinous material into the narrow subcupular space, where the stereocilia would then be deflected by a body of fluid whose pressure and velocity had been increased because of streaming from a large bore tube into a narrow slit (Fig 2.13).

Whatever the precise mechanism of physiological stimulation, the underlying principle remains fixed. As the head starts to rotate in one plane, that is, begins to accelerate, the endolymph of the semicircular canal tends to remain static because of its inertia. The crista within the ampulla moves with the head as it is directly attached to the bony labyrinth. Thus, there is relative movement between the endolymph and the stereocilia of the crista. Stimulation or inhibition occurs depending on the direction of fluid movement relative to the polarity of the sensory cells. Once rotation has reached a steady state (which is not often a physiological state, but which frequently occurs during testing procedures) the endolymph rapidly acquires momentum and rotates with the head. The deflection of the stereocilia ceases and they return to their resting position by their intrinsic elastic recoil. When the rotation slows then stops, the endolymph tends to continue moving because of its momentum and now the stereocilia are deflected in the other direction and the opposite output arises from the hair cells until all the momentum is lost.

Thus, the crista detect angular acceleration and deceleration. They do not respond to steady state rotation once the inertia or momentum of the

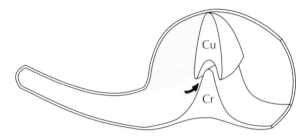

Fig 2.13 Dohlman's interpretation of subcupular flow. This diagram represents a longitudinal section through one of the semicircular canals. The crista (Cr) is located on the floor of the ampulla with its concavity towards the centre of the semicircle. Sitting astride the crista is the cupula (Cu), which in life extends to the limits of the ampulla. Dohlman envisages that as there is head movement, the endolymph of the semicircular canal is directed into the subcupular space and over the crest of the crista, where it deflects the stereociliary bundles, which in turn causes stimulation or inhibition of the associated nerve fibres.

endolymph has declined and then disappeared after each burst of acceleration or deceleration. On rotating chairs the system can be shown to be stunningly sensitive, responding to rotary accelerations of as little 0.1°/sec·sec⁻¹.

THE MACULAE OF THE SACCULE AND UTRICLE

Whereas the sensory cells of each crista are arranged with uniform polarity, no such arrangement occurs in the maculae. There is an extremely complex array within the utricle, with a complete reversal of orientation around the central divide called the striola. The pattern in the saccule is even more complicated. Movement can, therefore, induce opposite outputs – stimulation or inhibition from adjacent cells of certain parts of each maculae. The maculae themselves are nearly flat plates and in each ear lie almost perpendicular to each other. The output during linear motion must be complex and how this is deciphered centrally is not known. Nevertheless, the mechanism of stimulation is relatively straightforward. The stereocilia projecting from the surface of each of the macula are loosely enclosed in a fenestrated, fibrogelatinous matrix, which is called the otoconial membrane. Within this and embedded in the free endolymphatic surface of the membrane are the otoconia themselves. These have mass and when

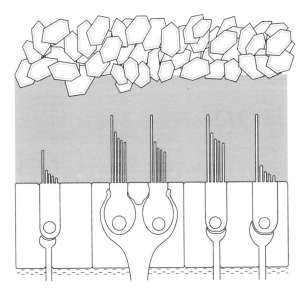

Fig 2.14 Highly schematic diagram of a cross-section of the sensory region of the macula of the saccule or utricle. The type-I and type-II sensory cells are surrounded by supporting cells. The stereocilia and single kinocilium of each cell extend into the fibrogelatinous matrix of the 'otoconial membrane'. Embedded within the endolymphatic surface of this structure are the calcium carbonate crystals that form the otoconial mass, which is essential for the detection of linear acceleration forces, including gravity.

the head accelerates in a straight line, the inertia of the otoconia causes them to lag behind the maculae, which move with the skull. This lag is transmitted to the otoconial membrane and in turn to the stereocilia of the sensory cells and continues while there is continuing acceleration. The deflec-tion results in the hair cells being stimulated or inhibited, depending on their polarity. When the acceleration is over and the head reaches a steady velocity the otoconia, in time, gain momentum and the elastic recoil of the otoconial membrane and stereocilia returns the system to its resting position. Deceleration causes the otoconia to move ahead of the maculae because of their acquired momentum and the reverse deflection of the stereociliary bundles occurs (Fig 2.14).

The pattern of output from the maculae, which have a range of lengths of individual stereociliary bundles and major variations in polarity of the hair cells and cells across the maculae, must give rise to complex neural firing patterns in even simple movements. It is easy to see that slight derangements of the system, whether it be in the maculae or the crista, can induce unusual patterns of firing that result in the sensation of movement when none is occurring.

Suggested reading

Baloh RW, Honrubia V. *Clinical neurophysiology of the vestibular system, 2nd ed.* Philadelphia: FA Davis, 1990.

von Békésy G. *Experiments in hearing.* New York: RE Kreiger, 1980.

Dohlman G. Critical review of the concept of cupular function. *Acta Otolaryngologica Supplementum* 1981; **376**:1–30.

More BCJ. *Perceptual consequences of cochlear damage.* Oxford: Oxford University Press, 1995.

Pickles JO. *An introduction into the physiology of hearing, 2nd ed.* London: Academic Press, 1991.

Webster DB, Fay RR, Popper AN. *The evolutionary biology of hearing.* New York: Springer–Verlag, 1992

CHAPTER 3

Clinical examination

HAROLD LUDMAN

Clinical examination entails examination of each ear, and in every patient, examination of the pharynx, postnasal space and larynx. Rarely should examination of the larynx be ommitted, as disease in that region may cause pain referred to the ear, and erosive diseases of the temporal bone may damage laryngeal innervation. Clinical tests of hearing, especially those using tuning forks, are components of the standard otological armamentarium, whereas clinical examination of facial nerve function and of vestibular function will often be indicated by the history.

The ear

Careful inspection of the ear is essential. Certain well established techniques yield better and more reliable information than others, and those to be described have stood the test of time.

Examination of the ear comprises that of the external ear, the pinna and external auditory meatus, and also the middle ear, as indicated by features of the tympanic membrane. This membrane is affected by almost all changes in the middle ear, and offers a window into the middle ear cleft. It is never possible to give an opinion on the state of the middle ear without a full account of the tympanic membrane.

ILLUMINATION

The better the ear is illuminated the easier departures from normal can be detected.

There is an inceasing and lamentable use of otoscopes by trainee otologists, which I noted and

regretted during my years as an FRCS examiner. Some otoscopes can give an excellent slightly magnified view, but, even if they have an occasional useful role, say at the bedside, or when chasing children, all real otologists must learn to examine ears with a separate head-worn light source and speculum, so that the hands are free to remove wax and discharge, and so that a pneumatic speculum can be used to best effect.

The separate light source can be from a lamp reflected by a concave head mirror with a central hole (Fig 3.1), or from an electric-powered head light, which is my preference. In either case the aim is to provide a bright light, coaxial with the line of vision, directed down the hand-held speculum. A head mirror and a head light need slightly different techniques, because the former provides direct coaxial access along the line of sight of the dominant eye, whereas the latter is between the two eyes, offering some degree of stereoscopic vision.

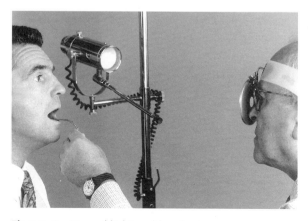

Fig 3.1 Position of light and head mirror.

For this reason it takes some practice to change from one form to the other. The heights of the chairs of patient and observer are adjusted to bring the ear to eye level, the light for a mirror being placed just behind and above the patient's head on the right of the examiner.

Otoscopes, if they are to be used, must be chosen with care. The worst is typified by dim light that is not accurately centred along the axis of the speculum. A good otoscope should offer bright, preferably halogen, lighting, delivered as a ring of light within the circumference of the speculum, together with a magnification of ×2–×6 (Fig 3.2). Pneumatic specular attachments are available for some, but they consist of a small stiff elastic bulb that does not deliver as controlled a pressure change as that available from a proper Siegle's speculum (Fig 3.3). This has a softish bulb usually made of rubber with a volume of about 150 ml connected by a flexible tube, trimmed to about 15 cm in length, to the specular attachment that contains a magnifying lens of ×2, canted by 30° across the optical axis of the speculum, in order to avoid obscuration of the view by the glare of light reflection. The precise character of a Siegle's speculum should be chosen with

care, and, when the ideal is found, it should be cherished and protected.

The use of a binocular microscope for inspection and manipulation of the ear canal is nowadays considered essential. The objective should have a focal length of 200, 225 or 250 mm and offer magnification within the range of ×6–×25. A microscope is used most comfortably with the patient lying on a couch, but can be managed in a near horizontal orientation with the patient sitting in a chair. A Siegle's speculum with clear glass is a valuable adjunct to the microscope, as it allows close inspection of the mobility of the tympanic membrane. For photographic purposes, or demonstration on a video screen, a short 4 mm Hopkin's telescope is useful.

The external ear is inspected, the pinna at one stage being folded forwards to display the retroauricular regions. The examiner should look for scars. Patients often fail to volunteer information about previous operations and, if a scar is missed, it is possible to mistake surgical changes for pathological lesions. The largest speculum that will fit into the external meatal opening with comfort is then selected. The pinna is held between the thumb and index fingers of the examiner's hand nearer the back of the patient's head. The pinna is gently but firmly retracted backwards and upwards by this grip, to straighten out the curve in the cartilaginous portion of the meatus, and to allow a more direct and efficient line of vision to the tympanic membrane (Fig 3.4). The forefinger and thumb of the other hand are used to hold the speculum and to manoeuvre it into position. The grip is then changed as necessary to release the right hand (of

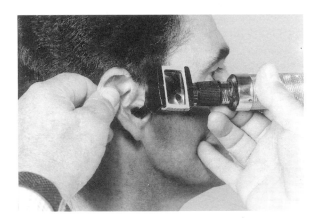

Fig 3.2 Examination of ear with an otoscope. Note protection by position of right little finger.

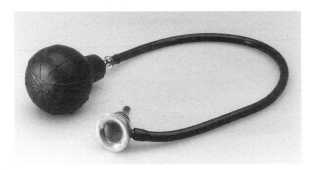

Fig 3.3 Siegle's pneumatic speculum.

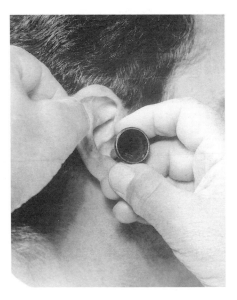

Fig 3.4 Speculum and handling for examination of right ear.

a right-handed observer) for removal of wax, debris or other foreign material and to perform other manipulations to be described.

REMOVAL OF WAX AND DEBRIS

The manual removal of material from the ear canal is an essential skill. Practice and experience are needed to learn how to do this without causing pain by abrasion of the deep meatal skin, which is exquisitely sensitive.

The choice of instrument at each stage requires experience of the way materials of different consistency respond. Hard lumps are best teased away from the skin wall of the meatus and rolled outwards with the ring end of a Jobson Horne probe (Fig 3.5), or a Cawthorne wax hook. Sheets of fairly dry material can be siezed with forceps; and it is often those with the largest blades like Tilley's Dressing Forceps that provide the best purchase. Small crocodile action forceps may be useful but often tear small pieces of the debris, making removal more difficult. So, for removal of the thin sheet of skin and its wax covering from a dry

mastoid cavity, I favour gentle separation of the peripheral edge with a flat dissector, which allows the development of a large surface to grasp and pull out. Moist debris, or liquefying wax, may yield to a sucker, but frequent clearance of obstructed tips is necessary. At all times the suction of the underlying living surface must be avoided to prevent pain and bleeding. Cotton wool may be twisted, or folded, onto the wool carrier end of a Jobson Horne probe or other wool carrier in order to create a tool, like a small paint brush (Fig 3.6), useful for mopping out wet material and the semi-liquid pultaceous mass of infected desquamating debris. These instruments have a roughened or screw-like surface (Fig 3.7). Practice is needed to learn how to attach or 'bend in' a cotton wool tip that will remain secure. A small piece of cotton wool is held between finger and thumb, and the wool carrier is laid onto one edge of the pledget and then twisted to invite the wool to wind round it (Fig 3.8). Early attempts will usually produce an instrument from which the wool easily separates when least wished. These are skills gradually acquired by patience and experience, and rank highly as indicators of the competence of a trained otologist. When infected

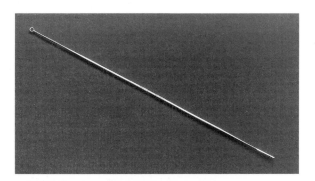

Fig 3.5 Jobson Horne probe. Note ring at one end and wool carrier at other.

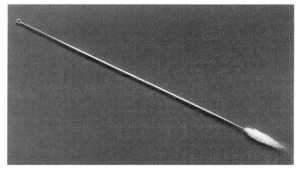

Fig 3.6 Cotton wool twisted onto end of Jobson Horne probe.

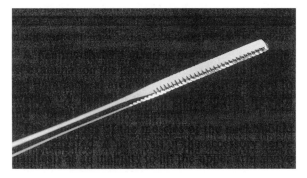

Fig 3.7 Enlarged view of serrated wool-carrier end of Jobson Horne probe.

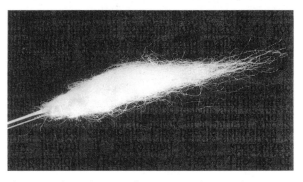

Fig 3.8 Enlarged view of cotton wool twisted onto serrated end.

material occupies the meatus, a sterile swab on a thin holder may be used to take a sample for bacterial and fungal culture and chemotherapeutic sensitivity analysis.

REMOVAL OF CERUMEN BY SYRINGING

Ear syringing must be one of the commonest minor procedures performed in general practice, or in the offices of primary care physicians. It is often delegated to practice nurses, and, inappropriately, seems often to be used as a diagnostic manoeuvre for any patient complaining of hearing loss. Considering the potential risks, and the frequency of its performance, it is surprising that accidents and subsequent litigation is as infrequent as it seems to be, at least in the UK. Syringing should never be undertaken in the presence of infection, when the ear is known to have a perforation, or is suspected from past history to have a vulnerable tympanic membrane. It should not be contemplated if there is any history of previous problems after syringing. Ideally, it should be conducted only if the tympanic membrane has been seen to be normal. The catch-22 nature of that requirement will not escape the astute reader.

The principle is to project a stream of fluid along the posterosuperior meatal wall, between the skin and the cerumen, so that the fluid jet, reflected from the tympanic membrane, will displace the obstruction outwards. Syringing may be accomplished with a bladder syringe, but more safely with a Higginson or Bacon rubber syringe (Fig 3.9), which does not allow the exertion of as much force. Dedicated syringing machines are available to deliver mechanically a stream of water at body temperature through an appropriate nozzle. The patient sits in a chair, holding a kidney dish receiver on the shoulder, protected with a waterproof cover. The syringing solution of sterile water or saline is warmed to just above body temperature and is drawn up into the syringe. Careful temperature control is vital to avoid caloric-induced vertigo. With one hand the operator draws the pinna upwards and backwards, to straighten the external meatus. With the other, the delivery tip of the syringing tool is inserted a few millimetres into the external ear canal under visual control, pointing its orifice slightly upward and backward. The contents of the syringe are discharged firmly, but without undue force. The ear canal is inspected with an otoscope, and, if the contained wax has not been delivered, the syringe should be refilled and used again. Syringing should never cause pain, and must cease if a patient has any complaints. Hard wax may be softened by the use of olive oil of domestic cooking quality, or by 5 per cent sodium bicarbonate drops instilled for a few days beforehand. Antibiotic/steroid drops can also be used before syringing. They will eliminate any otitis externa provoked by injudicious manipulation, and the preparation containing gentamicin 3 per cent and hydrocortisone 1 per cent is effective in softening wax.

Many proprietary ceruminolytics are skin irritants and should never be used for more than a day or so before wax removal. At best they may seal the edges of the wax to the surrounding skin surface with more marked obstruction to hearing, whereas occasionally they cause otitis externa, which against hard impacted wax causes severe pain that may be relieved only by removal under general anaesthesia.

When the meatus is clear, methodical inspection follows a set routine. The walls of the meatus are searched first; debris or foreign bodies, diseases of the skin, tumours and defects, especially of the posterior wall or outer attic wall are all excluded. Lumps within the meatus should be palpated with a probe to determine their texture and, by sweeping the probe around them, to define their possible attachment to the meatal wall. It is quite easy to recognize the bony hardness of an exostosis, for example. The view then follows the floor of the meatus to the tympanic membrane. This is the most certain way of identifying the membrane, for it makes a sharp angle with the floor. Posteriorly, the angle is obtuse and it is sometimes difficult to decide where the meatal wall ends and the membrane begins, especially if the latter is abnormally red. Above, the anatomy is more difficult with the pars flaccida often offering an irregular, indented appearance, whereas anteriorly it is often impossible to see the meatal–membrane junction when it lies beyond vision in the anterior recess, obscured

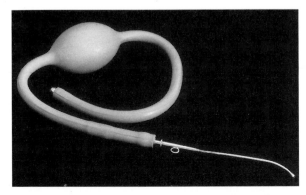

Fig 3.9 Higginson syringe, fitted with catheter for ear syringing.

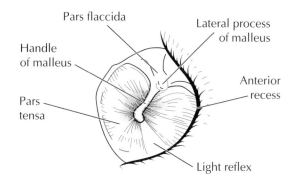

Pars flaccida

Lateral process
of malleus

Handle
of malleus

Anterior
recess

Pars
tensa

Light reflex

Fig 3.10 Normal right tympanic membrane.

by the bulge of the anterior meatal wall. Once the point of junction of the membrane and meatus inferiorly has been identified, the eye may then sweep round the circumference of the membrane and try to encompass and define its whole boundary.

The standard landmarks and features of the normal membrane must then be identified (Fig 3.10). First, the central portion and the handle of the malleus should be identified. This is visible in every normal membrane as an integral part of the middle layer of connective tissue. Next, the division between pars flaccida and pars tensa is defined, apparent as a slight fold (anterior and posterior malleolar folds). In transparent membranes it may be possible to see the long process of the incus and the stapedius tendon in the sector between the handle of the malleus and posterior meatal wall, but absence of visibility does not imply an abnormality. When a membrane has been severely deformed by disease, the most faithful feature, most resistant to obliteration, is the lateral process of the malleus, which appears as a yellow whitish knob. It will almost invariably provide an identifiable and reliable landmark.

Attention should then be directed towards the integrity of the membrane. Any breach of continuity is an important physical sign and perforations are frequently encountered. Perforations of the pars tensa are classified as marginal or central according to whether the rim of the tympanic membrane forms part of the circumference of the perforation (see Chapters 27 and 28).

Marginal perforations may therefore be described as anterior marginal, inferior marginal or posterior marginal, being qualified in addition as small, medium or large. Central perforations are also described as anterior, inferior or posterior according to their relation to the handle of the malleus, and similarly qualified as small, medium or large. Very large central perforations are described as subtotal and very large marginal perforations as

total. Defects of the pars flaccida are described as attic perforations and qualified as small or large.

The colour of the membrane must be considered. Normally it has the tint of mother of pearl, with a glistening appearance and a triangular sheen inferiorly (called the light reflex) where reflection of the examining light takes place. Loss of this reflex may indicate thickening of the membrane, for example, either by proliferation of the outer layers as in otitis externa or of the inner layer as in otitis media. Sometimes the middle layer of fibrous tissue undergoes hyaline degeneration and may become impregnated with deposits of calcium. Such patches of tympanosclerosis are not indicative of disease. In elderly people the degenerations due to age sometimes appear as a milky arcus senilis across the lower half of the membrane, or as a circumferential opacity.

The position of the membrane demands good judgement. Obstruction of the Eustachian tube prevents the constant replacement of air in the middle ear necessary to maintain atmospheric pressure. If not replaced the air becomes absorbed by the mucosa and a potential vacuum develops. This results in retraction of the membrane. The handle of the malleus is drawn inwards, and to the examining eye appears to adopt an increasingly horizontal position with the tip of the handle backwards. At the same time, the retraction of the membrane towards the medial wall of the middle ear tends to throw the handle and lateral process of the malleus into sharp prominence, so that in these circumstances the thing that strikes the examiner is the appearance of the malleus, unusually prominent, foreshortened and backward-pointing compared with normal. If retraction is especially marked, the posterior segment of the membrane may wrap itself round the long process of the incus and the head of the stapes. These structures may then stand out and deceptively suggest that the posterior part of the membrane is defective, allowing direct view of them. Again it is possible for retraction to be so complete that the membrane is plastered against the promontory. This is a fruitful source of error in diagnosis, as it may be very difficult to decide whether the promontory is being seen through a large perforation or whether it is, in fact, invested by the membrane. The reduction in the middle ear pressure relative to that of the atmosphere caused by Eustachian tube obstruction may not only cause the membrane to become retracted but may also promote serous exudation into the middle ear space (secretory otitis media). If this occurs a fluid level may be visible, typically as a hairline extending backwards from the umbo to the posterior margin. It may also be possible to discern air bubbles behind the membrane, a certain indication of fluid. Retraction of the pars flaccida and pars tensa may occur independently and from causes other than simple Eustachian tube blockage. An attack of otitis media can result in adhesions that may shorten and so distort the position. In particular, in view of the narrow approaches from the main chamber of the middle ear to the attic, the pars flaccida over the lower attic may become permanently retracted, the approaches having become sealed with denial of air replacement to the upper region. Traction on the pars flaccida in this event may be such as to cause a true invagination, possibly not without significance in the formation of cholesteatoma (see Chapter 28). All these abnormalities may be emphasized and more readily recognized by the use of a pneumatic speculum, as described below.

By contrast the membrane may bulge outwards into the meatus. It then presents a smooth convexity. If the bulge is due to raised air pressure in the middle ear it may be partial, not affecting the whole membrane. This is prone to occur if areas of the membrane have been weakened by loss of the connective tissue middle layer, such as by subjection to repeated pressure changes (e.g. players of wind instruments, excessive autoinflation or, perhaps, where a perforation has healed over). As a general rule, if the membrane is bulging but the colour and sheen are normal, this bulge is due to alteration in air pressure, but if the colour is changed or the sheen is absent, the inference is that the middle ear space has undergone expansion with abnormal fluid or solid contents. In acute suppurative otitis media, for example, in which the bulge shows the pressure of pus, the appearance may be of a bright cherry in the bottom of the meatus, with a matt surface and no normal landmarks. If the membrane is about to give way, a yellowish-looking nipple may be present, but it is the exception rather than the rule to be given the opportunity of inspecting a membrane at this momentary stage in the course of the disease.

Mobility of the membrane is tested clinically by two routine methods. The first is massage with a Siegle's pneumatic speculum, the second by the manoeuvres of Valsalva or Toynbee.

PNEUMATIC MASSAGE

The response of the visible tympanic membrane to the use of a pneumatic, or Siegle's, speculum is invaluable. The magnifying lens is fitted firmly into a speculum that fills the meatus, and the tympanic membrane is observed by illumination with the head-worn light, while the bulb of the apparatus is squeezed to raise intrameatal pressure and then relaxed to lower it and suck the membrane out-

wards towards the observer. The normal mobility can be recognized with experience, as can the immobility of an effusion in the middle ear. Some effusions are associated with a characteristic snap back of the displaced membrane as lowered pressure is released. Fluid in the middle ear may appear as a bead at a very small and otherwise unrecognized perforation. A very thin excessively flaccid drum can be recognized and often a thin drum that has been sucked into the middle ear can be sucked out again from its subjacent mucosa, allowing identification of a retraction pocket, and distinction between that and a perforation. The dusky red coloration of a glomus tumour may pale under raised pressure with the pneumatic speculum.

THE FISTULA SIGN (SEE CHAPTER 14)

This important physical sign depends on transmission of air pressure changes from the external ear canal to a fistula in the labyrinth causing endolymph movement (Fig 3.11). The raised air pressure may be produced by pressing with a finger on the tragus, but more reliably by the use of a pneumatic otoscope fitted with a speculum sufficiently large to fit securely into the meatus and produce an airtight seal. Recognizable and precise effects of pressure changes arise if the fistula test is positive. The nature of these positive findings has often been incorrectly described in textbooks. The sign is not simply one of nystagmus induced by the increased pressure. Raised pressure causes conjugate deviation of the eyes away from the the examined side. If the pressure is maintained, a jerk nystagmus develops beating towards the examined and affected ear. If the pressure is released the eyes return to the midline. Pulsation of pressure in the meatus causes repeated deviation of the eyes to the unaffected side with each pressure rise, and return to primary position of gaze when the pressure falls. The patient feels dizzy during these events, and accompanying head movements away from the examiner make continuous inspection of the eyes difficult. It is often useful, if not essential, to have an observer assisting while eliciting this sign. The direction of deviation of the eyes on raised pressure depends on the site of the fistula. The description of deviation towards the normal ear is the commonest finding, being associated with a fistula in the most usual site in the dome of the lateral semicircular canal. A lateral canal fistula anterior to the ampulla, which is rare, causes deviation towards the side of the fistula, however. Raised pressure on a fistula in the superior canal causes rotatory movement towards the normal ear. Finally, vertical deviation of the eyes suggests a fistula in the posterior

(a)

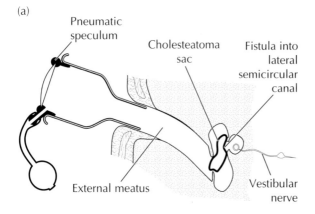

(b)

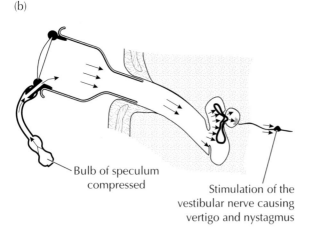

Fig 3.11 (a) and (b) Mechanism of the fistula sign.

canal. It is always important to seek a positive fistula sign in any vertiginous patient, and in any patient with chronic middle ear disease. There are, however, false positive and false negative results. The fistula sign may sometimes be positive in the presence of an intact tympanic membrane. This is described as Hennebert's sign, and traditionally in the literature had been attributed to syphilitic otic capsule disease. That explanation, however, is not satisfactory, and Hennebert's sign may be elicited in many other conditions associated with vertigo induced by raised or changing pressure, either in the air of the middle ear cavity or in the cerebrospinal fluid, during Valsalva manoeuvres. More important, however, is a false negative fistula sign, which may come about from inadequate sealing of the speculum in the meatus, because a mass of cholesteatomatous debris protects the inner ear from the transmission of the raised pressure or if the vestibular labyrinth has already succumbed to the disease and is unresponsive.

Valsalva's manoeuvre is the standard procedure of autoinflation of the middle ear. The subject pinches the nostrils between forefinger and thumb and then, with lips tightly compressed, blows out the cheeks while instructed to try to blow down the nose. If successful in inflating the ears a subjective sensation of fullness in the ears will be felt, and the observer will see a definite movement of the pars tensa, generally the posterior half. In *Toynbee's manoeuvre* the patient simply closes the mouth, pinches the nose and swallows, and the tympanic membrane moves outwards. About one-third of normal subjects cannot perform autoinflation. Failure by this method does not, therefore, indicate pathological obstruction of the Eustachian tube, but positive inflation indicates tubal patency, and is a useful sign.

PALPATION

Palpation of the ear and the region around it should not be omitted. Lymph gland enlargement may be detected either anterior to the tragus, over the mastoid or below the lobe. In pursuit of the principle of always considering the middle ear in an upper respiratory tract setting, the neck may profitably be palpated for any enlarged glands in addition to the immediate drainage areas of the external ear. Mobility and tenderness of the pinna are tested. Movement restricted by pain is often a sign of inflammatory disease in the cartilaginous portion of the external meatus. It is useful to become familiar with the feel of the normal mastoid bone. A sign of acute infection is oedema of the soft tissues overlaying it. As the infection of the mastoid approaches the surface there is increase in the swelling until finally a fully fluctuant subperiosteal abscess may form. Before the swelling becomes visible, however, a velvety feel may be detected, the normal bony characteristic being blurred, and firm palpation may perhaps elicit some tenderness.

Vestibular function

Clinical examination of vestibular function is discussed in detail in Chapters 5 and 14.

In any patient complaining of dizziness or vertigo, the eyes and their movements should always be examined under good illumination. They should be watched for several seconds both in the primary position of gaze – looking straight ahead – and on deviation of the eyes, but not too far, in each direction of gaze.

Nystagmus is an involuntary oscillating movement of the eyes, usually of both together. It may be classed as *pendular*, when the beats are of similar velocity in each direction, or *jerk*, if there is a slow movement in one direction with a quick return (see Chapters 5 and 14). Nystagmus associated with vestibular conditions is invariably jerking. Although the direction is traditionally labelled by that of the quick component, it is actually the slow movement that is evoked by the vestibular stimulus. Nystagmus visible when watching the eyes while the patient sits immobile under observation is defined as *spontaneous*. (Neurologists sometimes use this term to describe nystagmus apparent only in the primary position of gaze, using the name *gaze nystagmus* for spontaneous nystagmus visible when the eyes deviate in either direction.) As is described in other chapters, vestibular jerk nystagmus is always most marked when the eyes look in the direction of the quick component. The type of nystagmus is graded as first degree when it is visible only with the eyes looking in the direction of the quick component, second degree if it can be seen with the eyes looking straight ahead, in the primary position of gaze, and third degree if it beats with the quick component in the same direction, that is, while the eyes look towards the direction of the slow component. A third degree nystagmus must not be confused with one that beats, say, to the left on gaze to the left, and to the right on looking to the right. That would be a first degree nystagmus in each direction, changed in direction by change of gaze – a so-called bilateral jerk nystagmus or a direction-changing nystagmus, which is an indication of central brainstem disease.

Nystagmus may also be classified as spontaneous, as described above, or provoked, if it arises by physiological actions, such as head positioning. Induced nystagmus is that caused by unphysiological stimuli like the caloric test.

Examination of the eyes for spontaneous nystagmus should also be conducted while the patient wears Frenzel's glasses (Fig 3.12). These high dioptre ($\times$20) lenses remove a large part of the patient's ability to perform optic fixation, and give an indication of what might be expected from electronystagmographic examination of the eyes in darkness.

As a rule of thumb, spontaneous nystagmus cannot arise from a peripheral, labyrinthine cause if

- its direction changes (with time as one watches, or with head position, or change of direction of gaze);
- its direction is any other than horizontal (vertical, oblique, rotatory);
- it beats differently in the two eyes (dysjunctive or 'ataxic', see-saw);

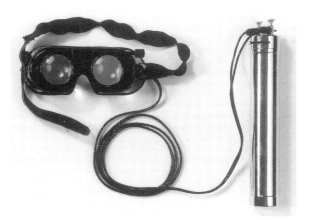

Fig 3.12 Frenzel's glasses.

- its amplitude is not increased by reducing optic fixation, or indeed if it is abolished by reducing optic fixation;
- it lasts unchanged over a period of more than 3 weeks; this is a difficult condition, as no one observes eyes continuously for 3 weeks, but its implication is that there is no central compensation for its cause.

Other aspects of the clinical examination of the dizzy patient include observation of stance and gait. Positional testing, which is a vital component of the examination of any patient whose complaints include vertigo, is also fully described in detail in Chapter 14.

Facial nerve function

A discussion of clinical examination of facial nerve function appears in Chapter 16.

The nasopharynx (epipharynx)

Examination of the ear is incomplete without inspection of the Eustachian tube openings. This is the portal of entry of many infective conditions of the middle ear. The cause of numerous cases of conductive deafness in children is Eustachian tube obstruction at the pharyngeal end. In adults the proportion is lower, but sooner or later, if this examination is overlooked, a serious cause of deafness due to obstructed Eustachian tube openings, for example, a carcinoma of the nasopharynx, will be overlooked. To obtain a good view of the nasopharynx is one of the most difficult skills in clinical practice. The instruments required are a Luc tongue depressor, St Clair Thompson postnasal mirror, a source of good head-worn illumination, a small flame to warm the mirror and a spray of lignocaine (lidocaine) 4 per cent. In patients with a sensitive pharynx it may be impossible to quieten the 'gag reflex' other than with the use of surface anaesthesia.

With the patient's mouth at examiner's eye level, and with good illumination, the examiner takes the Luc tongue depressor in the left hand and the postnasal mirror in the right. The patient is asked to lean slightly forward, tilt back the head and open the mouth (dentures having been removed and placed in a sterile dish). The glass side of the mirror is applied to the flame, until, when tested on the back of the hand, the back of the mirror feels hot but not uncomfortably so. It is a cardinal error to fail to test the temperature of the mirror before introducing it into the patient's mouth. The tongue depressor is then gently passed into the mouth until almost touching the uvula, allowed to drop quietly on to the tongue and very gently but firmly depressed so that the tongue is well separated from the soft palate. The mirror is then passed into the oropharynx into the space between the uvula, tongue and right pillars of the fauces. If the movement is made slowly, the patient may not anticipate discomfort. If it is made hurriedly or clumsily, an almost certain gag reflex will result. It is especially important when examining children never to make sudden movements. With care it is possible to obtain adequate views of the nasopharynx in any child old enough to be persuaded to open their mouth voluntarily. When the mirror is in position, behind and just below the palate, a rapid inspection of the nasopharynx must be made; rapid because even the most cooperative patient cannot resist the desire to swallow for very long, and once this has caused the mirror to touch the throat a gag reflex is inevitable.

If the palate is withdrawn towards the posterior pharyngeal wall, as sometimes occurs involuntarily despite every care, the view will be obscured. To obtain relaxation may be difficult, but sometimes the palate may be made to fall out of the way by asking the patient to sniff gently through the nose while still keeping the mouth wide open. While the examination is proceeding it is helpful to direct the patient's attention towards their breathing, by asking them to concentrate on regular inspiration and expiration through the mouth. If, despite all care, examination is frustrated by gagging, it may be successfully concluded after spraying the fauces with 4 per cent lidocaine (lignocaine) and waiting a minute or so for the anaesthesia to develop. If mirror examination is inadequate, a fibreoptic or Hopkin's rod nasopharyngoscope may be used. The instrument is passed along the floor of the nose (previously anaesthetized with local anaesthetic spray) and permits such visual examination of the nasopharynx as to avoid need for further examination under general anaesthesia. Occasionally, however, examination under general anaesthesia will be advisable, especially if biopsy material is needed.

The view of the nasopharynx obtained with a mirror is fleeting and often difficult to interpret. The appearance is built up as a composite of the small individual mirror views available as the angle and orientation are changed. A great deal of practice and experience is required before a confident judgement can be made. The first landmark to identify is the posterior end of the septum which, because the mucosa is stretched closely over bone, looks like a white dividing line down the middle of the image. Once the septum has been identified, the mirror is tilted to reveal the roof of the nasopharynx, then angled to bring the lateral wall, first one side then the other, into view. The Eustachian tube openings are seen as unmistakable openings in the lower lateral walls. They must be distinguished from the openings of the posterior choanae of the nose, to which they have a lateral and oblique relation. The gaze must be allowed to travel round each opening, and then, especially, to follow the bulge of the medial wall, the torus tubarii, backwards and upwards into the fossa of Rosenmüller. It is here that pathological lesions that cause compression of the tube may originate.

The nose

The Eustachian tube, middle ear and mastoid air cells constitute a continuous air space contained in bone, lined by epithelium, and in continuity with the atmosphere of the nose and nasopharynx. Apart from the function of conduction of sound evolved by the middle ear, this space, sometimes called the middle ear cleft, is, as an air space, comparable with the paranasal sinus in the frontal bone, save that for the ear the ostium is in the back of the nose whereas the frontal sinus opens into the nose nearer the front. The commonest disease of the nose is acute coryza, the common cold, and acute suppurative otitis media is one of the commonest complications of it. Chronic conditions of the nose and sinuses may also be aetiologically related to chronic conditions of the middle ear cleft. It is a mistaken concept mentally to isolate the middle ear cleft from the rest of the upper respiratory tract.

Pathological interplay between the whole area occurs. Chronic maxillary sinusitis may be the cause of a repeated otitis media, and a carcinoma of the laryngopharynx may cause intractable pain in the ear. The nose and larynx should therefore always be examined whenever the history of the symptoms suggests the possibility of a related condition in these areas.

The nose is usually inspected by means of a Thudicum spring speculum inserted into each nostril. The speculum is hung from the forefinger of the examiner's left hand, which points towards the examiner. The blades of the speculum are compressed between the middle and ring fingers and are allowed to separate inside the nostril. The floor of the nose is identified and the gaze then follows the septum from floor to roof and from front to back, noting spurs or other irregularities and estimating any impairment of the airway by deflection. The lateral wall of the nasal cavity is then inspected from below upwards, and study made first of the inferior turbinate then of the middle turbinate. Here, special care is taken not to miss the presence of purulent or mucopurulent discharge, as this is often the only clinical sign of a chronic sinus infection. Nowadays a fuller examination of the nasal cavity is often achieved with a Hopkin's rod telescope.

The larynx

Inspection of the larynx requires much skill and practice, and for fuller information on the clinical techniques involved in the clinical examination and interpretation of appearances of the larynx, nose, and sinuses, a textbook of diseases of the nose and throat should be consulted. The patient extrudes the tongue, which is held in a piece of gauze or linen between the examiner's left forefinger and thumb, the third finger being used to hold the upper lip out of the field of vision. A laryngeal mirror, warmed in a flame as described for the postnasal mirror, is then passed to the back of the mouth and pressed upwards and backwards against the soft palate, being centred over the uvula. The patient is then asked to make the sound 'E-E-E-E-E-E', which adducts the vocal cords and brings the larynx into a more prominent position.

CHAPTER 4

Basic acoustics and hearing tests

HAROLD LUDMAN

PART I – PHYSICS OF SOUND (ACOUSTICS)

Otologists need to understand the basic ideas of the physics of sound, increasingly so now that they often discuss issues with physicists and audiologists. They must learn to speak the same language and understand the precise meanings of terminology. Sound means the sensation associated with stimulation of the mechanism of the ear and also the physical events which cause that sensation. The external events arise from a vibrating system and are transmitted through air to the ear. The behaviour of the system in vibration, and the transmission of its vibrations through a so-called elastic medium observe the laws of physics.

The mechanical events of sound start with the vibration of a body that has the two properties – mass and elasticity. *Mass*, in Newtonian physics, implies the tendency to remain at rest, or in straight line motion at constant velocity, unless acted on by an outside force. This idea is embodied in the term inertia. *Elasticity* may be looked on as a force tending to return the mass to its resting position after displacement. It is the periodically changing magnitude of the relationships between the momentum of a mass in motion and the force offered by elasticity against the direction of that motion that makes these two properties fundamental requirements for vibration, and for the propagation of that vibration through air.

The vibrating system, from which the sound wave arises, may take many forms, but all have mass and elasticity. A stretched string, a column of air or a rod fixed at one end in the form of the prong of a tuning fork can all vibrate. The vibratory events are initiated by the displacement of a bit of the mass; a string under tension may be centrally displaced by the pull of a plucking finger or by the frictional drag of an applied bow. The initial displacement of the prong of a tuning fork is provided by a blow at right angles to its length. Let us consider the effect on a segment of that prong as its mass is accelerated in the direction of that applied force, while the whole prong, fixed at one end, bends. As the displacement of the segment increases, the force due to elasticity, directed against the direction of motion, rises in proportion to the size of the displacement, and so increasingly decelerates the mass moving away from its resting position. Progressively, the kinetic energy embodied in the moving mass is claimed as potential energy by the elasticity, until the movement ceases. The displacement is now at a maximum, and of course the velocity of the segmental mass is now zero. The elastic restoring force accelerates the segment on a return towards its resting position, and the force falls to zero when this position is reached. Now the segmental mass has regained the kinetic energy derived from the original displacing force, and is moving at maximum velocity in a direction opposite to that of its first displacement. Unresisted by any force in either direction, the segment overshoots its initial position of rest until it is displaced as far from it as at the end of its first movement, but now in the opposite direction. Once more it is halted by the force increasingly imposed by elasticity, and once again it is accelerated towards its position of rest. This alternating to and fro movement, or oscillation, to either side of the resting position involves the periodic exchange of kinetic for potential energy. It would continue indefinitely in the absence of a third property of any vibrating system – *frictional resistance*. As a result of the 'damping' effect of friction between adjacent 'segments' of the vibrating prong some energy is dissipated during each cycle of events and is lost as heat. Eventually all the energy is used up and vibration ceases.

The propagation of the vibratory activity as a sound wave involves the transfer of the kinetic energy of the vibrating source to the air, which, as one example of a so-called 'elastic medium', is endowed with the same basic properties of mass and elasticity. It is convenient to think of the air as consisting of 'particles', or small packets, each able to oscillate to and fro in the same manner as the vibrating sound source, and in accordance with the same physical principles. The particle adjacent to the vibrating source is accelerated away from the direction of vibration, and accelerated back towards its resting position by its inherent elasticity. When in motion its momentum is transferred to the next particle by collision, and that particle, when maximally displaced, is similarly returned towards its resting position by its inherent elasticity. In this way, by collision between adjacent particles, the mechanical disturbance of the sound wave is transmitted longitudinally through the air. The mechanical events affecting the particles are periodically repeated as the oscillations of the sound source impart repeated pushes on the propagating medium. When the particles become packed together, as the first in a bunch is maximally displaced, the ambient air pressure rises, and, when they become separated as the extreme members of a group reach positions most distant from one another, the ambient air pressure falls. So the sound wave can be considered as the movement through the air of a change in ambient air pressure. The 'velocity of sound' refers to the velocity of the transmission of that changing pressure, and this must be clearly distinguished from the velocity of the individual particles during their to and fro oscillations about their resting positions. Although the wave moves on as a mechanical disturbance, an individual particle moves no further than the bounds of its oscillation, and it rests in its original position when the wave has passed, and its motion has ceased. The description of a sound wave is expressed in terms of the periodically changing physical state, and in particular the air pressure, at a specific point in the propagating medium.

Types of vibrations and waves

The characteristics of a propagated sound wave are determined by the way in which the sound source (or sources) vibrate, and, as has been noted, these characteristics are defined by changing measurable quantities, such as pressure, during periods of time. If the events are regularly repeated, the wave is called *periodic*. The simplest form of periodic motion, and the form implicit to the discussion of quantitive characteristics later, is that of *simple harmonic motion*. This is the form of motion executed by the vibration of any body when the elastic force restoring the system when displaced is proportional to the distance through which it is displaced. This applies to a tuning fork, and the sound generated is a 'pure tone', or tone consisting of a note of a single frequency. It is also the form of oscillating motion of a pendulum swinging through a short arc. For reasons to be explained, the mechanical events of the transmission of simple harmonic motion can be portrayed as a sine wave. That is to say, the pressure changes in the transmitting air, the displacement of each particle of air, and the velocity of the movement of each particle when plotted on a graph against the time of occurrence exactly follow the shape of a sine wave. Mathematically, simple harmonic motion may be described precisely as the projection of uniform circular motion on to a straight line (Fig 4.1). It can be seen that the point is displaced from the horizontal at any time, as shown in the curve on the right, by an amount that is given by the formula:

$$\text{Displacement} = \alpha \sin \phi,$$
where α is the radius of the circle.

The maximum value is termed the *amplitude*, and corresponds, in the subjective aspect of sound, with

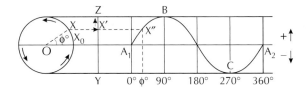

Fig 4.1 Simple harmonic motion. If a motion X describes a circle about a point O, with uniform angular velocity, the projection of X, or X', on the straight line YZ will move up and down in simple harmonic motion. If while oscillating in this way the point X' moves from left to right at constant velocity, the curve A_1BCA_2 will be described. This is a sine wave; the distance A_1A_2 is called a wavelength. The points along the abscissa are defined in terms of the number of degrees that the point X has rotated from the position X_0.

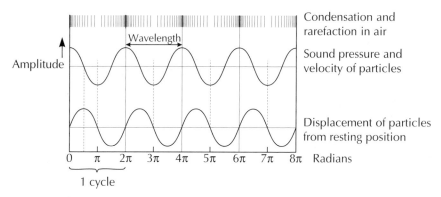

Fig 4.2 Events in transmission of a sine wave in air.

loudness. The number of times the events are repeated each second determines the frequency, which correlates subjectively with pitch. It is important to realize that the occurrence of the various events (particle velocity, air pressure and particle displacement) is not simultaneous (Fig 4.2). The distance between adjacent peaks is the *wavelength*. So-called *complex periodic waves* are made up of more than one sine wave. The actual form and shape of a complex wave depends on the contribution, in amplitude and phase, of each of the constituent sine waves, and the shape of the wave corresponds subjectively to the character or timbre of the sound. In a complex periodic wave the period of repetition of the overall cycle of events is called the *fundamental*. The constituent pure tones, with frequencies that are multiples of the fundamental, are termed *harmonics*. The individual characteristics of musical instruments are determined entirely by the proportionate contribution of different harmonics to the formation of the complex wave, whose fundamental defines the pitch of the note.

Non-periodic sound waves consist of random fluctuations of pressure, composed of numerous unrelated frequencies. Subjectively these produce what is meant by 'noise' in acoustic terms. Noise in which each frequency band 1 Hz wide contains sound with the same pressure is described as *white noise*.

Measurable attributes of sound waves

Many of the characteristics of sound waves can be expressed quantitatively. The metre kilogram second (mks) system of units, to which most SI units conform, is conventionally used. Some of the elementary relationships and measures must now be considered.

FREQUENCY

The frequency of a periodic wave is described in terms of the number of cycles of mechanical events in each second in units called hertz. If the wavelength is λ, and the frequency is f, then, during propagation, f wavelengths each λ in length will be passing a point in each second. The velocity of propagation, c, is clearly related to the frequency and wavelength by the formula

$$c = f \lambda$$

In air the velocity of sound at 15°C is about 340 m/s, and so it can be seen that a sound wave of frequency 1000 Hz has a wavelength of 0.34 m.

VELOCITY

The velocity of the wave in metres per second depends on the elasticity of the medium and the density, and the relationship between them is expressed by

$$V = \sqrt{E/\rho}$$

where V is velocity, E is elasticity, and ρ the density.

Elasticity or stiffness was described in the introductory comments to this section as a force tending to restore a displaced mass to its resting position. For quantitative treatment it must be more precisely defined. Elasticity is expressed in terms of the amount of force required to produce a particular amount of deformation. For solids the deforming force is termed *stress*, and the degree of deformation *strain*, and the relationship between them is Young's modulus of elasticity. For gases the equivalent measure is the bulk modulus of elasticity. The deforming force is expressed in terms of compressive force per unit area, and the amount of deformation as proportionate reduction in volume. When allowance is made for the rise in temperature that accompanies the compression of a gas with each phase of pressure rise, the elasticity is expressed as the so-called *adiabatic bulk modulus*.

The velocity of sound in air can, under certain limiting conditions, be shown to depend directly on the temperature (as this inversely determines density). At 20°C the velocity of sound in air is 343 m/s. At high altitudes the velocity is lower, despite the fall in density, because of the fall in temperature with increasing height. In solids the velocity of a sound wave is much greater than in gases, because the comparatively greater density is subordinated to a comparatively much greater elasticity. In fact in metals sound waves travel at over 5000 m/s.

MAGNITUDE OF SOUND

Of all the quantitative aspects none is more important to the otologist than measures of magnitude. The magnitude of disturbance caused by a sound wave depends on the rate of flow of energy through a unit area of the transmitting medium. Power, which is the measure describing energy flow rate (or production rate), is expressed in watts. The magnitude of the disturbance, defined as the average rate of flow of sound energy per unit area, is called the *sound intensity* and is expressed in watts per square metre (W/m^2). This sound intensity is related to the average sound pressure, and, as the ear is a pressure-sensitive mechanism and sound pressure levels are usually used when discussing magnitude, the relationship must be described. Under certain defined conditions the intensity of sound, I, is proportional to the square of the pressure, or

$$I \propto p^2$$

This relationship is valid only under specified relationships between the density of air and the velocity of the sound wave through it. The product of these two quantities, density and wave velocity, is called the characteristic impedance of the medium:

characteristic impedance = ρc (in rayls)

where ρ is density and c is velocity of sound and the square relationship holds when the characteristic impedance remains constant. As has been noted, in air the velocity depends on temperature, so the characteristic impedance depends on temperature and density. When this value, the characteristic impedance, is constant the relation between intensity, I, and average pressure, p, is given by the formula:

$$I = p^2/\rho c$$

The pressure in this relationship has been specified as the average pressure. This term refers to the average pressure throughout the cycle of pressure change. For sine waves, and indeed for other periodic waves, the average is defined as the root mean square (rms) pressure. This form of average allows the negative pressure of each half of a cycle to contribute in the same direction as the positive values and is approximately $0.7 \times$ the pressure level at the peak of the cycle.

PRESSURE MEASUREMENTS

Pressure measurements can be expressed in a number of different units. In the mks system the basic unit is the newton per square metre (N/m^2), which is called the pascal (Pa) in SI units. In acoustic practice, however, this is not always a convenient form of expression. There are two reasons. First, the range of pressures to be covered is so great – from those near the threshold of hearing to pressure levels 10^{13} (10 million million) times as high, at which level pain is caused in the ear. Second, the ear, like other sensory systems, does not respond equally to equal increases in sound pressure. Equal increments of loudness in the ear are provoked by sounds whose magnitudes are equal *multiples* of each other. Put another way, the ear responds subjectively in an arithmetical or linear fashion to sounds whose intensity (or pressure) increases geometrically. In mathematical parlance intensity is an exponential function of associated loudness. For these two reasons it is convenient to express a sound intensity or pressure level in the form of a ratio of that value to a so-called *reference level*, and, further, to express that ratio as an exponent of the number 10 (i.e. as its log to the base 10). This is the basis of the decibel system, which results in the expression of sound intensities and pressures in terms of reference levels in such a way that equal decibel increases are associated with equal subjective changes in the sensation of loudness. Let us start an examination of this system by first considering the application to measurements of intensity. The bel, which consists of 10 decibels, is defined as the log to the base 10 of the ratio of the intensity being measured to the reference intensity. The value in decibels is 10 times this log ratio. So

the sound intensity in decibels = $10\log_{10} I_m/I_{ref}$

where I_m is measured intensity and I_{ref} is reference intensity. Now sound intensity, as has been noted, is proportional to the pressure of the sound under certain conditions. Assuming the square relationship to be valid, the square of the sound pressure can be substituted in the above formula to give

sound pressure in decibels = $10\log_{10} P_m^2/P_{ref}^2$

where P_m is measured pressure and P_{ref} is reference pressure. By manipulating this formula in accordance with the usual principles of logarithms, we can say

$$\text{sound pressure in decibels} = 20\log_{10}P_m/P_{ref}$$

Obviously the expression of sound pressure in decibels is meaningless unless the reference level is stated. In acoustics the most usual pressure reference level is 2×10^{-5} N/m². This is the same as 2 Pa or 20 microPa. As we have seen, a related intensity level can be calculated when the characteristic impedance is known, and it is acoustic practice to express the reference level as a pressure measurement. For common conditions of temperature and density, the characteristic impedance of air is 400 rayls. With that value, a pressure of 2×10^{-5} N/m² corresponds to an intensity of sound of 10^{-12} W/m². With differing values of impedance, the numerical relationship is not precisely the same. (This poses a further problem. When making calculations, such as the effect of the addition of two sound pressures, the arithmetical operations must be performed on the corresponding intensity levels, and the result must then be converted back to the corresponding pressure level, to be expressed in decibels related to the reference level.)

From the formulae given, and the approximate value of 0.3 for $\log_{10}2$, it can be deduced that doubling a sound pressure represents an increase of 6 dB, whereas doubling a sound intensity corresponds to an increase of 3 dB. It may be useful to remember that an increase of about 10 dB creates a subjective impression of doubling the loudness sensation. This exemplifies the virtues of the decibel scale, for of course each 10 dB increase represents a 10-fold increase in the intensity of the sound.

Sound level measurement

If measurements of sound pressure are made with all frequencies using the same reference level of 2×10^{-5} N/m², which is the threshold of normal hearing at 1000 Hz, the levels are described as linear. Unfortunately the ear does not have the same threshold sensitivity at other frequencies, and so it is common practice to use scales of measurement using different reference levels for pressure measurement at different frequencies. The most familiar example is in ordinary pure tone audiometry. Audiometers are calibrated to use a different reference level at each frequency, corresponding to a 0 dB level (the reference level), that is, the pressure level of the normal threshold for hearing at that frequency.

Meters used for measuring sound pressure levels contain weighting networks to provide different sensitivities at different frequencies in order to account for the variation of sensitivity of the ear at different frequencies. Description of a measured *sound level* must always mention the weighting scale used in the measuring instrument, described as sound level 'A', 'B' or 'C', in order to indicate the reference levels to which the measurement relates. The 'C' scale closely approximates to the linear one, in which the same reference level is used for all frequencies. Meters using 'A' and 'B' scale weighting networks provide for different sensitivities of the ear at each frequency. On the 'A' scale, whose recorded measurements are referred to as dBA, sensitivity is reduced from the linear value at the low frequencies (and slightly at high ones). At all frequencies below 500 Hz the reference level used is greater than the standard 2×10^{-5} N/m². As an example, at 50 Hz the pressure level threshold is set 30 dB higher. This means that, at 50 Hz, 0 dBA would be a pressure level identical to 30 dB related to a reference of 2×10^{-5} N/m². This dBA scale approximates more closely than does a linear one to the sensitivity and hence behavioural responses of the human ear in normal environmental conditions.

Analysis of sound pressure by frequency involves the measurement of levels not only over the whole frequency spectrum, but, by the use of filters, in discrete bands of defined frequency width. The bands most commonly analysed are one octave wide, or one-third of an octave wide. The analysis of narrow bands 1 Hz in width produces what are called spectrum pressure levels.

When an elastic wave front meets an obstacle, the energy becomes involved in the processes of *diffraction, reflection* from the obstacle, and *transmission* into the substance of the obstacle. Diffraction involves scattering and breaking of the wave front around the edges of the obstacle, with diffusion of energy, and has a significant effect only when the dimensions of the obstacle are large in relation to the wavelength of the sound; the wave front reforms beyond small obstacles without casting a sound shadow. If the opposing surface is greater than 5 times the wavelength of an incident sound wave, a proportion of the energy in the wave is reflected and a proportion transmitted into the substance of the obstacle. The proportions undergoing reflection and transmission depend on the relationship between the characteristic impedance of the medium in which the wave is travelling and the impedance of the obstacle. When these are identical, all the energy is transmitted and none reflected. With increasing disparity, more and more energy is reflected until, as the difference between them approaches the theoretical infinite, all the incident energy is reflected. It may be useful to remember that at an air–sea water interface only about 0.1 per cent of the energy is transmitted (see Chapter 2).

Impedance

The concept of impedance has had increasing importance in otology with the increasing use of impedance measurements in audiology. Impedance is concerned with the idea of opposition to the flow of energy in a sound wave. It is not the same as the all too loosely used word 'resistance', which, as this chapter shows, has a precise and quite different meaning in physics. The properties of the sound transmitting system that contribute to this opposition are those we have already noted to be essential for a vibrating sound source, and for the medium (the air) through which the sound wave is propagated – namely *mass*, *elasticity*, and *frictional resistance*. Mass opposes the passing mechanical disturbance because of its inertia. Because the mass reacts against the force of the sound wave, without absorbing or dissipating energy, the contribution made by the mass to impedance is called a 'reactance', in this instance the *mass reactance*. Elasticity (or stiffness as it is sometimes called) expresses its opposition by imposing an increasing force against the increasing displacement of the moving mass. It may also be thought of as the opposition offered because energy is needed to compress an enclosed volume of air to a smaller volume. As with mass, this energy is not lost to the system, so the opposition imposed by elasticity is also called a reactance. For mathematical reasons it is convenient to use not the elasticity itself but its reciprocal, which is called *compliance*. The contribution of elasticity to impedance, expressed in terms of its reciprocal, is called the *compliant reactance*. The third component of impedance is friction and, as its effect does dissipate energy from the sound wave in the form of heat, its contribution is called *resistance*. The magnitude of these quantities, and of the impedance that is the result of the complex relationship between them, is expressed in mks acoustic ohms. Now these are all vector quantities as is impedance itself, and this means that the direction of the action must also be specified, just as it must with the more familiar vector quantities, such as force or velocity. This has to be clearly understood for a proper appreciation of the quantitative aspects of impedance measurement and the interaction between its components. The theories of acoustic impedance have been developed by analogies from the physics of electricity, and in particular from alternating current theory. In direct current theory, opposition to current flow is offered by resistance, and that resistance is defined, in the familiar Ohm's law, as the ratio of voltage (which is electrical pressure) to current flow (which is electrical energy flow rate). This simple relationship is valid only because the voltage and current in a DC circuit are in phase. In an AC system, which provides a model for acoustic impedance, the changing physical events are not in phase, and the principles of vector mechanics are needed to describe relationships. However, the opposition to energy flow can still be expressed as a ratio between voltage and current, but the complex ratio of one to the other is a vector quantity. In acoustics, sound pressure is equivalent to voltage, and the quantity corresponding to current flow is what is called volume velocity. This is the alternating rate of flow of air particles through a particular plane of measurement. It is the complex ratio of pressure to volume velocity that describes acoustic impedance. In what is called polar notation, the magnitude of the impedance is expressed in mks acoustic ohms, and the phase angle, indicating the direction, is specified in degrees.

We can now consider the contributions of mass reactance, compliant reactance and resistance to impedance. Mass reactance and compliant reactance act in opposite senses, and the algebraic sum of the positive mass reactance and the negative compliant reactance provides the overall acoustic reactance in a given plane, that is

acoustic reactance = mass reactance minus compliant reactance

If the mass reactance is greater than the compliant reactance, the system is said to be mass dominated; if the compliant reactance is the greater, the system is 'stiffness' dominated. The contribution of each in a given system depends on the frequency of the sound wave. In the middle ear, the system is stiffness dominated at low frequencies, below 500 Hz, with an increasing contribution from mass reactance with rising frequency. This is why impedance measurements using low frequency probe tones around 200 Hz are loosely spoken of as measures of compliance.

Now the frictional resistance operates at right angles to the acoustic reactance, and the relationship between these quantities (the acoustic reactance as defined above and the resistance) can be expressed as

$$Z = \sqrt{R^2 + X^2}$$

where Z is the acoustic impedance, R the acoustic reactance (the algebraic sum of mass reactance and compliant reactance), and X the resistance in acoustic ohms. Once again, the phase angle must be specified.

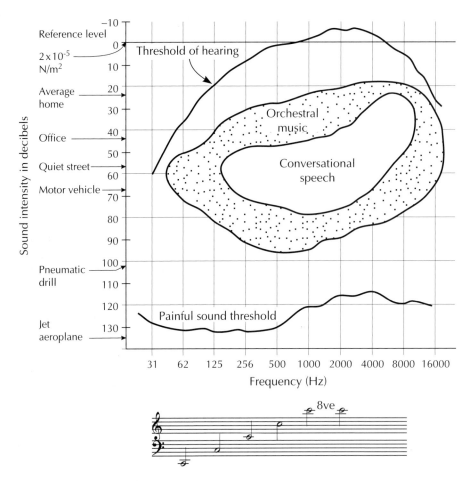

Fig 4.3 The range of human hearing.

Range of human hearing

The range of human hearing is indicated in Fig 4.3. It can be seen that the threshold is frequency dependent, with the greatest sensitivity around 2–3 kHz. As with intensities, the ear responds with subjectively equal increments of sensation to ratios between frequencies, rather than to the arithmetical difference between frequencies. Doubling the frequency of a presented tone produces a change in pitch sensation that is recognized as an octave. Indeed, all the intervals musically recognizable can be defined in terms of the ratios between the two frequencies. As long ago as 500 BC Pythagoras realized that the ratio between the wavelengths of sounds providing a recognizable relationship was always that of two small whole numbers. In audiological practice it is customary to use tuning forks and audiometric frequencies based on multiples of 256 Hz. It is worth noting that, with the international conventionally agreed frequency for the muscial note A established at 440 Hz in 1939, the actual frequency of middle C is a little over 261 Hz. The minimum increase in intensity detectable by the ear is about 10 per cent or 0.4 dB.

Middle ear sound conduction

A sound wave in air cannot be transmitted efficiently into the fluid medium that fills the cochlea. Without the special function of the middle ear, most of the sound energy would be reflected. A full description of the transformer mechanism that evolved to overcome this mismatch is found in Chapter 2.

PART II – HEARING TESTS

General impressions of a patient's hearing disability can be derived from spoken and whispered voice tests. These are not now regularly used to try to quantify hearing loss.

Tuning fork tests

Tuning fork tests are still the most valuable clinical tests of auditory function and should enable the clinician to distinguish a conductive from a sensorineural hearing loss with greater reliablility than pure tone audiometry. These tests are based on two physiological facts: first, the inner ear is normally twice as sensitive to sound conducted by air as to that conducted by bone; and second, in the presence of a purely conductive hearing loss, the affected ear is subject to less environmental noise, making it more sensitive to bone-conducted sound.

The most information may be obtained using tuning forks that vibrate naturally at 256, 512, 1024 and 2048 Hz. Tuning forks that vibrate at lower frequencies provide a tactile stimulus, which may confuse the result. Higher forks decay too rapidly for easy use. If, as is usually the case nowadays, one fork only is to be used, 512 Hz is the frequency to choose. The tests should be performed in a quiet room. The prong should be struck sharply against some resistant but elastic object, for example a mass of hard rubber or the forearm (of the examiner)

near the olecranon. The prong should be struck at a point about one-third of its length from the free end, thus keeping overtones to a minimum and producing a pure tone.

Because pure tone bone conduction audiometry is prone to technical errors, most experienced otologists rely on the tuning fork results in cases of ambiguity and disagreement. This is especially so when judging suitablity for operative improvement of hearing, as in stapedectomy.

RINNE TEST

The Rinne test was originally described by Rinne, a general practitioner in Gottingen, in 1855. The principle of the test is to compare the loudness of a tone perceived by air conduction (AC) with that perceived by bone conduction (BC). The fork is struck gently but firmly, as described previously, and held with its acoustic axis coincident with the anatomical axis of the external auditory meatus. The nearest tine should be within 1 cm of the entrance to the ear canal without touching protruding hairs. The fork is then immediately transferred so that the base is pressed firmly against the mastoid process, ensuring that no hair is caught between the base of the fork and the mastoid process (Fig 4.4). The fork is held for 2 seconds, with counter pressure applied to the opposite side of the head with the other hand. The patient is then asked whether the tuning fork was heard by AC and whether this sound was louder or quieter than that perceived by BC. When the sound perceived by AC is louder (>) than that heard by BC, the test result is referred to as *positive*. This is the result obtained

(a)   (b)

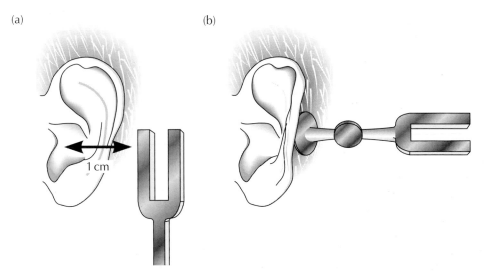

Fig 4.4 Rinne test (a) air conduction (b) bone conduction.

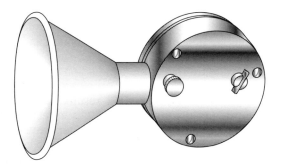

Fig 4.5 Barany noise box (courtesy of Down Bros Surgical plc).

from normal ears and the vast majority of patients with a unilateral sensorineural loss. If the sound heard by AC is quieter (<) than that heard by BC, then the test is termed a *negative* Rinne response.

Negative Rinne responses may be observed in association with an appreciable impairment of sound transmission in the affected ear, that is, a conductive hearing loss in excess of 15–20 dB hearing level (HL); or in cases of severe or total sensorineural hearing loss in the test ear, such that the bone conduction stimulus results in transmission of sound through the skull to the better cochlea on the non-test side. This latter situation is referred to as a *false Rinne negative* and may be

differentiated from a true Rinne negative by applying a masking noise to the non-test ear. A Barany noise box is a convenient clinical tool for this task (Fig 4.5). It is a clockwork device, which emits 'white noise' (wide frequency representation) and raises the threshold of hearing in the non-test ear to such a level that the tuning fork cannot be heard in that ear by cross hearing. Thus, if the Rinne test is repeated in this manner and no sound is heard, either by air conduction or bone conduction, a false negative Rinne response is confirmed. In a true negative Rinne response (i.e. in the presence of a conductive hearing loss), the bone conduction stimulus will still be perceived more loudly than the air conduction stimulus. It must be emphasized that erroneous true Rinne negative responses may be obtained with tuning forks of frequencies of 128 Hz and below due to vibrotactile stimulation.

WEBER TEST

The Weber test is performed in conjunction with the Rinne test and is of particular value in cases of unilateral hearing loss. The examiner applies a vibrating fork to the head in the midline, either the vertex or the forehead. The patient is asked to indicate if any sound is heard and whether it is in the middle of the head, in both ears equally, or directed towards the left or right. In a patient with

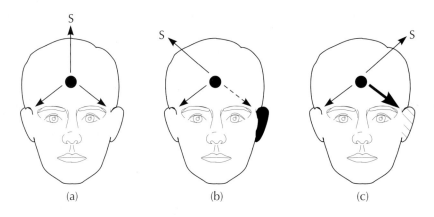

Key

S = Direction of perceived sound

● = Site of base of tuning fork

❩ = Sensorineural hearing loss

𝄄 = Conductive hearing loss

Fig 4.6 Weber Test (a) normal (b) sensorineural hearing loss (c) conductive hearing loss.

normal hearing, the tone is heard centrally. If the patient has a left-sided hearing loss and lateralizes the sound to that side, this is indicative of a conductive loss, whereas lateralizing the sound to the normal (or better) hearing ear indicates that the hearing loss is more likely to be sensorineural (Fig 4.6). It should be emphasized again that results obtained with the Weber test should be interpreted in the context of the results of a battery of hearing tests, as anomalous results are often obtained. For example, long-standing sensorineural hearing loss in one ear is commonly associated with a central Weber response, and bilateral hearing loss commonly gives rise to equivocal results.

Tuning fork tests may also be useful in suggesting the presence of a cochlear component, if a sensorineural loss has been defined. A vibrating tuning fork is presented to one ear, and then to the other, the patient being asked if the musical notes sound the same on both sides. If *dysacusis* is present, the patient will say that the sound is 'distorted', 'harder', 'harsher', 'rougher' or 'out-of tune' on one side or the other. Clinically, this phenomenon is characteristic of cochlear disorders and is commonly associated with diplacusis. Diplacusis may be monaural, when two tones are perceived from a vibrating tuning fork held beside one ear, or may be binaural, when a tuning fork of a given frequency is perceived as being of a different pitch in each ear. Diplacusis is also a feature of cochlear pathology and is commonly observed in endolymphatic hydrops.

The presence of a non-organic hearing loss may also be suspected on the basis of tuning fork tests, although for medicolegal or psychiatric purposes quantitative objective tests of auditory thresholds are essential.

Clinical audiometric tests

Despite the value of a clinical examination, precise quantification and identification of the site of pathology of an auditory deficit requires sophisticated audiometric investigation, which is aimed at

- identifying the presence or absence of auditory function
- differentiating a conductive from a sensorineural hearing loss
- differentiating a cochlear from a neural abnormality
- identifying central auditory dysfunction in the brainstem, midbrain or auditory cortex
- identifying any non-organic component.

Threshold assessment

PURE TONE AUDIOMETRY

Pure tone air conduction threshold assessment is the most widespread audiological measurement, in which the quietest sounds that a patient can perceive are recorded at different frequencies. The reference intensity level, which is designated 0 dB at each frequency, is the median value of the minimal audible intensity (threshold) of pure tones in a group of healthy, normally hearing, young adults, in accordance with standards set by the International Standards Organization (ISO).

An audiometer is an electronic instrument capable of delivering pure tone stimuli to the ear at frequencies between 125 and 8000 Hz at selected intensities. The instrument consists of a variable frequency pure tone oscillator, which produces stimulus tones; an amplifier; an attenuator, covering the range from 10 dB below average normal threshold to 110 dB or more above this level in 5 dB steps; a frequency selector and a signal key to switch the stimulus on and off. Specifications of pure tone audiometers in the UK are covered by a British Standard criterion, which defines acceptable limits of frequency and intensity accuracy and of the various forms of distortion of the pure test tones. A daily subjective calibration test should be carried out by the scientist or technician and a full objective calibration to the accepted standards must be carried out 6 monthly by a calibration centre or the manufacturers of the instrument.

A method of threshold assessment suitable for the majority of adults and children over 6 years of age, is now described. While operating the audiometer the tester should be able to see the patient, but care should be taken to provide no visual clues. The headphones are placed over the patient's ears, so that the centre of each transducer is at the entrance of the meatus without occlusion by pressure on the tragus and taking care that no hair is between the transducer and the ear. Women should remove earrings. The patient is instructed that the aim of the test is to establish the quietest sound that can be heard at each of several frequencies. It is helpful to describe the foghorn-like characteristic of a low frequency sound and the squeaky characteristic of a high frequency sound so that the patient may anticipate the quality of the sound. Tones should be presented for 1–3 seconds, with intervals of 1–3 seconds between each presentation. It is important to randomize the intervals and to avoid presenting the tones in a rhythmic fashion to facilitate the recognition of a true response. The patient responds as soon

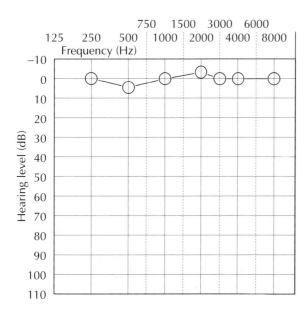

Fig 4.7 Normal air conduction audiogram, right ear.

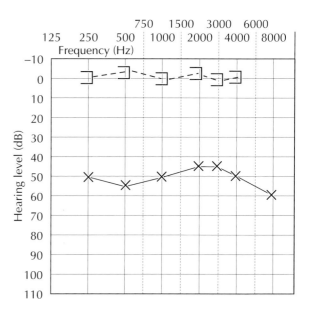

Fig 4.8 Air conduction and bone conduction audiograms in conductive deafness, left ear.

as the sound is heard, for example by raising a finger or pressing a button that lights a signal on the audiometer panel, and maintains the response as long as the sound is heard. It must be emphasized to the patient that the response should be made however faint the sound.

The various frequencies are presented in the following order: 1000, 2000, 4000, 8000, 250 and 500 Hz. The results at 1000 Hz should be rechecked at the end of testing each ear. For a given frequency, the initial presentation should be at a level sufficiently above threshold to allow easy recognition and identification. The intensity of the tone is then decreased by 10 dB steps until the patient ceases to respond, and then increased in 5 dB steps until it is heard again. This procedure is repeated until the patient has responded twice to the same intensity as the stimulus is increased in steps of 5 dB. Correctly, the threshold is statistically defined as 'the lowest intensity heard on 50 per cent of occasions on repeated crossings', but, in clinical practice, with steps of 5 dB, the faintest audible sound will be perceived, and the sound 5 dB quieter will never be heard. So, for practical purposes, the faintest audible intensity as established above is recorded against the test frequency on a standard audiogram chart as the threshold intensity (Fig 4.7). By convention, the symbols 'O' and 'X' are used for air conduction thresholds in the right and left ears, respectively, whereas the symbols '[' and ']' are used for right and left bone conduction thresholds, respectively (Figs 4.8 and 4.9). If the maximum sound intensity of the

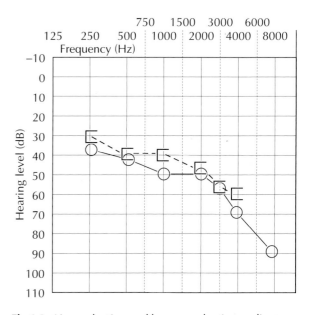

Fig 4.9 Air conduction and bone conduction audiograms in sensorineural deafness, right ear.

audiometer at a given frequency cannot be heard, this is indicated by a downward pointing arrow at the level of the maximum output on the appropriate frequency line.

Bone conduction thresholds are obtained in a manner identical to those described for air conduction, but the sound stimulus is produced by a bone vibrator placed on the mastoid process and held firmly by a head band. Care is taken to remove any intervening hair and contact with the cartilaginous external meatus or pinna is also avoided during the test, as these structures may carry air-conducted sounds. The vibrator should be placed on the mastoid process of the ear with the worse air conduction threshold. Measurements are restricted to the frequency range 250–4000 Hz and calibration standards do not generally give data for stimuli outside this range. The test is commenced at 1000 Hz, followed by 2000, 4000, 500 and 250 Hz. The patient is instructed to respond to sounds regardless of the side on which the sound is heard, and it must be emphasized that, without the use of masking, it is not possible to determine which ear is responsible for the detection of a 'non-masked' bone conduction threshold.

Bone conduction thresholds cannot be established with as great precision as air conduction thresholds. As the output level of bone vibrators rises, the distortion increases and the threshold measured may relate to second or third harmonics, rather than the fundamental frequency. At higher frequencies (2000–4000 Hz) airborne sound, radiated by the bone vibrator, may result in errors. Hence, an essential requirement of bone conduction testing is the exclusion of the non-test ear by an efficient masking sound, so that all threshold levels may be reliably attributed to the tested ear. The symbol 'Δ' is used to represent unmasked bone conduction.

Masking is the phenomenon by which one sound impairs the perception of another. The most effective sound to mask a pure tone is a narrow band of noise with a central frequency equal to the test tone (Fig 4.10). In commercially available audiometers, the masking band is automatically selected upon selection of the test tone frequency. Masking is mandatory for all bone conduction studies, whenever the unmasked bone conduction is 10 dB or more better than the worse air conduction; and air conduction studies when the difference between left and right unmasked air conduction threshold is 40 dB or more, and whenever the unmasked bone conduction is 40 dB or more better than the worse air conduction.

These requirements for masking may be readily understood considering certain facts regarding the transmission of air- and bone-conducted sounds across the head. An air-conducted sound is transmitted across the skull with an interaural attenuation of the order of 50 dB, whereas the attenuation for a bone-conducted sound is negligible. Hence an apparent threshold level may be a record of the sensitivity of the cochlea not under test.

In practice, a masking noise is applied to the ear opposite to that being tested in order to mask out sounds arriving at the non-test ear. The masking

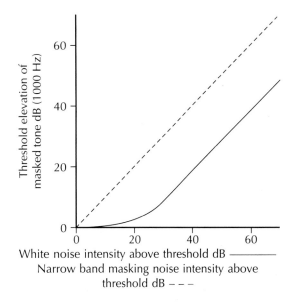

Fig 4.10 Diagram to illustrate efficiency of narrow band masking noise.

noise employed must be of high masking efficiency, but of minimal loudness to avoid crossover to the test ear and the phenomenon of central masking. (At high intensity levels a tone, or noise, presented in one ear can shift the threshold of a similar frequency in the opposite ear.) The 'shadowing' technique for determining the true auditory threshold is the most commonly used masking technique. The threshold of the masking stimulus is measured in the non-test ear and then the apparent pure tone threshold is measured in the test ear. The masking noise is then elevated by 10 dB and pure tone thresholds reassessed in the presence of contralateral masking noise. This procedure is repeated until the test threshold retains a constant value, despite further increases in masking intensity in the non-test ear. This plateau level represents a true auditory threshold for the ear under test and must be established at each frequency. For clarity, a chart may be plotted of intensity levels on the masking dial versus the pure tone threshold measure (Fig 4.11). Using this technique, it is possible to apply sufficient masking without the complication of overmasking mentioned above.

Under certain circumstances, for example a non-test ear with good cochlear function but a conductive hearing loss, it may prove impossible to obtain efficient masking as the audiometer may not generate a sufficiently intense masking output to exclude the non-test ear.

Masking for bone conduction audiometry is conveniently carried out using an insert earphone. This avoids the use of conventional earphones combined

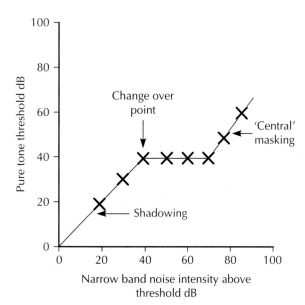

Fig 4.11 Masking chart.

with the bone conduction transducer, reduces the likelihood of cross masking and avoids the 'occlusion effect'.

Békésy audiometry is now rarely used, but has historical importance. The technique relies upon a specialized audiometer, which presents a continuous, or pulsed, tone sweeping from low to high frequencies. The patient adjusts the intensity of the test tone by depressing a button, which alternately reduces or increases the intensity of the signal. By this means, the patient maintains the signal at a level that is just audible. Using this technique, the entire frequency range is tested; there is some evidence that more sensitive thresholds are obtained, operator error is excluded and an automatic print out of the results is obtained. By using different test techniques, for example continuous or pulsed tones, forwards or backwards sweeps, it is possible to obtain not only threshold measurements, but also valuable diagnostic information about other auditory functions, including recruitment and abnormal auditory adaptation (see below). Specific configurations of the Békésy audiometric responses have been identified with specific kinds of hearing loss.

Acoustic impedance measurements

Audiology has been transformed by acoustic impedance measurements, which may provide information about middle ear, inner ear, VIIIth

nerve and brainstem function. The principles of impedance have been described earlier in this chapter.

The principle of an electro-acoustic impedance meter is outlined in Figure 4.12. A probe is placed in the external acoustic meatus so as to make an air-tight seal. The probe comprises three tubes: one connected to a pump, which alters the pressure in the meatus and measures that pressure with a manometer; a second, which delivers a continuous pure tone sound wave, called the 'probe tone', to the meatus; and a third, which transmits sound waves from the meatus to a microphone for conversion to electrical activity. This electrical signal is amplified and rectified to direct current, and represents the sound pressure level in the external meatus. It is compared with a reference voltage delivered by the impedance meter, and the comparison registered on a balance meter. By adjusting the intensity of the probe tone, it is possible to produce a voltage of the reflected sound equal to that of the reference voltage, such that the balance meter shows a null position of the needle. A rigid air-containing cavity acts as a pure acoustic compliance of a magnitude that depends on the volume of the cavity. Measures of compliance may be expressed as the volume of air in a rigid chamber, that would have an equal compliance. Most clinical instruments use the unit of an equivalent volume in cubic centimetres as the unit of measurement for compliance. The total compliance obtained using the probe in the meatus is the sum of that contributed by the volume of air in the meatus beyond the probe. Acoustic impedance measurements may be divided into *passive measures* of changes in acoustic impedance, or admittance, as a function of the pressure in the sealed external acoustic meatus, and *dynamic changes*, resulting from contraction of the stapedius muscle.

TYMPANOMETRY

Tympanometry is an important test of middle ear function, in which the compliance of the tympanic membrane is measured as a function of mechanically varied air pressure in the external canal. The ear insert is placed in the external auditory meatus and the air pressure within the canal slowly raised to 200 mmH$_2$O and then gradually reduced to –200 mmH$_2$O. Impedance, or admittance, values are recorded manually or automatically at various pressure conditions to produce a graph of compliance against air pressure with an XY plotter. By increasing or decreasing the external canal pressure to +200 or –200 mm H$_2$O, the tympanic membrane is stiffened and little energy is admitted and trans-

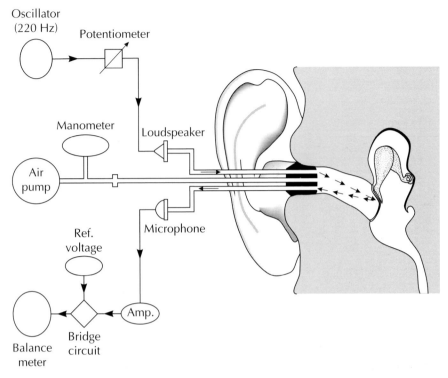

Fig 4.12 Diagram of components of electro-acoustic impedance bridge.

mitted to the inner ear. Readings taken at these pressures reflect the volume or compliance of the external ear canal. Between these two extremes, the compliance rises and reaches a maximum when the air pressure is equal on each side of the tympanic membrane. In patients with normal middle ears, this value is at or near atmospheric pressure. The magnitude of the maximum compliance allows calculation of the compliance attributable to the middle ear mechanism by subtraction of that attributable to the air in the external canal measured during pressure immobilization of the tympanic membrane. So, in a way, the tympanogram describes the 'flexibility' of the tympanic membrane (Fig 4.13), which is of the utmost importance as almost all middle ear disorders influence this function. For example, the absence of a peak with pressure changes suggests a middle ear effusion, whereas, in the presence of ossicular discontinuity the peak middle ear compliance is elevated, and in otosclerosis it may be reduced.

ACOUSTIC REFLEX MEASUREMENTS

Loud sounds directed into either ear cause bilateral contraction of the stapedius muscle in both ears. The middle ear, the cochlea and the auditory divi-

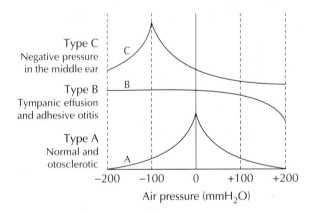

Fig 4.13 The three types of tympanometry curve.

sion of the VIIIth cranial nerve subserve the afferent limb of the reflex arc, whereas the efferent limb consists of the VIIth cranial nerve, the stapedial muscle and tendon and the stapes (Fig 4.14). Measurement of various features of the acoustic reflex, including threshold, latency, decay and amplitude, provides diagnostic information in the differentiation of cochlear, retrocochlear and brainstem pathology. The most widely used stapedial reflex measurement is that of the acoustic or stapedial

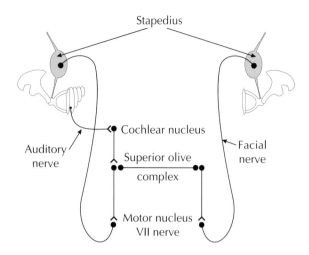

Fig 4.14 The acoustic reflex arc.

reflex threshold – the minimum sound intensity required to produce this response – normally 75–95 dB above the normal threshold. Ipsilateral threshold recordings are obtained by presentation of a tone and measurement of the compliance change produced by contraction of the stapedius muscle in the same ear. A normal ipsilateral stapedial reflex threshold provides evidence of integrity of the reflex arc, as outlined above, on that side. Contralateral stapedial reflex thresholds are of greater use. Here the tone is presented on one side and the compliance change produced in the contralateral ear recorded. A normal contralateral stapedial reflex threshold implies an intact afferent limb of the reflex arc on the side of the acoustic stimulus, an intact brainstem pathway and integrity of the efferent limb of the reflex arc in the opposite ear. Consideration of the various combinations of ipsilateral and contralateral stapedial reflex threshold findings provides a wealth of diagnostic information.

Many variables may affect the stapedial reflex measurements and must be considered in the interpretation of results. An ipsilaterally elicited acoustic reflex is rarely observed even in an ear with a minimal (5–10 dB) conductive loss. Furthermore, a contralateral acoustic reflex cannot be measured, even with the probe in a normal ear, if the sound intensity reaching the cochlea of the stimulated ear is attenuated to less than 70–90 dB by a conductive impairment. In addition, acoustic stimulation of an ear with a severe cochlear impairment (60–70 dB) or mild VIIIth nerve auditory impairment (0–40 dB) is unlikely to produce measurable acoustic reflex activity. VIIth cranial nerve dysfunction may also affect stapedial reflex measurements. Normal acoustic reflex activity, in the presence of a facial

nerve palsy, implies that the lesion is distal (peripheral) to the facial nerve branch innervating the stapedius muscle. Absence of measurable acoustic reflexes indicates gross facial nerve dysfunction proximal to the stapedial branch. Elevations of acoustic reflex threshold levels, abnormal decay or reduced reflex amplitude provide parameters for monitoring facial nerve function during progression or recovery of paralysis.

Assessment of cochlear versus neural hearing loss

Sensorineural hearing loss may result from cochlear, auditory nerve or central nervous system pathology. The most commonly encountered clinical problem is the differentiation of cochlear from neural lesions, which is often difficult because of the pathophysiological interdependence of the sensory and neural elements.

Before the availability of MRI scanning for possible acoustic neuromas, the results of tests for recruitment and abnormal adaptation were the main indications for neuroma suspicion, and they were of great otological importance. They are now used much less frequently, but a brief account of auditory phenomena and the techniques for investigating them is needed. It must be realized that none of these tests has high specificity or sensitivity. Their use in planning patient management in relation to supicions about acoustic neuromas needed experience and wisdom.

TESTS FOR RECRUITMENT

Loudness recruitment is defined as a more rapid than normal growth of subjective loudness sensation with increase in sound intensity. A patient with a sensorineural hearing loss with recruitment in one ear perceives a quiet sound to be of lower intensity in that affected ear, but a loud sound of 90–100 dB is perceived to be of equal intensity in the two ears; in other terms, the dynamic range of the affected ear is reduced compared with that of the normal ear (Fig 4.15).

Loudness recruitment is associated with disorders affecting the hair cells of the organ of Corti, and is characteristically absent in disorders affecting the auditory division of the VIIIth cranial nerve. The precise mechanisms subserving recruitment have not been fully elucidated but may be partly attributed to flattening of 'tuning curves' and partly to a steeper than normal increase of activity with

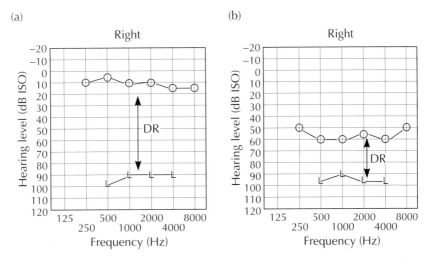

Fig 4.15 The dynamic range (DR) of auditory function in (a) normal subject and (b) a patient with right-sided recruiting hearing loss.

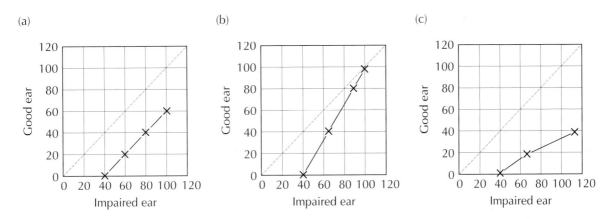

Fig 4.16 Loudness balance test records (a) non-recruiting hearing loss, (b) recruitment and (c) loudness reversal.

intensity exhibited by pathological cochlear nerve fibres. Among many tests of recruitment are the alternate binaural balance test, loudness discomfort level and stapedial reflex threshold measurements.

The *alternate binaural loudness balance test* (ABLB) is performed when only one ear is normal and the threshold in the impaired ear is less than 50 dB above normal, to avoid crossover of sound to the normal ear. A comparison of the intensity of a sound applied to the normal ear at a fixed frequency with the intensity of a sound required to create a sensation of equal loudness in the affected ear, is made. The results are plotted as shown in Figure 4.16 for each frequency selected.

The terms loudness discomfort level (LDL), uncomfortable loudness level (ULL), and threshold of discomfort may be used interchangeably. More

than 90 per cent of normally hearing patients can identify an intensity level between 90 and 105 dB above threshold, at which sounds feel unpleasant. In the presence of recruitment, loudness discomfort levels may be identified at similar levels to the normal population, despite the presence of reduced auditory thresholds. In the absence of recruitment, discomfort may not be experienced even at the maximum intensity output of the audiometer.

Assessment of ipsilateral and contralateral stapedial reflex threshold measurements is still of value in the differentiation of cochlear from retrocochlear hearing loss. If a sound stimulus of some 95 dB in an ear with an auditory threshold of say 45 dB produces a stapedial reflex response either ipsilaterally or contralaterally, it may be assumed that the hearing loss is of a recruiting nature.

TESTS FOR ABNORMAL AUDITORY ADAPTATION

Adaptation refers to the slow decline in discharge frequency with time observed following an initial burst of neural activity in response to an adequate stimulus applied to a receptor organ. Normally, VIIIth nerve discharges show little adaptation. In neural pathology, although the initial response may be normal or near normal, the response to a continuous stimulus cannot be maintained at the normal level. If a continuous tone is presented to an ear and the patient perceives that the tone fades over a given period, there is said to be *abnormal auditory adaptation* or, more commonly but inexactly, 'tone decay'.

As outlined above, the stapedial reflex threshold is commonly elevated or absent in auditory nerve pathology, even in the presence of normal or mild sensorineural hearing loss. In addition, acoustic reflex decay is well established as a screening procedure for retrocochlear dysfunction. The *stapedial reflex decay test* is usually administered by presenting an acoustic stimulus for 10 seconds at an intensity 10 dB greater than the reflex threshold level. The reflex related impedance change is recorded and then analysed for evidence of a decrease in amplitude. Slight decay is not uncommon in cochlear hearing loss and may occasionally be seen in normal ears, but significant decay (50 per cent in 3 seconds) is highly suggestive of retrocochlear pathology. This test is particularly sensitive at 500 and 1000 Hz.

Speech audiometry

Speech audiometry is concerned with the assessment of auditory discriminative ability, as opposed to the assessment of auditory acuity. Scores of auditory discrimination provide information about site of pathology, but are also of particular value in the assessment of handicap, hearing aid evaluation, preoperative and postoperative assessment and the detection of non-organic hearing loss. Speech sounds may be delivered either free-field or, more commonly, from pre-recorded tapes presented through earphones monaurally, with the application of masking to the non-test ear. In the UK phonetically balanced (PB) monosyllabic word lists (Boothroyd or Fry lists) are used most commonly, whereas in the USA, spondee words (e.g. cowboy, ice cream) are often preferred. Sentence lists are particularly appropriate for children, for example the Bamford–Kowal–Bench (BKB) standard sentence list. The material for speech testing must be selected with care, not only for content in the appropriate language, but also for enunciation and accent. Lists of words are presented at different intensity levels and the words are scored phonetically to give a percentage correct score, which is plotted against the sound intensity in dB of the presentation level (Fig 4.17). The highest score achieved is termed the *optimum discrimination score* (ODS). The *speech reception threshold* (SRT) identifies the sound level at which 50 per cent of the test stimuli are identified. This level was originally

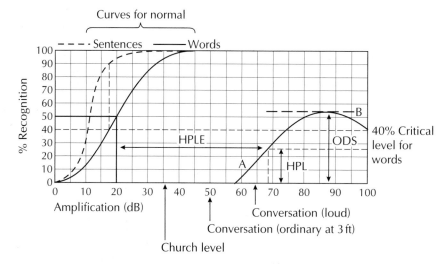

Fig 4.17 Speech audiogram. AB, speech audiogram of a sensorineural hearing loss; HPL, half peak level; HPLE, half peak level elevation; ODS, optimal discrimination score.

defined for spondees, and 20 per cent is usually described as a more appropriate level for phonetically balanced word lists. The most valuable diagnostic measures are the *half peak level* (HPL), which refers to the sound level at which the discrimination percentage is half the ODS, and the *half peak level elevation* (HPLE), which refers to the difference between the pathological and normal HPL.

Diagnostically, speech material is sensitive in distinguishing sensorineural from conductive hearing loss, as in a conductive loss, with sufficient amplification of speech material, the discriminative ability is excellent, whereas sensorineural pathology reduces not only auditory acuity, but also auditory discrimination. In the differentiation of sensory from neural hearing loss, speech discrimination is also useful. Neural dysfunction is often accompanied by more severe impairment of speech discrimination than would be anticipated from assessment of the pure tone thresholds alone. A patient with an acoustic neurinoma may present with an ODS of 20 per cent, despite apparently normal pure tone threshold levels. Nonetheless, caution in interpreting such results must be exercised, as it is well established that patients with cochlear lesions with recruitment may also present with low ODS scores. The results of speech audiometry, as with all audiometric tests, are therefore better interpreted in the context of a test battery than in isolation.

Auditory evoked potentials

Auditory evoked potentials may be recorded from many sites in the auditory pathways by varying stimulus and recording parameters. The responses evoked by auditory stimuli appear as minute electrical potential changes embedded in a continuous background of electrical activity. The separation of these potentials from background noise is possible only by the use of *averaging computer* techniques. The recording of the response to each stimulus is triggered by the stimulus, so that the physiological events are 'time locked'. Summation of individual responses provoked by repeated, successive stimuli results in growth of the stimulus response, whereas the fluctuating background noise, which is random, tends to be cancelled out. Mathematically, the signal to noise ratio grows in proportion to the square root of summed recordings.

The changes in electrical activity are detected by electrodes firmly held to the skin, and differential amplifiers, with good common mode rejection, are used to amplify the signal, which may be displayed on an oscilloscope. The record of each sweep of raw data may be stored in the computer memory, or on a disk or tape, for further analysis later, thus minimizing the patient test time. For convenience, a record of the average of several sweeps may be obtained by a pen recorder or by optical methods. Click stimuli are used most commonly and are produced by sending brief rectangular electrical pulses through a transducer. Each click stimulates the whole basal portion of the cochlea, almost simultaneously, and thus results in close synchrony of firing of the individual nerve fibres, giving a large clear evoked response. A pure tone, which produces a frequency-specific stimulus because of the low rise and fall time required to avoid scattering of the acoustic energy, results in loss of synchrony as individual nerve fibres fire at different moments during the use of the stimulus. This leads to a blurring of the evoked response. The number of clicks required to separate the response from background noise depends upon the stimulus strength and may vary from a few hundred to a few thousand. The stimulus may be delivered free-field or through earphones and, under certain circumstances such as the examination of young children or uncooperative patients of any age, sedation or anaesthesia may be necessary. Auditory evoked potential techniques are of value in the estimation of hearing, differential diagnosis and identification of site of lesion, and clinical monitoring of, for example, pharmacological effects and coma.

ELECTROCOCHLEOGRAPHY

Electrocochleography (ECochG) is the measurement of the electrical output of the cochlea and VIIIth cranial nerve in response to an auditory stimulus. The most reliable and largest amplitude responses are obtained by transtympanic placement of a thin needle electrode so that it lies on the promontory close to the round window niche. The response consists of the *cochlear microphonic* (CM), the *summating potential* (SP) and the *compound cochlear nerve action potential* (AP); the latter occurs during the first 5 milliseconds after the stimulus. Although the transtympanic approach is free from any serious risk, sedation or anaesthesia may be required for a particularly anxious adult or, but more importantly, for small children. Sedation does not appear to have any effect on these responses. Extratympanic techniques may be used, when the active electrode is placed close to the tympanic membrane in the meatus. In either method, the reference electrode is placed on the vertex, whereas the ground electrode is placed on the forehead. Click stimuli or tone pips are used and a few hundred sweeps are generally required to obtain an adequate response. High pass masking (i.e. masking that omits low frequency sound) has been used in conjunction with the click stimuli in order to obtain frequency-specific information. A 10 millisecond window and a band width of about 3 Hz to 3 kHz are used for recording.

The *cochlear microphonic* is an electrical wave form (Fig 4.18), which resembles the vibratory

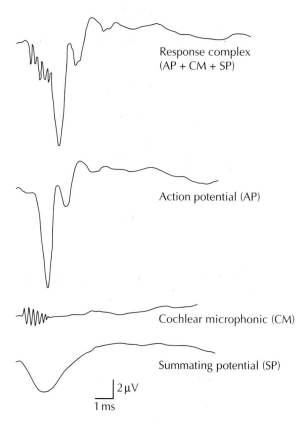

Fig 4.18 Electrocochleographic response complex, comprising the compound action potential (AP), cochlear microphonic (CM) and summating potential (SP).

pattern of the cochlear partition and shows as a deflection up or down depending on the polarity of the click stimulus. The mechanism of generation is not well understood, but the source of the potential is generally agreed to be in the hair cells. The presence of the cochlear microphonic indicates that the cochlear hair cells are physiologically intact, and experimental studies have shown that impairment of the cochlear microphonic parallels loss of hair cells in the spiral organ. Conversely, the retention of the cochlear microphonic in a patient with total hearing loss implies that the lesion is central to the cochlea.

There is no 'all or none' threshold for the cochlear microphonic, and the cochlear microphonic output grows linearly with the input of the acoustic stimulus until relatively high levels (greater than 90 dB hearing level) are reached.

The *summating potential* is the sum of various components, although only two are of importance, that is, a positive SP and a negative SP. In the normal cochlea the positive summating potential, like the cochlear microphonic, is primarily produced by the outer hair cells. In practice, the action potential may be separated from the summating potential by increasing the rates of stimulation; these higher rates result in a decrease in magnitude of the action potential but not the summating potential. Evaluation of the summating potential has proved of particular value in Menière's disease, in which a marked negative summating potential is commonly documented (Fig 4.19; also see Chapter 38). Unlike the cochlear microphonic, the *compound cochlear nerve action potential* exhibits an 'all or none' response and is independent of the polarity of the stimulus. Thus, by alternating the polarity of the stimulus, the cochlear microphonic may be cancelled, whereas the compound action potential grows in the direction of its deflection. However, precise superimposition of alternate action potentials does not occur, as the latency of the action potential is shorter for refraction than for

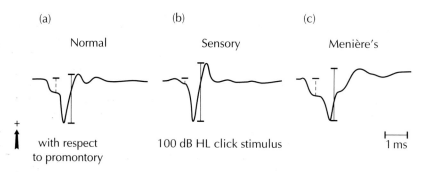

Fig 4.19 Electrocochleographic configuration of the compound action potential showing an SP : AP ratio greater than 50 per cent in (c) endolymphatic hydrops (Menière's disease) compared with a smaller ratio in the (a) normal and (b) other sensory hearing loss.

(a)

(b)

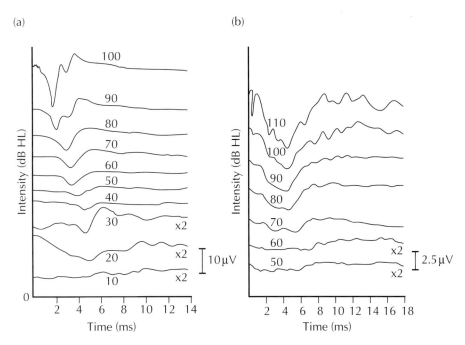

Fig 4.20 Electrocochleographic responses to threshold in (a) a normal subject; (b) the widened action potential and elevated threshold in a patient with an acoustic neuroma.

condensation clicks, at least for high stimulus levels. If earphones are used to deliver the stimulus, the observed AP may be contaminated by electrical artefacts, because the shortest AP latencies are of the order of 1 millisecond. This may be avoided by using a loud speaker as the signal source. The normal AP action potential is diphasic near threshold and has a latent period (the time from the stimulus to the start of the response) that decreases from 4 to 1.5 milliseconds as the stimulus intensity increases. In the assessment of threshold of hearing (Fig 4.20), it may be seen that in a normal patient, the AP becomes recognizable within 20 dB of the subjective threshold.

None of the evoked potentials are present in an ear that has been destroyed, for example by acute viral labyrinthitis. As outlined above, the presence of a cochlear microphonic with an absent AP indicates a lesion of the VIIIth cranial nerve, whereas the presence of an AP in the absence of a cochlear microphonic indicates an auditory lesion restricted to the hair cells. A prominent summating potential on the descending limb of the AP is a common finding in endolymphatic hydrops. A broad, trough-like AP with delayed recovery to the prestimulus level is suggestive of an acoustic neuroma. If this finding is associated with a clear cochlear microphonic and an AP, even when using stimulus intensities that are not audible to the patient, an VIIIth nerve lesion is suspected.

The advantages of electrocochleography are

- direct measurement of cochlear and VIIIth nerve function
- direct recording from the test ear and therefore masking is unnecessary
- highly reproducible results
- responses are unaffected by anaesthesia.

Brainstem auditory evoked potentials (BAEPs) are a series of neurogenic potentials that can be recorded using surface electrodes in response to click stimuli in the 10 milliseconds immediately after the stimulus. The waves are thought to arise from processing centres in the auditory system (Fig 4.21). The patient may be awake or asleep but should be relaxed to reduce myogenic activity, which tends to mask these tiny potentials. The active and reference electrodes are placed at the vertex and ear lobes, or mastoid processes, with a ground electrode on the forehead. The response may be satisfactorily obtained only by using a very brief stimulus with sharp onset characteristics. Clicks, filtered clicks and tone bursts are most commonly used. Stimuli are presented between 5 and 50 times per second depending on the aims of the test. Many summations may be needed before a clear response emerges.

The latency of each of the waves decreases with increasing intensity, but the interwave relationships

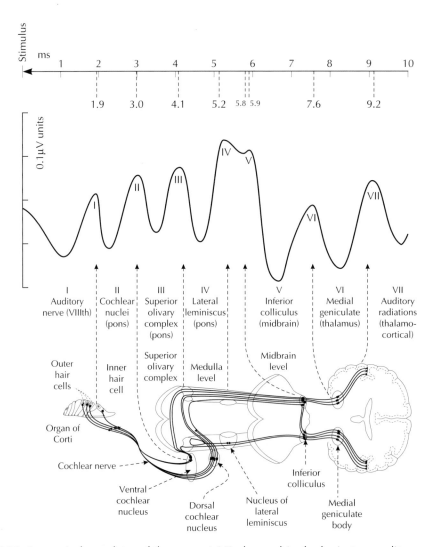

Fig 4.21 Anatomical correlates of the waves I–VII observed in the brainstem auditory evoked potentials.

remain constant. With decreasing intensity of stimulus, wave V is the most resistant and persists to a level that relates closely to psychoacoustic thresholds, although electrocochleography is the method of choice for obtaining threshold information. Thus, the main value of auditory evoked potentials is primarily in detecting lesions involving the auditory nervous system, particularly vestibular schwannoma and neurological conditions.

Various measures of brainstem electric response may be studied in order to establish dysfunction of the auditory pathways: absolute latency delay, interwave latency delay, latency–intensity function, absence of expected waves and deformation of individual wave forms. In general, latency abnormalities appear to be most consistent and several of

them have contributed to the development of brainstem evoked response criteria for the differential diagnosis of a retrocochlear lesion. Comparison of wave V latency after stimulation of each ear separately is of value in distinguishing cochlear from retrocochlear pathology (Fig 4.22). In cochlear lesions with loudness recruitment there is a progressive disappearance at high intensities of stimulation of the interaural difference in the latency of wave V, which may be observed consistently at low frequencies. In contrast, patients with a retrocochlear hearing loss exhibit a consistent interaural difference in the latency of wave V.

The value of interwave latency measurements, particularly the wave I–V interval, in evaluating disorders of the VIIIth nerve has been established. A

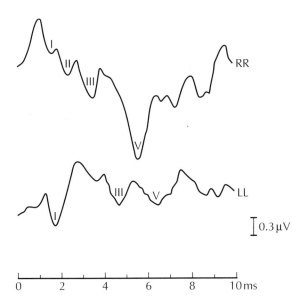

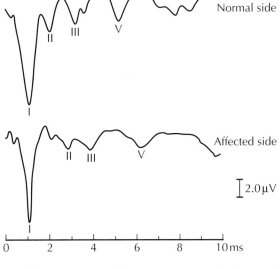

Fig 4.22 Brainstem auditory evoked potentials illustrating the interaural difference between a normal response from the right ear and an abnormal response from the left, in which there is an acoustic neuroma.

Fig 4.23 Combined brainstem auditory evoked potential and electrocochleograph showing the ease of identification of wave I and the prolonged I–V interval on the side affected by an acoustic neuroma.

major limitation has been the uncertainty involved in the detection of wave I, but this has been overcome by combining brainstem evoked potentials and electrocochleographic recordings (Fig 4.23). This combined technique greatly improves the detection rate of VIIIth nerve lesions.

MIDDLE LATENCY AUDITORY EVOKED POTENTIALS AND CORTICAL AUDITORY EVOKED POTENTIALS

The middle latency response occurs 12–50 milliseconds after the stimulus onset and is composed of a myogenic component, originating in the neck and postauricular muscles, and a neurogenic component, arising in the primary and secondary auditory cortex and possibly the upper brainstem. The precise value of middle latency auditory evoked potentials (MLAEPs) in audiological diagnosis has not been established, but the response may provide a useful objective measure of auditory thresholds.

The cortical auditory evoked potential (CAEP) refers to a series of potentials recorded between 30 and 100 milliseconds after the stimulus. The response is not well localized to one area, but may be recorded maximally at the vertex, whereas the reference electrode is usually sited on the chin or mastoid region. An important benefit is the possi-

bility of using pure tones at different frequencies, rather than click stimuli. A major disadvantage of the technique is that the response in sleep differs in many respects from the waking response, and so drowsiness or sedation interferes with the interpretation. The main application of the cortical evoked potential is in determining the threshold of hearing objectively, particularly if a non-organic hearing loss is suspected. In cooperative adults, the threshold based on this potential is usually within 10 dB of the psychoacoustic threshold, and in children within 20 dB. The CAEP can be elicited by pure tone stimuli, as well as clicks, so that a 'pure tone threshold audiogram' can be plotted.

Identification of non-organic hearing loss

Non-organic hearing loss (NOHL) implies an apparent auditory deficit that cannot be demonstrated upon full audiometric assessment. This condition is most commonly encountered in psychologically disturbed children, and in medicolegal cases of alleged hearing loss secondary to injury (e.g. industrial noise exposure, head injuries and exposure to ototoxic drugs). Regrettably, experience has shown that in every case of hearing loss that may prove financially advantageous to the patient, a non-organic component to the deficit must be excluded. The evaluation of cortical evoked potentials, which provides a non-invasive method of obtaining objective auditory thresholds, enables the clinician to define clearly the frequencies and intensities at which sounds can be perceived with minimal patient cooperation.

The diagnosis of NOHL depends primarily upon a high index of clinical suspicion, but certain audiometric inconsistencies may suggest the diagnosis.

CLINICAL ASSESSMENT

In an interview, the patient may appear to hear considerably better than would be expected from review of the audiogram. Nonetheless, the examiner must take care not to be misled by a severely, or profoundly, deaf patient who is a good lip-reader and, thus, can hold a near perfect conversation in the one-to-one situation of a medical consultation. An obvious inconsistency is revealed in a patient claiming to suffer a total unilateral hearing loss who alleges that they were unable to hear a tuning fork placed on the mastoid process of the affected ear. A patient with a genuine unilateral hearing loss would perceive the bone-conducted stimulus in the normal cochlea and report the perception of sound.

AUDIOMETRY

In patients with a fixed non-fluctuant hearing loss, repeated pure tone audiometry and speech audiometry reveal remarkably consistent results. Hence, disparate results upon repeated audiometry raise the suspicion of a non-organic component.

The *Stenger test* may be carried out using two audiometers, or a two-channel audiometer, with matched frequencies. The principle is that two tones of equal frequency and quality cannot be heard simultaneously if one is louder. A pure tone at, say, 1000 Hz is applied to the normal ear at 30 dB above normal and an identical tone is then applied to the allegedly affected ear at 60 dB above normal. If there is a genuine deafness of more than 30 dB in the affected ear, the patient will continue to perceive the sound in the normal ear. If the patient reports hearing nothing, it implies that the louder sound is perceived in the allegedly deaf ear, to which the patient is refusing to respond. The hearing threshold in the affected ear must be 29 dB or better. With genuine deafness the patient will be aware of and acknowledge the quieter sound in the good ear. An astute malingerer may be familiar with the test and report hearing sound in the good ear, despite a louder one in a normal ear alleged to be deaf. This deceit may be exposed by reducing and turning off the quieter stimulus in the acceptedly good ear. A patient truly deaf in the other will notice that the stimulus on the good side has vanished, but a malingerer will not and may continue to claim that the now absent stimulus, on the good side, is still present.

The threshold in the affected ear may be identified and may even be found to be normal by reducing the intensities of sound applied to the ears, until 5 dB is applied to the good ear and 10 dB to the 'affected' ear.

DELAYED AUDITORY FEEDBACK

The tone of the voice is normally regulated by the laryngeal–cochlear feedback system, operating both by the airborne and somatic routes. A system that allows a speaker to hear their own voice momentarily later than usual results in disturbance of the feedback system and confusion of speech results.

Part III – Otoacoustic emissions

BY DAVID T. KEMP

The existence and nature of stimulatable acoustic emissions from the human ear was first published in 1978. The term 'acoustic emission' is actually borrowed from Materials Science, in which it was well known that energy locked up in the internal stresses of a metal, for example after welding, could be released spontaneously or in response to physical excitation. The search for stimulated otoacoustic emissions (OAEs) was based on pyschoacoustical investigations of the unexplained peaks and valleys in the detailed structure of the normal audiogram, first noted by Elliot in 1958. Their orderly association with aural combination tones, subjective tonal tinnitus and other anomalies of normal hearing suggested a physical explanation. The model of these phenomena adopted at that time remains relevant today. It is that wave propagation in the cochlea is virtually loss free near threshold, and that a non-linearity at the peak of the travelling waves turns round or scatters back some of the travelling wave energy, thus returning both stimulus frequency and intermodulation signals to the middle ear. Reverse propagation of cochlear waves was unknown at that time. As with a reverberant room, in this scenario standing waves are set up within the cochlea that emphasize some frequencies and suppress others; this accounts for the microstructure of auditory threshold. In fact, the cochlea behaves more like a room with its natural acoustics enhanced by an imperfect acoustic amplification, hence the potential for spontaneous feedback howl or spontaneous otoacoustic emissions (SOAEs) and intermodulation distortion products or distortion product otoacoustic emissions (DPOAEs). These phenomena are observable because the oval window transmits internal cochlear vibrations on to the middle ear and so to the ear canal. Standing waves, SOAEs and DPOAEs recorded by an insert microphone were the first ever OAE observations and were made at the Institute of Laryngology and Otology, London in 1977. Publication proved difficult and a more compelling demonstration of the real behaviour of the cochlea was needed. This was achieved by borrowing a simple technique from Architectural acoustics. A single impulse is applied to reveal the strength and duration of reverberation and hence the 'quality factor' of the auditorium or the ear. These reverberations are called transient evoked otoacoustic emissions (TEOAEs).

The nature of OAEs – what are we looking at?

OAEs are sounds found in the external auditory meatus that originate from physiologically vital and vulnerable activity inside the cochlea. There is abundant experimental evidence that this activity is intimately associated with the hearing process. It happens that OAEs are generated only when the organ of Corti is in near normal condition and of course they can emerge (or at least can be detected) only when the middle ear system is operating normally as well. The sounds generated by the cochlea are small but potentially audible, sometimes amounting to as much as 30 dB SPL. They can emerge spontaneously, as sound already in the cochlea perpetually recirculates, but more commonly OAEs follow acoustic stimulation. No electrodes are needed to observe OAEs. They are not electrical in nature, rather they are vibratory responses. In fact, we use a microphone to detect them and then we convert them to an electrical analogue so that we can process them more easily.

The sounds – or ear canal pressure fluctuations – that we call OAEs are actually created by motion of the eardrum driven by the cochlea through the middle ear chain. Consequently, to record OAEs we need a healthy middle ear with good sound conduction. The cochlea itself does not significantly radiate sound through the air of the middle ear. At frequencies below 3 kHz the OAE vibration transmitted through the middle ear is undetectable without physically closing the ear canal during measurement. Closing the ear canal enables any oscillatory movement of the drum to compress (and rarefy) the air more efficiently, thereby creating sound. Amazingly the basilar membrane motions responsible for regular OAEs are subatomic in scale!

The need to close off the ear canal in order to maximize OAE levels reminds us that the specific sound level of an OAE is not an absolute physiological quantity, rather it is the product of the driving force within the cochlea: the conductive properties of the middle ear and the specific volume and acoustics of the air enclosed in the ear canal. If we were to keep the cochlea the same but change the fitting of the probe or the ear canal volume or the middle ear characteristics, then the OAE would change in intensity in much the same way that the recordable brainstem auditory evoked potential (BAEP) voltage changes with electrode positioning and resistance. No great clinical significance is attached to the absolute microvolt level of the BAEP and no great significance should be attached to the precise sound levels of OAEs.

A stronger OAE does nevertheless give us greater confidence that there is normal hearing in that ear, and there is a significant correlation between OAE strength and hearing threshold in a mixed population of normal and impaired ears. However, an individual's hearing threshold is only one of many factors that influence externally recordable OAE levels. Although it is certainly possible to establish norms of OAE levels under specific stimulus conditions for a population, it is not possible to translate an individual's OAE level into an audiometric threshold with any useful accuracy. Ears at the extremes of OAE levels can have a threshold of 0 dB and ears with average OAE levels can have thresholds of 20 or 30 dB. There are too many undefined sources of variance and intersubject differences in OAE levels for us to treat OAE dB SPL as a quantitative measure at present. A more physiologically meaningful measure, if it could be achieved, would be to assess the energy of the returned wave impinging on the stapes. However, even this measure would include the poorly understood and highly variable factors responsible for the return of energy from the cochlear travelling wave.

One thing that is certain is that healthy cochleas do contain a mechanism capable of returning sound to the middle ear, and significantly impaired cochleas normally do not. This makes OAEs a uniquely valuable clinical tool.

The basics of OAE technology – how are OAEs recorded?

In the most general terms an instrument for measuring OAEs consists of an acoustic ear canal probe assembly containing a loudspeaker to stimulate the ear; a microphone to record all the sounds in the ear canal and, finally, a signal-separating process that can discriminate between sounds emerging from the cochlea and other sounds, such as the stimulus and noise, so as to extract, analyse and display the uniquely cochlear sound – the OAE.

The probe must physically seal the ear canal to maximize OAE collection and also to exclude ambient noise. It must contain a sensitive microphone with low internal noise and wide bandwidth. It must also contain sound delivery transducers, one in the case of transient stimulus delivery and two in the case of two tone delivery for distortion product analysis. The latter is needed because feeding two tones in via a single transducer would introduce much more distortion than the cochlea itself produces.

Stimulation of the ear can be achieved in many ways and OAEs will always be generated. The choice of stimulation determines not only which portions of the cochlea are stimulated but also the form of processing needed for optimum OAE extraction. Cochlear biophysics teaches us that a pure tone stimulates a substantial portion of the cochlea simultaneously, not just one point as is often imagined. A pure tone stimulus is not a totally 'place-specific' stimulus. All of the cochlea up to the conventional 'frequency place' participates to some extent in advancing the travelling wave and hence participates in the detection of that tone. With two tone stimulation (as used for DPOAE measurement) an even wider portion of the cochlea is involved and, in the case of a transient stimulus, virtually the whole of the cochlea is stimulated.

Many find it difficult to accept that frequency-specific information can be obtained from OAEs elicited by non-frequency-specific stimuli such as transients. The fact is, however, that it is the cochlea that is frequency specific in its response and this frequency specificity is maintained in the case of transient or tonal stimulation. Each portion of the cochlea gives its strongest response at one specific frequency, and this applies to the OAE response. The unique feature of OAEs, which tends to confuse those more familiar with neural responses, is that the response of each portion of the cochlea can be separated from the OAE signal after it emerges from the ear by instrumental frequency analysis. In contrast, gross neurogenic electrophysiological signals cannot be retro-analysed for frequency specificity, hence the peculiar need for frequency-specific stimulation of an already frequency-specific cochlea in diagnostic BAEP work. Thanks to the cochlea and the nature of sound vibration, frequency-specific OAE recordings can be conducted with any stimulus, that is, clicks or tones. There is, of course, an operational difference between the use of wide-band (click) stimulation and narrow-band (tonal) stimulation. With tonal stimulation (e.g. DPOAE recording) only part of the cochlea is being tested at any one time, so that a series of measurements need to be made to cover the whole frequency range. With click-evoked OAEs data are collected from a substantial length of the cochlea simultaneously and the response is broken down into separate frequencies afterwards.

Once the desired stimulus is selected, the process of response extraction can be designed. This process is not trivial; many other sounds exist in the ear canal besides the stimulus and OAEs. There are those sounds entering from the outside world and those generated by motion and vibration in the head such as speech, breathing, swallowing and blood flow. So how can we be sure that a sound we record in the closed ear canal is a sound generated by the cochlea and not the stimulus or some other sound? This crucial question is at the very heart of all OAE technology and the effective use of OAEs.

The problem of response signal extraction is not unique to OAEs. The auditory brainstem response, for example, is but a small part (around 1/30th) of the total neurogenic electrical activity found on the scalp and an even smaller part of the possible myogenic and environmental interference present. Synchronous averaging and filtering can be employed to extract OAEs from noise as with BAEPs. In fact, in this OAEs have an advantage over BAEP responses. Their level (typically 10 dB SPL) is similar to the expected noise level in a good sound-treated room and with a quiet patient. It is possible to demonstrate OAEs without averaging, although with the typical patient this is never possible as the data collection time is too long. However, there is an additional problem to be overcome with OAEs. The stimulus and response are of the same nature (sound) and exist in the same place (the ear canal).

Fortunately, OAE responses can be identified and separated from the stimulus sound and the response of the middle ear system on the basis of unique properties associated with their cochlear origin. The key properties of OAEs that are used to extract them are the inherent delay of the OAE response and the non-linearity of the OAE generating mechanism. The delay of OAEs is, of course, associated with the slow cochlear travelling wave velocity, which is around 1 m/s, giving a time of 10 ms to travel 1 cm. The non-linearity is associated with the physiologically dependent nature of the mechanisms and forces encountered by the travelling wave as it engages with the hair cells of the

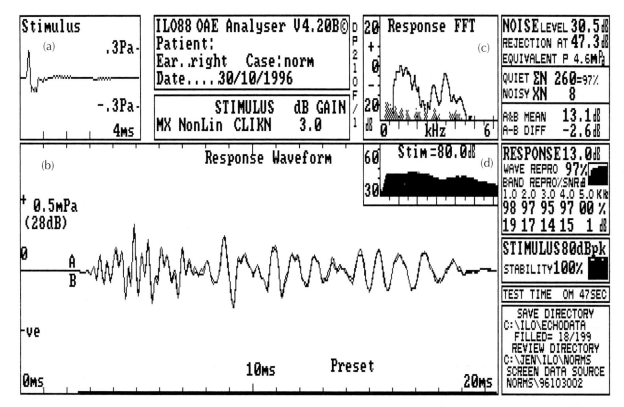

Fig 4.24 The print out from one type of oto-acoustic emission analyser, in this case the Otodynamic ILO88. The screen is rather 'busy' at first glance but the different boxes give all the information needed to make sense of this transient evoked oto-acoustic emission (TEOAE). (a) The stimulus waveform; (b) the response waveform; (c) the fast Fourier transformation of the response; and (d) the fast Fourier transformation of the stimulus. The other boxes give data relating to the stability of the system and the type of signal, in this case a non-linear click.

cochlea. Although delays and non-linearities can also be found in electro-acoustic instrumentation, these can normally be controlled to be much smaller than those found in the cochlea.

These are two major classes of OAE recording instruments. One measures the TEOAEs and the other DPOAEs, but in different ways. With tran-

sient stimulation, time-gating is very effective in separating the stimulus from the delayed OAE response. Most of the stimulus and middle ear response is over in around 3 ms and so this period is not included in the analysis (Fig 4.24). OAEs have latencies of up to 20 ms depending on the frequency considered. Nevertheless, a small component of the

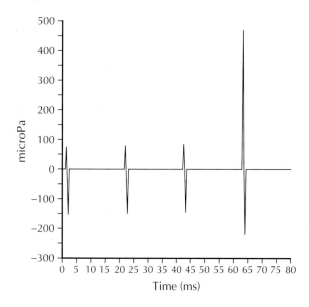

Fig 4.25 The click stimulus is represented diagrammatically. The wave forms represent the pressure changes produced by the loudspeaker in the ear canal insert. The first signal, which lasts 4 ms, has a small positive component and a larger negative component. There is then a delay of approximately 20 ms until the next stimulus, which is the same as the first. During the interstimulus interval the response occurs. The third stimulus is the same as the first and second stimuli, but the fourth stimulus is not only inverted but also three times the magnitude of the preceding signals. The use of this signal paradigm allows the extraction of non-cochlear signals by cancellation techniques that extract the non-linear cochlear output.

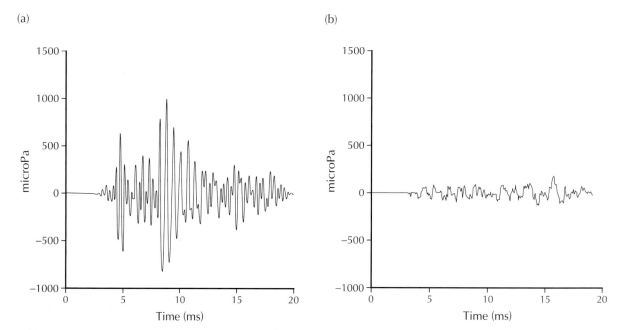

(a) (b)

Fig 4.26 (a) The response from the cochlea of a normally hearing newborn. The stimulus signal is not included and only the response is seen. This starts at about 4 ms and is over by 20 ms. (b) In this OAE recording from another neonate ear there is not obviously any clear cut response from the inner ear but a Fourier transformation, which abstracts the contributions made by various individual frequency responses of the cochlea, is necessary to confirm this. These fast Fourier transformations are shown in Figure 4.27.

probe and middle ear response spills over in the recorded post-stimulus period and can pose as a short latency OAE. It should also be noted that delayed echoes of the stimulus sound, from the walls of the test room a few feet away, would also show a latency greater than 3 ms. Fortunately, such reflections from insert probes are exceedingly small and are linear in behaviour, unlike biological responses. To protect from any acoustic artefact in TEOAE measurements the signal extracted by time-gating is further tested for genuine cochlear origin by alternating the level of stimulation (Fig 4.25). Cancellation processing can then easily eliminate any purely proportional acoustic responses or reflections leaving only the typically saturating biological response of the cochlea. In effect, regular TEOAE measuring instruments extract the distortion present in the delayed acoustic response found in the ear canal and identify this with the cochlea. In the process of non-linear extraction some genuine linear OAE response is lost, thus reducing the signal to noise ratio. To summarize, in TEOAE recording, OAE latency is the primary identifier and OAE non-linearity is the validator (Figs 4.26 and 4.27).

The other common method of OAE measurement uses the non-linearity of OAEs as the primary separator and is known as DPOAE recording. DPOAE processing is the reverse of TEOAE processing in that the non-linear response component is extracted first then tested for a cochlear origin. As with TEOAEs, the level of stimulation is varied, but with DPOAEs it is much more rapid, being many hundreds of times a second. This is achieved by applying two pure tones simultaneously, thus giving a frequency ratio that results in partial overlapping of the vibration fields in the cochlea. Stimulus level fluctuation occurs most strongly at the position in the cochlea where the two travelling waves [from stimulus frequency one (f1) and stimulus frequency two (f2)] are of equal size. The ratio of stimulus frequencies and levels determines where in the cochlea the maximum beating occurs. Cochlear travelling wave characteristics decree that for this to happen maximally at the place of reception of the higher of the two frequencies presented, the lower frequency tone must normally be stronger than the higher tone. It is not possible for the two tones to 'beat' at the place for the lower frequency tone because the higher frequency tone never reaches this place. Wherever the two tones meet, the OAE generator sees a vibration of fluctuating amplitude. Being a non-linear mechanism it fails to copy exactly the

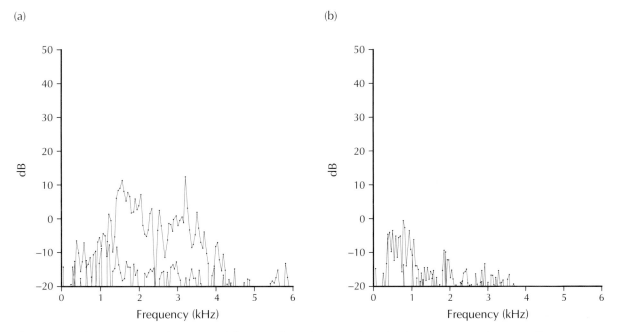

(a)   (b)

Fig 4.27 (a) The Fourier transformation of the OAE from the normal ear in Figure 4.26 (a). The upper line represents the contributions of various frequencies to the overall response. The lower line, which is shaded in the screen output shown in Figure 4.24 (c), represents the noise in the signal. There is thus a good signal to noise ratio and the response can be taken to indicate that the ear is hearing normally and that the cochlea is functioning well. (b) The Fourier transformation of the OAE from the neonate ear in Figure 4.26 (b). There is no output that is substantially different from the background noise so the hearing is suspect although the cause of the problem cannot be ascertained from this test alone.

dynamics of the waveform envelope returning an OAE signal comprised of an OAE response to each tone (the stimulus frequency emission) plus smaller OAEs at several new combination tones frequencies, including 2f1–f2, 3f1–2f2, 2f2–f1 etcetera. The new tones can be easily extracted from the ongoing stimulus tones by frequency analysis, but the stimulus frequency OAEs present are unfortunately lost in this method.

Overall, DPOAE and TEOAE techniques turn out to be rather complementary. First, they reveal cochlear status in two contrasting stimulus conditions: the one steady state, the other intermittent. TEOAEs are best at detecting threshold elevation below 3 kHz, DPOAEs are best above 3 kHz. TEOAEs are maybe a little too sensitive to the condition of the cochlea in adults whereas DPOAEs are perhaps a little too insensitive. TEOAEs present an averaged overview of cochlear activity. Distortion products are a 'snap shot' specific to one set of stimulus variables. TEOAEs provide a view of cochlear activity to light stimulation, DPOAEs can be obtained at moderate and (with care) higher levels of stimulation. Clearly a combination and comparison of the two seems ideal.

Suggested reading

Anonymous. Recommended procedures for pure-tone audiometry using a manually operated instrument. *Journal of Laryngology & Otology* 1981; **95**:757–61.

Anonymous. Recommended procedure for pure-tone bone-conduction audiometry without masking using a manually operated instrument. British Society of Audiology – technical note. *British Journal of Audiology* 1985; **19**:281–2.

Anonymous. Recommendations for masking in pure tone threshold audiometry. British Society of Audiology. *British Journal of Audiology* 1986; **20**:307–14.

Anonymous. Guidelines for screening for hearing impairment and middle-ear disorders. Working Group on Acoustic Immittance Measurements and the Committee on Audiologic Evaluation. American Speech-Language-Hearing Association. *ASHA* 1990; **32(suppl 2)**:17–24.

Browning GG, Gatehouse S, Swan IR. The Glasgow Benefit Plot: a new method for reporting benefits from middle ear surgery. *Laryngoscope* 1991; **101**:180–5.

Fearn RW, Hanson DR. Audiometric zero for air conduction using manual audiometry. *British Journal of Audiology* 1983; **17**:87–9.

CHAPTER 5

Vestibular investigations

CLIODNA F OMAHONEY AND ROSALYN A DAVIES

Introduction

In humans, balance is maintained by the integration within the central nervous system (CNS) of information from the vestibular labyrinths, the eyes and the proprioceptive systems. Damage to any of these three systems, or to the ability to integrate the information, may lead to dysequilibrium. Although this chapter is mainly confined to investigation of the vestibular system, it must be emphasized that a systematic approach to the assessment of 'dizziness' must include evaluation of each of these three peripheral systems and of the 'central processing unit' itself.

Furthermore, an understanding of the functions of the integrated systems that maintain balance and visual stability is necessary in order to understand the relevance of vestibular tests and to interpret the results. The roles of the balance system include

- the maintenance of gaze stability during head movements. This is achieved by the vestibulo-ocular reflex (VOR), which is the eye movement response to movements of the head, detected by the labyrinth and transmitted to the extra-ocular muscles
- the maintenance of visual fixation on a moving object in the absence of head movement. The movement of an image across the retina results in compensatory eye movements, which, in turn, keep that image fixed on the fovea. This is the optokinetic reflex, which can be separated into the response to slowly moving objects that remain within the visual field, when the term 'smooth pursuit' is used, and the response to objects that move out of the visual field when a restorative movement of the eyes (i.e. a

'saccade') returns them to a central position; this is optokinetic nystagmus (OKN)
- the preservation of appropriate muscle tone to avoid falling when the environment is moving and the maintenance of posture during head or eye movement. These responses are mediated by the vestibulospinal pathways.

The contribution of the vestibular system to gaze stability via the VOR is relatively well understood and forms the basis of many of the tests of vestibular function (caloric and rotation tests, see below). Smooth pursuit and optokinetic responses (OKN) are assessed by the use of visual stimuli moving across the visual field. The role of posturography in providing information about the relative contribution of the vestibulospinal connections is being reassessed.

The control of eye movements

NYSTAGMUS

The anatomy and physiology of the vestibular system is discussed in detail in Chapters 1 and 2. In the horizontal semicircular canals the kinocilia on the hair cells are orientated on the ampullary side of the cristae, thus ampullopetal movement of the endolymph and consequently of the stereocilia, increases the spontaneous impulse rate, and ampullofugal flow decreases it. However, the strength of the response to ampullopetal stimulation is greater than that to ampullofugal stimulation. The cristae of the semicircular canals are connected, via the vestibular reflex arc, to the appropriate eye muscles so as to bring about eye movement in the plane of stimulation of that canal (Ewald's law[1]); the direction of eye movement is opposite to that of the head movement, so preserving gaze stability.

Each individual semicircular canal can respond to rotation in either direction in the plane of the canal, that is, for the right lateral canal, horizontal rotation of the head to the right causes ampullopetal stimulation (increasing the spontaneous firing rate), whereas rotation to the left causes ampullofugal stimulation, so decreasing its spontaneous firing rate. The response to ampullopetal stimulation is, as mentioned above, stronger than that to ampullofugal stimulation. Thus the loss of function of either canal of any of the pairs will lead to an imbalance of the response, which will give rise to abnormalities of eye movement called nystagmus, which persist until compensation occurs. Nystagmus is defined and described below.

The above description of the VOR is, however, an oversimplification. Many other influences from the cerebellum, brainstem, cortex et cetera may modify it. For example, in normal subjects the VOR can be totally suppressed by asking the subject to fixate on a target that is moving in time with their head. By this means, visually generated impulses in the CNS inhibit the VOR via the pursuit pathways and override the movement induced by the vestibular system. This, in essence, is optic fixation and implies the ability of the visual system to override labyrinthine information provided the central pathways are normal.

An abnormal VOR may arise from either labyrinthine (peripheral) or central pathology, that is, unilateral hypofunction of the VOR suggests peripheral pathology, but an increased gain of the VOR implies central pathology.[2] The separate assessment of eye movement not generated by the vestibular system but by visually induced ocular stabilizing mechanisms in the CNS including the optokinetic system, will help to elucidate the site of the lesion, and to differentiate between peripheral and central pathology.

Testing the balance system is, as you might have guessed, almost like trying to assess a can of worms. Touch one and the whole collection moves. The tests of balance try to dissect out the particular contributions of labyrinthine, visual, proprioceptive and central functions to the overall problem. The simplest way to do this is to monitor eye movements in response to a series of stimuli and then deduce whether there is a problem and where it might be located. We hope that it is also clear from this introduction that vestibular testing is unlikely to diagnose the specific cause of a problem but may contribute significantly to siting the lesion.

The cornerstone of balance tests is the observation of nystagmus. 'A rhythmic, oscillating, involuntary and conjugate movement of the eyes' is a working definition of nystagmus suitable for a practising otorhinolaryngologist. This is commonly seen as a slow drift of the eyes in one direction followed by a fast flicking movement in the opposite direction (jerk nystagmus). The slow phase is the vestibular or visually induced component of the movement whereas the quick flick – a saccadic movement – is a centrally generated movement to restore eye position. Paradoxically the direction of the nystagmus is named in relation to the direction of the fast, saccadic phase (see also Chapter 3). Nystagmus is derived from the Greek word meaning tired or sleepy and relates to the nodding head movements of someone about to fall asleep as they read a particularly tedious chapter on nystagmus. From our point of view, this description is adequate, although it must be admitted that there are some neurological manifestations of nystagmus that do not quite fit this definition.

Nystagmus can be horizontal, rotatory or, more uncommonly, vertical. Nystagmus can be physiological; it can induced by an unphysiological stimulus such as the caloric test or by specific manoeuvres in the presence of disease or it can be the result of disease, when it is often spontaneous.

Physiological nystagmus

Physiological nystagmus can be seen by looking at the eyes of someone who is staring out of the windows of a railway carriage as it is passing by a line of telegraph poles. The eyes drift slowly to one side (depending on the speed of the train) then flick back rapidly in the horizontal plane to somewhere near the central position. What happens is that vision is fixed first on one of the poles and lateral movement of the eyes keeps this image steady until the eyes reach the limit of their movement when a quick flick – the saccade – returns them more or less to the centre and the eyes fix on the next pole. During the saccade, vision is suppressed so that a blurred image is not seen. This form of physiological nystagmus is not a product of the labyrinthine system but is one form of OKN.

Induced nystagmus

As well as arising spontaneously, nystagmus can be induced by several test procedures. These tests are described below. One particular form of induced nystagmus, the positional nystagmus of benign positional paroxysmal vertigo (BPPV), is described and depicted in Chapter 14.

Spontaneous nystagmus

Spontaneous nystagmus nearly always indicates disease when properly observed (see Chapter 3) as there are only a very few individuals who can produce nystagmoid eye movements at will. The patient is asked to look at the examiner's finger, which is held in front of the patient's face beyond the focal point so that it can be clearly seen. The patient is then asked to follow the finger as it is moved from side to side. The finger must not be moved so that the edge of the iris passes the angle at the corner of the eyes as there may be a slight physiological nystagmus at the extremes of gaze. Has any horizontal or rotatory nystagmus been seen? If it has, is the direction of the fast phase the same in each direction of eye movement, that is, does it flick in the same direction on looking both to the left and to the right or does the direction change (likely to be central)? Are both eyes doing exactly the same thing or are their movements dissociated, that is, dysconjugate. Is the nystagmus only present when the patient is looking in the direction of the fast phase – when it is called first degree – or when looking straight ahead – second degree – or when looking in the direction opposite to the fast phase, that is, in the direction of the slow phase – third degree (see Chapter 3).

The same manoeuvres and observations need to be made in the vertical plane, moving the eyes up and down.

The differentiation between peripheral and central disease can often be made by simple observation of the features of any spontaneous nystagmus. The features that distinguish central from peripheral disease are described in Chapter 3.

Spontaneous nystagmus is not always present despite an underlying defect, and it is often the case that damage to the balance system can only be detected by some form of test procedure that results in the production of eye movements. Thus, some system of recording eye movements is extremely helpful as it allows analysis of the variables associated with these movements and the production of a permanent record.

Recording eye movements – principles of electronystagmography

A potential difference exists between the retina and the cornea, the retina being negative with respect to the cornea. An electrode placed near the eye will become more positive when the eye rotates towards it, that is, when the cornea moves closer to it, and negative when the eye rotates away from the electrode (Fig 5.1). Usually, recording of these eye movements using electronystagmography (ENG) is carried out using three electrodes: two active and a ground electrode. The most common method of recording used clinically involves placing an active electrode on each outer canthus (to record conjugate horizontal eye movements) and the ground electrode at some remote point such as the vertex. Thus deviation of the eyes in the horizontal plane will cause a potential difference between the two active electrodes that is proportional to the magnitude of eye movement. This voltage difference activates a pen-recording system on paper moving at a predetermined rate and provides a tracing of the

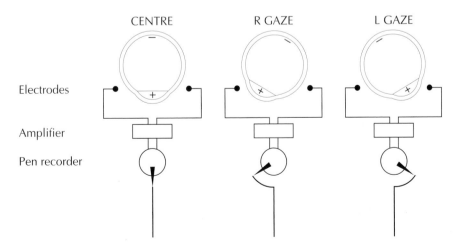

Fig 5.1 Corneoretinal potential. The electrode lateral to the eye becomes more positive when the eye rotates towards it, and more negative when the eye rotates away. The voltage change represents the change in eye position. (Adapted from Baloh and Honrubia[3] with permission.)

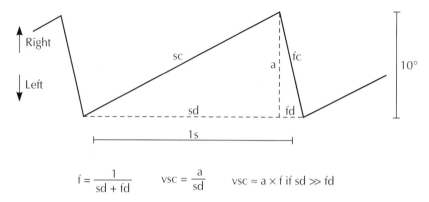

$$f = \frac{1}{sd + fd} \qquad vsc = \frac{a}{sd} \qquad vsc \approx a \times f \text{ if } sd \gg fd$$

Fig 5.2 Single nystagmic beat recorded with ENG, showing how the slow phase velocity (vsc, velocity of the slow component) is calculated. a, amplitude; f, frequency; fc, fast component; fd, fast duration; sc, slow component; sd, slow duration. (Reproduced from Baloh and Honrubia[3] with permission.)

eye movement. By convention the pen moves upwards with movements of the eye to the right and downwards for movements to the left. Alternative placements of the electrodes, such as on the medial and lateral canthus of each eye, or above and below the eye, and the use of a multichannel ENG machine will record horizontal movements of each eye individually or vertical movements, respectively, and so allow detection of dysconjugate eye movements and vertical nystagmus.

Figure 5.2 shows a recording of a beat of nystagmus (to the left). If one knows the speed of the paper (x axis), typically chosen to be 10 mm/s, and one has calibrated the pen recorder so that a known amplitude of upward or downward deflection corresponds to a known angle of eye movement away from the centre (y axis), one can calculate variables such as the velocity of the slow phase of nystagmus, frequency and duration of nystagmus.

In addition to nystagmus, ENG can be used to record any other eye movement such as saccades, smooth pursuit and OKN.

A laser-generated light that remains the same size regardless of the distance from the subject is used as the target when the subject's ability to perform saccades or track a small object is being evaluated, or when the patient's eye movements while they attempt to maintain their gaze in the midline, or to the right or the left, are assessed.

Although expensive, ENG is a means of obtaining an accurate, quantifiable and permanent record of eye movements, both spontaneous and in response to visual and vestibular stimuli. With clinical examination, the direction and duration of the nystagmus are the only variables easily assessed but with the use of ENG variables such as the slow phase velocity, frequency and duration can be evaluated. Some specific forms of nystagmus, such as rebound nystagmus, are more easily recognized using ENG. On the other hand, low amplitude nystagmus, such as that often seen in spontaneous nystagmus, may be detected clinically but be missed on ENG. In addition, vertical nystagmus is difficult to measure using ENG because electrical activity from the eye lids will be in the same plane as the corneoretinal potentials and thus the observed potential change will include elements of both.

Greater detail on the technical aspects of ENG recording, importance of correct electrode placement, the differences between AC and DC recording, et cetera is beyond the scope of this book and the reader is referred to Baloh and Honrubia.[3]

Other systems of detecting eye movements use infrared and electromagnetic and video recording techniques. However, these are not widely available and will not be further discussed. Advances in computer technology have led to the replacement of rolls of recording paper by storage on magnetic media and observation of the eye movements on a television monitor. The principles, however, remain the same.

Vestibular tests

Initial assessment of balance disorders – as with all symptoms – comprises history and clinical examination. This chapter concentrates on the principles, application and interpretation of vestibular investigations. The aims of vestibular testing are to assess whether there is vestibular disease to account for the patient's complaints; to ascertain whether the lesion is peripheral (labyrinthine or VIIIth nerve, or both) or in the CNS (e.g. brainstem, cerebellum, basal ganglia or cortex); and to establish the side of the lesion. However, abnormalities discovered during vestibular testing, although they will site the lesion if one exists, will not directly establish the aetiology of that lesion; but, the pattern of abnormality taken in conjunction with the history and clinical examination will often suggest a specific aetiology.

CALORIC TEST

The cornerstone of vestibular testing is the caloric test, first described in 1906 by Bárány.[4]

Procedure

A widely accepted method of performing the caloric test is that described by Fitzgerald and Hallpike.[5] Testing is carried out with the patient supine with their head elevated to 30° (Fig 5.3). This brings the horizontal semicircular canal into the vertical plane. Each ear is then irrigated with cool and then with warm water. It is thought that the decrease and increase in temperature causes changes in the specific gravity of the endolymph in that part of the canal nearest to the middle ear and thus induces convection currents in the endolymph (in opposite directions for the cool and warm irrigations) thereby stimulating the hair cells of the crista (Fig 5.4); other

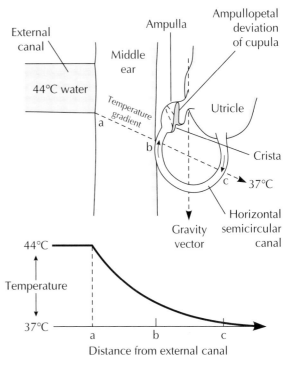

Fig 5.4 The mechanism of stimulation of the horizontal canal during caloric testing, showing the temperature gradient across the canal and the ensuing convection current and endolymph flow. (Reproduced from Baloh and Honrubia[3] with permission.)

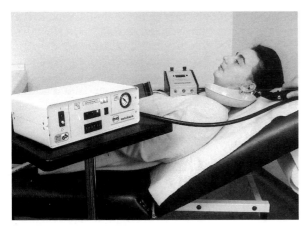

Fig 5.3 Patient undergoing caloric testing. The patient's head is inclined at 30° to bring the horizontal canals into the vertical plane. (Reproduced from Davies and Savundra[6] with permission.)

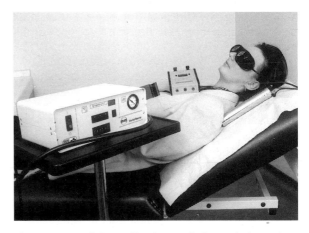

Fig 5.5 Use of Frenzel's glasses during caloric testing. The effect of removing optic fixation on the end-point of nystagmus duration can be observed in a darkened room using Frenzel's glasses once nystagmus has disappeared with optic fixation. (Reproduced from Davies and Savundra[6] with permission.)

possibilities such as direct thermal stimulation of the afferent nerve have been suggested. After the inspection to exclude aural pathology, each ear is irrigated for 40 seconds with water, first at 30°C and then at 44°C, and the response observed. Ideally, a gap of at least 5 minutes should be left between each irrigation and the tympanic membrane inspected for presence of a red flush after warm irrigation. In many centres the test has been modified so that for each irrigation the effect of optic fixation is evaluated. If direct observation of the nystagmus is being made, then the duration of response is measured from the start of irrigation until the nystagmic response ends while the patient is fixating (in the light). When the nystagmus ceases, Frenzel's glasses are applied (Fig 5.5) and the the time taken for the nystagmus to re-emerge is noted. Figure 5.6 shows the recording of a normal response for which the duration of nystagmus was the variable assessed. If the maximum slow phase velocity is being used as the measure of assessment, then soon after what seems to be the most active period of nystagmus as shown on the recording paper, computer screen or other device, the lights are switched off or Frenzel's glasses applied so that the response in the absence of fixation can be measured. The calculation of the optic fixation index is given below.

If no response is detected to the above standard irrigations at 44°C and 30°C on one or both sides, the affected ear(s) should then be irrigated with water at 20°C, to see whether a response can be detected with this stronger stimulus.

Response assessment

Variables such as the duration of the evoked nystagmus (either by direct observation or using the ENG recording technique described above), or the maximum velocity of the slow component of the nystagmus (i.e. the vestibularly induced component), the frequency of nystagmic beats or the subjective response of the patient, are used to quantify the 'response'. Use of each variable has advantages and disadvantages. For a detailed discussion of response assessment see Luxon.[7]

Interpretation of results

Several aspects of the caloric test are important to appreciate the significance of test results

Before the formal evaluation of the caloric responses, any spontaneous nystagmus must have been recognized and assessed. This assessment should be made before any test procedure other than calibration is performed. If the maximum slow phase velocity is used to assess the caloric responses, then the value of this measure should be

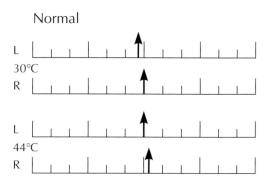

Fig 5.6 Graphic record of a set of normal responses (using duration as the response variable) to caloric irrigations as described in the text. Each tall bar on the horizontal line indicates a period of 1 minute and the shorter bar an interval of 20 seconds. The arrows indicate the duration of the response in each ear at either temperature.

derived from any spontaneous nystagmus and added to or subtracted from the caloric results, depending on the direction of the induced nystagmus, for any calculations.

Stimulation of the horizontal semicircular canals as a result of temperature changes induces nystagmus via the connection in the brainstem between the vestibular afferent nerve fibres and the nerves supplying the ocular muscles (VOR) in the same way as fluid movement caused by angular head acceleration is the normal physiological trigger of the VOR. The response should be symmetrical when both horizontal semicircular canals are intact.

Increase in temperature above body temperature causes nystagmus in one direction whereas a lower than body temperature leads to nystagmus in the opposite direction. (Note 'direction' of nystagmus, by convention, refers to the direction of the fast phase). The mnemonic *COWS* is helpful – **c**old irrigation gives nystagmus to the **o**pposite side and **w**arm irrigation gives nystagmus to the **s**ame side as the irrigation. An alternative is *ACTH* – **a**way **c**old – **t**owards **h**ot.

Irrigation of each ear individually, first with cool water (or air) and then with warm, gives the most accurate information. Irrigation at only one temperature, sometimes advocated as a 'screening' or 'shortened' test, can be misleading as it may fail to detect a combination of a directional preponderance and a canal paresis (see below). Nonetheless, if a poor response is anticipated and if the patient is unlikely to tolerate all four irrigations, a hot water only test is likely to give most information.

The most common abnormalities found are canal paresis, directional preponderance, or a combination of the two.

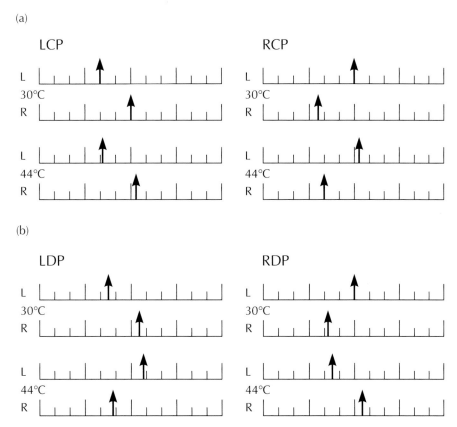

Fig 5.7 (a) Caloric response showing a left and right canal paresis (CP), whereby stimulating one ear with either hot or cold water elicits a weaker response (i.e. shorter duration nystagmus) than the same stimulus applied to the other ear. (b) Directional preponderance (DP), that is, the stimuli that cause a nystagmus beating in one direction elicit a stronger response than those that cause nystagmus beating in the other.

Unilateral canal paresis denotes that the response of one side to hot and cold stimuli is reduced or absent compared with the opposite side (Fig 5.7). Such a finding almost always implies a lesion of the peripheral vestibular system, more specifically of the horizontal canal or vestibular nerve on that side, that is, peripheral vestibular pathology. Exceptions to this include patients with lesions at the vestibular nerve root entry zone of the brainstem, for example multiple sclerosis or lateral brainstem infarction, in which there is central vestibular pathology and also a canal paresis.

A directional preponderance implies that the nystagmus evoked in one direction is 'stronger' than that evoked in the opposite direction. Remembering the COWS mnemonic, irrigation of the left ear, for example with cool water, will give rise to right-beating nystagmus, as does irrigation of the right ear with warm water. If these two irrigations evoke a stronger response than irrigation of the left

with warm and the right with cool (both of which give rise to left-beating nystagmus), then a right directional preponderance is said to exist (Fig 5.7). Similarly, a greater response to irrigation of the left ear with warm water and the right ear with cool water implies a left directional preponderance.

Unlike a canal paresis, which implies the presence of vestibular pathology (usually peripheral, see above) and the side of this pathology, a directional preponderance suggests pathology but is usually non-localizing. It may occur with peripheral vestibular disorders (either end organ or VIIIth nerve) or central disorders anywhere from the cortex to the brainstem or cerebellum (i.e. involving the central vestibular connections). With peripheral lesions, directional preponderance is usually directed away from the diseased ear, and in that instance has localizing value.

Any combination of canal paresis and directional preponderance may also be seen (Fig. 5.8).

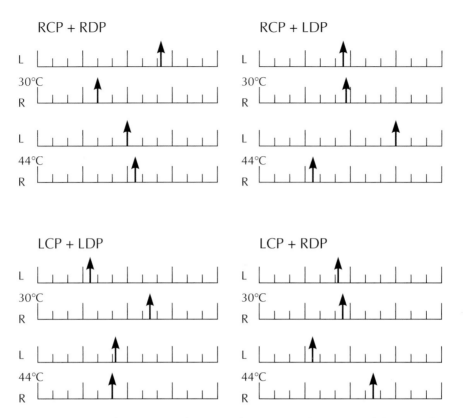

Fig 5.8 Caloric response showing a combination of various canal pareses and directional preponderances.

The degree of canal paresis and directional preponderance can be calculated as a percentage by the following formulae (a negative result implies a left canal paresis or directional preponderance and a positive result a right canal paresis or directional preponderance):[8]

Canal paresis (%)

$$\frac{(L30 + L44) - (R30 + R44)}{L30 + L44 + R30 + R44}$$

Directional preponderance (%)

$$\frac{(L30 + R44) - (R30 + L44)}{L30 + R44 + R30 + L44}$$

where the values are the duration of the response in seconds or degrees per second for each irrigation when the response variable is duration of nystagmus or maximum slow phase velocity, respectively.

Canal pareses and directional preponderances in the region of 20–25 per cent or more are usually deemed significant, but each centre needs to establish its own normative data, depending on the type of response measured. The variance of canal paresis is always much less than that of directional preponderance; so canal paresis is a more useful and significant abnormality than directional preponderance.

Bilateral symmetrically increased or decreased caloric responses are difficult to detect because of the wide range of normal values. Assuming there is no reason to suspect impaired temperature transfer (e.g. bilateral middle ear effusions), response duration of less than 90 seconds without optic fixation, even if symmetrical, is suggestive of bilateral depressed peripheral vestibular function, and clearly the absence of any response to standard irrigations or to irrigation at 20°C implies bilateral vestibular hypofunction. Serial measurements on a individual will help to detect early bilateral vestibular hypofunction, and as such may be a useful means of monitoring the effects of ototoxic drug treatment.

Bilateral increased responses can result from lesions of the cerebellum; these are thought to be caused by loss of the normal inhibitory influence that the cerebellum exerts on the vestibular nuclei.

When the caloric test is carried out with and without optic fixation, the re-emergence of nystagmus when fixation is abolished (e.g. in darkness or with Frenzel's glasses) implies that the patient was suppressing the nystagmus when allowed to fixate. An inability to suppress the nystagmus during fixation suggests impaired central, visually generated pursuit movement pathways and thus central nervous system dysfunction, particularly brainstem or cerebellar.

$$\text{Fixation index} = \frac{\text{Maximum slow phase velocity without fixation}}{\text{Maximum slow phase velocity with fixation}}$$

Above is an example of one of the many formulae for calculating the optic fixation index. This index will be normal (i.e. greater than one) in those with no pathology or a peripheral vestibular disorder but abnormal (i.e. a value of one) in patients with central nervous system lesions.

In patients with perforations of the tympanic membrane, in whom irrigation with water is contraindicated, bithermal air caloric testing under controlled pressure conditions can be carried out. The variability of the results obtained using the air caloric technique is greater than that with water caloric tests, but the principles of interpretation are the same.

The reader is referred to Luxon[7] for further information on the applications and assessment of the caloric test.

ROTATION TESTS

Rotation testing, as the name suggests, involves stimulating the vestibular system by rotating the subject in the horizontal plane and observing the eye movement response that occurs as a result of stimulation of the VOR; the response is proportional to the stimulus.[9]

Although valuable information can be obtained simply by observing the nystagmic response to rotation in an office swivel chair in the clinic, the advent of ENG and sophisticated computer-driven rotating chairs means that a very consistent and accurate rotatory stimulus can be delivered and the resultant response analysed in detail.

In specialist centres rotational tests are carried out using such motorized rotational chairs. Two types of rotational stimuli – sinusoidal and impulsive – are the most common used in clinical practice. Sinusoidal rotation involves oscillation to the right, followed by oscillation to the left at a given frequency, peak velocity and angle of displacement. The peak slow phase velocity of the generated nystagmus is compared with the peak slow phase velocity of the chair, and the gain is calculated. In

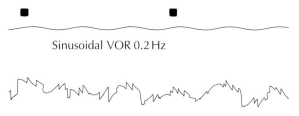

Fig 5.9 Nystagmus generated by the VOR in response to sinusoidal rotation, showing the change in direction of the nystagmus with change in direction of rotation.

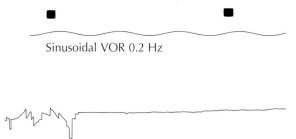

Fig 5.10 VOR suppression. Abolition of nystagmus with optic fixation while sinusoidal rotation continues.

addition, the symmetry of the responses to right and left rotation can be assessed and the presence of a directional preponderance, with the same implications as discussed under the caloric test, ascertained (Fig 5.9). In patients in whom vestibular responses are absent at one frequency, rotation can be repeated at several frequencies to establish the 'threshold' of response and to detect any residual function.

Suppression of induced nystagmus can also be tested by asking the subject to fix on a target that is moving in unison with the chair. The ability to override the VOR and suppress nystagmus (using pursuit pathways, see below) is a function of the CNS (Fig 5.10).

Impulsive rotation involves a single rotation to one side followed by the same rotatory stimulus in the opposite direction. These two rotations each include two stimuli, that is, an initial acceleration followed by deceleration, once the induced nystagmus subsides. The rate of change of velocity (angular acceleration) is very rapid, and is a powerful though brief stimulus to the semicircular canals. Comparison of the response (e.g. using variables such as the duration of nystagmus or slow phase velocity) in each direction determines the presence of a directional preponderance.

Procedure

The patient sits in the rotational chair and is connected to an electro-oculograph recording instrument, usually with three electrodes, two active (bitemporal) and one ground (see above). Rotational testing is generally carried out in conjunction with assessment of the integrity of visually induced eye movements – smooth pursuit, saccades and OKN and the presence of pathologic nystagmus (see below) – as the same eye movement recording techniques are used. Several oscillations of sinusoidal rotation are carried out, initially in the dark, to observe the gain and symmetry of the induced nystagmus. Then, in the light, the effect of fixation is recorded by asking the patient to fix on a target sited approximately 30 cm directly in front of the patient's eyes and moving with the chair. After sinusoidal rotation, impulsive rotation may be carried out, and once more the gain and symmetry of the response recorded and analysed. Throughout testing the patient must be kept alert as drowsiness affects the nystagmic response and the ability to suppress it.

Interpretation

Abnormalities of the vestibulo-ocular response to rotation may arise from pathology affecting the peripheral vestibular system or its central connections. Asymmetry (as discussed above) of the response will occur in unilateral peripheral lesions in the acute stage, although this asymmetry decreases with time as compensation occurs.

Although there is a range of 'normal' responses to rotational stimuli, the variance is less than that seen in the caloric test. This, in conjunction with the fact that rotational tests assess both horizontal canals simultaneously, means that bilateral peripheral lesions will be detected earlier. Also, the ability to give graded stimuli (e.g. different frequencies of sinusoidal rotation) allows vestibular function to be assessed in greater depth. Patients showing no response at one frequency of stimulation may show response at a different frequency, thus suggesting some residual function, which will have important implications for their rehabilitation.

Central vestibular dysfunction may lead to similar changes (altered gain and asymmetry) to those described for peripheral lesions, in addition to other abnormalities. The gain may be increased in patients with cerebellar lesions or the whole pattern of nystagmus may become disorganized (dysrhythmic nystagmus). Absence of nystagmus may result from an inability to generate the fast component of the nystagmus (saccade) because of CNS dysfunction. As the slow component, generated by the vestibular system remains intact, a 'to and fro' tonic deviation of the eyes occurs. Probably the easiest feature to detect on glancing at an ENG tracing is the inability to suppress nystagmus during sinusoidal rotation (Fig 5.10). Assuming the patient was kept alert and correctly instructed, such an abnormality suggests impairment in the pursuit pathways resulting from CNS dysfunction.

STRENGTHS AND LIMITATIONS OF CALORIC AND ROTATION TESTS

Rotation tests and the caloric tests are, by different methods, assessing the same aspect of vestibular system function, that is, the VOR. It must be remembered that in both tests only the horizontal semicircular canal input to the VOR is being assessed, so pathology in the other canals or otolith organs may be overlooked.

Unlike rotation tests, the stimulus in the caloric test has been criticized on the grounds that it is not a physiological stimulus and thus the results may not be valid physiologically. In addition, the caloric test is often less well tolerated by patients than are rotation tests.

Each labyrinth is assessed separately by the caloric test but simultaneously with rotation testing. Although the former is an advantage to detect unilateral, particularly long-standing lesions for which compensation has occurred (and asymmetry on rotation testing may have resolved), the testing of each canal separately in conjunction with the wider intersubject variation of results in normal people makes the caloric test less suited, and rotation tests more suited, to detect bilateral peripheral vestibular dysfunction, particularly in the early stages.

With modern rotational chairs the accuracy of the rotational stimulus is easier to control. It does not depend on the symmetry of ear canals, the thickness of the temporal bone, the absence of middle ear disease, et cetera. Clearly, however, this equipment, the laboratory to house it and the expertise of the personnel needed to operate it is more expensive and less widely available than caloric testing. In skilful hands the caloric test gives reliable and reproducible results.

As caloric tests and rotational tests have different strengths and limitations, they should be thought of as complementary rather than mutually exclusive tests. It is known that the vestibular stimulation brought about by the caloric test is akin to a lower frequency of stimulation (i.e. 0.04 Hz) than standard rotation tests, so although both are testing the VOR, they are testing different aspects of it. As noted above for testing different frequencies of sinusoidal rotation, a lack of response to the caloric test may not necessarily imply a total absence of vestibular function. Responses may be seen at the frequencies of stimulation assessed in the rotational tests and have implications for rehabilitation.

AUTOROTATION TEST

The autorotation test, described by O'Leary and Davis[10] provides an alternative approach to VOR testing. The caloric and rotation tests stimulate the vestibular system at relatively low frequencies (0.01–0.5 Hz), but the autorotation test provides stimuli at frequencies of the order of 0.2–6 Hz, more akin to the frequencies of natural stimulation during walking, running, et cetera. Above approximately 2 Hz the smooth pursuit system is ineffective at maintaining gaze stability, thus the vestibular system is tested in isolation by this method. Vertical and horizontal canal function can be assessed, and the total time taken for the test is only a matter of minutes. The subject is asked to oscillate their head up and down (to test the vertical canals) or side to side (to test the horizontal canals) at frequencies of between 0.2 and 6 Hz. These oscillations are detected by a sensor attached to a head strap. The resultant nystagmus is detected by the ENG technique described above. Abnormalities have been detected in patients with vertigo, even when caloric and conventional rotational tests were normal.

Visually induced eye movements

As well as eye movements controlled by the labyrinth, three kinds of eye movements are controlled by the visual system interacting with the CNS:

- smooth pursuit (slow optokinetic responses without nystagmus)
- optokinetic nystagmus (OKN)
- saccades

The object of each of these systems is to maintain gaze stability in a variety of situations, as outlined below. Normal smooth pursuit, saccades and OKN depend on the integrity of the visual pathways and the CNS connections to the VOR.

Thus, in order to ascertain whether pathologic eye movements are due to peripheral vestibular (labyrinth or VIIIth nerve) or central pathology, assessment of each of these three systems in isolation as well as of the VOR makes it possible to tease out the site of lesion causing the abnormal eye movement and hence the dizziness/balance disorder.

SMOOTH PURSUIT (TRACKING EYE MOVEMENTS)

The smooth pursuit system allows gaze to be maintained on a moving target and the image of that target to be kept on the fovea, assuming the velocity and frequency of the target remains within certain limits. The pursuit pathways include the cortex, brainstem and cerebellum and also depend on adequate foveal vision. Smooth pursuit is usually tested by asking the patient to track a target moving sinusoidally (Fig 5.11). Eye velocity and target velocity should be the same, that is, the gain of the smooth pursuit system should be 1 with sinusoidal rotation at frequencies of 0.1–0.3 Hz (depending on age) and target velocities of 30°/s. If the frequency or velocity of the target is too great, the eyes will be unable to follow the target smoothly and several 'catch up' saccades will be interspersed; this type of pursuit is said to be 'broken'. Similarly, intrusion saccades will occur at normal frequencies and velocities in patients with CNS disease.

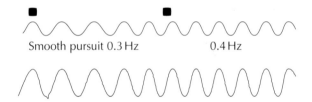

Smooth pursuit 0.3 Hz   0.4 Hz

Fig 5.11 Normal smooth pursuit. The upper tracing shows the sinusoidal movement of the target. The lower tracing shows the patient 'tracking' the target.

OPTOKINETIC NYSTAGMUS

OKN is thought to be a cruder system of tracking moving objects, which keeps the image on the whole retina, rather than specifically on the foveal region (as in the smooth pursuit system). Stimulation of the optokinetic system leads to a slow tracking eye movement followed by a saccade in the opposite direction (Fig 5.12). In normal subjects, OKN is seen when targets are tracked across a structured background, for example, the familiar jerking eye movements seen when a subject is looking at the landscape from a moving vehicle. The nystagmus, that is the fast phase, is in the opposite direction to that of the target.

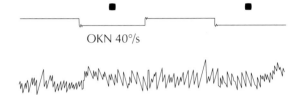

Fig 5.12 Normal optokinetic nystagmus. The upper trace indicates change in OKN target direction i.e. right = up, left = down. The speed of the rotating visual surround is 40°/s. The lower tracing is taken from a normal subject.

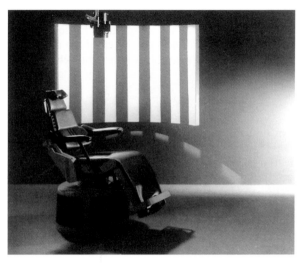

Fig 5.14 Full field OKN. The patient is seated in front of a moving field of parallel bars. The stripes are rotated to right and left, reversing direction every 9 seconds. (Reproduced with permission of Jaeger Toennies, Wurzberg, Germany.)

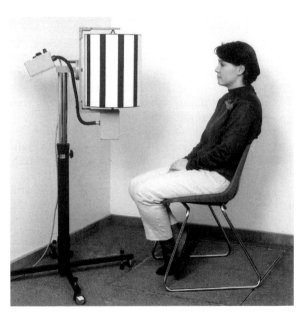

Fig 5.13 Mechanically driven OKN drum. The patient is seated 30 cm from a mechanically driven OKN drum that can be rotated either through a vertical or a horizontal axis. The tester stands behind the drum to observe the patient's nystagmic response. (Reproduced from Davies and Savundra[6] with permission.)

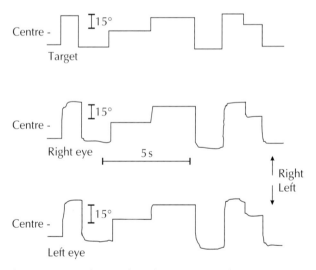

Fig 5.15 Normal saccades. The top tracing shows a target moving rapidly 15° to the right and left. The bottom two tracings show the right and left eyes following the target accurately.

It is thought that there are two main pathways subserving the optokinetic system, one depending on foveal vision, the cerebral cortex and overlapping with much of the pursuit pathways (active OKN), and the second subcortical pathway separate from the pursuit system and depending on an intact brainstem (passive OKN). The former is stimulated by a small striped drum (foveal vision) as well as a full field target (Figs 5.13 and 5.14), whereas the latter occurs only with full field optokinetic stimulation.

Up to a target velocity of 60°/s, the slow phase velocity of the active OKN should match that of the target, that is, a gain of 1. The direction of the nystagmus reverses with reversal in target direction, and should be symmetrical. For further details see Yee *et al.*[11]

SACCADES (FAST EYE MOVEMENTS)

Saccades are very rapid eye movements with velocities between 350 and 600°/s, which serve to bring the image of an object onto the fovea as quickly as possible. Normal subjects can generate accurate saccades to either side of up to 30° from the midline (Fig 5.15). Their generation, either voluntary or involuntary (as in the fast phase of nystagmus), depends on activity in the midbrain and brainstem, in particular the parapontine reticular formation, with projections to the oculomotor nuclei on both sides via the medial longitudinal bundle. The speed, accuracy and latency of saccades are all parameters that may be affected by CNS disease.

Other eye movement disorders

The integrity of the visually controlled eye movements – smooth pursuit, saccades and OKN – can be accurately tested in the horizontal plane using computer-driven stimuli and ENG recording.

A comprehensive test battery includes recordings of

- Spontaneous nystagmus: in each direction of gaze and at rest the eyes must be assessed for spontaneous nystagmus as its presence alters the interpretation of the results of the other test procedures
- Saccades: the eye movement response to a target moving rapidly and randomly from the midline to between 10° and 30° in both (horizontal) directions (Fig 5.15)
- Smooth pursuit: the eye movement to track a target moving sinusoidally in the horizontal plane at frequencies ranging from 0.1 to 0.4 Hz (Fig 5.11)
- OKN: the nystagmic response to movement of large portions of the visual field (Fig 5.12). It is usually tested by moving stripes across the field of vision first clockwise then anticlockwise using either an optokinetic drum (Fig 5.13), testing active OKN (see above), or a full field optokinetic stimulus (Fig 5.14), which tests active and passive OKN pathways. In the latter the patient's chair is surrounded by a striped curtain or screen, which is rotated in each direction at velocities ranging from 20° to 40°/s.

INTERPRETATION

Abnormalities of saccades imply CNS pathology, assuming the ocular muscles are intact. Abnormalities of accuracy include overshooting (hypermetric

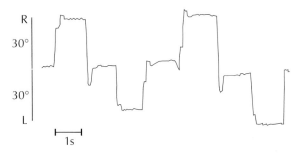

Fig 5.16 Saccadic dysmetria. ENG recordings of saccadic eye movements in a patient with cerebellar dysmetria. The patient has been asked to look at a target 30° to his right (deflection upwards), back to midline and then to look at a target 30° to his left (deflection downwards) and back to centre. The trace shows examples of both under-shooting (hypometria) and overshooting (hypermetria).

saccades) or undershooting (hypometric saccades) the target, hypermetria being suggestive of cerebellar disease and hypometria occurring in lesions of the brainstem or basal ganglia (Fig 5.16). In degenerative conditions such as Huntington's chorea, multiple system atrophy and the Shy–Drager syndrome the latency (reaction time) may be prolonged and velocity of saccades reduced.

An inability to generate saccades, either voluntary or involuntary (as in the fast phase of OKN or in association with spontaneous vestibular nystagmus), usually arises from a lesion in the brainstem. Absent saccades will thus affect the observed response to vestibular stimulation. Tonic deviation of the eyes without the fast 'resetting' component occurs (i.e. only the slow, vestibularly induced phase remains intact) instead of the expected nystagmic response. This absence of nystagmus on either side may be misinterpreted as being bilateral vestibular failure if it is not appreciated, by testing the saccadic system separately, that a central lesion is causing failure of generation of saccades.

Impaired pursuit suggests CNS pathology, but has limited localizing value. Bilaterally impaired pursuit is most commonly caused by certain drugs such as psychotropic drugs, sedatives, including those used as anti-emetics in acute vestibular pathology, for example prochlorperazine (Stemetil), anticonvulsants, even in therapeutic doses, and alcohol, or it can be associated with poor concentration or drowsiness. Unilateral broken pursuit is more indicative of an ipsilateral structural lesion in the CNS. As the pursuit pathways involve the cortex, brainstem, basal ganglia and cerebellum, pathology in any or all of these areas can give rise to 'broken pursuit' (Fig 5.17). Failure to suppress

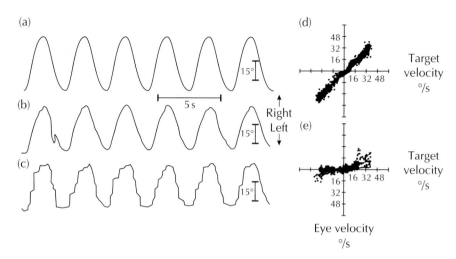

Fig 5.17 (a) Target moving with a sinusoidal waveform. (b) Eye movements of a normal subject tracking the target, and (c) of a patient with cerebellar atrophy tracking the target. (d) and (e) The eye velocity is plotted against target velocity after saccades have been removed for the normal subject and the patient, respectively. (Reproduced from Baloh and Honrubia[3] with permission.)

Table 5.1 Protocol for assessment of eye movements using ENG

Calibration
Eyes centre 0°
Eyes right 30°
Eyes centre 0°
Eyes left 30°

Detection of pathologic nystagmus

Gaze held in midposition:	with fixation (10 s)
	eyes open in the dark (20 s)
Gaze held 30° right:	with fixation (10 s)
	eyes open in the dark (20 s)
Gaze held 30° left:	with fixation (10 s)
	eyes open in the dark (20 s)

Recording of visually induced eye movements

Saccades:	Random presentation of laser targets 10–30° to the right and left of centre
Smooth pursuit:	Target velocity of 20–40°/s 0.1, 0.2, 0.3 and 0.4 Hz in the horizontal plane
Optokinetic nystagmus:	Curtain/drum velocity 20–40°/s in each direction

Rotation tests

Sinusoidal rotation:	Chair rotation from 0.1 to 0.4 Hz, maximal velocity 40°/s
VOR suppression:	Chair rotation from 0.1 to 0.4 Hz, maximal velocity 40°/s
Impulsive rotation:	Acceleration from 0 to 60°/s in <1 s; clockwise followed by anticlockwise rotation

Bithermal caloric test	Each ear in turn irrigated with water at 30°C followed by water at 44°C, with and without fixation

vestibularly induced nystagmus (as in the rotation and caloric tests) is a manifestation of impaired pursuit, as it is the pursuit system that normally brings about this suppression.

Bilateral symmetrical abnormalities of OKN, that is, decreased slow component velocity, may occur in diffuse disease of the cortex, brainstem or cerebellum. Unilateral disease gives rise to impaired OKN when the stimulus is moving towards the damaged side.

As the neural pathways subserving the slow component of active OKN overlap with those of the

Table 5.2 Site of pathology indicated by abnormalities of vestibularly induced eye movements (caloric/rotation tests) and visually induced eye movements

	Peripheral	Central
Canal paresis	++	Rarely may occur with lesion at vestibular nerve root entry zone
Directional preponderance (on caloric or rotation)	+	+
Abnormal nystagmic response to rotation (VOR)	+ (↓ gain)	+ (↑ gain)
Impaired VORs	–	++
Impaired pursuit	+ Transiently in acute lesions	++
Unilateral	No abnormality	Ipsilateral structural lesion of CNS – often cerebellum
Bilateral	No abnormality	Drugs; alcohol
Impaired saccades	–	++
Hypometria	No abnormality	Brainstem/basal ganglia/cerebellum
Hypermetria	No abnormality	Cerebellum
Impaired OKN	+ Transiently in acute lesion. Rarely seen with full field OKN testing	++
Spontaneous nystagmus	+ Obeys Alexander's Law	+ May change direction e.g. congenital nystagmus
Positional nystagmus	+	+
Latency	20 s	None
Fatigability	Usual	Unusual
Duration	<30 s	>30 s
Gaze-evoked nystagmus	–	++
Symmetric	–	Drugs; metabolic disorders
Asymmetric	–	Cerebellum/brainstem
Rebound	–	Cerebellum
Dysconjugate	–	Medial longitudinal bundle

+, typical; –, atypical.

pursuit system, and those subserving the fast phase are part of the saccadic system, abnormalities of OKN may coexist with abnormalities of the pursuit or saccadic systems, or both, and imply CNS pathology.

Some exceptions to the above need to be remembered. In the section on pathologic nystagmus it has been pointed out that a recent acute peripheral vestibular lesion causes spontaneous nystagmus even with fixation for the first few weeks after the vestibular insult. Generally inability to suppress the nystagmus by fixation implies a disorder of the pursuit pathways. In acute peripheral vestibular disorders, transient impairment of contralateral smooth pursuit (and occasionally also of OKN stimulated by a small drum but very rarely with full field optokinetic nystagmus) that does not imply CNS disease may be seen. It will resolve in a matter of weeks, in tandem with the disappearance of spontaneous nystagmus with fixation, although spontaneous nystagmus in the dark, due to vestibular tone asymmetry, may persist for many years.

'Broken pursuit' (intrusion of saccades) may merely reflect poor attention or fatigue, despite the tester's best efforts to keep patient alert and concentrating. If the velocity of the eye movement between saccades is the same as the target velocity, that is, the gain is 1, then it is more likely that the saccades are spurious (i.e. due to poor attention) and that the pursuit system is in fact intact despite the saccadic intrusions. However, if the gain is decreased then the saccades are necessary to 'catch up' with the target and reflect a true impairment of smooth pursuit (Fig 5.17).

A typical ENG test battery assessing eye movements is shown in Table 5.1, and a summary of the abnormalities seen in peripheral and central pathology is outlined in Table 5.2.

Vestibulospinal function

Apart from the maintenance of gaze stability during head motion, it has been noted above that the preservation of normal posture during head movement and in the gravitational field (via the vestibulospinal pathways) is another important function of the vestibular system, although, as yet, it is less well understood than the vestibular control of eye movements.

The vestibulospinal tracts carry information about the position of the head with respect to gravity, mainly from the gravitational receptors – the maculae of the saccule and utricle – to the brainstem and from there to innervate the anti-gravity muscles, that is, extensor and flexor muscles of the neck, trunk and lower limbs, which maintain the upright posture. The push–pull system that operates to control these muscles is similar to that which controls the VOR.

However, the lack of knowledge about the precise organization of the neural pathways involved and the difficulty of isolating the role of the vestibulospinal tract from that of the other systems involved in preserving equilibrium (chiefly vision and proprioception) has hampered the development of specific tests of vestibulospinal function.

The advent of more sophisticated computerized force plate technology allowing objective quantification of sway and the ability to control stimuli accurately (in dynamic posturography, see below) has led to a renewed interest in posturography as a means of objectively analysing this aspect of vestibular function.

Two main forms of posturography exist: static and the more recently developed dynamic posturography. A small amount of postural sway is normal (Fig 5.18), that is, physiological sway; this degree of sway is detected by the visual, vestibular and proprioceptive (especially proprioceptive input from the ankle joints) systems and appropriate righting action is taken to avoid falling. However, patients with balance disorders will sway beyond normal limits, even to the point of falling in severe cases. In simple static posturography, the subject stands upright on a platform that has a force transducer in each corner. The amount of postural sway is assessed by measuring the centre of pressure of the subject's body as detected by the force transducers. The sensitivity of posturography has been increased by the advent of dynamic posturography. In essence, dynamic posturography attempts to 'stress' the ability to preserve equilibrium by removing or altering the information normally available from the visual and proprioceptive systems. A feedback system (known as sway referencing)[12] is incorpo-

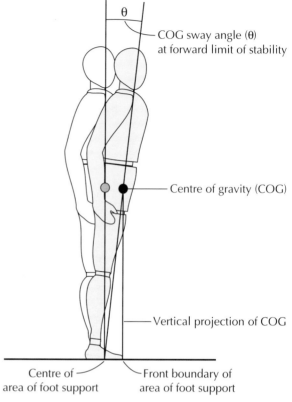

COG sway angle (θ) at forward limit of stability

Centre of gravity (COG)

Vertical projection of COG

Centre of area of foot support

Front boundary of area of foot support

Fig 5.18 The centre of gravity (COG) and sway angle in a normal subject on a balance platform.

rated whereby the subject's sway during testing is detected, and the platform is tilted so as to keep the angle between the foot and lower leg constant thus removing the proprioceptive information from the ankle joint, (i.e. platform sway referencing). Likewise, movement of the visual field can be separately or simultaneously coupled to body sway thus removing just visual or proprioceptive and visual information, respectively (i.e. visual sway referencing). Thus, theoretically, with both visual and proprioceptive information removed the subject's balance under these conditions should reflect vestibular function alone. However, this is an oversimplification of the true situation as factors other than those that are controlled during posturography, including proprioceptive information from other joints, are important in maintaining balance. Despite early work suggesting characteristic patterns of response in patients with vestibular, cerebellar and basal ganglia disorders, the American Academy of Neurology has concluded in 1993 that posturography, static or dynamic, was not useful in the localization of lesions in the nervous system or vestibular system.

In addition to removing information from the visual or proprioceptive systems, or both, another

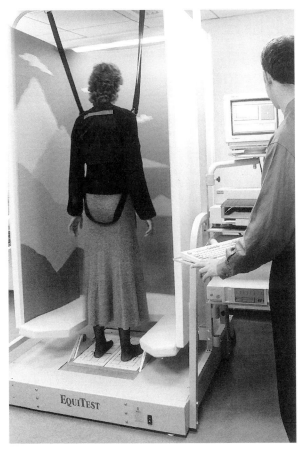

Fig 5.19 'Equitest' (Neurocom International Inc, USA) balance platform. Computerized dynamic posturography (CTD) allows sway referencing of both the platform on which the patient stands and the visual surround.

way of using dynamic posturography involves delivering conflicting information to the subject from these various systems. For example, the platform may be tilted upwards so that the proprioceptive information from the ankle suggests the body is tilting forwards, while at the same time the visual field is moved away from the subject simulating backward sway (Fig 5.19). The degree to which balance is maintained in the face of these conflicting clues is an indication of the individual's reliance on the various systems. For example, one subject may rely more heavily on visual clues to maintain balance whereas another uses vestibular information. This does not necessarily imply site of pathology as such, but gives information about the strategies that the subject uses to preserve equilibrium and provides valuable data in the planning of rehabilitation.

It thus appears that the true value of posturography lies not in the specific diagnosis of the cause of imbalance but in the objective demonstration of imbalance (and of the improvement in balance with treatment as positive feedback to the patient), and in the evaluation of how individuals depend differentially on visual, vestibular and proprioceptive information to achieve perfect balance. With this information, the planning, execution and evaluation of the efficacy of rehabilitation programmes (see Chapter 15) can be carried out in a more systematic and scientific way than was previously possible.

Miscellaneous tests

GALVANIC TEST

The galvanic test attempts to differentiate between pathology affecting the end organ from that affecting the vestibular nerve, in much the same way as auditory brainstem evoked responses, stapedial reflexes et cetera differentiate between cochlear and retrocochlear disorders. A current is applied to the labyrinth via a saline pad applied to the tragus, external auditory canal or mastoid process with the second electrode on the sternum. In normal subjects, the application of a current of between 1 and 2 mA increases postural sway away from the cathode (the excitatory electrode). With higher levels of stimulation nystagmus may be seen with the fast phase towards the cathode. However, these levels of stimulation may be painful for the subject. A normal postural (or nystagmic) response is thought to indicate normal function of Scarpa's ganglion and the vestibular nerve central to it, and has been shown to be preserved after destruction of the vestibular end organ. Thus patients with end organ damage only and those with VIIIth nerve disease will show a pattern of results from other tests described above suggestive of 'peripheral vestibular disorder' but those with end organ damage only will have normal galvanic responses, whereas a patient with VIIIth nerve disease will have abnormal galvanic responses.

Galvanic testing had fallen into dysfavour because of the discomfort caused by the stimulation. In addition, the electrical currents necessary for testing gave rise to interference with ENG recording and led to difficulties in interpreting the traces. However, with the availability of more sophisticated and sensitive body sway platforms, it is possible to observe significant changes in posture with lower levels of stimulation, and galvanic testing may become a feasible and acceptable test in the future.

AUDITORY TESTS

In conjunction with the vestibular tests described above – those most useful for routine clinical practice being shown in Table 5.2 – all patients undergoing vestibular assessment should have evaluation of their auditory function (Chapter 4). Clearly there is a close relationship, both anatomically and physiologically, between the vestibular and auditory labyrinth, and between the vestibular and auditory divisions of the VIIIth nerve. As more becomes known about central auditory function and its neural pathways, and as clinically applicable tests develop, without doubt such information will also be valuable in determining the precise site of lesions causing vestibular disturbance.

It needs to be appreciated that the severity of symptoms and degree of disability or handicap experienced by the patient do not necessarily run in parallel with the degree of vestibular dysfunction as judged by the above tests. A unilateral abnormality of the vestibular system, of even a relatively minor degree, will cause a mismatch between the left and right responses and lead to a sensation of imbalance or dizziness, whereas paradoxically, a bilateral, symmetrical severe or even complete loss of peripheral vestibular function may be entirely asymptomatic.

The emphasis in this chapter has been on the use of vestibular tests in the assessment of the patient with dizziness or imbalance. However, as well as assessing patients with such complaints, it needs to be pointed out that the assessment of vestibular function, despite the patient having no vestibular symptoms, can be crucial to the correct diagnosis of the aetiology of sensorineural hearing loss, such as in acoustic neuromas, and in the differentiation between types I and II of Usher's syndrome; such a distinction, once made, has very significant prognostic implications. Thus, detailed vestibular assessment should form part of the routine investigation of all patients with sensorineural hearing loss.

In conclusion, the tests of vestibular function outlined above, taken in conjunction with a full history, general medical examination (with particular emphasis on the cardiovascular and neurological systems, including proprioception and vision), and audiovestibular assessment provide information on the presence or absence of vestibular pathology, the site of the lesion, the degree to which the patient has compensated, and a tool by which to monitor progress (or deterioration) and provide positive feedback to the patient as part of their rehabilitation programme (see Chapter 15). Although the most likely aetiology of the identified lesion may often be apparent from the history and the coexistence or otherwise of auditory dysfunction, the test results do not define specific aetiologies. Further investigations, such as blood tests and radiology are needed to achieve this end.

References

1. Ewald JR. *Physiologische untersuchungen uber das enorgan des nervus octavus*. Wiesbaden: Bergmann, 1892.
2. Hood JD, Korres S. Vestibular suppression in peripheral and central vestibular disorders of the brain. *Brain* 1979; **102**:785–804.
3. Baloh RW, Honrubia V. Electronystagmography. In: *Clinical neurophysiology of the vestibular system*. Philadelphia: FA Davis, 1990:130–52.
4. Bárány R. Untersuchungen uber den vom Vestibularapparat des Ohres reflektorisch ausgelosten rhythmischen Nystagmus und seine Begleiterscheinungen. *Monatschrift für Ohrenheilkunde* 1906; **40**:193–297.
5. Fitzgerald G, Hallpike CS. Studies in human vestibular function. I. Observation on the directional preponderance of caloric nystagmus resulting from cerebral lesions. *Brain* 1942; **65**:115–37.
6. Davies RA, Savundra PA. Diagnostic testing of the vestibular system. In: Stephens SDG ed. *Adult audiology*. London: Butterworth–Heinemann 1997 (Kerr A ed. *Scott-Brown's Otolaryngology*, 6th ed; vol 2.)
7. Luxon L. Comparison of assessment of caloric nystagmus by observation of duration and by electronystagmographic measurement of slow-phase velocity. *British Journal of Audiology* 1995; **29**:107–16.
8. Jongkees LBW, Maas JPM, Philipzoon AJ. Clinical nystagmography. *Practica Otolaryngologica* 1962; **24**:65–93.
9. Van Egmond AAJ, Groen JJ, Jongkees LBW. The turning test with small regulable stimuli. *Journal of Laryngology and Otology* 1984; **62**:63–9.
10. O'Leary DP, Davis LL. Vestibular autorotation with active head movements. In: Jackler RK, Brackmann DE eds. *Neurotology*. St. Louis, Missouri: Mosley, 1994:229–40.
11. Yee RD, Baloh RW, Honrubia V, Jenkins HA. Pathophysiology of optokinetic nystagmus. In: Honrubia V, Brazier M eds. *Nystagmus and vertigo. Clinical approaches to the patient with dizziness*. New York: Academic Press, 1982:251–75.
12. Horak FB, Nashner LM, Diener HC. Postural strategies associated with somatosensory and vestibular loss. *Experimental Brain Research* 1990; **82**:167–77.

Suggested reading

Brandt T. Downbeat nystagmus/Vertigo syndrome. In: *Vertigo: Its multisensory syndromes*. London: Springer–Verlag, 1991.
Rudge P. *Clinical neuro-otology*. Edinburgh: Churchill Livingstone, 1983.
Sharpe JA, Barber HO. *The vestibulo-ocular reflex and vertigo*. New York: Raven Press, 1993.

CHAPTER 6

Diagnostic imaging of the ear (normal and congenital)

PETER D PHELPS

Conventional radiography

Although polytomography is now obsolete, plain film views of the petromastoid still have a minor role in the imaging investigation of the petrous temporal bone. The *lateral view* is obtained by placing the head in the true lateral position and angling the tube caudally 15° thus preventing superimposition of the mastoid processes. The incident beam is centred so that it will emerge through the external meatus on the affected side. The state of translucence of the mastoid air cells is demonstrated as is the position of the bony plates overlying the sigmoid sinus and the middle fossa dura and tegmen of the middle ear (Fig 6.1). The *Stenver's oblique posteroanterior projection* demonstrates the whole length of the petrous bone by placing it parallel to the X-ray film with the incident ray passing at right angles to it. When a skull table is used the patient sits erect facing the film. With the radiographic baseline horizontal, the sagittal plane of the skull is rotated through 35° and tilted 15° away from the side to be examined (Fig 6.2). The incident ray is inclined at an angle of 12° cranially and is centred on a point 2 cm medial to the tip of the mastoid process. A radiograph in Stenver's position should demonstrate the petrous tip and internal auditory (acoustic) meatus (IAM), the semicircular canals (superior and lateral), the middle ear cleft, the mastoid antrum and the mastoid process.

PERORBITAL VIEW

The perorbital view is the best one of the IAM by plain films and should be done in the posteroanterior

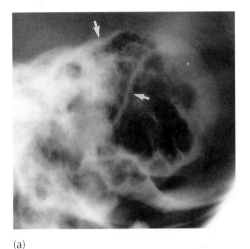

(a)

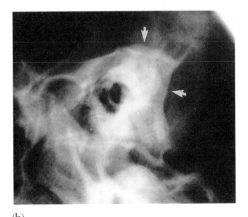

(b)

Fig 6.1 Plain lateral view of the mastoid, (a) well pneumatized and (b) sclerotic. The arrows point to the dural plate (higher arrow) and sigmoid sinus plate (lower arrow).

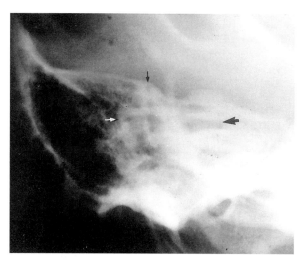

Fig 6.2 Stenver's view. The large arrow points to the IAM, the smaller arrows indicate superior and lateral semicircular canals.

position to reduce radiation to the eyes. The orbito-meatal line is at right angles to the film. The tube is angled 5–10° caudally, centring between the orbits. The petrous pyramids and IAMs are thus projected through the orbits. The apical and middle coils of the cochlea are superimposed on the lateral part of the IAM but the basal turn may be identified below it and the vestibule. Deformity of the labyrinth can be shown in infants in whom there is little surrounding ossification (Fig 6.3).

Computed tomography

High resolution computed tomography (CT) is now the investigation of choice for the petrous temporal bone. Initially CT was a major advance because great improvement in contrast resolution compared with conventional imaging made it possible to

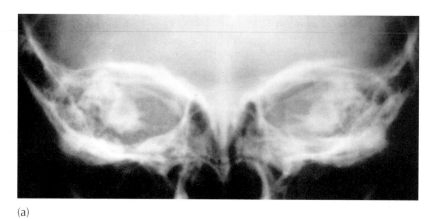

(a)

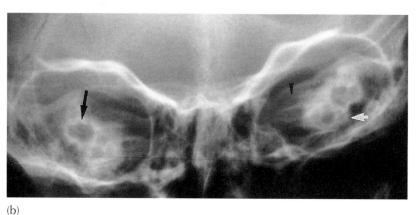

(b)

Fig 6.3 (a) Perorbital view: note the labyrinths and IAMs seen outlined by the orbital rims. (b) A similar view in a child with congenital ear deformities. The white arrow points to the basal turn of cochlea, the black arrow to an enlarged vestibule continuous with a dysplastic lateral semicircular canal. The left IAM (arrow head) appears narrow.

demonstrate intracranial lesions such as tumours or the complications of suppurative ear disease. Spatial resolution on these early machines was poor, however, but greatly improved technology has enabled thin sections to be made by using a narrower X-ray beam and a greater number of detectors. A choice of optimum spatial or density resolution lies to some extent with the operator; however, with poor results from attempts to assess tissue characterization and the advent of magnetic resonance imaging (MRI) proving superior for soft-tissue discrimination few attempts are now made at densitometric assessment. Partial volume averaging makes it impossible to differentiate fluid from soft tissue in the petromastoid. An exception, however, is the use of densitometry for the labyrinthine capsule. Otospongiosis and other bone dysplasia can be usefully assessed by taking densitometric readings from selected areas in the petrous temporal bone. Generally, however, CT is only used when there is a high relative contrast, as for demonstrating the situation and extent of a small soft-tissue mass in an otherwise air-containing middle ear cavity. Optimum assessment of fine bone detail can be made as for the ossicles in the middle ear and fine canal and tracts in the petrous pyramid. The pictures are viewed on a wide window setting of 4000 Hounsfield Units (HU) using the bone algorithm and in this mode CT can be used for the study of the middle and inner ears. Thin sections 1 or 2 mm thick are obtained. Contrast enhancement is almost never used if lesions are confined to the petrous pyramid.

The success of CT can be attributed to its great sensitivity for very small changes in X-ray attenuation. This is known as contrast resolution. The quality of the CT image, however, depends on a complex relationship between radiation dose, spatial resolution, contrast resolution and noise. Noise is the mottling or granularity that affects the image when there is insufficient information from the detectors available for assessment. In practice, most scanners have two options for image production: standard resolution for optimum density discrimination, as when demonstrating brain tumours, And high resolution for fine detail discrimination, especially that of small bony structures in sinus and temporal bone. With new rotate-only scanners it is possible to obtain images in soft tissue and bone resolution using the same raw data but, inevitably, the reprocessing increases the length of examination.

Twenty years ago the demonstration of fine detail in the ear was considered the ultimate achievement of polytomography. In some respects the same is now true of high resolution CT, and a brief consideration of some of the limiting factors of this technique for the examination of regions such as the middle ear seems desirable.

Partial volume averaging is a phenomenon that occurs with CT when the dimensions of the object being imaged are smaller than the slice thickness of the individual voxel (the smallest separable volumes, made up of pixels and the slide thickness). Non-representative attenuation values may be generated when all the densities within an individual voxel are averaged to produce a single attenuation coefficient. Bone or air in a voxel depicting soft tissue will significantly alter the averaged attenuation reading of that voxel.

Soft-tissue silhouetting is the outlining of small dense structures, which may happen when soft tissues such as normal adjacent brain, haemorrhage, tumour or fluid envelope are contiguous with a structure usually bordered by air. The difference between the density of the structures and the background may be insufficient for their visualization.

The routine CT examination of the petrous temporal bone begins with a lateral scout view showing the sections required for the examination in the axial plane (Fig 6.4). This is the natural plane for CT and the most comfortable for the patient. It also gives the maximum information about the middle and inner ear, especially the coils of the cochlea.

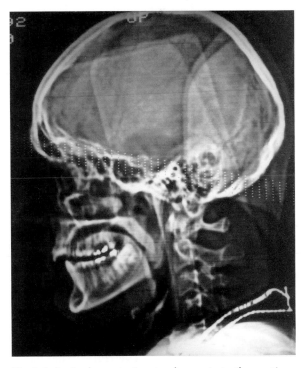

Fig 6.4 Sagittal scout view to demonstrate the sections necessary for an axial CT study of the petrous temporal bone.

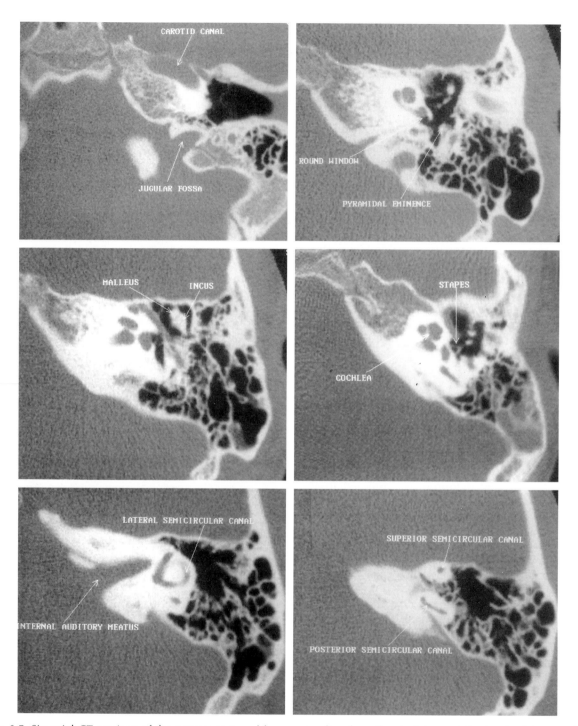

Fig 6.5 Six axial CT sections of the petrous temporal bone extending from the skull base at the level of the carotid canal and jugular fossa to the labyrinth and the superior and posterior semicircular canals in the highest section (i.e. that nearest the top of the head).

The plane is not strictly speaking a true axial but a plane at 30° to the radiographic baseline, which is the orbitomeatal line, drawn from the centre of the external meatus to the outer canthus of the eye. This is to limit the radiation dose to the eye as, although some sections will pass through the orbit, the centre of the globe is not in the direct X-ray beam.

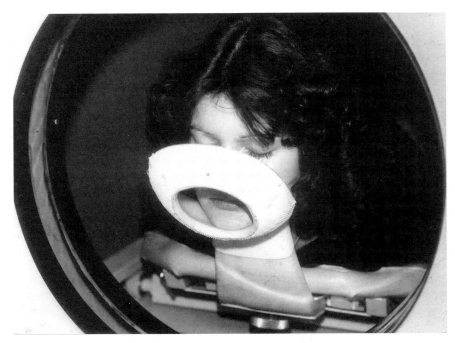

Fig 6.6 The position for coronal sections of the petrous temporal bone from the coils of the cochlea in front to the jugular fossa and posterior semicircular canal behind.

Sections in the axial plane start just below the external auditory (acoustic) meatus (EAM) and show the basal turn of cochlea and round window niche; the mid-modiolar section shows the individual coils of the cochlea and incudostapedial region; the section passes through the vestibule and loop of the lateral semicircular canal, at right angles to each other. Sections at the level of the vestibule best show the EAM. Head of the malleus and body and short process of incus are also shown at this level. The three parts of the facial nerve canal can be identified, although the base plane is least satisfactory for the descending portion, which is seen in cross-section behind the middle ear cavity. Other important features in the axial plane are the round window niche and the pyramid on the posterior wall of the middle ear and the jugular fossa (Fig 6.5). Coronal sections 1–2 mm thick are obtained as nearly as possible in the coronal plane aided by gantry tilt (Fig 6.6). Either the 'chin up' or head hanging position may be used. The radiation dose to the eyes from coronal sections is very low as they are not in the X-ray beam.

Coronal sections (Fig 6.7) begin at the level of the carotid canal and curl of the central bony spiral of the cochlea; the malleus is well shown at this level. Further back the section at the level of the vestibule shows the IAM and the stapes and oval window.

Further back still at the most prominent part of the lateral semicircular canal the pyramidal eminence is shown between facial recess and sinus tympani. The descending facial canal and jugular fossa are assessed and the examination finishes at the posterior semicircular canal, although further sections may be necessary to show the mastoid antrum and air cells.

Reformatted images

Reformatted images can be obtained from multiple thin contiguous base sections. They can be made in any plane but the quality is always poorer than a direct examination and depends on two factors:

- the number of sections and therefore the amount of raw data available for the reconstruction process
- the absolute immobility of the patient while these sections are being obtained.

Sagittal reformatted views are useful for assessing a large vestibular aqueduct (Fig 6.8) and may also be used to show the descending facial canal and disruption between malleus and incus (Fig 6.9).

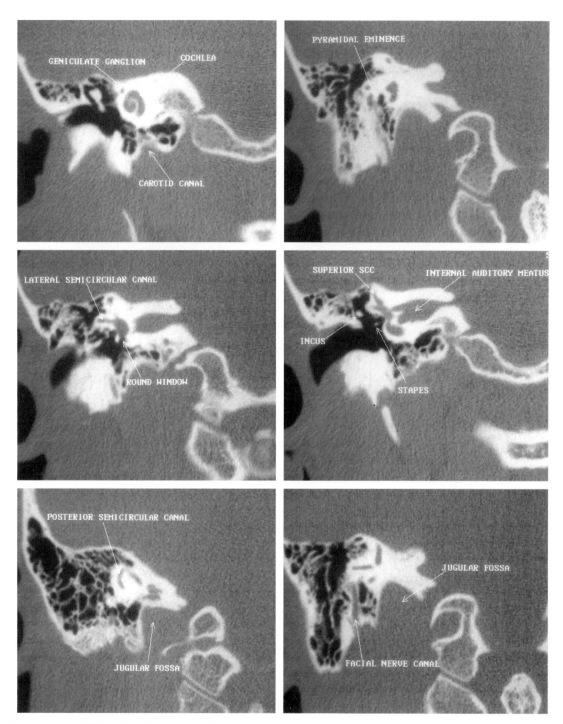

Fig 6.7 Six coronal CT sections from the cochlea anteriorly to the posterior semicircular canal.

DEMONSTRATION OF THE FACIAL NERVE CANAL

The facial nerve runs a complicated course through the temporal bone. From the lateral end of the IAM to the stylomastoid foramen, the facial canal is divided into three parts on the basis of the direction of each part. These are difficult to demonstrate with conventional radiography and the Stenver's view, which may show the descending part, is probably the only projection of value.

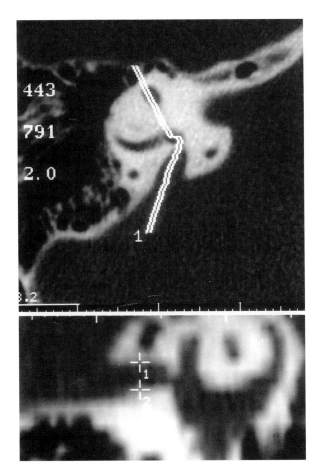

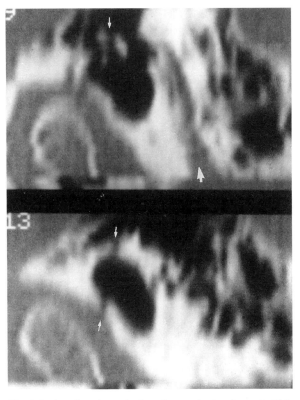

Fig 6.8 Large vestibular aqueduct. The upper figure shows the targeted axial CT view of the foreshortened vestibular aqueduct and the lateral semicircular canal. The lower figure is a sagittal reformat with a measurement at the midpoint of the descending limb of 2.0 mm.

Fig 6.9 Another lateral view by sagittal reformat. This shows in the upper section a dislocation between malleus and incus (small arrow) and the normal descending facial nerve canal (large arrow). The lower section shows the fracture line through the roof and floor of the EAM (arrows).

Labyrinthine part

Starting at the anterosuperior aspect of the lateral end of the IAM, this short segment swings anteriorly above the cochlea to the pit for the geniculate ganglion, where the nerve turns sharply backwards to become the second part (Fig 6.10), but the sulcus for the geniculate ganglion is well demonstrated in coronal sections (Fig 6.7).

Tympanic part

From the geniculate ganglion to the second bend, the nerve runs backwards above the oval window and below the lateral semicircular canal, which overhangs it. It is surrounded by a thin bony sheath that may be dehiscent. Its course is somewhat oblique and the bony canal is, therefore, best seen in cross-section on the axial projection (Fig 6.10).

Mastoid or descending part

The third part of the nerve runs downwards from the second bend at the level of the pyramidal eminence to the stylomastoid foramen. Its length is partly dependent on the shape of the temporal bone and partly on the extent of pneumatization of the mastoid. Its width varies considerably. The bony canal is best demonstrated by coronal section and sagittal CT views (Fig 6.9). Recognition is easy where the nerve passes through solid bone, but may be difficult where there is much pneumatization. In children with congenital ear lesions, it is important not to confuse the facial nerve canal with other dehiscences such as the tympanic fissure.

Spiral or helical CT scanners are capable of approximately 1 cm isotropic image resolution; both the minimum collimation and the minimum table increment are 1 mm. The image quality of

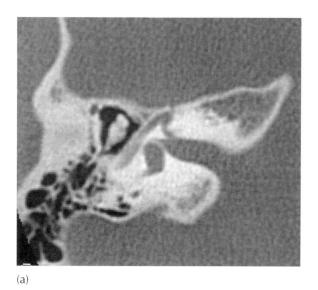

(a)

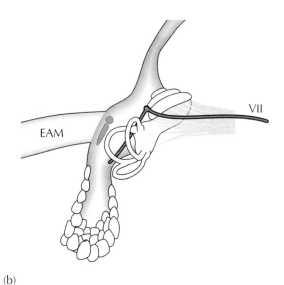

(b)

Fig 6.10 Axial images of the first and second parts of the facial nerve: (a) the CT section shows the first and second parts of the facial nerve canal; (b) a complementary diagram; (c) a similar gadolinium-enhanced T1-weighted MR section shows enhancement of the second part of the facial nerve (arrows).

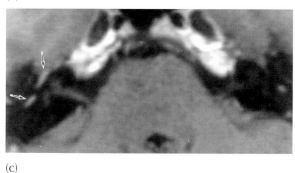

(c)

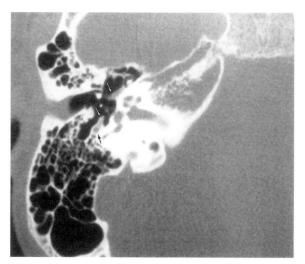

Fig 6.11 Axial CT section at the level of the coils of the cochlea showing the two muscles in the middle ear cavity (white arrows). The tensor tympani passes back to be inserted into the malleus, and the stapedius passes forwards to the stapes. The descending facial nerve canal is shown behind the stapedius (black arrow).

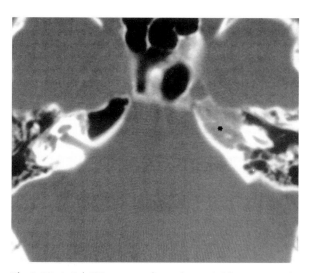

Fig 6.12 Axial CT scan to show the variable anatomy in the petrous apex. On one side there is a large air cell, on the other bone marrow (asterisk). This had caused some confusion on a previous MR scan when the high signal from the bone marrow on the T1-weighted sections was wrongly interpreted as pathology.

spiral CT has been shown to be roughly equivalent to that of conventional CT, but with greatly reduced data acquisition time.

Other important features can be shown by axial CT scans (Figs 6.11 and 6.12).

Magnetic resonance

The continuing development of new MR techniques means that the standard protocols for investigating deafness and lesions affecting the petrous temporal bone and posterior cranial fossa are subject to change. Clinical tests can usually give some idea of whether the abnormality is primarily in the petrous bone or the posterior cranial fossa. Objective audiometry, in particular the brainstem auditory evoked potentials (BAEPs), can help to decide whether sensorineural deafness is cochlear, that is, end organ in type, or retrocochlear, that is, from lesions of the central nerves or their central connections. MR is the imaging investigation of choice for the retrocochlear type, but is secondary to CT for the assessment of the cochlear type of deafness. The protocols used for different pathologies will be described subsequently.

Bone produces a negligible signal on MR scans, and so both the bone of the petromastoid and the air in the middle ear cleft and mastoid cell system appear as black areas on the scan, devoid of any of the bone detail so well demonstrated by high resolution CT. Thus, only soft-tissue structures within the petrous temporal bone are imaged and this can be an advantage for the demonstration of the cranial nerves passing through the skull base, as the nerve itself will be shown rather than the canal in which it lies. In contrast to the non-signal of compact bone, marrow spaces, which are very variable in extent but occur mostly in the petrous apex, give an intense signal because of their large fat content on T1-weighted images. The diagnostic protocol for MRI of the temporal bone and posterior fossa uses axial sections with long and short repetition time (TR) spin-echo sequences after a short sagittal localizer. These repetition times are combined with long and short echo times (TEs) to give T1-weighted and T2-weighted images. The region of interest is portrayed in 4 mm thick slices (Fig 6.13).

Recently a new technique of *fast spin echo* (FSE) has been introduced. This gives greatly improved spatial resolution and allows the individual nerves and vascular loops to be identified in the IAM as bands of low signal (Fig 6.14). A method that uses spin echoes and altered k-space filling, k-space being the amount of space that must be filled with

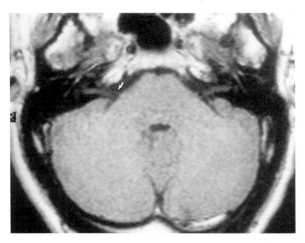

Fig 6.13 Axial T1-weighted section through the posterior cranial fossa showing the cranial nerves crossing the cerebellopontine angle (arrow). Note the high signal from marrow fat in the petrous apex and basisphenoid.

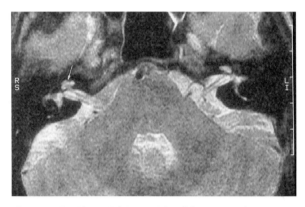

Fig 6.14 Similar axial T2-weighted fast spin echo section showing the cranial nerves in the IAMs and the cochlea on each side (arrow).

information (raw data) to create an image, FSE is designed to provide more conventional spin-echo-type contrast in a shorter time. In the fast spin echo pulse sequence the initial 90° pulse is followed by the acquisition of 2–16 spin echoes. Each echo is acquired with a different phase-encode gradient, meaning that this information can be collected 16 times faster than normal spin echo. The number of echoes selected is called the echo train length and the time between each echo is called the echo space. This not only shortens the examination time but enables a finer matrix to be used. Thinner sections (3 mm instead of 5 mm) can also be made and the greatly improved spatial resolution using four acquisitions means that it is possible to demonstrate the individual nerves in the IAM. Although gadolinium-enhanced T1-weighted images have proved the gold standard for demonstrating all acoustic neuromas large and small, this is not an entirely non-invasive procedure because an intravenous injection is necessary.

Sections of the temporal bone as thin as 1 mm can be acquired by a three-dimensional Fourier transformation (3DFT) technique using a small receiver coil, a low flip angle with short TR and gradient reversal instead of 180° radio frequency (RF) refocusing. Images in any plane can be reformatted from the data acquired in the axial plane. However, some of the earlier gradient echo 3DFT sequences, although giving high signal from fluids at flip angles of around 50°, were very sensitive to flow of fluids producing artefacts. To overcome this disadvantage Casselman in 1994 introduced the 3DFT-CISS (constructive interference in steady state) protocol, which ensures that not only the fluid in the membranous labyrinth and IAM but also the fast flowing fluid around the brainstem always has a high signal and remains white.

Contrast enhancement using the paramagnetic agent gadolinium DTPA has tended to replace the T2-weighted sequences. Most tumours show a significant degree of enhancement but studies with gadolinium are especially valuable for the demonstration of acoustic neuromas (*vide infra*).

Magnetic resonance angiography (MRA) can now be used as part of the MR examination, especially for vascular lesions such as glomus tumours or for vascular anomalies like a high jugular bulb, if this is not differentiated convincingly by routine CT and MR protocols. Obstruction of the sigmoid sinus with demonstration of multiple venous collaterals can be usefully shown by MRA after arterial saturation. Occasionally, selective arterial MRA with elimination of venous flow may be useful for showing the blood supply to the tumour, usually from posterior auricular pharyngeal arteries. Digital subtraction and catheter angiography should now only be required for therapeutic embolization techniques to reduce the blood supply to glomus tumours preoperatively.

Congenital vascular anomalies

The jugular fossa and intrapetrous carotid canal are well shown by tomographic techniques. Very rarely an ectopic internal carotid artery, or more commonly a large jugular bulb, may appear in the middle ear and cause not only symptoms but problems in differential diagnosis (Fig 6.15) from glomus tumours. An aberrant carotid artery in the middle ear becomes apparent on CT if comparison is made

with the course of the normal artery on the opposite side. Vascular anomalies are usually discovered in late childhood or adulthood. The differential diagnosis and their distinction from vascular neoplasms is almost entirely dependent upon radiology. Angiography has been considered the definitive investigation and in many cases is mandatory when there appears to be a vascular mass behind the eardrum. Rare abnormalities are a persistent stapedial artery or an aneurysm of the internal carotid artery. This discussion concerns aberrations in position of the internal carotid artery and jugular bulb.

The anatomy of the jugular bulb is variable, the right usually being larger than the left. Not infrequently, it extends above the inferior rim of the bony annulus, with or without a bony covering. The anatomy has been comprehensively reviewed by Graham,[1] who quoted dissections by other authors showing the jugular bulb extending above the inferior rim of the annulus in 6 per cent of specimens, and a similar percentage showing dehiscence in the bony floor of the middle ear cavity.

When the jugular bulb is small, it is separated from the floor of the middle ear by a comparatively thick layer of bone, which is usually compact but may contain air cells. Anterior to the bulb is the internal carotid artery. A spur or crest of bone separates the jugular fossa from the carotid canal. When the jugular bulb is very large, it can extend up into the mesotympanum with a thin bony covering, which can easily be damaged at surgery (Fig 6.15). When there is dehiscence of this bony covering, the exposed jugular bulb is at even greater risk. The soft-tissue mass of a dehiscent jugular bulb cannot be shown adequately by conventional imaging, but is well shown by CT, especially in the coronal plane.

Another aspect of the large jugular bulb is encroachment on inner ear structures. The IAM, vestibular aqueduct and posterior semicircular canal may be affected, especially if there is an associated diverticulum from the bulb.

Aberrations in the course of the internal carotid artery through the petrous temporal bone are extremely rare. Normally the artery ascends vertically, medial and anterior to the middle ear cavity, before bending sharply anterior and medially below the Eustachian tube and cochlea; it then passes through the foramen lacerum into the cranial cavity. A thin bony septum separates the artery from the hypotympanum. There is said to be dehiscence in 1 per cent of people, but the true incidence is probably much less than this. If the ascending part of the artery is more posteriorly placed than usual with a very acute bend, it is more likely to be dehiscent, although the spur between the carotid and the jugular bulb remains intact. In more severe

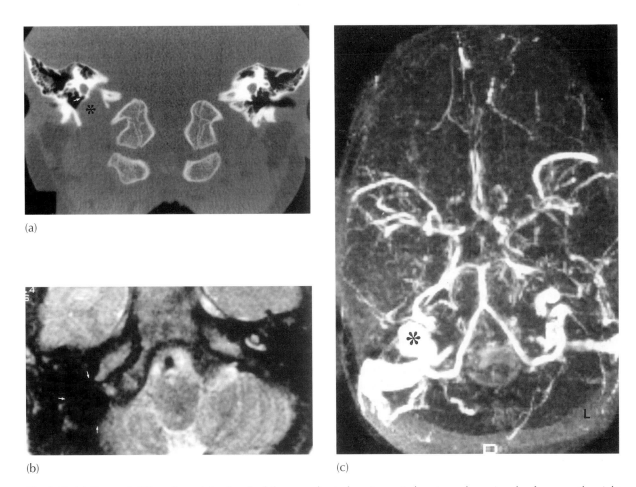

(a)

(b)

(c)

Fig 6.15 (a) Coronal CT section at the level of the round window (arrow) showing a large jugular fossa on the right with diverticulum (asterisk). (b) Axial T1-weighted MR section showing the jugular bulb appearing black from flowing blood (white arrows). The MR scan was undertaken to be sure that this was no space-occupying lesion, although this would have been highly unlikely in view of the smooth bony outline shown on CT. (c) Time-of-flight MRA showing the sigmoid sinus and large jugular bulb (asterisk). Note how small the venous return is on the left side.

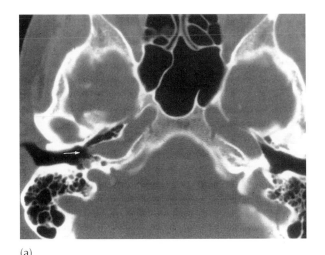

(a)

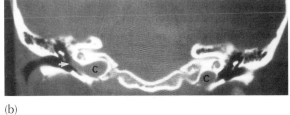

(b)

Fig 6.16 Aberrant internal carotid artery extending into the middle ear cavity: (a) axial section; the arrow points to the soft-tissue mass in the middle ear. Note the accompanying stapedial artery just posterior to the carotid artery and compare with the normal bony covering on the opposite side. (b) Coronal CT section showing the carotid artery (C) extending into the middle ear cavity (arrow) at the level of the cochlea and malleus.

aberrations, a soft-tissue mass will be shown in the middle ear by CT (Fig 6.16) but the important differentiating feature on coronal CT is absence of the normal carotid canal and a laterally and more posteriorly placed vertical canal. These features need to be confirmed by angiography and no attempt at surgical interference should be made.

Congenital ear deformities

Congenital abnormalities of the ear can be shown in great detail by CT if there is osseous deformity, but MRI is now providing evidence of soft-tissue lesions in some cases.

Structural abnormalities of the inner, middle and external ear can be shown in considerable detail by tomographic techniques. Unfortunately, affected children are usually referred between the ages of 2 and 4 years, when the deafness is first confirmed, and sedation or a general anaesthetic is required for the examination. If, after careful consideration, it is felt that the results of the investigation are unlikely to affect patient management, it may be reasonable to defer the examination until the child can cooperate. In the neonatal period a few sections can usually be obtained after a large feed, and this is recommended for those infants with relevant external deformities or syndromes of which temporal bone abnormalities are a feature. Plain films will also give some information at this stage, when full ossification of the petrous pyramids has not yet occurred, but at a later stage are only really useful for showing the degree of pneumatization.

Congenital abnormalities of the middle and external ear are seen much more often than deformities of the inner ear, although combined deformities occur in about 20 per cent of patients. The study of the outer ear relates to the prospects for surgical intervention to improve the sound-conducting mechanism, and is mandatory before any exploration of congenital atresia. Surgery is now, however, rarely performed for unilateral lesions, but in bilateral atresias the radiological examination is crucial to indicate the best side for exploration, especially the all-important assessment of the presence, state and size of the middle ear cavity, but in fact the success of bone-anchored hearing aids has meant that only the most minor deformities of the conducting mechanism now warrant surgical exploration.

INNER EAR DEFORMITIES

Congenital malformations of the bony labyrinth, IAM and vestibular aqueduct, which vary widely in severity from minor anomalies with normal cochlear function to severe deformities that preclude any

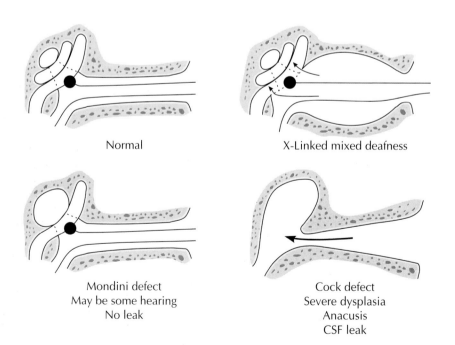

Normal

X-Linked mixed deafness

Mondini defect
May be some hearing
No leak

Cock defect
Severe dysplasia
Anacusis
CSF leak

Fig 6.17 Three important types of congenital cochlear deformity based on axial CT sections. (From Neuroradiology 1991, with permission.)

level of hearing whatsoever, may be suggested by audiological assessment. Traditionally two eponyms are enshrined in accounts of congenital deafness and so need to be defined.

- Michel[2] defect: complete lack of development of any inner ear structures.
- Mondini[3] defect: a cochlea with one and half turns and the apical coil replaced by a distal sac. Although the subject of Mondini's dissection had been completely deaf, the normal basal turn of the true Mondini defect means that some hearing is possible. Mondini's patient also had very dilated vestibular aqueducts.[4]

Line drawings of some examples of labyrinthine deformities are shown in Figure 6.17. A primitive sac with one or more appendages is more common than a Michel deformity.

The semicircular canals may be missing or dilated in varying degree, but the commoner inner ear anomaly, namely a solitary dilated dysplastic lateral semicircular canal, is often associated with normal cochlear function. Dilatation of the vestibular aqueduct often accompanies minor abnormalities of the bony cochlea and vestibule and congenital hearing loss. The deafness may by fluctuant or progressive, or both, giving rise to speculation that endolymphatic hydrops is also a feature.

Anomalies of the IAM include the bulbous type, which is usually of no significance; unusual direction, which is the result of skull base aberrations; and a very narrow or double IAM, which usually indicates severe or total deafness.

INNER EAR LESIONS ASSOCIATED WITH CEREBROSPINAL FLUID FISTULA

Congenital cerebrospinal fluid fistula into the middle ear cavity is a rare but potentially fatal condition that is frequently misdiagnosed. When the fistula occurs spontaneously it usually appears in the first 5 or 10 years of life as

- cerebrospinal fluid rhinorrhoea, if the eardrum is intact; cerebrospinal fluid passes down the Eustachian tube causing a nasal discharge
- cerebrospinal fluid otorrhoea, if there is a perforation in the eardrum, or if myringotomy has been performed for presumed serous otitis media
- attacks of meningitis that are usually recurrent; at times meningitis is the sole presenting manifestation of a cerebrospinal fluid fistula.

Deafness is usually severe or complete, but it is difficult to diagnose and assess, especially in a young

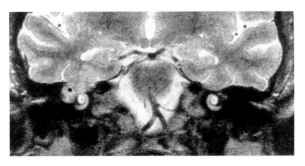

Fig 6.18 Coronal FSE section through the petrous temporal bones at the level of the cochlea showing an encephalocoele (asterisk) extending into the upper middle ear cavity.

child. It is frequently unrecognized if unilateral. The conductive and sensorineural components of the deafness are also hard to define.

Spontaneous cerebrospinal fluid fistulae from the subarachnoid space into the middle ear cavity may be classified as perilabyrinthine or translabyrinthine. Those in the very rare perilabyrinthine group, through bony defects close to but not involving the labyrinth, usually have normal hearing initially (Fig 6.18). The commoner translabyrinthine type is nearly always associated with anacusis, severe labyrinthine dysplasia and a route via the IAM. The labyrinthine deformity is more severe than the type classically described by Mondini,[3] and evidence of a dilated cochlear aqueduct in these patients is also unconvincing.

I have discussed the perilabyrinthine and translabyrinthine routes elsewhere (Fig 6.19).[4] The most important route is via an abnormally shaped IAM that usually tapers at its lateral end (Fig 6.20). The cochlea is an amorphous sac that lacks a modiolus or central bony spiral. The cochlear sac may be bigger or smaller than a normal cochlea. No proper basal turn can be recognized as in a true Mondini deformity, and there is a wide communication between the cochlear sac and the vestibule, which is itself abnormal and enlarged, especially in the horizontal plane. This important congenital ear deformity was first described by Cock in 1838 from a postmortem study of a child who died of otogenic meningitis.[5] The semicircular canals, especially the lateral canals, may be dilated to a varying degree.

The labyrinthine malformation is often accompanied by a defective stapes – usually a hole in the footplate – and the exit route of cerebrospinal fluid into the middle ear is via the oval or, less commonly, the round window. It should be stressed that the fistula is usually spontaneous or the result of a minor head injury.

(a)

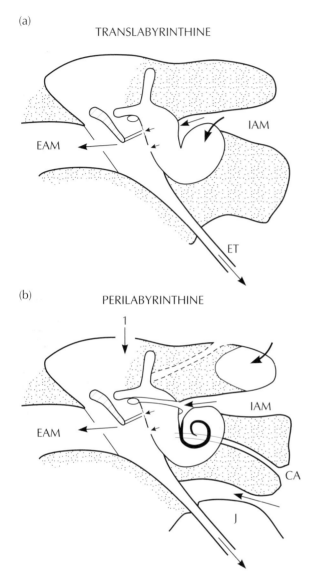

Fig 6.19 The routes of cerebrospinal fluid fistula through the petrous temporal bone. (a) The translabyrinthine type: note the wide communication between vestibule and cochlear sac. These diagrams are based on coronal section CT. (b) The commonest perilabyrinthine route is through the tegmen tympani (1). Routes through large apical air cells, Hyrtl's fissure, petromastoid canal and via the facial nerve canal are very rare. EAM, external auditory meatus; IAM, internal auditory meatus; ET, Eustachian tube; CA, cochlear aqueduct; J, jugular fossa. (Reproduced with permission.[4])

Congenital fixation of the stapes footplate is likely to be associated with a profuse perilymph or cerebrospinal fluid leak after stapedectomy. The surgical results of stapedectomy for congenital stapedial fixation are not very satisfactory.

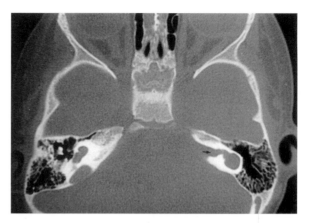

Fig 6.20 Axial CT section of the temporal bones of a child with severe bilateral dysplasia of the labyrinth (Cock's deformity). The child had several attacks of meningitis.

X-LINKED DEFORMITY

An association of X-linked mixed deafness with a stapes gusher (a profuse flow of perilymph or cerebrospinal fluid if the stapes is disturbed) has been recognized for 20 years. However, it is only recently that a distinct type of deformity has been recognized by imaging in some severely deaf men.[6] It would seem that the most important aspect of the deformity is deficient bone between the lateral end of the bulbous IAM and basal turn of the cochlea (Fig 6.21). This would preclude the insertion of a multichannel electrode as the deficient bone would almost certainly mean that the electrode would enter the IAM rather than staying in the cochlear coils. However, genetic studies have shown that there are at least two types of X-linked deafness[7] some of which have normal inner ears as shown by CT and are therefore suitable candidates for implantation.

The management of cerebrospinal fluid fistulae into the middle ear depends on a high degree of clinical suspicion. Perilabyrinthine fistulae are extremely rare and usually associated with normal hearing. Bone defects around the labyrinth may be shown by sophisticated bone imaging, but tracer cerebrospinal fluid contrast studies may be necessary to confirm the aural route. The commoner translabyrinthine type is almost always associated with labyrinthine dysplasia. Sensorineural deafness, or two unexplained attacks of meningitis, make CT study of the temporal bone mandatory. When a basal turn of normal calibre is associated with a distal sac, that is, a true Mondini deformity, then some hearing is possible and there is no risk of meningitis or a fistula (Fig 6.22). The 'large vestibular aqueduct syndrome' was a term first used by

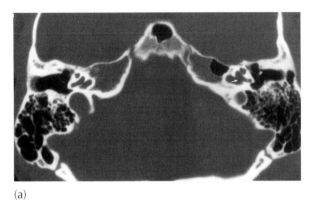 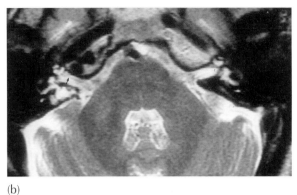

(a)   (b)

Fig 6.21 X-linked deafness deformity. (a) Axial CT section showing deficient bone between the end of the IAM and the basal turn of the cochlea (arrow). (b) Similar T1-weighted MR section showing the bilateral bony deficiency at the end of the IAM but demonstrating that the cochlear nerve is present (arrow).

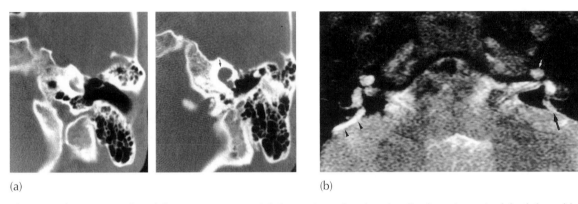

(a)   (b)

Fig 6.22 The true Mondini deformity. (a) Two axial CT sections showing the distal sac (arrow) of the left cochlea. (b) Axial FSE MR section showing the cochlear sac (white arrow), the normal nerves in the IAM and bilateral large vestibular aqueducts (black arrow). Note the enlarged endolymphatic sac (arrowheads).

Valvassori and Clemis[8] in 1978 to describe a condition of audiometric and vestibular symptoms in association with an abnormally wide vestibular aqueduct as demonstrated by sectional imaging, although the first description of a wide vestibular aqueduct was by Carlo Mondini in 1791[3] from the account of his dissection of the temporal bone of a boy born deaf. Valvassori and Clemis had been using polytomography for the investigation of sensorineural deafness. Their examination included sagittal sections that showed the vestibular aqueduct in its whole length. The measurements of the aqueduct were obtained in the midpoint of the post-isthmic segment, or halfway between the external aperture and common crus. An aqueduct was considered enlarged wherever its anteroposterior diameter was 1.5 mm or more. The usual way to assess a large vestibular aqueduct is now by multiple thin axial CT sections and pretargeted reformatting (Fig 6.8). Such measurements have little value from a management point of view except for the prognostic aspects for future cochlear implantation when progression of the deafness seems likely. We have shown recently that a large vestibular aqueduct is a more constant feature than a Mondini cochlea in Pendred's syndrome.

MIDDLE EAR DEFORMITIES

Radiology of congenital deformities of the middle and external ear relates almost exclusively to the prospects of improvement of conductive deafness. The size and shape of the middle ear cavity is the most important assessment to be made, especially if there is atresia of the EAM.

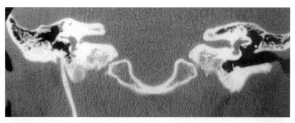

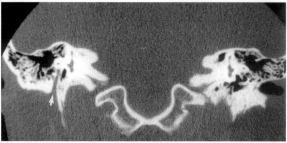

Fig 6.23 Typical unilateral atresia of the EAM. Two coronal CT sections showing the thick bony atretic plate, the air-containing middle ear cavity and anterior descending facial nerve canal (arrow).

In the majority of unilateral atresias with associated deformity of the pinna but no other congenital abnormality, there is a normally formed mastoid with good pneumatization and the middle ear cavity is of relatively normal shape (Fig 6.23). Even in the most severe deformities there is rarely complete absence of the middle ear and usually at least a slit-like hypotympanum can be shown lateral to the basal turn of the cochlea. The middle ear cavity may be reduced in size by encroachment of the atretic

plate laterally, by a high jugular bulb inferiorly or by descent of the tegmen superiorly. In craniofacial microsomia and mandibulofacial dysostosis, the attic and antrum are typically absent or slit-like, being replaced in varying degrees by solid bone or by descent of the tegmen.

If the middle ear cavity is air-containing, its shape and contents are relatively easy to assess. Frequently, however, the middle ear in congenital abnormalities contains undifferentiated mesenchyme, a thick glue-like substance that is radiologically indistinguishable from soft tissue or retained mucus. Thin bony septa may divide the middle ear cavity into two or more compartments.

Facial nerve

The next most important structure from a surgical point of view is the facial nerve. It is very rarely absent, although it might be hypoplastic. The main problem is aberration in the course of the nerve.

In early embryonic life, the developing VIIth cranial nerve lies anterior to the otocyst, so if development is arrested at this stage, a tract for the facial nerve is found anterior to a primitive otic sac. If development is arrested at a later stage, after the cochlea has formed to some extent, then the first part of the facial nerve is found in its usual situation above and lateral to the cochlea. The facial nerve is, therefore, relatively unaffected by developmental abnormalities of the labyrinth, and aberrations of the first part of the facial nerve canal are most unusual.

The course of the second and third parts is, however, dependent on normal development of the

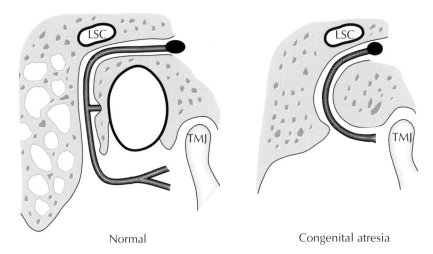

Normal   Congenital atresia

Fig 6.24 Line drawing based on sagittal section imaging of the course of the facial nerve in congenital deformities. LSC, lateral semicircular canal; TMJ, temporomandibular joint. (Reproduced with permission.[9])

branchial arches, the facial nerve being the nerve of the second arch. During its development and migration, the facial nerve curves behind the branchial cartilage to reach the anterior aspect of the same cartilage. At the same time, part of the cartilage adheres to the otic capsule to form the Fallopian canal. If, during development, the external pharyngeal groove of the first branchial arch is active, and atresia is only due to maldevelopment of the tympanic ring, then the second and third parts of the facial canal follow a relatively normal course (Fig 6.24).

The greater the deformity the more marked is the tendency for the facial nerve to follow a more direct route out into the soft tissues of the face. Exposed facial nerves in the middle ear cavity are the most common abnormalities recorded at surgery for congenital malformations. Usually the Fallopian canal is dehiscent but the descending segment may also be exposed, and overhang of the facial ridge with absence of the second genu is a usual finding in the Treacher Collins syndrome, making access to the oval window difficult for the surgeon. A short vertical segment of the facial canal and high stylomastoid foramen mean that the nerve turns forwards into the cheek in a high position.

In the preoperative radiological assessment the descending facial canal and its relationship to other structures must be demonstrated, preferably in lateral and coronal sections. Axial CT sections will show the descending canal in cross-section and identification is less certain. Grossly displaced nerves that cross the middle ear cavity are more difficult to identify, but there are two useful signs of aberrant pathways through the middle ear cavity.

- An exit foramen through the floor of the middle ear cavity or lateral atretic plate may be identified.
- Absence, at the back of the middle ear cavity, of the pyramidal eminence, which normally contains the stapedius muscle and tendon, is good presumptive evidence of an exposed facial nerve. Bifurcation of the descending portion of the facial nerve is far commoner with congenital malformations than in normal patients. The descending facial canal is often short (Fig 6.23).

Ossicles

A normal ossicular chain is rarely found when there is atresia of the external ear, but complete absence of the ossicles is also unusual. In most cases at least some vestige of the ossicular chain is evident. The ossicles are often thicker and heavier than normal or, less frequently, thin and spidery. They may be fixed to the walls of the middle ear cavity by bosses

of bone but the more usual deformity discovered at surgery is a fusion of the bodies of the malleus and incus. The ankylosis varies in degree and may be bony or fibrous. The radiological recognition of this ossicular union is difficult but is, in any case, not of great practical importance, and an irregular lump of bone in the middle ear cavity usually represents an ossicular mass.

Because of the partial or complete replacement of the tympanic membrane by a bony plate, the handle of the malleus is not surprisingly the part of the chain that is most often abnormal and most easily recognized. If the handle is absent, the 'molar tooth' appearance of the ossicles will no longer be evident in the lateral projection, and a triangular appearance of the ossicular mass will be seen. Often, the handle of the malleus is bent towards the atretic plate to which it may be fixed and this gives a typical L-shaped appearance to the ossicular mass. A slit-like attic so typical of Treacher Collins syndrome or an overhanging facial ridge may obstruct the free movement of the ossicular chain.

EXTERNAL AUDITORY MEATUS

In congenital deformities of the external ear, the EAM may be narrow, short, completely or partially atretic or it may run in an abnormal direction. It often slopes towards the middle ear and in such cases it may be curved in two planes, becoming more horizontal at its medial end. The obstruction in atresia may be due to soft tissue or bone but usually both are involved. The tympanic bone may be hyperplastic (rarely), deformed or absent.

The so-called atretic plate may therefore be composed partly of a deformed tympanic bone and partly of downwards and forwards extension of squamous temporal and mastoid bones, in which case it may be pneumatized.

Syndromes

It is not intended to discuss the radiological features of syndromic ear deformities except for the commonest and most important.

HEMIFACIAL MICROSOMIA

The ear lesions are usually bizarre and severe. The pinna is often represented by a small tag. Meatal atresia and middle ear abnormalities are almost constant findings and there may be gross descent of the tegmen to, or even below, the level of the lateral

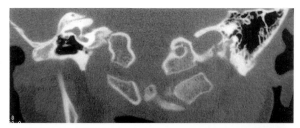

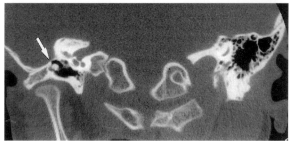

Fig 6.25 Hemifacial microsomia. Two coronal CT sections showing the gross descent of the tegmen, the deformed posteriorly placed temporomandibular joint and ossicular mass (arrow).

semicircular canal (Fig 6.25). Occasionally, some degree of hyperplasia of external ear structures, particularly the tympanic bone, occurs, but the mastoid is hypoplastic, and unpneumatized. The middle ear cavity is usually small, being encroached upon by the low tegmen and thick atretic plate. The ossicles in such case are absent or hypoplastic and malformed. Three of my patients had an ossicular mass displaced laterally, far from the oval window. This anomaly is only seen in cases of facial microsomia. The condition is not exclusively unilateral and often involves the bones of the skull base. Although if bilateral, there is always considerable dissymmetry between the two sides. This dissymmetry distinguishes the syndrome from Treacher Collins syndrome, with which it has often been confused in the past. There is no hereditary factor in craniofacial microsomia. It is the most common of the otocraniofacial syndromes.[10]

TREACHER COLLINS SYNDROME (MANDIBULOFACIAL DYSOSTOSIS)

The middle ear abnormalities in Treacher Collins syndrome are symmetrical and characteristic, although they may vary in severity.[11] The mastoid is unpneumatized and the attic and antrum are often reduced to slit-like proportions (Fig 6.26). Atresia of the EAM is a less constant feature and in 50 per cent of patients the meatus may be patent, although it tends to be curved, running upwards in

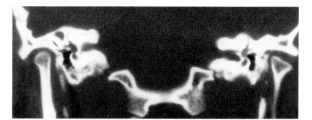

Fig 6.26 Coronal CT in Treacher Collins syndrome showing virtual absence of mastoid aeration.

its lateral part. Ossicular abnormalities are common and, in nearly all the operated ears in our series, the facial nerve followed a more direct path with opening out of the bends. It usually appeared at surgery as an overhanging facial ridge.

BRANCHIO-OTO-RENAL SYNDROME

Pedigrees of families with this distinctive syndrome indicate an autosomal dominant disorder with a high degree of penetrance. Any of the following anomalies may be present: auricular deformities, pre-auricular pits or sinuses, branchial fistulae or clefts, external meatal atresia and conductive or mixed hearing loss.[12] Lachrymal duct aplasia occurs rarely, but urinary tract anomalies are common. The base of the skull and petrous pyramids are somewhat distorted in this syndrome. Generally speaking, the petrous pyramids are short and point

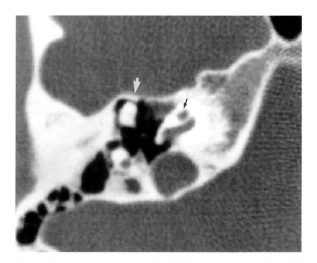

Fig 6.27 Branchio-oto-renal (BOR) syndrome. Axial CT section showing typical inner and middle ear deformities of BOR syndrome. The black arrow points to the small two-turn cochlea, the white arrow to the ossicular mass fixed to the anterior wall of the middle ear cavity.

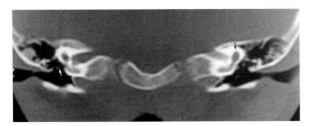

Fig 6.28 The CHARGE association. Coronal CT section at the level of the oval window and stapes (white arrow) showing absence of the semicircular canals (black arrow).

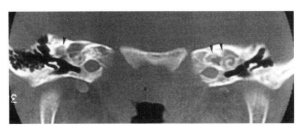

Fig 6.29 Osteogenesis imperfecta. Coronal CT section showing the patches of bone rarefaction in the petrous pyramid (arrow head).

upwards at their medial end, giving an upwards and backwards slant to the IAM, which appears rather short and bulbous. There is often dysplasia of the lateral semicircular canal, but of more importance is the small cochlea. This seems to have a reduced number of turns, but is not a truly Mondini-type deformity (Fig 6.27). The middle ear cavities are usually of reasonable size and air-containing, although bony atresia of the EAM may occur. The malleus and incus are usually mobile, though coarse and clumsy in shape. Minor anomalies of these ossicles are frequent, but the stapes is the ossicle usually affected, often with one crus only and fixation in the oval window, which may appear to be absent. The ossicles also appear to be more anteriorly situated than normal.

In theory such cases with a conductive hearing loss should be amenable to surgical improvement of the sound conductive mechanism, but unfortunately the results have been disappointing.

THE CHARGE ASSOCIATION

In 1981 Pagon *et al*.[13] applied the acronym CHARGE to an association of congenital defects that includes coloboma, heart disease, atresia of the nasal choanae, retarded development or CNS abnormalities, or both, genital hypoplasia and ear anomalies. There are now several published reports of the external ear malformations and hearing impairment in CHARGE association. The most characteristic feature is absence of the semicircular canals (Fig 6.28).[14]

BONE DYSPLASIAS

Deafness is a common childhood feature of the rare congenital generalized bony dysplasias. Only a brief account of the radiological features of osteogenesis imperfecta and of the dysplasias with increased bone density is given here.

Deafness in osteogenesis imperfecta tarda may be conductive, sensorineural or mixed.[15] The radiological appearance consists of demineralization in the labyrinthine capsule indistinguishable from otospongiosis but, in contrast to otospongiosis, which only affects the capsule, deficient ossification occurs in other sites in the petrous pyramid (Fig 6.29).

The osteopetroses are a group of uncommon genetic disorders that are characterized by increased skeletal density and abnormalities of bone modelling. Common to all of these disorders is a proclivity for involvement of the calvarium and skull base. An associated constellation of neurotological symptoms may result, presumably secondary to bony encroachment on the cranial foramina. Sectional imaging of the petrous temporal bones shows generalized sclerosis and narrowing of the IAM (Fig 6.30). Encroachment by bosses of bone in the attic may also be revealed.[16]

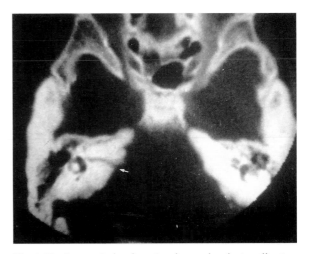

Fig 6.30 Congenital sclerosing bone dysplasia affecting the petrous pyramids and causing gross narrowing of the IAM (arrow). Note that the labyrinth is not affected.

References

1. Graham MD. The jugular bulb: its anatomic and clinical considerations in contemporary otology. *Archives of Otolaryngology* 1975; **101**:560–4.
2. Michel M. Memoire sur les anomalies congenitale de o'orielle interne. *Gazette Medicale de Strasbourg* 1863; **4**:55–8.
3. Mondini C. Anatomica surdi nati section. Bononiensi scientarium et artium instituto atque academic commentarii. *Bononiae* 1791; **VII**:419–28.
4. Phelps PD. Congenital cerebrospinal fluid fistulae of the petrous temporal bone. *Clinical Otolaryngology* 1986; **11**:79–92.
5. Phelps PD, Michaels L. The common cavity congenital deformity of the inner ear. *Journal of Oto-Rhino-Laryngology* 1995; **57**:228–31.
6. Phelps PD, Reardon W, Pembrey M, Bellman S, Luxon L. X-linked deafness, stapes gushers and a distinctive defect of the inner ear. *Neuroradiology* 1991; **33**:326–30.
7. Reardon W, Middleton-Price HR, Sandkuijl L, Phelps P, Bellman S, Luxon L, *et al.* A multipedigree linkage study of X-linked deafness: linkage to Xq13–q21 and evidence for genetic heterogeneity. *Genomics* 1991; **11**:885–94.
8. Valvassori GE, Clemis JD. Large vestibular aqueduct syndrome. *Laryngoscope* 1978; **88**:723–8.
9. Phelps PD, Lloyd GAS. *Diagnostic imaging of the ear, 2nd ed.* London: Springer–Verlag, 1990.
10. Phelps PD, Lloyd GAS, Poswillo D. The ear deformities in craniofacial microsomia and oculo-auriculovertebral dysplasia. *Journal of Laryngology and Otology* 1983; **97**:995–1005.
11. Phelps PD, Poswillo D, Lloyd GAS. The ear deformities in mandibulofacial dysostosis (Treacher Collins syndrome). *Clinical Otolaryngology* 1981; **6**:15–18.
12. Slack RWT, Phelps PD. Familial mixed deafness with branchial arch defects (earpits-deafness syndrome). *Clinical Otolaryngology* 1985; **10**:271–7.
13. Pagon RA, Graham JM, Zonana J, Yong S-L. Coloboma, congenital heart disease and choanal atresia with multiple anomalies: CHARGE association. *Journal of Paediatrics* 1981; **99**:223–7.
14. Morgan D, Bailey M, Phelps P, Bellman S, Grace A, Wyse R. Ear-nose-throat abnormalities in the CHARGE association. *Archives of Otolaryngology – Head and Neck Surgery* 1993; **119**:49–54.
15. Bergstrom LA. Osteogenesis imperfecta: otologic and maxillofacial aspects. *Laryngoscope* 1977; **87(suppl 1)**:87–9.
16. Beighton P, Sellars S. *Genetics and otology.* Edinburgh: Churchill Livingstone, 1982:80.

PART II

Principles of management

Section A

Hearing impairment

CHAPTER 7

Epidemiology of hearing impairment

ADRIAN DAVIS

Introduction

The drive towards establishing evidence-based medical practice has two main foci: establishing the burden of different pathological conditions and obtaining the evidence for cost-effectiveness of the interventions or services provided to remedy those conditions. Evidence-based medicine is an ideal that every practitioner might agree with to some extent, but it is not a panacea that can be used when needed and then discarded. The effort required to establish the evidence base is considerable and constantly needs updating. That effort is very worthwhile and will be seen as one of the major steps forward in establishing effective health care in the UK and throughout the world by means of the International Cochrane Collaboration.[1] This collaboration is named after Archie Cochrane, a doctor and an epidemiologist, whose insights into the effectiveness and efficiency of the health service in the UK two decades ago[2] have been the basis of the international drive to pool resources for randomized trials of effectiveness of treatments.

One of the substantive areas that interested Cochrane was that of the provision of hearing aids for those people who had a hearing problem.[2] This arose partly out of personal interest, but also because he had been involved in one of the first systematic epidemiological studies of hearing impairment in the UK.[3] Cochrane wrote about the tremendous gap between need for hearing aid services and the supply of services, particularly for elderly people with impaired hearing. He concluded that hearing aid services were 'inefficient because they were under-applied' and suggested that 'carefully designed

randomised control trials (RCTs) should be started to discover which old people benefit from which kind of help'. In the 25 years that have elapsed since then, the hearing aid service has improved, but these initial studies and those detailed below provide the current public health context in which services for those with hearing disability are still substantially underprovided.

The public health context needs a thorough consideration of the epidemiology of hearing impairments and disabilities as well as good independent information on the current service provision for those with a genuine health need. To inform public health priorities for prevention, early identification of need and rehabilitation, a national and a local epidemiology of hearing impairment and disability are required.

That epidemiology should have information on

- the prevalence and incidence of hearing impairment and disability as a function of severity and demographics
- the natural history of hearing impairment and its consequences
- the distribution of aetiology, and its change over time
- potential risk factors
- current service indicators, for example, the proportion of adults aged 60–69 years with a hearing aid, the outcome of intervention for tinnitus or the age of identification of permanent childhood hearing impairment.

This chapter divides the epidemiology of hearing impairment into three parts. Some of the concepts and terms used in the epidemiology of hearing impairment and disability are discussed. Then the five types of information that are needed for an informative epidemiology are discussed, first for adults and then for children.

The data that are presented here are taken from studies that the Institute of Hearing Research of the Medical Research Council of the UK has undertaken.[4–9] These studies include information from work done at other centres, but to keep the presentation simple in terms of its message, I will refer to other published work that has reviewed this literature.[10]

Terminology, definitions and methodology

The terminology and definitions used here are taken from the Audiological, Epidemiological and Genetic Definitions agreed by the European Union study group on the genetics of hearing impairment.[11] The major conceptual distinction I would like to emphasize is between the *prevalence* of hearing disorders and the *incidence* of hearing disorders. The *prevalence* of hearing impairment is the total number of instances of a specified degree and type of hearing impairment, for example an average air conduction hearing threshold in the better ear (over the frequencies 0.5, 1, 2 and 4 kHz) that is equal to or greater than 25 dB hearing loss (HL), in a given population at a specific time. *Prevalence* is often used to denote *prevalence rate*, that is, the percentage (or proportion) of the given population who have the defined characteristic. On the other hand the *incidence* of the defined degree of hearing impairment is the number of new cases of the defined condition occurring in the given population per unit time, for example 1 year. The incidence is not the number of new cases seen per year. Too often the term *incidence* is used when *prevalence* is meant.

A second emphasis is the need for population studies of hearing disorders. A population study is the study of a whole collection of units from which a sample may be drawn. Usually the population is a collection of individual people, but it could also be households, hearing aid clinics or hospitals. For instance, if we study a random sample of 1000 adults taken from the population of adults aged 71–80 years and we determine that 603 of this sample reach our criterion for hearing impairment (e.g. as stated above) then the *prevalence (or prevalence rate)* would be 60.3 per cent. We would try to quantify the accuracy in that prevalence rate by calculating the confidence interval[12] for the given sample. For the sample used in Davis[6] the *95 per cent confidence interval* for the estimated prevalence rate of 60.3 per cent was 52.9–67.3 per cent, using a stratified random sample of 272 people aged 71–80 years. This means that in a 100 replications of the work conducted on this population, with the same sample size and sampling method, we would expect 95 of the replications to have a prevalence estimate falling in the range 52.9–67.3 per cent.

It is useful to distinguish between the concepts of pathology, impairment, disability and handicap.[13–15] *Pathology* should be considered as an abnormality of the structure such as the middle ear, the cochlea, the stria vascularis et cetera. An *impairment* is a defect or abnormality of function of the auditory system that is normally measured by psychoacoustic or physiological function, for example pure tone hearing threshold, otoacoustic emission and brainstem response threshold to clicks. *Disability* is often a consequence of impairment and is the problem(s) that a person experiences or reports in basic tasks, for example difficulty communicating in a noisy environment or knowing who is speaking in a group conversation. *Handicap* arises from the disadvantage resulting from an impairment or disability that limits or even prevents a person from fulfilling a 'normal' role for that person, for example social isolation or extra effort in communicating. An indicator of handicap may be obtained by using a questionnaire to measure an individual's quality of life.

In talking and writing about hearing disorders it is often useful to distinguish between two types of hearing impairment. The majority of permanent impairments are *sensorineural*, that is they are related to disease of deformity of the cochlea or cochlear nerve. In these individuals there is no 'air–bone gap' (over the average thresholds for the frequencies 0.5, 1 and 2 kHz). It is suggested that if the difference between the air conduction and the bone conduction average thresholds is less than 15 dB, and the average hearing impairment on the ear is 25 dB HL or greater (over the frequencies 0.5, 1, 2 and 4 kHz) then an individual can be presumed to have a *sensorineural* pathology, whereas if the air–bone gap is 15 dB or greater the individual has a significant *conductive* pathology contributing to the impairment. This is a working definition rather than a prescriptive one, because the extent to which the middle ear might be involved in any impairment depends on a number of factors. Thus the air–bone gap tells us something important, but not everything. The pathology is important because *conductive* impairments may be amenable to surgical intervention to ameliorate the pathology and reduce the impairment. On the other hand, *sensorineural* impairments of a mild to severe type are not yet amenable to surgical or medical intervention, and the intervention of choice is rehabilitation centred around the use of a personal hearing aid, which aims to reduce the disability (and therefore, one would hope, handicap) and increase the quality of life. Profound or total hearing impairment may be amenable to intervention using cochlear implants.[16]

In considering health care provision (e.g. interventions through which patients or their families benefit) and the concepts given above, there is a need to distinguish three further concepts: need, demand for services and supply of services. Furthermore we should not consider that everyone who demands a service actually needs it, or that all services that are provided actually benefit those in need.[17] A pragmatic definition of need[18] used here is the ability of groups in the population to benefit from intervention (usually health, social or educational). So those with a substantial conductive impairment may have a need for surgery to improve the middle ear's conduction of sound, those with annoying tinnitus may have a need for tinnitus counselling, those with a sensorineural hearing impairment may have a need for rehabilitative training using a personal hearing aid, the whole population may have a need to be screened at around birth for sensorineural hearing impairment, and the list could be extended very easily. Providers of health care have to enter into dialogue with society (usually through those who purchase health care) to decide the priority given to the hearing health care needs of the population. The major inputs into these priority decisions should be the epidemiology (i.e. distribution and determinants) of hearing disorders, which will be modified by the national and local realities, such as the configuration of present services and the cost-effectiveness of the different services provided. The rest of this chapter concentrates on the general epidemiological data.[6,9]

Prevalence of hearing disorders in adults

About 20 per cent of the total adult population (18 years and over) of the UK has a hearing impairment of 25 dB HL or greater in the better hearing ear (using an average threshold over the frequencies 0.5, 1, 2 and 4 kHz). This figure is true for the population profile in 1993[6] and is similar to previous estimates.[2,3] Thus there are 8.580 million people in the UK with impaired hearing at this level and beyond, of whom about one-quarter are over 80 years of age and three-quarters over 60 years of age. For moderate hearing impairments (45 dB HL or

greater) there are 2.94 million people of whom 45 per cent are over 80 and 84 per cent are over 60 years of age. For more severe levels of impairment, there are probably about 898 thousand people with severe hearing impairments (65 dB HL or greater) and about 150 thousand adults with profoundly impaired hearing (95 dB HL or greater), of whom about one-tenth may have had the profound impairment from childhood, but nine-tenths acquired their impairment in adulthood.

In terms of self-reported disability, 26 per cent of the population said that they had great difficulty hearing what was said against a background noise, whereas only 10 per cent reported some difficulty in a quiet environment on the better ear, with 19 per cent reporting some difficulty in quiet on their worse ear. This compares with 30 per cent who have at least one ear hearing impaired, 20 per cent with two ears impaired, 12 per cent with their better ear at 35 dB HL or worse and 7 per cent with their better ear at 45 dB HL or worse (all average thresholds as defined above).

Incidence of hearing impairments

There are very few studies on the incidence of hearing impairment in the population.[19] But from the cross-sectional data in Great Britain the derived incidence of mild hearing impairment (25 dB HL or worse) is 1 per cent per annum in middle age (45–55 years) increasing to about 1.5 per cent per annum in older ages. The incidence of moderate impairments (45 dB HL or worse) is about 1 per cent per annum between ages 65–75 years in the British and Danish populations. The natural history of sensorineural hearing impairment in the adult population is also difficult to establish, but most longitudinal studies suggest that it is slow erosion of hearing functions that occurs, although in a small proportion of people there can be catastrophic impairments in a short period of time, for example corresponding to acute vascular incidents.

Aetiology of hearing impairments

Table 7.1 shows the prevalence of hearing impairment as a function of the pathology, and give some impression of the different major aetiologies of hearing impairment and how they change with age

Table 7.1 The prevalence (%) of different types and degrees of hearing impairment as a function of age group

Age group (years)	Impairment criterion ≥25 dB HL			Impairment criterion ≥45 dB HL		
	SNHL	Conductive	Percentage conductive	SNHL	Conductive	Percentage conductive
18–40	1.5	0.4	21%	0.2	0.1	33%
41–60	10.7	3.1	22%	1.6	1.3	45%
61–80	42.0	3.8	8%	7.8	2.8	26%
18–80	13.8	2.1	13%	2.4	1.1	31%

Note that data only report on those aged 18–80 years. HL, hearing loss; SNHL, sensorineural hearing loss. (Reproduced with permission.[6])

or time. Two severities of hearing impairment have been chosen to show that the distribution of aetiology changes not only with age but also with severity of impairment that is considered. Overall, 13 per cent of the hearing impairments that are mild or worse have a conductive component, in which the conductive component is defined as at least 15 dB air–bone gap. It is hardly surprising that the percentage in those with a moderate degree of impairment or worse is greater at 31 per cent. Conductive impairments are therefore a considerable burden on the population of people with greater degrees of hearing impairment, although the older the cohort the smaller the contribution from the conductive pathologies. Thus although 7.8 per cent of the 61–80 years age group had a sensorineural hearing impairment, there were 2.8 per cent who had an impairment with a conductive component of at least 15 dB air–bone gap. The question as to whether surgery or a hearing aid rehabilitation regime is the most cost-effective is one that has not yet been appropriately investigated.

Risk factors

The major factor affecting the prevalence of hearing impairment is age, with smaller contributions coming from gender, occupational group and occupational noise exposure.[4] Table 7.2 shows the effect of age on the prevalence of hearing impairment at three degrees of severity and also on tinnitus prevalence. The prevalence of profound hearing impairment is a difficult quantity to measure accurately as even with a sample of 10 000 one might expect, from Table 7.2, only 34 such people, of whom maybe 14 would be over 80 years of age. The potential for biases to be present in these types of studies is quite high, because it is

possible that not only are such people reluctant to come to an institute of hearing research to have their hearing tested, but they may not live randomly in the population. The older profoundly impaired people may live in sheltered housing and the younger may live in particular geographical areas. A different sort of study might be needed to enumerate this particular population fully. However, our study can be presumed to show the lower limit of the estimate for profound impairments and, despite variability in estimates over the 18–80 year olds, these impairments do seem to be greater in those over 80 years old. For the 18–80 year age group the 95 per cent confidence interval for the prevalence of profound bilateral impairments was 1–5 per thousand.

In terms of mild and moderate impairments, the estimates are probably less biased and more valid. These show that the major increases in prevalence start at 50 years of age and above. There is a 10 per cent increase in prevalence of ≥25 dB HL impairments between the 41–50 years age group and the 51–60 years age group and each successive age group increases at a greater rate. A similar pattern is seen with the ≥45 dB HL impairments, with one in 13 people having this degree of impairment at age 61–70 years.

The prevalence of tinnitus, which is here defined as noises in the head or ears lasting for over 5 minutes and not only after loud noise (reported elsewhere as prolonged spontaneous tinnitus – PST), including those who have undefined tinnitus that usually lasts for over 5 minutes, is also shown in Table 7.2. Tinnitus prevalence increases with age, although not as relentlessly as hearing impairment, and becomes a stable 20 per cent at about 60 years. The major predictors of tinnitus are concerned with the hearing impairment,[20] and tinnitus and hearing disability are found to influence quality of life adversely.[21,22]

Table 7.2 The prevalence (%) of different degrees of hearing impairment in the better ear averaged over the frequencies 0.5, 1, 2 and 4 kHz as a function of age in the GB population

Degree of impairment in the better hearing ear	Age group (years)							
	18–30	31–40	41–50	51–60	61–70	71–80	81+	Overall
≥25 dB HL	1.8	2.8	8.2	18.9	36.8	60.3	93.4	19.8
≥45 dB HL	0.2	1.1	1.7	4.0	7.4	17.6	63.6	6.8
≥95 dB HL	0.0	0.6	0.1	0.1	0.6	0.1	3.7	0.34
Possess a hearing aid	0.5	0.8	1.9	3.0	6.6	13.7	25.6	4.0
Tinnitus report	6.4	8.4	11.3	14.8	19.8	19.9	19.7	12.3

Service indicators

Table 7.2 also shows the proportion of the population who possess a hearing aid. This figure reflects the product of effort given by providers such as general practitioners, ear, nose and throat surgeons and audiologists and is not necessarily the best index of the rehabilitative benefit. Overall, just under 4 per cent of the population say that they have (or have had) a hearing aid compared with the 6.8 per cent who have a moderate hearing impairment, which is about one-fifth of those who have any hearing impairment. Davis *et al.*[23] and Stephens *et al.*[24] show that those who are fitted with a hearing aid in a proactive manner (through screening programmes) and those with a hearing impairment of ≥25 dB HL do get material benefit from a hearing aid. Thus there is substantial under-provision of hearing rehabilitation centred around personal hearing aids. The cost of providing hearing aids even for only a small proportion of those who would benefit is substantial. Furthermore, the overheads in maintaining an enlarged pool of hearing aid users would also be substantial, as two-thirds of hearing aid centre activity is concerned with maintaining current users.[25]

There is considerable 'need' in the adult population as a result of hearing impairment. Although only 1.1 per cent per annum of the adult population consult a hospital specialist about their hearing, about one-quarter of these people are offered an operation and another quarter are offered a hearing aid. Almost one in five people who consult at this level are very dissatisfied with the outcome of their appointment. This compares with only one in 20 who consult their family doctor about a hearing difficulty.

Prevalence of hearing impairment in children

This section will be concerned only with permanent childhood hearing impairment (PCHI) and not with fluctuating impairments due to acute and chronic secretory otitis media.[26] A major study of PCHI has recently been completed in the Trent region of the UK. This region has about 4.8 million people and a typical distribution of ethnic minorities and occupational groups. Fortnum *et al.*[9] report the prevalence of hearing impairment. Their data are shown in Table 7.3, which indicates the prevalence rate per 100 000 live births for all impairments ≥40 dB HL (i.e. including acquired, progressive and late-onset losses) and

Table 7.3 Prevalence per 100 000 live births of permanent hearing impairment ≥40 dB hearing loss (HL) for birth cohorts from 1985 to 1990, for all impairments and for congenital impairments only, for three degrees of severity of congenital impairment (moderate, 40–69 dB HL; severe, 70–94 dB HL; and profound, ≥95 dB HL) and for congenital sensorineural impairments

Impairment type and severity	Prevalence per 100 000	95% confidence interval
All ≥40 dB HL	133	122–145
Congenital ≥40 dB HL	112	101–123
40–69 dB HL	65	56–73
70–94 dB HL	23	19–29
≥95 dB HL	24	20–30

for congenital losses alone (i.e. equivalent to incidence) for four degrees of severity of impairment: ≥40 dB HL, 40–69 dB HL (moderate), 70–94 dB HL (severe) and ≥95 dB HL (profound). The confidence intervals have been calculated according to the logistic distribution model because of the very low values of the prevalences.

The prevalence of all PCHI ≥40 dB HL is 133 per 100 000 and for congenital impairments only is 112 per 100 000. The prevalence of profound impairments that are congenital is of the order of one in 4000 births.

For congenital impairments the incidence is equivalent to the prevalence. However, there are a number of children, 21 per 100 000, who have either a progressive or an acquired hearing impairment. By the age of about 5 years the proportion of the profoundly hearing impaired that have acquired impairments, mostly through meningitis, is about 20 per cent. The proportion of children with a progressive hearing impairment is not known very accurately, but may be up to 15–25 per cent of those who have a PCHI at the age of 5 years;[27] however, the present study only finds about 10 per cent of PCHI to be progressive.

Aetiology of childhood hearing impairments and major risk factors

The major aspect concerning the aetiology of congenital PCHI is that there are a considerable number of cases with no ascribed aetiology (41 per cent). The proportion of children who have an aetiology with no genetic cause is 19 per cent, which leaves 40 per cent with an aetiology that has been given a genetic cause. Of the total number of children with a stated genetic cause, a dominant genetic inheritance is found in only about 6 per cent and 30 per cent have a stated syndrome.

There were three major risk factors associated with the hearing impairments. The first and most important was a history of staying in the neonatal intensive care unit (NICU), which was 29 per cent. The second was a family history of hearing impairment (after excluding those who had an NICU history) at 26 per cent, and the third was the presence of a craniofacial abnormality noticeable at birth (after excluding those with an NICU or family history), which was 4 per cent. Altogether 59 per cent of those with PCHI had a risk factor that might be used as the basis of a targeted neonatal screen. Others have found a higher proportion[5,8,28] and so this may be something that varies over districts, regions or countries.[7]

Service indicators for PCHI

There are very few studies that look at the overall benefit derived from identifying children with congenital hearing impairments and starting them on a programme of habilitation. The major focus over the past 20 years has been concerned with reducing the age of identification and hearing aid fitting. The National Deaf Children's Society (NDCS) quality standard guidelines[29] apply to children with an average hearing impairment of bilateral ≥50 dB HL (0.5, 1, 2 and 4 kHz) and suggest that 40 per cent of the children with PCHI should be identified by 6 months of age and 80 per cent by 12 months. In the current study only 14 per cent (95 per cent confidence interval 8–18 per cent) were identified by the age of 6 months and only 42 per cent by the age of 12 months.

Table 7.4 shows the distribution of ages for significant events in the rehabilitation chain: referral, confirmation of the hearing impairment and hearing aid fitting. For overall severities the age referral was 10 months at the median, with 30 per cent aged less than 8 months at referral and 10 per cent aged 2 months at referral. It can be seen that the severe and profound impairments are referred earlier and 'diagnosed' earlier than moderate impairments; for those with moderate impairments the median age at referral is 18 months, and age at hearing aid fitting is 43 months. The data are reasonably encouraging, but for the higher percentiles there are still 30 per cent of children with hearing impairments who have not been referred before about 23 months and a similar number who are almost 4 years of age before they are fitted with a hearing aid. The delays between referral and fitting are indicative of the long time it takes for some children to be 'diagnosed'. Some of these delays are inevitable. However, many children are kept without amplification while a conductive impairment is ruled out and inevitably this leads to considerable delays that could be reduced considerably by having a hearing aid while waiting for the operation.[9]

The age at referral reflects the service reality that during 1985–90 the targeted neonatal screening services in the region were starting up and that the mainstay of identifying children with permanent childhood hearing impairment was the health visitor distraction test (HVDT). The performance of these tests is discussed elsewhere,[30,31] with the yield coming from the HVDT being much lower than expected and the sensitivity very dependent on the severity of the hearing impairment.[9] The more systematic use of neonatal hearing screening may substantially improve the age at referral, 'diagnosis'

Table 7.4 The mean and selected percentiles of the distribution of the age (months) of referral, confirmation of hearing impairment ('diagnosis') and hearing aid fitting, as a function of severity of the hearing impairment, for birth cohorts between 1985 and 1990 who have a congenital hearing impairment

Age at key points in identification and rehabilitation	Severity group	Mean	Percentiles				
			10	30	50	70	90
Age at referral	Overall	19	2	8	10	23	47
Age at 'diagnosis'	Overall	26	5	11	17	37	59
Age at aid fitting	Overall	32	9	16	27	44	63
Age at referral	40–69 dB HL	25	3	9	18	39	55
Age at referral	70–94 dB HL	13	3	7	9	12	34
Age at referral	≥95 dB HL	9	1	5	8	10	19
Age at 'diagnosis'	40–69 dB HL	35	9	16	35	46	65
Age at 'diagnosis'	70–94 dB HL	17	3	8	11	19	42
Age at 'diagnosis'	≥95 dB HL	11	3	7	10	13	21
Age at aid fitting	40–69 dB HL	42	14	29	43	51	70
Age at aid fitting	70–94 dB HL	24	8	14	18	29	50
Age at aid fitting	≥95 dB HL	14	6	9	12	17	24

and fitting of hearing aids for those with congenital PCHI. Children with substantial other risk factors, such as parental anxiety concerning language development or meningitis ought to seek a diagnostic appointment at the first opportunity.[32]

Summary and implications for service provision

The public health priority of hearing impairments and tinnitus in adults should be substantially higher than it presently appears, because hearing disorders constitute the most prevalent chronic impairment in the population, with over 8 million people in the UK (i.e. about 20 per cent) having an impairment. The situation has not changed substantially since Cochrane's assessment in 1971.[2]

The major factor associated with this high prevalence is age, with noise being the chief preventable factor, especially in young people. Because age is the major factor, the whole population prevalence of hearing impairments will increase over the next 20 years by up to 20 per cent because of the demographics of the population.[17]

Early identification of those with chronic but progressive impairment is not currently being achieved, even of those with substantial impair-

ments, by the mainly reactive hearing services and hence provision of services substantially lags behind need. Furthermore, the service is not inspiring people to use their hearing aids, as only about 40–50 per cent are used most of the time.

The implications of this global epidemiology are that, in the UK and almost certainly in every developed country, there is a substantial underprovision of services for hearing disabled people. This could be met by the use of a proactive screening service.[2,11,23] People with hearing disability and tinnitus have a significantly worse quality of life,[21] which can be ameliorated by the appropriate use of rehabilitation, such as the use of a hearing aid for most of the time.[22]

For children the public health priority stems on the one hand from the high burden that the condition confers on a relatively small proportion of the population (about 850 children per year in the UK) with a prevalence of 112 per 100 000 births for the congenital hearing impaired with average thresholds of 40 dB HL or greater, and on the other from the very high cost of interventions such as cochlear implants and educational training for the profoundly impaired (24 per 100 000 births).

We are still considerably in the dark with respect to the full story of the aetiology of hearing impairments in children; however, three risk factors (NICU history, family history of childhood deafness and craniofacial abnormalities) cover over 50 per cent of the population of congenitally hearing impaired children. There are very few children with rubella as an aetiology (<5 per cent) and so the main scope for prevention may be in understanding why children with an NICU history develop hearing impairment. The understanding of genetic impairments should also be a major priority.

In terms of service development, the wider use of neonatal screening to identify and habilitate hearing impaired children with the least delay should be given urgent public health attention.[33]

Although both adult and child epidemiology have come out in favour of systematically screening the population for congenital and then later acquired hearing impairment, the precondition for this screening to be successful is that an appropriately staffed and cost-effective service is available for those who do not pass the screen. These important diagnostic and rehabilitative services are discussed elsewhere in this book (Chapters 8 and 9).

References

1. *The Cochrane Collaboration, vol 1 [CD].* London: British Medical Journal, 1996.
2. Cochrane AL. *Effectiveness and efficiency. Random reflections on Health Services.* London: The Nuffield Provincial Trust, 1971.
3. Hinchcliffe R. Prevalence of the commoner ear, nose and throat conditions in the adult rural population of Great Britain. *British Journal of Preventative and Social Medicine* 1961; **15**:128–40.
4. Davis AC. The prevalence of hearing impairment and reported hearing disability among adults in Great Britain. *International Journal of Epidemiology* 1989; **18**:911–7.
5. Davis AC, Wood S. The epidemiology of childhood hearing impairment: factors relevant to planning of services. *British Journal of Audiology* 1992; **26**:77–91.
6. Davis AC. *Hearing in adults.* London: Whurr, 1995.
7. Davis AC, Parving A. Towards appropriate epidemiological data on childhood hearing disability: a comparative European study on birth cohorts 1982–88. *Journal of Audiological Medicine* 1994; **3**:35–47.
8. Davis A, Wood S, Rowe S, Webb H, Healey R. Risk factors for hearing disorders: epidemiologic evidence of change over time in the UK. *Journal of the American Academy of Audiology* 1995; **6**:365–70.
9. Fortnum HM, Davis A, Butler A, Stevens J. *Health Service implications of changes in aetiology and referral patterns of hearing-impaired children in Trent 1985–93. Report to Trent Region NHS Executive.* Nottingham: MRC Institute of Hearing Research, 1996.
10. Davis AC. Public Health aspects of paediatric audiology relevant to screening children's hearing. In: B McCormick ed. *Paediatric audiology 0–5, 2nd ed.* London: Whurr, 1993:1–41.
11. Stephens D, Davis A, Reed A. *Audiological, epidemiologiccal and genetic definitions. Report on workshop of European Working Groups I and II on genetics of hearing impairment.* Ferrara: HEAR European Union Concerted Action, 1996.
12. Gardner MJ, Altman DG. *Statistics with confidence.* London: British Medical Journal, 1989.
13. World Health Organization: *International classification of impairments, disabilities and handicap.* Geneva: World Health Organization, 1980.
14. Davis AC. Hearing disorders in the population: first phase findings of the MRC national study of hearing. In: Lutman ME, Haggard MP eds. *Hearing science and hearing disorders.* London: Academic Press, 1983.
15. Stephens D, Hetu R. Impairment, disability and handicap in audiology: towards a consensus. *Audiology* 1991; **30**:185–200.
16. Summerfield AQ, Marshall DH. *Cochlear implantation in the UK 1990–1994. Report by the MRC Institute of Hearing Research of the evaluation of the National Cochlear Implant Programme.* London: HMSO, 1995.
17. Davis A. Epidemiology. In: Stephens SDG ed. *Adult audiology.* London: Butterworth-Heinemann, 1997. (Kerr A ed. *Scott–Brown's Otolaryngology, 6th ed*; vol 2.)
18. Doyal L, Gough I. *A theory of human need.* Basingstoke: Macmillan Education, 1991.
19. Davis AC, Ostri B, Parving A. Longitudinal study of hearing. *Acta Otolaryngologica* 1991; **482 (suppl)**:103–9.
20. Davis A. The aetiology of tinnitus: risk factors for tinnitus in the UK population – a possible role for conductive pathologies? In: Reich GE, Vernon JA eds. *Proceedings of the Fifth International Tinnitus Seminar.* Portland, OR: American Tinnitus Association, 1996.
21. Davis AC, Roberts H. Tinnitus and health status: SF-36 profile and accident prevalence. In: Reich GE, Vernon JA eds. *Proceedings of the Fifth International Tinnitus Seminar.* Portland, OR: American Tinnitus Association, 1996.
23. Davis AC, Stephens SDG, Rayment A, Thomas K. Hearing impairments in middle age: the acceptability benefit and cost of detection (ABCD). *British Journal of Audiology* 1992; **26**:1–14.
24. Stephens SDG, Callaghan DE, Hogan S, Meredith R, Rayment A, Davis AC. Hearing disability in people 50–65: effectiveness and acceptability of early rehabilitative intervention. *British Medical Journal* 1990; **200**:508–11.
25. Davis AC. Costing an adult hearing aid service. *British Society of Audiology News* 1996; **19**:4–6.
26. Haggard MP, Hughes EG. *Screening children's hearing.* London: HMSO, 1991.
27. Stevens J, Webb H. Targeted hearing screening in neonates – comparison of follow-up with neonatal results. *Audiens (BACDA Newsletter)* 1995; **April**:4.
28. Sutton GJ, Rowe SJ. Risk factors for childhood sensorineural hearing loss in the Oxford Region. *British Journal of Audiology* 1997; **31**:39–54.

29. *Quality standards in paediatric audiology, vol 1.* London: NDCS, 1994.

30. Lutman ME, Davis AC, Fortnum HM, Wood S. Field sensitivity of targeted neonatal hearing screening by transient otoacoustic emissions. *Ear and Hearing* 1997; [In press].

31. Wood S, Davis AC, McCormick B. Changing performance of the health visitor distraction test when targeted neonatal screening is introduced into a health district. *British Journal of Audiology* 1997; **31**:55–61.

32. *Quality standards in paediatric audiology, vol 2.* London: NDCS, 1996.

33. Davis A, Bamford J, Wilson I, Ramkalawan T, Forshaw M, Wright S. A critical review of neonatal screening in the detection of congenital hearing impairment. *Health Technology Assessment* 1997; **1**(10).

CHAPTER 8

Principles of treatment of hearing impairment

DAFYDD STEPHENS

Introduction

Although hearing loss in adults is very common (see Chapter 7), only a very small proportion of those cases seen in audiological and otological clinics are amenable to medical or surgical treatment that will restore normal hearing. Audiological rehabilitation is therefore the normal choice of management for such individuals. Even in patients who do show some improvement in their hearing after surgical or pharmacological intervention, the residual hearing loss usually found will require rehabilitative management, either in relation to the intervention or sometime later.

The reasons for this lack of success of medical or surgical treatment are various. Most hearing loss is of cochlear origin and, at present, established cochlear damage is usually irreversible, although work on hair cell regeneration may alter the picture in the future. Many causes of such hearing loss are not identified, although the proportion for which a cause can be found is greater with increased attention to the personal and family history and to some general medical investigations.

Much hearing loss is caused by irreversible damage from noise and physical trauma, viral infections and chemotherapeutic agents. It is also commonly caused by genetic factors, often with late onset or progressive hearing loss. Here, however, molecular genetics is advancing rapidly in terms of gene identification, although in due course we are more likely to be dealing therapeutically with the prevention of the development of the condition or arresting its progress rather than reversing established hearing loss.

Perhaps the biggest problem is that the onset of most hearing loss is insidious, slowly progressive and associated with a stigma in most societies. Consequently, the patient generally does not present to the clinician until some 10–20 years after the onset of the loss, by which time even most potentially treatable conditions have become largely irreversible. Finally, the average age of patients presenting for the first time to clinics with hearing loss is 70 years, many of whom have systemic diseases that may preclude surgical or pharmacological intervention for their hearing loss. Consequently, although I shall briefly consider some aspects of pharmacological treatment of hearing loss, aspects of surgical treatment (middle ear surgery, bone-anchored hearing aids and cochlear implants) are dealt with in other chapters of this book, and I shall largely concentrate on the rehabilitative management of hearing impaired individuals.

From a rehabilitative standpoint we must first consider what we are trying to achieve. Audiological rehabilitation can be defined as 'a problem solving process aimed at the minimising of disability and handicap consequent to the hearing loss'. Our patients are not concerned whether we achieve a good surgical or pharmacological result in the treatment of their hearing loss if it does not reduce the problems from which they suffer. They rarely come to a clinic complaining of a specific hearing loss (impairment) unless they have failed a screening test at work. What makes them consult a doctor is the handicap experienced – the effect of their hearing loss on their life.

Within this chapter I shall follow the World Health Organization[1] definitions of disablements as applied to audiology by Stephens and Hétu.[2] In these, *impairment* is the abnormal function of the hearing mechanism that can be measured psychophysically (e.g. pure tone audiograms) or electrophysiologically (e.g. brainstem auditory evoked potentials). *Disability* encompasses the hearing difficulties experienced by the patient in their life (e.g. a problem hearing in noisy places) and is usually tapped by interview and questionnaire. *Handicap* describes the effects of the hearing loss on the patient's life (e.g. social withdrawal, loss of employment) and again is determined by interview of the patient and by questionnaire, which may be supplemented by questioning the patient's 'significant others'. Significant Others are those people – spouse or partner, children, parents, carers – who play an important part in the patient's life. In some cases, particularly in those of children and of dependent adults, the significant others may play a dominant role.

The development of handicap through the interactions between the patient, their Significant Others, their environment, their occupation and their lifestyle has been discussed at length elsewhere.[3] In this context it must be borne in mind that Significant Others may have both alleviating and aggravating roles in the context of the development of handicap. There will be interactions, too, with the patient's underlying personality, which may furthermore lessen the handicap through the patient's perception of positive experiences arising from the hearing loss (such as not hearing disturbing sounds such as traffic at night or providing an excuse to avoid activities they dislike).

This development of handicap is summarized in Figure 8.1 which also includes a feedback loop by which changes in handicap, such as changes in a work, family or social situation, can lead to a behavioural change that results in a change in disability. It must be emphasized that development of handicap is a dynamic process that alters all the time with changes in the individual's life. Thus it can be aggravated by increased hearing loss, onset of tinnitus, working in a noisy environment, stress, et cetera and ameliorated by factors such as rehabilitative intervention, improved environment or new caring relationships.

The starting point

The first clinician to see a patient referred with hearing difficulties is confronted with the patient's problems: 'Why do I have hearing problems? Will it get worse? What can be done about it? Do I need a hearing aid?'

The evaluation of the patient will endeavour to answer these questions. They will not necessarily be evaluated separately, there being a large overlap between the elements of the evaluation for diagnostic and rehabilitative purposes, particularly for the onset and progress of the hearing loss and its measurement. There is also an important interaction between the two. Generally speaking, individuals are better prepared to accept the presence and irreversibility of their hearing loss if they know its cause.

Arriving at a specific diagnosis will be achieved using a variety of approaches: careful history taking, examination and audiometry, together with haematological, microbiological, immunological and biochemical investigations and appropriate imaging. In some cases the results will be clear cut. In others the best that can be achieved is the balance of probability of a cause, and it has been argued that this is important for the patient's acceptance, even if it is not as definite as would be liked from a medicoscientific standpoint. By this means

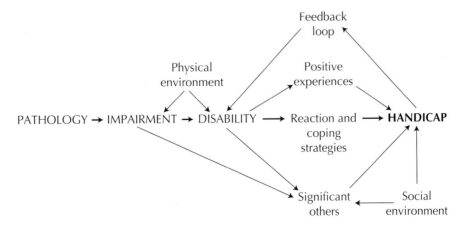

Fig 8.1 Simplified mechanism of the development of handicap.

the patient can be given a better idea of the likely prognosis, even though audiological prognostics is a crude art. If the aetiology is not clear, often the best we can offer are the results from the longitudinal component of the British Medical Research Council's National Study of Hearing (see Chapter 7), which indicates a mean progression of hearing loss of 0.8 dB/year, although there is much variability.

The approach to patient's questions about rehabilitation depends very much on the patient themself. As was stated earlier, rehabilitation with or without a hearing aid depends upon the patient's disability and handicap and should not be attempted should the patient be resistant to such an approach or deny any disability.

Should the patient be uncertain and the clinician feel sure that rehabilitative intervention would help, some gentle persuasion may be used, but care must be taken that the individual patient does not feel threatened by this nor feel obliged to accept intervention 'to keep the doctor happy'.

Pharmacological treatment

Drugs have been used in the treatment of hearing loss that stems from problems in the outer ear (wax), middle ear (otitis media and otosclerosis), inner ear and brainstem (vertebrobasilar ischaemia). The generally disappointing results in inner ear conditions have recently been reviewed by McKee[4] and will be discussed below. The role of drugs in otitis media with effusion are considered elsewhere in this book, as is the possible role of fluoride in the management of otosclerosis.

Cerumen, or wax, as a possible but exaggerated cause of hearing loss is generally seen and dealt with by primary physicians (general practitioners). A variety of softening agents ranging from olive oil and sodium bicarbonate to proprietary cerumenolytics have been assessed in a variety of studies and there appears to be little to choose between them. Furthermore, as dissolving agents, aqueous solutions, such as 0.5 per cent decussate sodium and 5–10 per cent sodium bicarbonate, again each have their advocates with little difference in their effectiveness.

The medical treatment of acute auditory failure or sudden hearing loss (usually cochlear) has followed a variety of approaches, including glucocorticoids (steroids), carbogen (5 per cent CO_2 in 95 per cent O_2), vasodilators, anticoagulants and plasma expanders, each having its supporters. There are several problems here. First, sudden hearing loss is not a disease in itself, but the consequence of a variety of conditions such as infections, vascular, immunological or neoplastic disease, endolymphatic hydrops or labyrinthine window rupture. Treatment is often initiated before reasonable attempts have been made to arrive at a definitive diagnosis.

Second, as sudden hearing loss is rarely regarded by the patient or their primary physicians as a medical emergency, days or weeks may elapse before the patient is seen in the clinic and appropriately investigated and managed. This means that the likelihood of effective treatment is reduced in those cases amenable to such treatment.

Third, response rates will depend on the severity of the hearing loss, with a poorer prognosis for those patients with a more severe hearing loss. Many studies fail to control for this. This is perhaps because any individual physician or surgeon sees only small numbers of these patients.

Finally, the natural remission rate is high, reportedly up to 65 per cent in some studies, although this again depends on the severity of the hearing loss.

Because of all these complicating factors, no consistent results have been found across the reported controlled studies, and there is a need for a well controlled multicentre study accompanied by publicity to primary physicians to ensure early and rapid referral.

Treatment of treponemal hearing loss caused by syphilis involves therapy with antibiotics in the early stage or with a combination of antibiotics and steroids in the late stage. This approach may prevent progress of the disease but rarely results in a significant improvement in hearing. One of the difficulties faced in current studies is the often concomitant HIV infection, which may in itself cause a hearing loss. On the other hand, Lyme disease (caused by *Borrelia burgdorferi*), which can also result in a hearing loss, is more amenable to antibiotic therapy, which can result in an improvement in hearing thresholds.

In most other infectious conditions, such as forms of meningitis, drugs may be used in the prophylaxis of the conditions but are rarely effective once the hearing loss is established.

Pharmacological treatment of the Menière's disorder is at best a controversial area and is usually focused on the control of vertigo. There is little evidence of improvement in the hearing in controlled studies.

Hearing loss may occur in a variety of autoimmune conditions, including polyarteritis nodosa, Behçet's disease, Cogan's syndrome and temporal arteritis, as well as the poorly defined autoimmune sensorineural hearing loss. In general, the hearing loss may improve with the improvements in the systemic condition with early treatment with steroids and appropriate immunosuppressive therapy, but such benefits rarely occur with well established hearing loss.

Rehabilitation – an overview

Audiological rehabilitation, aimed at minimizing disability and handicap, must be approached in a broadly pragmatic way with an open mind and preparedness to improvise. The framework described below is meant to be broad and applicable to any kind of hearing loss in any sociomedical setting. Essentially it was developed to provide a structure to the problem-solving exercise to ensure that all relevant factors are taken into account in a coherent manner.

Within the different sections of the management model outlined below the various components that need to be taken into account are mentioned. The important point is to consider each of these components briefly, even if only to dismiss some of them immediately. Thus, for example, manual communication skills will not be relevant to an elderly person with a mild hearing loss, but should be considered if there is a deaf child.

Different approaches to assessing relevant factors are outlined in Table 8.1, which covers the broad categories of observation, questioning and testing, which may be approached in different ways in different circumstances. Even in a well equipped clinic, although hearing levels will be assessed by standardized formal systematic quantitative multiply variable testing, non-verbal communication may be evaluated by informed direct observation. Again, the speech-reading abilities of a patient with a mild hearing loss can be assessed by direct observation or a short informal test, whereas those of someone with a profound acquired hearing loss may be assessed in the same clinic using formal systematic quantitative

testing. In a poor Third World society, in which resources are limited and hearing aids available only for individuals with severe or profound hearing loss, a binary screening test of hearing, perhaps non-standardized, will be used to determine whether it is justified to proceed to further testing that would lead to the provision of amplification.

Again, within the framework specified here the individual personnel involved in different parts of the assessment and management are not specified. Indeed, whereas in a well staffed department different components may be conducted by different professionals, including doctors, hearing and speech therapists, scientists, technicians and psychologists, in a local direct referral service almost everything will be performed by the technician, so emphasizing the need for one with appropriate training and experience. However, even in the largest department it is important that one individual retains responsibility for an overview and management decisions for any individual patient.

The overall approach to the rehabilitative process is a comprehensive one that includes all elements rather than focusing on a hearing aid or cochlear implant. Whereas in many cases these may have pivotal role, in other cases they are inappropriate. Even when they have an important role, this is generally dependent on other aspects of rehabilitative support for its enhancement and on appropriate patient evaluation to ensure that the correct form of instrumentation for the particular individual is selected. In all cases the rehabilitation process comprises the four sections of *evaluation, integration and decision making, remediation* and *outcome assessment* (Fig 8.2).

Table 8.1 Methods of evaluation

Observation	Direct
	Video-recorded
Questioning	Direct
	Questionnaires
	Open set
	Closed set
	Computer administered
Testing	Subjective
	Objective

All may be approached in a formal or informal, quantitative or qualitative, standardized or non-standardized manner.

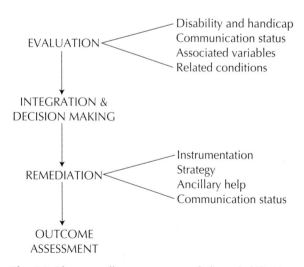

Fig 8.2 The overall components of the rehabilitation process.

EVALUATION

Within the process of rehabilitation we are determining what the patient's problems may be and how they can best be approached and overcome. It is essential that we have an effective overview of the patient's strengths and weaknesses, their needs and their feelings rather than limiting our approach to performing an audiogram.

The process of evaluation is summarized in Figure 8.3. It may be seen to consist of four major sections, each of which comprises a number of important components.[3,5] Each of the main sections has a specific relevance to the rehabilitative process.

Thus the first component 'Disability and handicap' defines the specific problems that are important to the patient. 'Communication status' provides the information on the communicative capacities of the individual on which the rehabilitative approach can be built. 'Associated variables' deals with attitudes of the patient and those around them, and so defines the particular strategy that will need to be adopted by the professionals. Finally, 'Related conditions' draws together other elements of the patient that can have a modifying effect on the details of the approach to be adopted.

Disability and handicap

Disability and handicap are the problems that bring the patient to the clinic and for which they

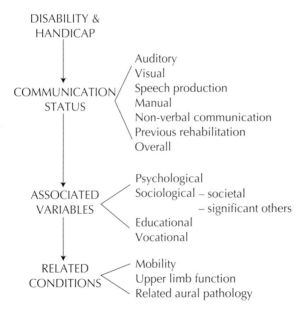

Fig 8.3 The components of evaluation.

seek help. They are most commonly tapped by simply asking the patient about the problems that they experience as a result of their hearing loss. However, for many a clinic appointment may be a stressful experience and useful information can be obtained by sending the patient, along with their appointment letter for the clinic, a questionnaire asking them to list the problems they have because of their hearing loss.[6] Further useful information can be obtained by asking their Significant Others to complete a similar questionnaire that asks about the problems experienced by the patient, and also about the impact of the patient's hearing loss on them (the Significant Other). This questionnaire is often more usefully administered while the patient is being tested during their clinic appointment.

The patient-problem questionnaire focuses the patient's attention on their difficulties and provides a useful starting point for discussions with them and their Significant Others. The patient can also be asked to rate the importance of each of their problems for them on a 10–100 point scale, providing a quantitative base for subsequent outcome measures.

The most commonly listed problems are hearing the television, general conversation, door and telephone bells and speech in noisy situations. The handicaps generally reported are social isolation, loneliness, embarrassment and loss of confidence.

In addition to such an open-ended approach, there are a plethora of scales of disability and handicap. Although these measure a variety of aspects of the disablements, they cannot focus in on what is particularly important for the specific individual and their most important role is as 'before and after' measures for evaluating the effectiveness of a particular rehabilitative programme. As such they will be discussed later.

Communication status

Communication status includes the audiometry, which all too often is the only component of the rehabilitative evaluation taken seriously by the clinician. However, this is only one aspect of the *auditory* component of communication status, others being measures of dynamic range (e.g. uncomfortable loudness levels), speech discrimination, binaural processing, et cetera. These tests are those that will have relevance to different aspects of the rehabilitative process, particularly in the context of hearing aid selection.

Visual elements of communication are important, particularly because the high frequency components of speech, which will be most affected by the commonest patterns of hearing loss, are those that are generally the easiest to read on the lips. Such speech-reading is much affected by impaired visual acuity so that provision of appropriate spectacles can often have a dramatic effect on the individual's receptive communication skills even if they are unaware that they lip-read. The use of spectacles may have a bearing on the type of hearing aid that is fitted, particularly in sociomedical systems in which behind-the-ear hearing aids are the norm.

Finally, the assessment of speech-reading ability will depend on the degree of hearing loss of the patient. In most patients a simple clinical measure is enough to focus attention on the problem and reassure them that they are able to lip-read, whereas in patients with severe and profound hearing loss detailed testing to determine the optimal training approaches will be necessary using appropriate video-recorded materials such as consonant confusion lists and sentence lists.

Speech production skills, as usually informally assessed during the clinical interview, are rarely problematical except in patients with a prelingual hearing loss or a profound acquired hearing loss. In these cases, marked deviations from the norm should lead to appropriate assessment by speech therapists or phoniatricians.

Another matter that arises in this context is the question of the dominant language of the patient. As far as possible any evaluation and therapy should be conducted in that language, through an interpreter if necessary.

Manual communication (sign language) skills are on the whole assessed only in individuals with profound hearing losses, usually the congenitally deaf. Enquiry should be made about them, however, in all patients. It is important when dealing with prelingually deaf patients that a member of the rehabilitative team should have sign language skills to ensure effective communication with the patient.

Non-verbal communication skills are generally assessed informally in the context of the patient interview and usually need to be considered more extensively in prelingually deaf young adults who may not have developed appropriate skills.

It is important to know what *previous rehabilitative* help the patient has had in order to build on the positive components and help overcome any hangups the individual may have because of inappropriate previous rehabilitation, such as an unsuitable hearing aid.

Finally, in this section it is apparent that the *overall* totality of the patient's communication skills may be more or less than the sum of the individual components. In this section it is important to measure communication ability in the optimal mode of communication in order to assess the real needs of the patient in their own environment.

Associated variables

Associated variables comprise predominantly the psychosocial factors that govern the patient's approach to their hearing loss. These will stem largely from the patient's own attitude and understanding, those of the people close to them, and the overall approach to hearing impaired people of the society in which the patient lives. In addition, the patient's educational background and experience together with the attitudes of workmates and employers will also have an important role.

The attitude of the patient is critical to the success of any rehabilitative programme. They should have a positive but realistic approach, not expecting too much but, on the other hand, anticipating some benefit; without this they will not persist sufficiently with the rehabilitative process. They must have some enthusiasm and motivation to receive help, as only some 50 per cent of patients seen in rehabilitation clinics are self-motivated, the figure being even lower among older individuals.

This brings us to the central role of Significant Others in influencing the attitude and approach of the patient, and helping the patient overcome the stigma of the hearing loss and the added stigma of a hearing aid in most societies. Involvement of the Significant Others in making decisions jointly with the patient is particularly important, although care must be taken that they are not allowed to make the decisions for the patient.

In interviewing the patient, one of the most important and revealing questions that can be asked is: '*What made you decide to do something about your hearing now?*' This, followed by some gentle probing, can provide invaluable information about the attitudes of the patient and their Significant Others.

Related conditions

Related conditions cover three particular areas that can influence the details of the rehabilitative process and how it is provided for the patient. These are the patient's mobility, their upper limb function and whether or not they have any related aural pathology.

Mobility governs whether the rehabilitation should be provided on a domiciliary basis, as in very immobile individuals; consideration that also highlights the importance of outreach clinics for predominantly elderly populations who find it difficult to travel long distances. Furthermore, the individual's mobility will govern the balance between personal hearing aids and environmental aids (assistive listening devices) in the rehabilitative process.

This balance is also affected by the individual's *upper limb function*, that is, their tactile sensitivity and manipulative skills, which are influenced by tremor, cerebrovascular accidents and degenerative conditions. Most commonly, this will have a bearing on the choice of hearing aid, when vanity will make the patient press for the smallest possible device, which they are never going to be able to fit or manipulate. A reasonable balance has to be achieved in this context between what the patient will accept and what will help them, and it is often best to allow them to try an unrealistically small device in the first instance, on the basis that they will be happy to change to a more realistic fitting on follow-up.

Related aural pathology covers tinnitus, otorrhoea, the Tullio phenomenon and sensation of pressure in the ears. Tinnitus can generally be helped by an appropriate hearing aid fitting, particularly using open earmoulds or moulds with large vents. Vents are important in ensuring that the feeling of pressure in the ears due to Eustachian tube problems or endolymphatic hydrops is not exacerbated. The presence of the Tullio phenomenon together with sensitive uncomfortable loudness levels will lead to care in limiting the maximum output of the hearing aid by compression, peak clipping or other techniques.

Otorrhoea may be caused by otitis externa or chronic suppurative otitis media. The former may be aggravated by poor hygiene associated with earmoulds or, more rarely, by a true allergy to the mould. This emphasizes the need for appropriate instruction of the patient and allergy testing, leading to the use of low-allergenic earmoulds. Chronic suppurative otitis media can be exacerbated by the fitting of earmoulds and if possible vents should be used. Failing this the patient should alternate aids between ears and in some cases may be considered to be a candidate for bone-anchored hearing aids.

INTEGRATION AND DECISION MAKING

Before starting the rehabilitation process it is important to pull together all the information acquired in the evaluation process and to make decisions about the management of the patient. In particular it is important to assess their attitude towards the process, their understanding of what is involved and their expectations of the outcome. On the basis of this, and some immediate changes to these elements made in a brief discussion with the patient aimed at inducing as realistic an approach as possible, the patient should be categorized.

The aim of this *categorization* is to facilitate as appropriate an organization of the rehabilitative services for the patient as possible. It serves to ensure that excessive rehabilitative resources are not put into patients who do not need them, and that an optimal approach is devised for those requiring more complex management.

We have broadly defined four categories of patients, the first two of which encompass some 90 per cent of those seen.[5]

Type-I patients are highly motivated with no complicating factors. They should pass quickly through the rehabilitative system and use relatively little in the way of manpower resources; they are fitted with hearing aids, advised about appropriate hearing tactics and environmental aids, and given appropriate but relatively brief counselling at fitting and follow-up.

Type-II patients are positively motivated but either they or the clinician anticipates complicating factors. They may have very mild or very severe hearing loss or an audiometric configuration likely to create difficulties. They may have otorrhoea or disturbing tinnitus, be confused or have particular handling difficulties. Whatever the case, it can be anticipated that they will require more and longer sessions before they are optimally rehabilitated compared with the type-I patients, and appropriate plans should be made. The ratio of type-II to type-I patients increases with age, particularly in those over 75 years.

Type-III patients genuinely want rehabilitative help but are opposed to one or more parts of the normal rehabilitative process, usually hearing aids or in-depth counselling. With these individuals it is often necessary to proceed in a somewhat roundabout (or even devious) way, offering the necessary but undesired intervention in a non-threatening way at a later stage of the rehabilitative process, by which time they have become more aware of its importance or relevance.

The final group, *type-IV*, deny any disability or handicap and attend the clinic as a result of pressure from their Significant Others. If after a brief discussion they persist in their approach or if such a hidden denial emerges in those previously pretending to accept intervention, they should be discharged from the clinic with it being made clear that they are free to return should they change their mind. At the same time advice on communication tactics and environmental aids should be offered to their Significant Others.

Finally, some *preliminary goal setting* should be approached at this stage, considering with the patient what they want to achieve from the rehabilitative process and how best this can be accomplished. Clinicians may lead the focus of the

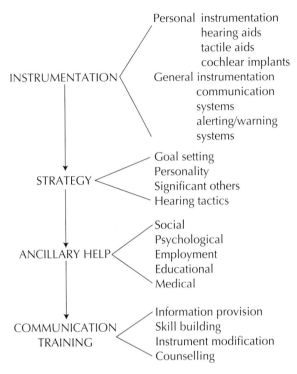

Personal instrumentation
  hearing aids
  tactile aids
  cochlear implants
General instrumentation
  communication
  systems
  alerting/warning
  systems

INSTRUMENTATION

STRATEGY
  Goal setting
  Personality
  Significant others
  Hearing tactics

ANCILLARY HELP
  Social
  Psychological
  Employment
  Educational
  Medical

COMMUNICATION TRAINING
  Information provision
  Skill building
  Instrument modification
  Counselling

Fig 8.4 The components of remediation.

approach towards environmental aids and hearing tactics in some individuals, with a major concentration on hearing aids in others.

REMEDIATION

The components of remediation are outlined in Figure 8.4. Again, as with evaluation, each section covers a different aspect of the process. The first three, *instrumentation, strategy* and *ancillary help* refer to short-duration actions taking only a few sessions, whereas the last, *communication training*, may be brief or may last for days, weeks, months or even years.

It is important, again, to consider each section for its relevance to the individual patient, even if superficially it would appear not be necessary.

Instrumentation

Instrumentation is for many the key section of remediation, for others the sum total, but in reality is only one part of a complex whole. It may be broadly divided into two sections, 'personal instrumentation' and 'general instrumentation', each accompanied by appropriate instruction of the patient and Significant Others.

Personal instrumentation deals with instruments selected to fit the needs of the individual concerned and, for the vast majority of hearing impaired patients, entails hearing aids. However, cochlear implants (see Chapter 9) and tactile aids are also considered here for the small minority of individuals with profound or total hearing losses.

In recent years it has become apparent that it is important for the characteristics of hearing aids to be matched to the hearing loss of the individual; in most patients this entails broadly following a variation on the 1/2-gain rule, that is, the hearing aid should be used to give a gain equivalent to about one-half the hearing loss in decibels. It is, however, important to measure the actual gain in the ear fitted either by measuring changes in the thresholds as a result of the fitting or by use of an appropriate insertion gain system by which the sound pressure levels at the eardrum can be measured with and without the hearing aid in place. A variety of formulae for calculating the exact gain needed have been proposed, but the most widely used now is the National Acoustics Laboratory (NAL) system developed by Byrne and Dillon.[7]

A further point is that patients may take up to 6 months to habituate to a new amplification system and obtain optimal benefit from it.[8] They may initially reject a frequency response that will ultimately give them most benefit preferring a response giving sound more similar to that to which they are used, and will require to be weaned onto the optimal system.

Hearing aids have gradually become smaller and body-worn aids are now used generally only for individuals with profound, often mixed, hearing losses, or those requiring aids with large controls. Most are fitted with a variety of behind-the-ear, in-the-ear and in-the-canal aids.

The ultimate choice will depend on the patient (cosmetic, ergonomic and acoustical factors) the sociomedical system and the experience of the individual fitting the patient. In general, it is still true that the more electronically sophisticated aids are normally found in behind-the-ear casings for reasons of size and lack of feedback. Despite rapid change, most sophisticated new processing technologies are being initially applied to behind-the-ear aids.

The auditory system is a binaural system and a binaural fitting of aids should always be considered. However, many people will choose not to use two, will find it difficult to cope with two, or may not derive much additional benefit from the use of two aids so that, in most good audiological departments, only some 25–33 per cent of patients are usually fitted binaurally.

The earmoulds are a critical link that can make or break a good hearing aid fitting. Our understanding of this has progressed rapidly in the past decade with the work of Killion[9] and others. Moulds can modify the acoustical characteristics of the hearing aid system, any occlusion effect, feedback and the fit and quality of sound. More hearing aids are probably rejected because of the earmoulds than because of the aids themselves. The choice of aids and moulds have been discussed elsewhere by Gatehouse.[8]

Patients with congenital atresia of the external meatus or with uncontrollable chronically discharging ears may be fitted with bone-anchored hearing aids[10] unless their bone conduction hearing loss is too severe. In such devices a titanium screw is inserted into the skull behind and above the pinna and a hearing aid producing a mechanical vibratory output connected to this. Results with this approach are generally very encouraging provided that the patients are carefully selected.

These devices have largely superseded the Xomed aid, in which the attachment and transducer were separated by a layer of skin, and which was contraindicated if there was more than 25 dB bone conduction hearing loss. The bone-anchored hearing aids exist in several versions. The postaural version may be used for patients with bone conduction hearing levels of up to about 45 dB and body-worn devices for up to 60 dB bone conduction thresholds.

Apart from the patients with congenital meatal atresia (e.g. Treacher Collins syndrome), the main group of patients to be fitted with such aids are those with chronic suppurative otitis media resistant to medical and surgical treatment and who cannot tolerate appropriate air conduction hearing aids, which exacerbate their infections.

Cochlear implants are generally used only with patients with profound bilateral hearing losses and are discussed in Chapter 9. For patients unable to benefit from hearing aids and unable or unwilling to undergo cochlear implants a variety of tactile aids are now available, which can provide information to the patient by way of monitoring their own speech and environmental sounds, and may help with speech-reading.[11]

General instrumentation covers instruments that may be used by more than one hearing impaired patient at a time and are often referred to as environmental aids or assistive listening devices. The range of devices available is shown in Table 8.2, which indicates that they broadly cover the domains of electronic speech and of alerting and warning signals.

The principle of those instruments dealing with speech is generally based on improving the signal

Table 8.2 Types of environmental aids

Electronic speech

Telephones	Amplifiers, induction coils, additional receiver, videophones, text telephones
Television	Headphones, extra speaker, loop systems, additional amplifers and speakers, subtitling, simultaneous signing
Public address systems	Loop, visual announcements

Alerting/warning systems

Doorbells or telephone bells	Buzzers, louder bells, extension bells, visual systems
Alarms	Low frequency buzzers, radio alarms, flashing lights, vibrators, fans
Baby alarms	Amplification with loudspeakers, visual systems
Smoke alarms	Louder alarms, visual systems

to noise ratio to the patient or the quality of the sound. Increasingly, however, visual supplements in terms of subtitling and parallel signing are being incorporated and this will be further enhanced with the development of video telephones. In general, the selection of such a device is normally delayed until the patient has been fitted with a hearing aid system and their subsequent needs assessed.

Warning signals are enhanced with either a change in the frequency or loudness of the signal (e.g. using a low frequency buzzer instead of a high frequency bell) or by sensory substitution, generally involving the use of visual signals.

Strategy

Strategy entails initially *defining* desirable and realistic *goals* in discussion with the patient and Significant Other. Once appropriate goals have been decided upon, the clinician will need to make a further assessment of the patient and Significant Other and their *personalities* to decide on appropriate hearing tactics to be used to achieve these goals.

Hearing tactics are techniques devised for the patient to manipulate their environment (human and physical) and their reaction to it in order to optimize the communication system. Hearing tactics have been classified into manipulating social interaction, manipulating the physical environment and tactics involving observation. However, improving one's ability to hear may also have costs from the patient's point of view and, although earlier workers have criticized avoidance tactics and 'pretending that they have heard', these may be useful from the patient's overall relational standpoint under certain circumstances. More assertive tactics entail 'interrupting and taking over conversations' and 'asking for repetition', with 'positioning oneself optimally' being a more neutral approach.

Ancillary help

Many of the problems that the audiologist and otologist encounter cannot be dealt with adequately within the domains of such departments. It is thus important when, for example, the patient highlights psychological, employment, social, educational or other medical problems arising from their hearing loss that appropriate professional referrals are made. Social workers for the deaf and hearing impaired play a particularly important role in this context in their provision of sign language support and environmental aids. Employment training advisors also have an important role in assisting hearing impaired people of employment age.

Communication training

As mentioned earlier, this is an ongoing element of rehabilitation that may last as little as a few minutes or as long as several years, particularly in some patients with profound hearing loss or severe central auditory dysfunction. In all cases it consists of four components: *information provision, skill-building, instrument modification* and *counselling*.

Information provision is ensuring that the patient and Significant Other is aware of the causes of the hearing loss and its prognosis, its implications and what can be done to help, including some details of the technical help. Such an understanding is necessary to the acceptance of the hearing loss and its global consequences by both the patient and Significant Other.

Skill-building entails training the patient in the new skills necessary in order to function optimally. Although these are normally thought of in terms of audiovisual communication or use of alternative communication systems, they also entail such basic factors as learning to fit a hearing aid in the ear, which will be crucial for many elderly individuals, and appropriate hearing tactics.

Instrument modification comprises adjustments made once the patient has had a chance to use their initial instrumentation in their real-life environment. Thus, as mentioned earlier, the frequency characteristics of the hearing aid(s) may need to be adjusted as the patient adapts to the new auditory input. Environmental aids such as television or tele-phone aids may need to be considered in the light of any residual problems found with these after hearing aid fitting.

Counselling is a key problem-solving component involving professional and patients with or without Significant Others. The patient needs to discuss their initial experiences and residual problems or anticipated problems, and various counselling techniques have been advised for dealing with these.[12]

OUTCOME ASSESSMENT

If rehabilitation is concerned with the reduction of disability and handicap, it follows that it is best assessed by measuring this. The problem is how to do so in a relevant way.

A plethora of scales of such disablements have been proposed and 'before and after' outcome measures described. The difficulty is to choose relevant measures for the population and, ideally, for the individual under consideration. As different patients will have different disablements the best that can normally be achieved is a consideration of changes in terms of group effects on disabilities and handicaps commonly reported. Even then, it is essential to select a scale short enough and psychometrically robust enough to be completed and scored easily, and some progress in this respect has been made with the hearing disability and handicap scale.[13] Other scales may be useful for specific groups of patients, such as one of the many speech hearing disability scales in King Kopetzky syndrome (obscure auditory dysfunction or auditory disability with normal hearing). However, even in this group, there is also a need to tap the emotional handicap component highlighted by several authors.

An individual-based measure has been used in cochlear implant patients in a preliminary study in which after listing their problems the patients are asked to rate the severity of each of these problems on a 100-point scale. These measures can be repeated at different stages after the rehabilitation to track relevant changes.

More general *quality of life* measures have also been used in hearing aid and cochlear implant patients and can provide a means of comparing the benefits of these and other types of interventions. There is often a large overlap between the specific questions posed in such quality of life measures and handicap scales.

Patient satisfaction has always been approached in a variety of ways. I have opted for a simple approach, merely asking the patient to list the benefits and shortcomings that they have experienced as a result of the rehabilitative approach under consideration. This may further be quantified by asking the patient to rate each of these benefits or shortcomings.

Specific outcome measures have been used, especially in the assessment of effectiveness of particular instrumentation (e.g. hearing aids) in terms of speech, auditory and audiovisual recognition skills. A great variety of approaches have been used but probably the most useful one in repeated monitoring is the measure of connected discourse tracking[14] by which the number of words per minute that can be correctly repeated by the patient when presented to them either visually or audiovisually by the tester reading from an appropriate text is measured.

References

1. World Health Organization. *International classification of impairments, disabilities and handicaps.* Geneva: World Health Organization, 1980.
2. Stephens D, Hétu R. Impairment, disability and handicap in audiology: towards a consensus. *Audiology* 1991; **30**:185–200.
3. Stephens SDG. Hearing rehabilitation in a psychosocial framework. *Scandinavian Audiology* 1996; **25(suppl 43)**:57–66.
4. McKee GJ. Pharmacological treatment of hearing and balance disorders. In: Stephens SDG ed. *Adult audiology.* London: Butterworth–Heinemann, 1997: (Kerr A ed. *Scott-Brown's Otolaryngology, 6th ed*; vol 2.)
5. Goldstein DP, Stephens SDG. Audiological rehabilitation: management model I. *Audiology* 1981; **20**:432–52.
6. Barcham LJ, Stephens SDG. The use of an open-ended problems questionnaire in auditory rehabilitation. *British Journal of Audiology* 1980; **14**:49–54.
7. Byrne D, Dillon H. The National Acoustic Laboratories (NAL) new procedure for selecting the gain and frequency response of a hearing aid. *Ear and Hearing* 1986; **7**:257–65.
8. Gatehouse S. Hearing aids. In: Stephens SDG ed. *Adult audiology.* London: Butterworth–Heinemann, 1997: (Kerr A ed. *Scott-Brown's Otolaryngology, 6th ed*; vol 2.)
9. Killion MC. Earmould design: theory and practice. In: Hartvig-Jensen J ed. *Hearing aid fitting.* Copenhagen: Danavox, 1988:155–72.
10. Tjellstrom A, Granstrom G. Long-term follow-up with the bone-anchored hearing aids. *Ear Nose and Throat Journal* 1994; **73**:112–4.
11. Summers IR ed. *Tactile aids for the hearing impaired.* London: Whurr, 1992.
12. Erdman SA. Counselling hearing impaired adults. In: Alpiner JG, McCarthy PA eds. *Rehabilitative audiology: children and adults, 2nd ed.* Baltimore: Williams and Wilkins, 1993:374–413.
13. Hétu R, Getty L, Philibet L, Desilets F, Noble W, Stephens D. Mise au point d'un outil clinique pour la mesure d'incapacités auditives et de handicaps. *Journal of Speech-Language Pathology and Audiology* 1994; **18**:83–95.
14. de Filippo CL, Scott BL. A method for training and evaluating the reception of ongoing speech. *Journal of the Acoustical Society of America* 1987; **63**:1186–92.

CHAPTER 9

Cochlear implants

GRAEME M CLARK

Introduction

A cochlear implant is a device to restore some hearing in severely–profoundly deaf people when their organ of Corti has not developed, or is destroyed by disease or injury, to such an extent than no comparable hearing can be obtained with a hearing aid. When the organ of Corti is grossly malfunctioning or absent, sound vibrations cannot be transduced into temporospatial patterns of action potentials along the auditory nerve for the coding of frequency and intensity, and a hearing aid, which amplifies sound, is of little or no use. A cochlear implant should at least partially reproduce the patterns of action potentials required for the coding of sound, so that speech and environmental sounds can be recognized and understood. This is done by placing electrodes along the scala tympani of the basal turn of the cochlea so that residual auditory nerves can be excited using electric stimuli.

Studies have demonstrated that multiple-electrode systems giving multiple-channel stimulation can provide more information for speech understanding than single-electrode systems.[1] Furthermore, the average speech perception scores in profoundly deaf adults with a postlinguistic hearing loss,[2] and profoundly deaf young children with postlinguistic and prelinguistic hearing losses,[3] who are using the current University of Melbourne/Cochlear Limited multiple-channel cochlear implant, are now better than the average scores obtained by severely–profoundly deaf persons with some residual hearing using a hearing aid.

Principles

Some cochlear implants have had a single electrode to excite auditory nerves, in particular devices developed in Vienna[4] initially and in Los Angeles[5] and London.[6] Single-electrode implants can be placed extracochlearly or intracochlearly and provide global stimulation of auditory nerve fibres. They are simpler and cheaper to construct than multiple-channel systems, but should no longer be used as speech perception results for multiple-channel systems are superior. The reason is that speech is processed by the brain through the reception of information along a number of channels.

To achieve multiple-channel stimulation speech can be filtered into a number of frequency bands and the variations in voltage from appropriate filters presented to electrodes around the basal turn of the cochlea (Fig 9.1). However, in our initial research we found that channel interactions due to current flowing along the cochlea produced unpredictable variations in loudness.[7] Consequently, multiple-channel stimuli should not be presented simultaneously. Furthermore, because of the difficulty in presenting a lot of speech information through what is effectively an electro-neural 'bottle neck' we found it necessary to select the speech information providing the greatest intelligibility and coding this on a place basis. This meant encoding the second formant, and subsequently the first formant and other frequency bands, as place of stimulation. Voicing was coded as rate of stimulation and intensity as current level. Recently, improved results have been obtained by selecting

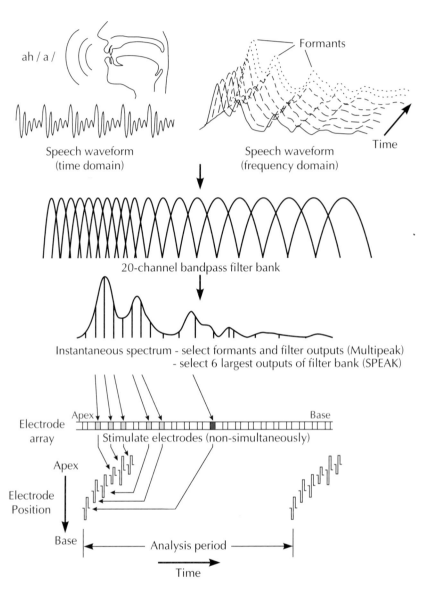

Fig 9.1 Speech is a mixture of frequencies at different amplitudes, and has concentrations of frequency energy or formants caused by resonances in the oropharynx. The sounds are normally filtered by the cochlea into a number of information channels for the brain to decode. With a cochlear implant speech processor, sound is filtered into frequency bands, and the outputs of the filters can be selected and used to excite electrodes at sites along the cochlea corresponding to the centre frequency of the filter. The rate of stimulation may vary with the voicing frequency, in the case of the Multipeak strategy, or be at a constant rate, as with the SPEAK strategy.

6–10 spectral maxima and presenting the amplitude variations from the filters to electrodes at a constant rate, as illustrated in Figure 9.1.

Multiple-electrode arrays that provide multiple-channel stimulation have been implanted either on the surface or within the cochlea. Although surface arrays will produce less trauma to the membranous structures of the cochlea, they are not very effective in providing multiple-channel stimulation because

the high impedance of bone restricts the delivery of current to the auditory nerves, and their distance from the spiral ganglion cells prevents localized stimulation of groups of neurons. On the other hand, with care intracochlear electrodes can be inserted along the scala tympani of the basal turn of the cochlea without significant damage or loss of neurons to provide the necessary multiple-channel stimulation.

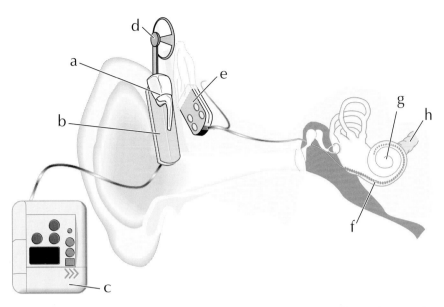

Fig 9.2 The Nucleus multiple-channel cochlear prosthesis. a, microphone; b, speech processor (behind-the-ear); c, body-worn speech processor; d, transmitter coil; e, receiver stimulator; f, electrode array; g, cochlea; h, auditory nerve.

The information transmitted to the electrode array may be sent percutaneously or transcutaneously. Percutaneous transmission is via an opening in the skin and requires a plug and socket. Although there have been improvements in the biocompatability of the materials used for the connectors, there is still a risk of infection around the socket, it can be fractured, it is not practicable for children, and it is not aesthetically pleasing. Transcutaneous transmission through the intact skin is preferable, and is most effectively achieved by transmitting signals electromagnetically using an inductive transmitting coil externally and receiving coil internally.

The overall design concept of a multiple-channel intracochlear implant is illustrated in Figure 9.2, which is a diagram of the system developed by University of Melbourne/Cochlear Limited and known as the Nucleus system. It consists first of a directional microphone worn above the ear, which transforms sound into a voltage waveform. This voltage is applied via a small cable to a speech processor, which can be a separate unit worn behind the ear or a more versatile unit, worn in a pocket. The speech processor filters this waveform into frequency bands. The output of the filters are referred to a map of the patient's electric current thresholds and comfortable listening levels for the individual electrodes. A code is produced for the stimulus parameters (electrode site and current level) to represent the speech signal at each instant in time. This code, together with power, is transmitted inductively via a circular aerial through the intact skin to the receiver–stimulator. This receiver–stimulator directs current pulses to the appropriate electrodes on an array lying close to the auditory nerve fibres within the basal turn of the cochlea. The current pulses excite populations of auditory nerve fibres to simulate the pattern of auditory nerve activity in response to sound, and provide a meaningful representation of speech and environmental sounds.[8]

Historical perspectives

Initial operative studies on profoundly deaf patients to see when speech perception could be achieved using electrical stimulation were carried out in the 1950s and 1960s.[9–12] In these studies, although the patients could recognize some stimuli as speech-like, they were not able to understand what was said. For this reason basic research to understand better how the central auditory nervous system would process speech information via electrical stimulation was commenced by Clark,[13,14] and Clark et al.[15,16] and others.[17]

Our research showed that rate of stimulation could not adequately code the high frequencies required for speech understanding on a temporal coding or single-channel basis, and a fully implantable multiple-channel receiver–stimulator was needed for the place coding of frequency. A prototype fully implantable multiple-channel receiver–stimulator was developed at the University of Melbourne and implanted in our first patient in 1978. With this device we were able in 1978 to develop our inaugural speech processing strategy,[18,19] which when evaluated using standard audiological tests was found to give the patient considerable help when used in combination with lip-reading. It also gave some open-set speech understanding for electric stimulation alone when the patient was tested with open-sets of monosyllabic words and Central Institute for the Deaf (CID) sentences.[20,21] The inaugural strategy extracted the second formant frequency (F2) and presented this to an appropriate electrode in the cochlea on a place coding basis. The second formant frequency is a concentration of energy in the midspeech frequency range (750 to 2300 Hz). The voicing or fundamental frequency (F0) was presented to each electrode being stimulated as a rate code. The fundamental frequency is low: on average 120 Hz for men, and 225 Hz for women. It distinguishes voiced from unvoiced phonemes and questions from statements. The amplitude of the sound energy of F2 was used to set the current level of the stimulating electrode.

Studies also took place in other research centres to see whether speech perception could be achieved with a multiple-electrode cochlear implant. Primarily, fixed filter rather than speech feature extraction schemes were explored at Stanford,[22] in Salt Lake City,[23] San Francisco,[24] and Paris.[25] Except for one patient in San Francisco, no open-set speech understanding was reported for these fixed filter strategies. While the above multiple-electrode studies were being undertaken, research was also carried out in Los Angeles,[5] London,[6] and Vienna,[4] to see whether it was possible to use single-electrode systems to provide closed or even open-set speech understanding. In these studies some closed-set but no open-set speech perception was reported for electrical stimulation alone. A more detailed review of the results of the above systems is provided by Millar *et al.*[26]

Subsequently, improvements to our F0/F2 speech processing strategy were made when it was found in 1985 that as more formant information (in particular the first formant F1) was extracted and coded on a place basis (F0/F1/F2 speech processor), speech perception improved not only in quiet (Fig 9.3), but especially in noise. A further improvement in speech perception in quiet and in noise occurred in 1989 when the spectral energy in the frequency bands 2.0–2.8 kHz, 2.8–4.0 kHz and 4.0–6.0 kHz was extracted; for voiced sounds the energy in the first two bands, together with F1 and F2, was used to

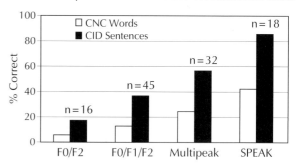

Mean open-set scores for electrical stimulation alone

Fig 9.3 Open-set CID sentence and Consonant–Nucleus (vowel)–Consonant (CNC) word scores for electrical stimulation alone for the F0/F2, F0/F1/F2, Multipeak and SPEAK strategies on unselected patients at the Royal Victorian Eye and Ear Hospital Cochlear Implant Clinic less than 6 months postoperatively.[27,28]

stimulate four electrodes sequentially on a place-coding basis. For unvoiced sounds the energy in the above frequency bands, together with only F2, was used to stimulate the cochlea on a place-coding basis. The first formant frequency was not used, as energy in this region is minimal with unvoiced sounds. This speech processing strategy, called Multipeak, was implemented in a speech processor called MSP (miniature speech processor). The improvement in speech perception in quiet is shown in Figure 9.3.

Further research to improve speech processing by extracting more frequency information and coding it on a place basis was limited by channel interaction caused by the spread of current along the cochlea. To overcome this difficulty two strategies – the Spectral Maxima Sound Processor (SPEAK)[29] and the Continuous Interleaved Sampler (CIS)[30] – used constant rate of stimulation on all electrodes and provided timing information by allowing the amplitude variation on each filter output to produce changes in the current on the corresponding electrodes. In this way there is an interaction in current level but not in pulse rate. The difference between these two strategies is that SPEAK has roving filters and selects the 6–10 maximal outputs from a bank of 20 filters and CIS has eight fixed filters. These differences are reflected in the patterns of electrodes stimulated (electrodograms) for acoustic stimuli, and are illustrated in Figure 9.4 for the word 'choice'.

The SPEAK strategy has shown better results than Multipeak in quiet and in noise, and the comparative results in quiet from patients at our clinic are shown in Figure 9.3. The Multipeak strategy and MSP processor were compared with the SPEAK strategy and Spectra-22 processor in a field trial on

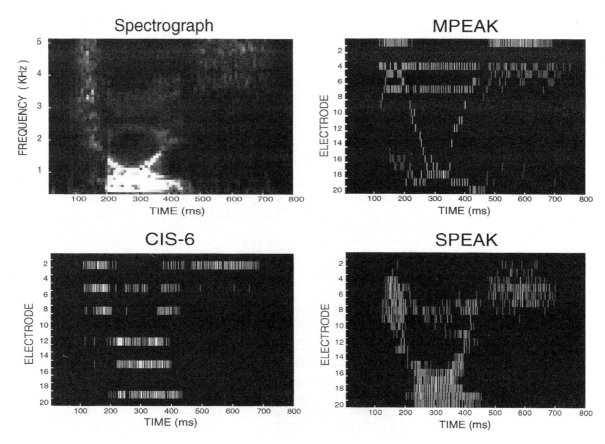

Fig 9.4 Spectrogram for the word 'choice' and the electrode representations (electrodograms) for this word using the Multipeak, CIS stimulation (six fixed filters) and SPEAK (six spectral maxima) strategies.

63 postlinguistically deaf adults at eight centres worldwide.[3] The patients in the comparative study all had some open-set speech recognition with the Multipeak–MSP system with scores from 5 per cent and above before using the SPEAK–Spectra-22 system. The mean score for vowels was 75 per cent for SPEAK and 70 per cent for Multipeak, for consonants 69 per cent for SPEAK and 57 per cent for Multipeak, for words 34 per cent for SPEAK and 25 per cent for Multipeak, for words in sentences 76 per cent for SPEAK and 67 per cent for Multipeak. For the 18 patients who had the special sentence tests at a signal-to-noise ratio of 5 dB the mean score for words in sentences was 60 per cent for SPEAK and 32 per cent for Multipeak. The above results were all statistically significant at the 0.0001 level.

The mean open-set City University New York (CUNY) and CID sentence score of 76 per cent for 63 profoundly deaf adults tested 3 months after changing from the Multipeak to the SPEAK strategy[2] is also very similar to the 77 per cent CID sentence score for a group of 41 severely–profoundly deaf people converted from the Multipeak to SPEAK

strategy. The data from this latter study were presented to the US Food and Drug Administration (FDA) on 30 June 1995. In addition, the mean CID sentence score for 51 unselected profoundly deaf patients using the SPEAK–Spectra-22 system for the first time and tested 2–26 weeks after start up was found to be 71 per cent. The mean open-set sentence score for the CIS strategy on 64 patients with the Clarion speech processor was reported by Kessler *et al.*[31] to be 60 per cent. These data were presented by the Advanced Bionics Corporation to the FDA on 21 July 1995. Published results for the SPEAK–Spectra-22 and Advanced Bionic CIS systems are shown graphically in Figure 9.5. The development of speech processing for cochlear implants in adults is discussed in more detail elsewhere.[32,33]

In the early 1980s, the Los Angeles/3M single-electrode implant was inserted for the first time in a child. Subsequently, the results for the single-channel device on 49 children (aged 2–17 years) were reported;[34] the children could discriminate syllable patterns, but only two could obtain any open-set speech understanding. The University of

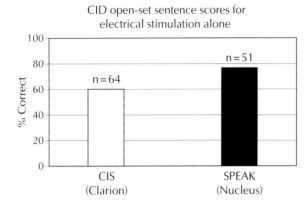

CID open-set sentence scores for electrical stimulation alone

Fig 9.5 The mean open-set CID sentence score of 71 per cent for the SPEAK (University of Melbourne/Cochlear Limited) strategy on 51 patients (data presented to the FDA January 1996) and 60% for the CIS (Advanced Bionics) strategy on 64 patients.[31]

Melbourne/Cochlear Limited multiple-electrode prosthesis was first implanted in children in 1985,[35,36] once the FDA trial on postlinguistically deaf adults had been completed, and the device about to be approved for use in such patients. The F0/F1/F2 speech processing strategy was evaluated on 142 children for the FDA, and was approved on 27 June 1990. The results showed that 51 per cent of the children had significant open-set performance with their cochlear prosthesis using electrical stimulation alone compared with 6 per cent preoperatively. In addition, 68 per cent of the children could perceive some spectral cues for speech perception with their cochlear prosthesis compared with 23 per cent preoperatively. Performance also improved over time, with significant increases in open-set and closed-set speech perception between 1 and 3 years postoperatively. When the test results on 91 prelinguistically deaf children in the study were examined separately it was found that improvements were comparable with the postlinguistic group in many areas, however, performance was poorer on the open-set measures for the prelinguistic group.[37]

The latest SPEAK speech processing strategy has been compared with Multipeak on 12 children from centres in Melbourne and Sydney. The children in the trial all had more than 1 year of experience with the Multipeak–MSP system, and had some open-set speech understanding for electrical stimulation alone. The results of the study[3] showed that in quiet their mean open-set sentence scores for electric stimulation alone were 60 per cent for SPEAK and 53 per cent for Multipeak. At a 15 dB signal-to-noise ratio the scores were 58 per cent SPEAK and 48 per cent Multipeak. These results indicate that

children's central auditory nervous systems are adaptable or plastic enough to process new patterns of stimulation. That the new SPEAK strategy also better enables the children to comprehend speech in the presence of background noise is important, as this ability is needed in everyday situations, including the classroom. The development of speech processing for cochlear implants in children is discussed in more detail elsewhere.[27,28,33]

How does the cochlear implant system work?

The external section of the Nucleus multiple-channel cochlear implant system, shown in Figure 9.2 and illustrated diagrammatically in Figure 9.6, has a directional microphone placed above the pinna to help select the sounds coming from in front of the patient, particularly in noisy conditions. The sensitivity of the microphone increases from 0.151 kHz to approximately 5.0 kHz at 6 dB/octave before dropping off, to emphasize the high frequencies of speech that are important for intelligibility but low in intensity. The energy of the component frequencies in the speech signal, or environmental sound, is amplified with a preamplifier, low pass filtered to remove any high frequency energy that would interfere with the conversion of the analogue signal to a digital one by an A-to-D converter. With the Nucleus-24 behind the ear speech processor (ESPrit) the signal is filtered by a bank of filters, and with the Nucleus-24 body worn speech processor (SPrint) a digital signal processor (DSP) enables a fast Fourier transform (FFT) to provide the filtering. The output voltages from the filter bank and FFT are selected. These are referred to a 'map' where the thresholds and comfortable loudness levels for each electrode selected are recorded and converted to stimulus levels. An appropriate digital code for the stimulus is produced and transmitted through the skin by electromagnetic waves from a transmitter coil worn behind the ear. The transmitter coil is linked inductively to a receiver coil that is part of the implanted receiver–stimulator. The transmitting and receiving coils are aligned through magnets incorporated in the centres of both coils. The transmitted code is made up of a digital data stream representing the sound at each instant in time, and is transmitted by pulsing the radio-frequency carrier. The receiver–stimulator decodes the information into instructions for the selection of the electrode, mode of stimulation (i.e. bipolar, common ground or monopolar), current level and pulse width through

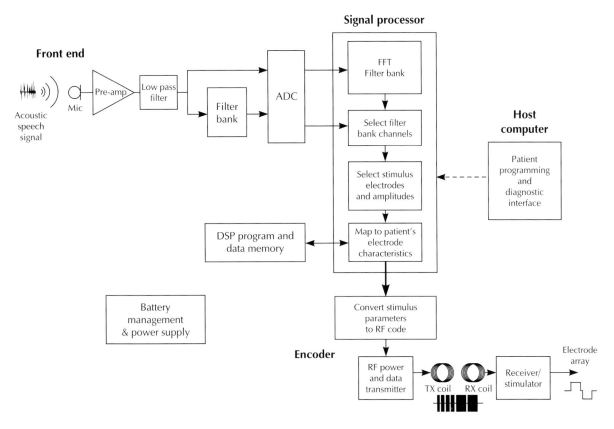

Fig 9.6 The Nucleus behind-the-ear and body-worn speech processors are implemented using either a standard filter bank or fast Fourier transform (FFT) filter bank, respectively. The front end sends the signal to a signal processor chip via a filter bank or to a digital signal processor (DSP) chip, which carries out an FFT and signal processing. The signal processor selects the filter bank channels and the stimulus electrodes and amplitudes, and maps these to the patient's requirements. An encoder section converts the stimulus parameters to a code for transmitting to the receiver–stimulator on a radio-frequency (RF) signal together with power to operate the device. ADC, A-to-D converter; RX, receiver; TX, transmitter.

controlling the opening and closing of gates or switches. The stimulus current level is controlled via a digital-to-analogue converter. Power to operate the receiver–stimulator is also transmitted by the radio-frequency carrier.

Is the multiple-electrode intracochlear implant safe?

Our studies on implanting the cochlea in the experimental animal have demonstrated that there is no significant loss of ganglion cells if an electrode is inserted without tearing the basilar membrane or producing a fracture of the spiral lamina,[38] as Figure 9.7, a monkey cochlea implanted for 24 months, illustrates.[39] However, a fracture or even abrasion of the endosteal lining may lead to increased new bone formation. Insertions without trauma to the basilar membrane or spiral lamina result in hair cells being preserved distal to the electrode array, but the hair cell population opposite the array is usually depleted or absent. The loss of inner hair cells correlates with the number of remaining peripheral processes (dendrites). The University of Melbourne/Cochlear Limited banded array is very flexible, and can be inserted along the scala tympani with minimal trauma. If the University of Melbourne/Cochlear Limited smooth free-fitting banded electrode array needs to be removed and a similar array inserted, this can also be done with minimal damage to the cochlea or loss of spiral ganglion cells.[39]

If infection invades all scalae and turns of the cochlea, there will be early and extensive loss of hair cells and spiral ganglion cells.[38] New bone formation can be seen as early as 2 weeks after the onset of the infection.[40] This is relevant to the

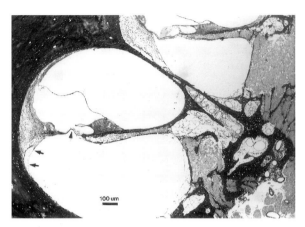

Fig 9.7 A photomicrograph of the upper basal and upper middle turns of the cochlea of the Macaque after a free-fitting banded array had been implanted for 24 months. The minimal tissue response evoked by the electrode is indicated by the arrows. Hair cells were absent adjacent to the array but present apicalwards.[39]

shown that if an otitis media due to *Staphylococcus aureus, Streptococcus pyogenes* and *Strep. pneumoniae* occurs when an electrode sheath has had time to form, there is no significant risk of labyrinthitis.[41] A fascial graft around the electrode entry point may facilitate the development of a sheath and protect the cochlea. Care must always be taken to ensure that the operation is not carried out when an otitis media is developing. In addition, the surgery should be covered with systemic and topical antibiotics, and a postoperative course given as well. It should also be noted there is a risk of infection developing even if the operation is carried out 6 or more months after a chronically infected ear has been made clean by surgery.

timing of a cochlear implant for patients with a profound sensorineural hearing loss after labyrinthitis. Animal experimental studies[40] have shown that acute labyrinthitis is more likely to develop post-operatively before there has been time for a fibrous tissue sheath to have formed around the electrode and the electrode entry point. Our studies have also

Not only may trauma and infection damage spiral ganglion cells, but choosing inappropriate stimulus parameters, for example those that have a high charge density or are not charge-balanced, may do the same. Our chronic electric stimulation studies on cats have shown that charge-balanced biphasic stimuli up to 500 pulses/s with charge densities up to 52 μC/cm^2 geom. per phase were safe.[42,43] Although the safe upper limit for charge density has not been established, it should be kept as low as possible, and below 52 μC/cm^2 geom. per phase. Using electrodes like the University of Melbourne/Cochlear Limited banded array will keep the charge density low as they have a large surface area but can still stimulate discrete groups of auditory nerve fibres for the place

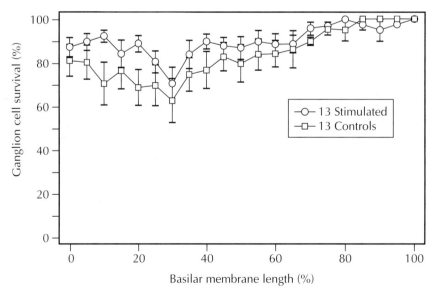

Fig 9.8 The mean ganglion cell populations and their standard errors in 13 cats after up to 2100 hours of continuous bipolar stimulation at 2000 pulses/s and monopolar stimulation at 1000 pulses/s compared with controls. The stimulator had circuitry which modelled that of the CI-22M and CI-24M receiver–stimulators. The ganglion cell populations were plotted for corresponding distances along the length of the basilar membrane.[46]

coding of speech frequencies. The electrical stimuli should not only have a low charge density, but be charge-balanced biphasic pulses. The Nucleus-22 and Nucleus-24 receiver–stimulators produce biphasic pulses that are charge-balanced to less than 0.1 per cent asymmetry. The stimulator is also shorted between pulses to ensure that there is no significant charge imbalance. If the two phases of the pulse are not adequately balanced, a damaging direct current can occur. A direct current of 2.0 μA has been shown to produce a marked reduction in the spiral ganglion cell population, and extensive new bone formation.[44] Although the safe upper limit for a direct current has not been established, it is desirable to keep it below 0.1 μA, the level known to be safe from our chronic stimulation studies. High rates of stimulation (1000–2000 pulses/s) can also produce loss of neural function independent of charge imbalance. The damage caused by high stimulus rates can be the result of direct effect on the cell biochemistry, and principally occurs at high current levels.[45] However, with current levels in the normal operating range our chronic studies at rates of 1000 and 2000 pulses/s in the experimental animal with the Nucleus receiver–stimulator have shown no loss of neuron function or damage (Fig 9.8).[46]

Who will benefit?

Originally the multiple-channel cochlear implant was only recommended for people who were postlinguistically deaf with a profound–total hearing loss and did not obtain any useful hearing with a well fitting hearing aid. That meant they had an average pure tone air threshold in the better ear for 0.5, 1 and 2 kHz of 90 dB sound pressure level (SPL) or greater, and zero speech perception for hearing alone for open-sets of monosyllabic words and words in sentences. In addition, they had no significant improvements in word and sentence scores when using hearing combined with lip-reading compared with lip-reading alone.

As the perception of speech and environmental sounds by profoundly deaf adults has continued to improve with the development of speech processing strategies,[2,37] as seen in Figure 9.3, patients can now be considered for a cochlear implant if they have some residual hearing (i.e. if they are severely–profoundly deaf). The average results from profoundly deaf people for open-sets of CID, CUNY and SIT sentences (scored as words correctly identified) for electrical stimulation alone, using the most recent University of Melbourne/Cochlear Limited (SPEAK) speech processing strategy has varied from 71 to 86 per cent.

As a result, it is recommended that the Nucleus cochlear implant system can be used in patients 18 years and older who have bilateral, postlinguistic, sensorineural hearing impairment and obtain limited benefit from appropriate binaural hearing aids. Limited benefit from amplification is defined by test scores of 30 per cent correct or less in the best listening condition for open-sets of tape-recorded words in sentence tests.

The factors that indicate which postlinguistically deaf adults will benefit most from an implant have been assessed in a number of studies. The findings have varied, and have been reviewed by Blamey.[47] Duration of deafness was most consistently correlated negatively with speech scores. Age at implantation also correlated negatively with speech scores for durations of deafness less than 10 years, but not for longer durations when the effect of duration was accounted for. Increased implant usage gave better results because of learning. The study by Blamey *et al.*[48] also showed that speech perception scores were better if there was good gap detection and frequency discrimination for preoperative promontory testing, and larger numbers of electrodes in use (indicating the need for an adequate depth of insertion).

It is more difficult to decide whether a child will benefit from an implant than it is for an adult. First, it is necessary to use speech tests that are language appropriate to assess their speech perception ability. For example, the perception of speech in a young child is tested by a picture vocabulary test, and in an older child using phonetically balanced kindergarten (PBK) words. It is also important to remember that a deaf child's language will be below that of a group of normally hearing children of the same chronological age. The results for age- and language-appropriate tests need to be interpreted in the light of the unaided and aided pure tone thresholds and the child's ability to use their hearing in communication tasks. It is then a matter of clinical judgement whether the child has too much useful hearing for a cochlear implant operation.

Factors that may predispose to good speech perception also need to be considered before advising surgery. These factors vary according to whether the child is postlinguistically or congenitally deaf. Analysis of results in our clinic[49] has shown that for both postlinguistically and congenitally deaf children speech results correlate negatively with duration of deafness. However, congenitally deaf children do better when they are young at the time of operation, but age at operation per se is not a factor for postlinguistically deaf children. Children also get better results if there is a progressive hearing loss, some residual hearing and they are in an oral–aural education programme.

How are patients selected preoperatively?

Children and adults should be assessed at a clinic that specializes in cochlear implants. When they are diagnosed as having a severe–profound hearing loss they also need to be reviewed to see whether a hearing aid or cochlear implant is preferable. The clinic should be led by an otologist with a good knowledge of audiology and the development of speech and language in children, as the cochlear implant is an invasive procedure and the otologist is ultimately responsible for its success. The other members of the clinic need to be professionals in audiology, speech pathology and education of the hearing impaired. Ideally, however, the field requires a human communication specialist with expertise in hearing, speech and language.

When the patient presents for the first time they should have an initial otological consultation to determine the cause of the hearing loss; the extent of the disability; previous medical, surgical or hearing aid assistance; and previous or intercurrent ear, nose, and throat disease or general medical conditions that may be relevant to their management. The expectations of the patient or their parents from a cochlear implant are also important. For suitable patients an audiological assessment should follow and include a complete history of the onset, severity, and nature of the hearing disability. Particular attention must be given to the type and fitting of any hearing aids. An initial audiological examination includes pure tone air and bone thresholds and speech perception scores, both aided and unaided, and impedance audiometry. Children will require behavioural testing with an age-appropriate procedure. At this stage it is best if the patient's further management is reviewed by the cochlear implant team in the light of the initial otological and audiological consultations, as they may have too much hearing, other clinical contraindications, unreasonable expectations or not wish to proceed.

If a decision is made with the patient or parents to assess suitability for a cochlear implant further, plain X-rays of the temporal bones, and CT scans of the cochleas will be required. These will indicate whether there are any congenital deformities or mastoid and middle ear disease and the condition of both cochleas. If the results do not clearly show which ear could receive a multiple-electrode array because of ossification then a three-dimensional reconstruction of a standard or helical CT scan may be required to give a better overall view. If there is any doubt about the presence of fibrous tissue in the scalae then an MRI will also be needed. When the CT is required in a child an anaesthetic is given, and at the same time an objective assessment of hearing such as steady-state evoked potential (SSEP)[50,51] or electrocochleography can be made. With adults it is also necessary to stimulate the promontory of the cochlea electrically to determine the perceptual response to global electrical stimulation of the auditory nerve. The test involves determining thresholds and comfortable levels, whether the patient can perceive pitch or only loudness, and whether pitch varies with stimulus rate. A single-channel speech processor extracting voicing is then connected to assess closed-set syllable identification.

If an adult or child has some useable hearing and has not been optimally fitted with a hearing aid, this will need to be done, and the aid tried for at least 3 months in an adult and longer in a child. With children it is also very important to assess their speech production, receptive and expressive language and general communication skills. Sociological issues need careful examination to ensure that there is good support from the family, as rehabilitation in the home and at work is just as important as the training sessions provided at the clinic or school. With children their educational management is critical, and it is essential with those of school age for the clinic staff to have close contact with their teachers before proceeding with surgery.

How is the surgery performed and what are the complications?

The cochlear implant surgery should be carried out with care to prevent infection. This requires good aseptic procedures and theatre routine. When implanting a foreign body there is an increased risk of postoperative infection, and with cochlear implants this has been 1.2 per cent in adults and 0.73 per cent in children.[52] This has been a factor in flap necrosis, for which the rate has been 0.84 per cent for adults and 0.37 per cent for children. Postoperative infection is a largely preventable complication that can be reduced to a minimum with preoperative skin swabs to exclude any pathogens, attention to the details of asepsis and haemostasis.

The hair should be shaved 5 cm beyond the proposed skin incision to avoid compromising sterility when the drapes are applied. An inverted J incision is recommended. The inverted J incision commences at the junction of the middle and upper thirds of the postauricular sulcus, and then sweeps in a curve upwards and backwards to a point that is 5 cm above and behind the external auditory meatus. It is preferable to take the incision even higher and further back than have it lie over the edge of the package when there is a greater chance of a wound breakdown. A modification of the inverted J incision is one that commences as an endaural incision and then extends above and behind the ear canal. The C incision has been abandoned in favour of the inverted J incision as the latter has good dependent venous drainage, and does not cut the branches of the occipital artery. The posterior branches of the superficial temporal artery are at risk, however, and when maximum blood supply is needed the combined endaural approach should be considered.

The skin and superficial fascia are elevated together as an inferiorly based flap. The deep fascia and periosteum are then dissected forward as an anteriorly based flap. Some surgeons raise all the tissue together, but we prefer to create two flaps so that the deeper one can if necessary be rotated to prevent the incision lying directly over an exposed package. The deep layer can also be useful for suturing over the package to hold it in place.

Sufficient mastoid air cells need to be drilled away to provide access for the posterior tympanotomy (Fig 9.9). Before undertaking the posterior tympanotomy it is important to identify the landmarks for the vertical segment of the facial nerve, so that the nerve itself can be identified and not injured when carrying out the procedure. The landmarks of importance are the short process of the incus, the fossa incudis and the lateral semicircular canal. The largest convenient diamond paste burr must be used to expose the facial nerve, but a thin layer of bone should be left over it to reduce further the chance of damaging it during the posterior tympanotomy. An accompanying artery and the pink colour of the nerve will help with its identification. The position of the facial nerve is not always predictable, and it is important not to assume that the first nerve encountered is the facial, because if it is the chorda tympani, the drill will soon enter the ear canal. Only when the posterior surface of the vertical segment of the facial nerve has been exposed should the bone leading into the middle ear be drilled away. The posterior tympanotomy is facilitated when there are sentinel cells beneath the floor of the antrum, as they can be followed to the middle ear. However, the tympanotomy can be difficult when there is solid bone in the region, in which case the chorda tympani and the posterosuperior margin of the annulus of the tympanic membrane need to be identified and preserved. This will then define the limits of the approach. Occasionally, especially in children, and

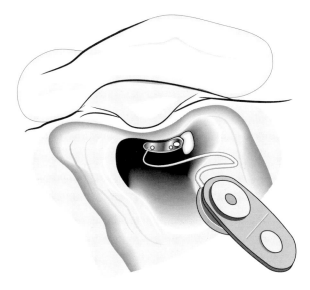

Fig 9.9 A drawing of the surgical implantation of the Nucleus CI-24M and CI-22M receiver–stimulators showing the left mastoid exenteration, posterior tympanotomy, bed for receiver–stimulator, electrode array inserted, and receiver–stimulator package about to be placed in its bed.

when there is an anteriorly placed lateral venous sinus, the access for a posterior tympanotomy is very restricted. In this situation the posterior wall of the osseous ear canal should be thinned, and the view through the microscope changed to be more medial. Rarely will it be necessary to drill away the posterior canal wall or approach the middle ear down the ear canal.

Having entered the middle ear (Fig 9.9), it is important to identify the round window niche and membrane. Locating the round window helps in the correct siting of a cochleostomy, which should lie close to the anteroinferior margin of the round window niche. The round window can be difficult to see, in which case bone anterior to the vertical section of the facial nerve should be drilled away. Sometimes the infracochlear air cell looks like the round window niche, and on occasions the electrode array has been inserted into it. It can only be distinguished if the surgeon is very familiar with the anatomy of the first part of the scala tympani of the basal turn of the cochlea. The scala tympani has a distinctive inferolateral curvature that distinguishes it from an air cell. Occasionally the round window is absent, especially with otosclerosis and labyrinthitis ossificans, when the centre of its superior margin can be estimated as 2.7 mm inferior to the centre of the inferior margin of the oval window, or footplate of the stapes. Originally most electrode placements were made through the round window membrane; now it is preferable to create a cochleostomy as this allows a better view along the scala tympani. This enables the Nucleus free-fitting banded electrode to be directed more easily along the scala tympani, resulting in a deeper and less traumatic insertion.

Once access has been obtained for a cochleostomy, the next stage of the operation is to create a bed in the mastoid for the receiver–stimulator package. Alternatively, the package bed can be created before the posterior tympanotomy is completed. The Nucleus-22 (CI-22M) receiver–stimulator (Fig 9.9) should be placed in a bed so that its anterior edge lies 35 mm behind the ear canal. This will prevent the microphone case, or arm of spectacles, pressing on the anterior edge of the receiver–stimulator and causing discomfort or even skin erosion. The Nucleus-24 (CI-24M) receiver–stimulator needs to be placed so that the anterior edge of the receiver coil is 45 mm above and behind the ear canal. With the CI-24M this placement will avoid limiting access to the transmitting coil, especially when using a behind-the-ear speech processor. In fashioning the bed for the CI-22M receiver–stimulator a template will help to make it the correct size and it should have vertical sides. If necessary, in thin skulls and especially in children, the bone overlying the dura can be drilled away, and the dura depressed 1–2 mm by the device. As the CI-24M is thinner than the CI-22M and has a smaller protruding section, a bed may not need to be created or it may be part of the mastoid cavity.

When the bed for the package has been made the next step is to place a platinum wire around the floor of the mastoid antrum for tying the lead wire down once the electrode is inserted into the cochlea. Then the cochleostomy should be created. This is best done by drilling from below upwards so that the scala tympani can be entered away from the spiral lamina to minimize any risk of damage to the latter structure. If possible the endosteal lining should be preserved during the drilling to protect the inner ear structures, and then an opening made with a fine needle. If the scala is being entered through the round window membrane, this should be incised anteroinferiorly to avoid damage to the spiral lamina. In this case, to achieve a good exposure along the scala, the crista fenestra should also be reduced. If there is new bone or fibrous tissue in the initial part of the scala tympani, this will need to be dissected away to provide adequate access to the more distal section of the scala, if shown on X-ray to be patent. Drilling along the scala should not be carried further than 8 mm, otherwise the inter-

nal carotid may be pierced. Commencing the drilling close to the round window helps to ensure the correct orientation so that the scala tympani is entered and a channel is not made tangential to the scala. If a patent scala is not present, or cannot easily be created, an attempt should be made to enter the scala vestibuli, as it can be patent but not clearly seen on the CT scans. This will involve drilling into the scala vestibuli 1.5 mm anteroinferior to the centre of the inferior margin of the oval window. A variant of this procedure is to drill along the basal sections of the scala tympani and vestibuli separately and then join up the two channels, preserving overlying bone to hold the electrode array in place. If the middle and apical turns of the cochlea are patent, a cochleostomy in the middle or apical turns can be made with anterograde or retrograde insertion.[53] Finally, if the CT scans and MRIs show that the turns in the cochlea are obliterated, it will be necessary to drill out the bone overlying the basal turn. This will require a permeatal approach to the middle ear with the elevation of an endomeatal flap. In drilling the bone over the scala tympani care will be required to avoid damaging the spiral lamina, the horizontal section of the facial nerve and the internal carotid artery.

In the uncomplicated case the electrode array can usually be inserted for a distance of 21 mm on average; the range is 15–27 mm. A deeper insertion has been reported if the electrode array is coated with Healon, which reduces the friction between the array and the outer wall of the scala. The surgery for children is basically the same as for adults. The incision will appear relatively larger because of the reduced head size, but must not be reduced in extent.

Consensus has still not been reached on the best method of fixing the electrode. However, it must be fixed close to the round window in children so that head growth does not pull it out of the cochlea. We have found a Silastic grommet slid along the electrode and into the cochleostomy to could an effective solution.[54]

What is the postoperative management and auditory training of patients?

The patient is normally discharged 3 days postoperatively. The wound should be inspected daily, and a tight bandage maintained to avoid a haematoma. If this develops it may need aspiration. An aerocoele arising when air is forced up the Eustachian tube will also normally resolve with a compression bandage. Wound infection, in addition to topical antiseptics, will require further systemic antibiotics according to the sensitivity of the organism. In a proportion of patients the wound will require exploration, especially if there is exposure of the receiver–stimulator. In some patients debridement of tissue and administration of long-term antibiotics (3 months) will avoid having to remove the device. If infection is extensive the package will have to be removed.

In most patients the surgical outcome is uneventful and the receiver–stimulator can be 'fired up' when the scalp is healed 3 weeks postoperatively. The first task then is to establish thresholds and maximum comfortable levels for each electrode pair for bipolar stimulation, and each electrode for common ground and monopolar stimulation. Thresholds are obtained by an ascending technique. The maximum comfortable level is arrived at by first reaching the minimum discomfort level and reducing the stimulus current a small amount. The stimuli are then swept across groups of electrodes to ensure that they are of equal loudness and that the levels have been correctly set. When it has been established that they are of equal loudness, the stimuli should then be swept across all the electrodes to determine whether there is adequate pitch scaling for the place coding of frequency or pitch information. The thresholds and maximum comfortable levels are programmed into the map of the patient's speech processor.

Auditory training exercises involve listening to speech and repeating what is heard. The speech material may be sentences, words or vowels and consonants. The exercises allow the audiologist to assess the performance of the patient and at the same time provide training. The task must not be too difficult or the patient will be discouraged. The patient is also counselled on how to use the device, for example what to expect if the batteries become flat. Later, training is given in the use of the telephone, and this may vary from the use of a code when the patient has limited speech perception ability to interactive conversations for the best performers.

Auditory training for children will not only concentrate on improving their ability to perceive and understand speech and environmental sounds, but also their speech production, receptive and expressive language and communication. The speech material used for the training will need to be age-appropriate. The training should be integrated into the child's educational programme which will be at either a preschool or school level. They will need to be taught by auditory–oral or auditory–verbal methods to take advantage of the new auditory information they are receiving. In certain situations the use of total communication in which signed English is combined with an auditory stimulus will be required. Sign language for the deaf should not be used because it does not have the grammatical structure required for communicating with normally hearing people, and is not appropriately combined with a cochlear implant.

References

1. Gantz BJ, McCabe BF, Tyler RS, Preece JP. Evaluation of four cochlear implant designs. *Annals of Otology, Rhinology and Laryngology* 1987; **96(suppl 128)**:145–9.
2. Skinner MW, Clark GM, Whitford LA, Seligman PM, Staller SJ, Shipp DB, *et al.* Evaluation of a new spectral peak coding strategy for the Nucleus 22 channel cochlear implant system. *The American Journal of Otology* 1994; **15**:15–27.
3. Cowan RSC, Brown C, Whitford LA, Galvin KL, Sarant JZ, Barker EJ, *et al.* Speech perception in children using the advanced SPEAK speech processing strategy. *Annals of Otology, Rhinology and Laryngology* 1995; **104(suppl 166)**:318–21.
4. Burian K, Hochmair E, Hochmair-Desoyer I. Designing of and experience with multichannel cochlear implants. *Acta Otolaryngologica* 1979; **87**:190–5.
5. House WF, Luetje CM, Campos CT. The cochlear implant: performance of deaf patients, practicality in clinical practice, co-investigator experience. *Hearing Instruments* 1981; **32**:12–30.
6. Fourcin AJ, Rosen SM, Moore BCJ. External electrical stimulation of the cochlea: clinical, psychophysical, speech-perceptual and histological findings. *British Journal of Audiology* 1979; **13**:85–107.
7. Laird RK. *A sound encoder for an implantable hearing prosthesis* [MEngSc Thesis]. Melbourne: University of Melbourne, 1979.
8. Clark GM. Electrical stimulation of the auditory nerve: the coding of frequency, the perception of pitch, and the development of cochlear implant speech processing strategies for profoundly deaf people. *Journal of Clinical and Experimental Pharmacology and Physiology* 1996; **23**:766–76.
9. Djourno A, Eyries C. Prothése auditive par excitation électrique a distance du nerf sensoriel a l'aide d'un bobinage inclus a demeure. *Presse Medicale* 1957; **35**:14–7.
10. Simmons FB, Monegeon CJ, Lewis WR, Huntington DA. Electrical stimulation of acoustical nerve and inferior colliculus. *Archives of Otolaryngology* 1964; **79**:559–67.
11. Doyle JH, Doyle JB, Turnbull FM. Electrical stimulation of eighth cranial nerve. *Archives of Otolaryngology* 1964; **80**:388–91.
12. House WF, Berliner K, Crary W, Graham M, Luckey R, Norton N, *et al.* Cochlear implants. *Annals of Otology, Rhinology and Laryngology* 1976; **85(suppl 27)**:3–6.

13. Clark GM. *Middle ear and neural mechanisms in hearing and in the management of deafness* [PhD Thesis]. Sydney: University of Sydney, 1969.

14. Clark GM. Responses of cells in the superior olivary complex of the cat to electrical stimulation of the auditory nerve. *Experimental Neurology* 1969; **24**:124–36.

15. Clark GM, Nathar JM, Kranz HG, Maritz JS. A behavioral study on electrical stimulation of the cochlea and central auditory pathways of the cat. *Experimental Neurology* 1972; **36**:350–61.

16. Clark GM, Kranz HG, Minas HJ. Behavioral thresholds in the cat to frequency modulated sound and electrical stimulation of the auditory nerve. *Experimental Neurology* 1973; **41**:190–200.

17. Merzenich MM. Studies on electrical stimulation of the auditory nerve in animals and man: cochlear implants. In: *The nervous system, vol 3: Human communication and its disorders*. New York: Raven Press, 1975:537–48.

18. Clark GM, Tong YC, Bailey QR, Black RC, Martin LF, Millar JB, *et al.* A multiple electrode cochlear implant. *Journal of the Otolaryngological Society of Australia* 1978; **4**:208–12.

19. Tong YC, Black RC, Clark GM, Forster IC, Millar JB, O'Loughlin BJ, *et al.* A preliminary report on a multiple-channel cochlear implant operation. *Journal of Laryngology and Otology* 1979; **93**:679–95.

20. Clark GM, Tong YC, Martin LFA, Busby PA. A multiple-channel cochlear implant. An evaluation using an open-set word test. *Acta Otolaryngologica (Stockh)* 1981; **91**:173–5.

21. Clark GM, Tong YC, Martin LFA, Busby PA. A multiple-channel cochlear implant. An evaluation using open-set CID sentences. *Laryngoscope* 1981; **91**:628–34.

22. Atlas LE, Herndon MK, Simmons FB, Dent LJ, White RL. Results of stimulus and speech-coding schemes applied to multichannel electrodes. Cochlear Prostheses, an International Symposium. *Annals of the New York Academy of Sciences* 1983; **405**:377–86.

23. Eddington DK. Speech discrimination in deaf subjects with cochlear implants. *The Journal of the Acoustical Society of America* 1980; **68**:885–91.

24. Michelson RP, Schindler RA. Multichannel cochlear implant: preliminary results in man. *Laryngoscope* 1981; **91**:38–42.

25. Chouard CH. The surgical rehabilitation of total deafness with the multichannel cochlear implant. Indications and results. *Audiology* 1980; **19**:137–45.

26. Millar JB, Tong YC, Clark GM. Speech processing for cochlear implant prostheses. *Journal of Speech and Hearing Research* 1984; **27**:280–96.

27. Clark GM. Advances in cochlear implant speech processing. In: Clark GM ed. *Cochlear Implants. XVI World Congress of Otorhinolaryngology Head and Neck Surgery Sydney (Australia) March 2–7 1997*. Bologna: Monduzzi Editore, 1997:9–15.

28. Clark GM. Historical perspectives. In: Clark GM, Cowan RSC, Dowell RC eds. *Cochlear implantation for infants and children. Advances.* San Diego: Singular Publishing, 1997:9–28.

29. McKay CM. McDermott HJ, Clark GM. Preliminary results with a six spectral maxima speech processor for the University of Melbourne/Nucleus multiple-electrode cochlear implant. *Journal of the Otolaryngological Society of Australia* 1991; **6**:354–9.

30. Wilson BS, Finley CC, Lawson DT, Wolford RD, Eddington DK, Rabinowitz WM. Better speech recognition with cochlear implants. *Nature* 1991; **352**:236–8.

31. Kessler DK, Loeb GE, Barker MJ. Distribution of speech recognition results with the Clarion cochlear prosthesis. *Annals of Otology, Rhinology and Laryngology* 1995; **104(suppl 166)**:283–5.

32. Clark GM, Tong YC, Patrick JF. Introduction. In: Clark GM, Tong YC, Patrick JF eds. *Cochlear prostheses*. Edinburgh: Churchill Livingstone, 1990:1–14.

33. Clark GM. Cochlear implants: historical perspectives. In: Plant G, Spens K-E eds. *Profound deafness and speech communication*. London: Whurr, 1995:165–218.

34. Luxford WM, Berliner KI, Eisenberg MA, House WF. Cochlear implants in children. *Annals of Otology, Rhinology and Laryngology* 1987; **96**:136–8.

35. Clark GM, Blamey PJ, Busby PA, Dowell RC, Franz BK, Musgrave GN, *et al.* A multiple-electrode intracochlear implant for children. *Archives of Otolaryngology* 1987; **113**:825–8.

36. Clark GM, Blamey PJ, Busby PA, Dowell RC, Franz BK, Musgrave GN, *et al.* Preliminary results for the Cochlear Corporation multi-electrode intracochlear implants on six prelingually deaf patients. *American Journal of Otology* 1987; **8**:234–9.

37. Clark GM, Dowell RC, Cowan RS, Pyman BC, Webb RL. Multicentre evaluations of speech perception in adults and children with the Nucleus (Cochlear) 22-channel cochlear implant. In: Portmann M ed. *Proceedings of the Third International Symposium on Transplants and Implants in Otology, Bordeaux, June 1995*. The Netherlands: Kugler, 1996; 353–63.

38. Clark GM. An evaluation of per-scalar cochlear electrode implantation techniques. An histopathological study in cats. *Journal of Laryngology and Otology* 1977; **91**:185–99.

39. Shepherd RK, Clark GM, Xu SA, Pyman BC. Cochlear pathology following reimplantation of a multichannel scala tympani electrode array in the Macaque. *The American Journal of Otology* 1995; **16**:186–99.

40. Clark GM, Shepherd RK. Cochlear implant round window sealing procedures in the cat. An investigation of autograft and heterograft materials. *Acta Otolaryngologica (Stockh)* 1984; **410**:5–15.

41. Dahm MC, Clark GM, Franz BK, Shepherd RK, Burton MJ, Robins-Browne R. Cochlear implantation in children: labyrinthitis following pneumococcal otitis media in unimplanted and implanted cat cochleas. *Acta Otolaryngologica* 1994; **114**:620–5.

42. Shepherd RK, Clark GM, Black RC. Chronic electrical stimulation of the auditory nerve in cats. Physiological and histopathological results. *Acta Otolaryngologica (Stockh)* 1983; **399**:19–31.

43. Ni D, Shepherd RK, Seldon HL, Xu S, Clark GM, Millard RE. Cochlear pathology following chronic

electrical stimulation of the auditory nerve 1: normal hearing kittens. *Hearing Research* 1992; **62**:63–81.

44. Shepherd RK, Matsushima J, Millard RE, Clark GM. Cochlear pathology following chronic electrical stimulation using non charge balanced stimuli. *Acta Otolaryngologica (Stockh)* 1991; **111**:848–60.

45. Tykocinski M, Shepherd RK, Clark GM. Acute effects of high-rate stimulation on auditory nerve function in guinea pigs. *Annals of Otology, Rhinology and Laryngology* 1995; **104(suppl 166)**:71–5.

46. Xu J, Shepherd RK, Millard RE, Clark GM. Chronic electrical stimulation of the auditory nerve at high stimulus rates: a physiological and histopathological study. *Hearing Research*. [In press].

47. Blamey PJ. Factors affecting audiology performance of postlinguistically deaf adults using cochlear implants: etiology, age and duration of deafness. In: *Abstracts of the 100th NIH consensus development conference: cochlear implants in adults and children.* Washington D.C. National Institutes of Health, 1995.

48. Blamey PJ, Pyman BC, Gordon M, Clark GM, Brown AM, Dowell RC, *et al.* Factors predicting postoperative sentence scores in postlinguistically deaf adult cochlear implant patients. *Annals of Otology, Rhinology and Laryngology* 1992; **101**:342–8.

49. Dowell RC, Blamey PJ, Clark GM. The potential and limitations of cochlear implants in children. *Annals of Otology, Rhinology and Laryngology* 1995; **104(suppl 166)**:324–8.

50. Burton MJ, Cohen LT, Rickards FW, McNally KI, Clark GM. Steady-state evoked potentials to amplitude modulated tones in the monkey. *Acta Otolaryngologica* 1992; **112**:745–51.

51. Cohen NL, Rickards FW, Clark GM. A comparison of steady-state evoked potentials to modulated tones in awake and sleeping humans. *Journal of the Acoustical Society of America* 1991; **90**:2467–79.

52. Hoffman RA, Cohen NL. Complications of cochlear implant surgery. *Annals of Otology, Rhinology and Laryngology* 1995; **104(suppl 166)**:420–2.

53. Singh RS. Ossified cochlea and its impact on cochlear implants. In: Clark GM ed. *Cochlear implants. XVI World Congress of Otorhinolaryngology Head and Neck Surgery. Sydney (Australia) March 2–7 1997.* Bologna: Monduzzi Editore, 1997:201–3.

54. Pyman B, Clark GM. Siting the receiver-stimulator of the CI-24M model of the Cochlear Limited multiple-channel cochlear implant, and fixation of its electrode array. In: Clark GM ed. *Cochlear implants XVI World Congress of Otorhinolaryngology Head and Neck Surgery. Sydney (Australia) March 2–7 1997.* Bologna: Monduzzi Editore, 1997:211–5.

CHAPTER 10

Childhood deafness

SUSAN SNASHALL

Introduction

Childhood deafness presents special problems in terms of assessment and habilitation as it is usually present before language has been acquired (prelingual). Children do not complain of impaired hearing, and even parents and carers are known to be unaware of the deficit in at least 30 per cent of affected children. If a permanent effect upon language development is to be avoided, children with hearing loss must be found and treated promptly, before the critical period for language acquisition has passed. Children born with sensorineural hearing loss may never acquire normal speech and language, but their chances are improved if habilitation begins before the age of 6 months. Children with conductive deafness due to otitis media with effusion suffer more subtle effects upon language, attention and behaviour.

One of the special problems of childhood deafness is that it is frequently accompanied by other impairments and disabilities. Up to 30 per cent of children born with sensorineural deafness have other defects, and conditions such as Down's syndrome and cleft palate increase the likelihood of conductive hearing loss. Otitis media is also prevalent in disadvantaged and learning disabled children who are already at risk of language delay. Early intervention in chronic secretory otitis media has become an area of controversy, but hearing loss in the presence of language or development delay requires treatment.

The management of hearing impairment in children is most effective if undertaken by a consultant-led multidisciplinary team, including audiology, paediatrics, genetics, otolaryngology, plastic surgery, education, speech therapy, mental health, social services and voluntary bodies. This approach is best delivered in a hospital-based centre because of the special needs of hearing impaired children and the rarity of sensorineural hearing impairment and craniofacial defects in the child population.

Assessment, diagnosis and management of the hearing impaired child is best undertaken in a child friendly environment. This means that the clinic and waiting area need to be specially designated for children. The clinic rooms must be larger than those used for adults as the child is always accompanied by at least one other person and needs freedom to move around.

Development of the auditory system and speech

Awareness, recognition and discrimination of sound, particularly speech, and the expressive counterpart, communication, language and speech production all develop gradually from birth. Communication is the interactive exchange of feelings and needs between two individuals and may be excellent without any speech or language, as in the communication between infant and parent. Language involves the expression of ideas and concepts using common rules, and may not necessarily be spoken, for example sign language. Speech involves the production of specific sounds, sometimes referred to as articulation. A child may have problems in any of these aspects and in any combination. Speech and language delay describes a child who has the speech and language appropriate to a younger child. A speech or language disorder describes a situation in which the speech or language has deviated from the normal sequence of development. Children with sensorineural hearing loss may have deviant as well as delayed speech and language and may have a coexisting aphasia or dyspraxia unrelated to the hearing impairment.

FIRST SIX MONTHS

The neonatal response to sound is reflexive. Very loud sounds will give rise to the full Moro response, but the startle reflex may be limited to eye blinking only (the auropalpebral reflex). Reflex responses to sound at this age are present at approximately 60–70 dBA and include sucking, head turning, stilling, moving, eye widening, frowning, change in breathing pattern, change in heart rate and eye movements. Within a few weeks the infant will recognize family voices and will respond to different tones of voice such as anger or loving care. Certain sounds are more likely to elict a reaction such as familiar voices or toys, musical boxes, bells and narrow bands of noise rather than pure tones. A quiet voice is more interesting than a louder voice. By 4 months turns to sounds at 45–55 dBA may be obtained. Behavioural responses to sound during the first 6 months are extremely variable and are influenced by non-auditory factors such as comfort, tiredness, hunger and levels of alertness. Lack of response at this stage does not necessarily mean hearing impairment. During this period speech develops from vocalizations associated with physical discomfort to early communication and turn taking. Infants attempt to mimic lip patterns and sound from the first weeks of extrauterine life, and discover that they can produce noises for pleasure around 3–4 months. The first meaningful communication is gesture, soon followed by word precursors.

SECOND SIX MONTHS

Providing vision is intact the normal child will be able to localize sounds and respond consistently by head turning by 6–7 months. Sounds originating at close range are located earlier than sounds coming from further away. By 7 months the majority of normal children will turn to soft (30–35 dBA) sounds presented in the plane of the ear at a distance of 1 metre. They then learn to localize above and below the plane of the ear, and by 10 months can localize sounds in the vertical plane. At this time sounds may also be located at a distance of 3 metres. These skills do not appear in blind or partially sighted infants, and are delayed in children with development delay or attention deficits such as autism. Motor difficulties will also limit head turning

and localization, an example being *preferred head turning*, which may cause confusion with unilateral hearing impairment. Hearing impaired children become visually aware during this period, and have been shown to have enhanced peripheral vision.

During the second 6 months the child's babble becomes more tuneful as the rise and fall of speech is imitated. Precursors of words and phrases may be recognized. By the first birthday there will be a small number of intelligible words with meaning, such as family names and familiar objects. The hearing impaired child loses the reflexive utterance of the first 6 months and becomes silent.

In some children the auditory pathways have delayed myelination and the infant behaves as if severely hearing impaired. Auditory evoked potentials will also give abnormal responses if the problem is in myelination. This condition is known as *delayed auditory maturation* and is equivalent to the well recognized *delayed visual maturation*, which can manifest as apparent blindness. In both cases myelination and migration of neural tissue catches up and the child develops completely normal vision and hearing. For hearing this is usually before the first birthday.

SECOND YEAR

The vocabulary expands steadily during the second year, towards the end of which the child is beginning to join two or more words together and use situational phrases. By 18–24 months a child will fetch two items from another room without contextual clues or lip-reading. The cooperative test utilizes the child's ability to identify parts of the body or to 'give it to mummy'. *If there are no recognizable words by the age of 16 months prompt investigation is required.* During this period the child is aware of sounds at a distance and is capable of categorizing sounds according to their source and meaning. From the age of 18 months there is increasing reluctance to turn to sounds that are not meaningful. This inhibition of response to sound can be overcome by techniques such as *visual reinforcement audiometry* using warble tones to which turning responses may be obtained at 5–25 dBA. As sounds become better recognized they become more relevant and the child's attention increases. In consequence reactions are obtained to quieter sounds than in early infancy.

THIRD TO FIFTH YEARS

Speech and language expand rapidly during the third year. The development of speech will be related to the breadth of the child's environmental experience and opportunities for interacting with others. If hearing is partially impaired at this age, the effect is reduced by increasing the level of language stimulation. The child can name specified toy items and identify them on request in the absence of lip-reading and at minimal levels. The child will describe pictures with gradual improvement in vocabulary and grammar and should be understandable to strangers by the age of 3 years. Language development in the preschool years is crucial for subsequent educational achievement as language delay will affect reading ability.

From the age of 2 years children may be *conditioned* to respond to warble tones in soundfield using toy material that must be well within their motor capabilities. Earphones may be used from the age of 3½ years and bone conduction from around 3 years. Masking of the good ear in suspected unilateral loss is not possible until at least the age of 6 years. Threshold responses improve by 3–4 dB hearing level (HL)/year at high frequencies up to the age of 7 years. This is over and above the learning effect that improves responses by 2 dBHL at low frequencies and up to 8 dbHL at high frequencies, demonstrated by repeated testing of children aged 6–18 years. Minimum behavioural response levels mature as a result of attention, test design and test environment, as children are more easily distracted than adults. This means that the conditions of the test environment must be more stringent than for adults.

Prevalence of the problem

CONGENITAL HEARING IMPAIRMENT

Congenital conductive hearing impairment is uncommon and is associated with congenital defects of the outer and middle ear (Chapters 18 and 19). Middle ear defects, such as congenital stapes fixation with or without the oto-brachio-renal syndrome or osteogenesis imperfecta, are easily overlooked in the absence of visible stigmata. Hearing impairment in children with craniofacial abnormalities poses particular management problems because of the psychological effects upon the child and the parents.

Sensorineural hearing impairment is present in 1–1.5/1000 children and can be congenital or of early onset. Early onset hearing loss can begin at any time during the first year and is progressive during the preschool years. Progressive deafness accounts for 15–20 per cent of preschool children with sensorineural hearing loss. These children may

not be detected by a neonatal hearing screen. The prevalence of hearing loss varies between populations. Those in which consanguineous marriages are common may have a prevalence of 12/1000 children, and graduates of special care baby units or neonatal intensive care have a prevalence of approximately 15/1000. Precise rates will be individual to a particular community. Factors that increase the prevalence of hearing impairment are a family history of deafness, congenital abnormalities of the head and neck, prenatal and perinatal infection, prematurity, low birth weight, anoxia, high bilirubin concentrations and parents who are first cousins. The mumps, measles and rubella vaccination programme has reduced the prevalence of congenital deafness due to these infections, but cytomegalovirus, herpes and meningitis from any organism are also associated with congenital and perinatal deafness. High bilirubin accounts for much less hearing loss than previously, but such cases are still seen. Risk factors are present in up to 70 per cent of children with sensorineural hearing loss, but are not always recognized at birth. Neonatal screening is targeted at these groups. In 30–40 per cent of children no cause is found and the deafness is presumed to be due to a recessive gene, with considerable implications for genetic counselling.

ACQUIRED HEARING IMPAIRMENT

The commonest type of acquired hearing impairment in children is a *conductive* loss due to chronic secretory otitis media, a self-limiting disease with peak prevalence in the second and third years and again at school entry. It is more common in deprived children, learning disabled and syndromic children, atopic children and children exposed to passive smoking. It is much more prevalent in the winter, when up to 30 per cent of preschool children may be affected for at least part of the season. The high prevalence of this disorder places enormous demands upon children's audiology services as it is necessary to test the hearing of affected children in order to determine the need for intervention and the possibility of coexisting sensorineural loss. Up to 50 per cent of parents will be unaware of their child's problem. Chronic secretory otitis media is more common in the population who fail to attend clinic appointments, so that intervention does not always reach the worst affected. This is one reason for the variable rate of surgical intervention between geographical locations. In one unselected cohort of routine child health clinic attenders 8 per cent of children had surgery for this condition before they were 4 years old and a further 4 per cent by the time they were 8 years of age.

The commonest cause of acquired *sensorineural* hearing loss is meningitis, particularly meningococcal. All children suffering from meningitis should have a hearing test within 4 weeks of fitness to test. The loss can improve or deteriorate in the months after the illness, a fact to be considered when planning the management of a child with postmeningitis hearing impairment. Children deafened by meningitis also lose almost all vestibular function and will be temporarily off balance after the illness. Head injury is another important cause of acquired hearing loss in children. In the case of minor congenital abnormalities of the temporal bones, such as a wide vestibular aqueduct, sensorineural hearing loss results from minor head trauma. Affected children may be born with normal hearing and suffer a stepwise deterioration in hearing and balance after such trauma. Viral infections such as mumps cause unilateral cochleovestibular failure, which may go unnoticed in a young child. Sudden, progressive and fluctuating hearing loss is uncommon in children, but is investigated and treated as in adults. Acoustic schwannoma is less common in children than adults but does arise *de novo* and in children from families with NF2 syndrome.

Causes of hearing impairment in childhood

The causes of ear disease and deafness are fully described elsewhere and it is only necessary to emphasize those causes of hearing impairment that occur specifically in childhood.

CONGENITAL HEARING IMPAIRMENT

Congenital hearing impairment has genetic and non-genetic causes. The mumps, measles and rubella vaccination programme is reducing hearing loss attributable to these infections. Hearing impairment due to intrauterine infections usually progresses during the first 2 years of life, but may be delayed until the second or third decade, as is seen in congenital syphilis. In many of these cases the cause of the hearing loss will also cause other developmental problems such as speech and language disorders, development delay, learning disability, cerebral palsy and visual impairment. This is why up to 30 per cent of hearing impaired children have other disabilities. The only cause of 'congenital deafness' that improves is delayed auditory maturation. Non-genetic causes are given in Table 10.1.

Table 10.1 Non-genetic causes of congenital hearing loss

Intrauterine	Environmental hazards, diabetes, toxaemia, ototoxic drugs, teratogenic chemicals
Infections	Rubella, cytomegalovirus, measles, chickenpox, herpes, toxoplasma, syphilis, parvo, HIV
Perinatal factors	Low birth weight, hyperbilirubinaemia, anoxia
Neonatal infections	Meningitis, encephalitis, septicaemia
Developmental	Delayed auditory maturation

Genetic hearing impairment may be syndromal, or non-syndromal, recessive or dominant. Genetic inner ear disease is usually confined to the cochlea, but syndromal hearing impairment and progressive losses are commonly associated with vestibular deficit, for example Usher syndrome type-II. Craniofacial abnormalities are particularly associated with hearing impairment, both conductive and sensorineural. This applies to even minor defects such as ear pits or tags, for example ear pits syndrome and oto-brachio-renal syndrome. Some syndromes may not manifest until the second or third decade such as Usher and Refsum (with retinitis pigmentosa), Alport (with renal failure), NF2 and Pendred (with hypothyroidism and goitre). Other syndromes may be manifest early but progress during the first two decades, for example Waardenburg, Marshall Stickler and Down's syndrome.

Children with a wide vestibular aqueduct may be born with normal hearing and lose it progressively, with or without minor head trauma. Non-syndromic dominant genetic hearing impairment may be early onset, that is, normal hearing at birth and rapid progression of hearing loss during the first years of life. Approximately 30 per cent of congenitally hearing impaired children will have non-syndromic recessive cochlear hearing impairment and many of these will be progressive during the first two decades.

ACQUIRED HEARING IMPAIRMENT

Inner ear infections cause permanent hearing loss, but if this is unilateral it may go undetected until school screening. Deafness due to infection, viral or meningococcal, is likely to be accompanied by vestibular deficit as the mechanism is labyrinthitis. The accompanying vestibular deficit may cause ataxia during the acute illness, but central compensation is rapid in children and is forgotten. This creates diagnostic difficulties for the clinician when presented with unilateral hearing loss in a school-child. The deafness caused by meningitis may improve or deteriorate during the first year after the illness, but later than this the only changes will be deterioration. Cochlear implantation after meningitis should not therefore be undertaken too soon after the illness (except if osteoneogenesis is suspected). In some cases inner ear hearing loss is a sequel to chronic suppurative otitis media. *Perilymph leak and Menière's syndrome* produce sudden or fluctuating hearing loss and vestibular disturbance in children with Mondini defect or a wide vestibular aqueduct. If these symptoms arise after minor head trauma or Valsalva manoeuvre, a perilymph leak should be suspected, but is very difficult to prove. Menière's disorder is uncommon in childhood and tends to be atypical. Response to treatment is very poor and headache is often a feature. *Central deafness* can result from inflammation, such as Reye's syndrome, or may be part of progressive neurological disorder.

Functional hearing loss is common and arises for very different reasons in children than those that cause the disorder in adults. A proportion of these children may be called *iatrogenic* as they have only arisen because of poor and repeated audiometric testing, sometimes in relation to 'watchful waiting' for secretory otitis media. This leaves the child believing there is something wrong and confused over the correct way to respond to audiometry. It is for this reason that testing of children, whether for school screening or clinic diagnosis, must be undertaken by staff thoroughly trained in audiometry and in handling children. Others will be under pressure to perform well at school or at home, and are either lacking in confidence or attempting to find a way out of a difficult situation. In this context Munchausen syndrome should also be considered. Many of the children presenting with functional hearing loss will be suffering abuse, and it is for this reason that functional hearing loss is so important and requires close collaboration with other agencies, especially the school health service. The age of presentation and gender distribution at each age mimics that of sexual and physical abuse (predominantly boys of 8–9 and girls of 12–13 years). These children require careful handling and it may be inappropriate to remove this mechanism of 'crying for help', as the child will then have to invent another. *For any child found to have functional hearing loss the possibility of abuse should be considered.*

Screening

Congenital and acquired hearing impairment in children may not be noticed until speech and lan-guage fail to develop. The average age of detection of congenital deafness was found to be around 3 years in the European Community and 2 years in the UK, with some children not being discovered until the age of 8 years. The age of detection is gradually improving, but the median remains closer to 2 years than 1 year. The targets set by the UK National Deaf Children's Society in 1994 are for 40 per cent to be found by 6 months and 85 per cent by the first birthday, with hearing aids fitted within 4 weeks of diagnosis. For a 1980–86 cohort in the UK, 17 per cent were fitted with hearing aids by the first birthday.

To improve detection neonatal hearing screens are being established, whereas infant surveillance and screening aims to detect those not found at birth. Neonatal hearing screening is either *universal* or, if resources are more limited, *selective*. A selective screen is targeted at those neonates with the highest risk of congenital deafness. In the USA a universal neonatal hearing screen was piloted in Rhode Island. The outcomes of the Rhode Island study resulted in a National Institutes of Health consensus statement recommending that all US children should be screened in the neonatal period using transient evoked otoacoustic emissions (TEOAEs). A neonatal screen is insufficient on its own as 15–20 per cent of children with prelingual hearing loss will develop that loss in the first 2 years of life.

Subsequent universal screens are the 8-month distraction test and the school entry audiometric sweep. Subsequent selective screens are those after meningitis or head injury. Screening or surveillance is required for acquired hearing impairment as children do not complain of hearing loss.

Although many parents are not aware of their child's hearing loss, some do recognize the problem within the first 2 weeks of life. Any concern by parents should be taken seriously and the hearing assessed as a matter of urgency. In many localities parents receive information on normal infant hearing and speech development as a component of parent-held records so that hearing loss may be suspected before language fails to develop. Such a scheme is presented in Table 10.2 and has been of proven benefit. Properly informed parents do not become unduly anxious or ask for unnecessary referral.

NEONATAL PERIOD

Goals

The goal of neonatal hearing screening is to detect all hearing loss present at birth so that training can

Table 10.2 Hints for parents

"Can your baby hear you?"

Here is a checklist of some of the general signs you can look for in your baby's first year:

Shortly after birth   **YES/NO**
Your baby should be startled by a sudden loud noise such as a hand clap or a door slamming and should blink or open his eyes widely to such sounds.

By 1 month
Your baby should be beginning to notice sudden prolonged sounds like the noise of a vacuum cleaner and he should pause and listen to them when they begin.

By 4 months
He should quieten or smile to the sound of your voice even when he cannot see you. He may also turn his head or eyes towards you if you come up from behind and speak to him from the side.

By 7 months
He should turn immediately to your voice across the room or to very quiet noises made on each side if he is not too occupied with other things.

By 9 months
He should listen attentively to familiar everyday sounds and search for very quiet sounds made out of sight. He should also show pleasure in babbling loudly and tunefully.

By 12 months
He should show some response to his own name and to other familiar words. He may also response when you say 'no' and 'bye bye' even when he cannot see any accompanying gesture.

Your health visitor will perform a routine hearing screening test on your baby between 7 and 9 months of age. She will be able to help and advise you at any time before or after this test if you are concerned about your baby and his or her development. If you suspect that your baby is not hearing normally, either because you cannot answer yes to the items above or for some other reason, then seek advice from your health visitor.
(Courtesy of Prof. B McCormick)

be instituted early enough to allow the child to achieve speech and language that is as normal as possible. In the babbling period the infant makes perceptual and productive categorizations of the speech signal, and treatment should ideally be implemented before this period, that is, 3–6 months. This makes universal neonatal hearing screening highly desirable if resources are available for assessment and management of all infants failing the screen. If these resources are not available, a selective screen of those most at risk should be undertaken. Screening should be monitored for coverage and outcome. Neonatal screening programmes are part of an overall screening programme, not tests done in isolation from other surveillance systems.

Procedures: children at risk of congenital hearing loss

The risk factors for hearing impairment enable paediatricians and primary care staff to select those children requiring special screening and surveillance. For selective screening to be efficient coverage of the at-risk population must be at least 90 per cent and have a prevalence rate of 14 times greater than the general population. Lists of risk factors are a compromise between a detailed list of all known factors and a simplified check list that is easy to remember. Prenatal factors (family history, consanguinity, infections in pregnancy and congenital defects of the head and neck) are universally accepted. Perinatal factors can be too detailed and have less well defined cut-off points. Examples are low birth weight, high bilirubin levels, anoxia, prematurity, infections and ototoxic antibiotics. For this reason the National Deaf Children's Society has recommended a stay of more than 48 hours in a special care baby unit. The risk criteria selected will alter the size of the selected population, and this can vary between 6 and 18 per cent of the birth cohort. However comprehensive an at-risk list is, it will not account for all children born hearing impaired as 30–40 per cent have no identifiable cause. Nor will risk factors always be apparent at the time of birth. In a cohort of 10 000 births screened selectively in the neonatal period and followed for 5 years, only 43 per cent of children with congenital hearing impairment were detected by the screen, the remainder being detected by subsequent screens and surveillance. The most important risk factor is parental concern.

The startle response

The startle response can be elicited by a loud sound such as a shout and is either a whole body startle (Moro response) or little more than a blink (auropalpebral reflex). The startle response does not fulfil the criteria of a screening test but is nevertheless a useful part of the neonatal examination and should alert the clinician to a possible hearing problem.

Brainstem auditory evoked potentials

The principles of evoked potential audiometry when used for determination of auditory threshold are presented in Chapter 4. For neonatal screening a fixed level is used (30–50 dB) and the latency of wave V determined. The failure rate of this screen can be as low as 2 per cent. If a pass is not obtained the screen is repeated 2–4 weeks later as delayed maturation or myelination of the auditory pathways can contribute to a fail, as can other central nervous system disease. Pathology in the brainstem may cause absence of wave V despite an identifiable wave I. Screening by brainstem auditory evoked potentials alone will miss that small proportion of congenital hearing impairment in which the loss is confined to the low frequencies.

Transient evoked otoacoustic emissions (TEOAEs)

Recording otoacoustic emissions is a very quick procedure, taking only a few minutes in sleeping neonates. It also has the advantage of testing cochlear function at all frequencies. For emissions to be present hearing must be better then 30 dBHL, thus this screen is more sensitive than other methods. Persistent fluid in the middle ear prevents emissions being recorded. In a cohort of 18 000 children in Rhode Island the failure rate was 26 per cent, of which 11 children were found to have congenital sensorineural hearing loss at the second stage of the screen. Of these only six would have been detected by a selective screen. Because of the high failure rate, neonates who fail emissions are retested using the auditory brainstem response. Despite these disadvantages TEOAE is an extremely useful method of neonatal screening.

Auditory response cradle

The auditory response cradle measures changes in head turn, body movement, and respiration in babies of less than 5 kg weight in response to bursts of high pass noise at 90 dBHL. This level is required as neonates do not produce repeatable behavioural responses to sound at less than 70–80 dBHL. Mild–moderate recruiting cochlear hearing loss may be missed, but non-recruiting conductive loss may produce a fail.

SCREENING AND SURVEILLANCE IN THE FIRST YEAR

Goal

The goal is to detect congenital deafness and early onset hearing loss that may have been missed by selective neonatal screening or have deteriorated after screening took place.

Procedure

The 8-month distraction test

The distraction test, described in the next section, is performed at the age of 8 months, corrected for prematurity, by two trained health visitors. Normal infants turn reliably to sounds presented in the plane of the ear at this stage, and those with hearing impairment have not yet become so visually aware that they can easily pass the test. The intensity used for screening is 35 dB and the stimuli are a high frequency rattle (6 kHz), a sibilant 'S' (4 kHz), low frequency voice (250–500 Hz) and warble tones of 1 and 2 kHz. There is a failure rate of 20–25 per cent, attributable to a combination of poor testing conditions and hearing loss due to otitis media with effusion. Failures are retested 2 weeks later, and 5–10 per cent will require referral on to audiology services. Of children born with sensorineural hearing loss of more than 50 dB, at least one-half are detected for the first time by this screen but up to 35 per cent falsely pass. For this reason the test has been abandoned in some health authorities, and others use automated visual reinforcement.

Structured surveillance

Authorities that have abandoned the distraction test have substituted specific surveillance at 8 months using a questionnaire administered by health visitors. This follows on from the surveillance undertaken at the 6 and 10 week postnatal visits and builds upon the information already given in the parent-held records. The cost in professional time is similar to the distraction test, as is the coverage (around 95 per cent). This is the last specifically hearing-orientated surveillance, although speech development will be monitored throughout the preschool period. Children missed by infant screening and surveillance commonly present in the second year with parental concerns related to development of speech and language.

Monitoring infant screening

In order to evaluate the effectiveness of any hearing screening or surveillance procedure the following outcomes require evaluation: coverage, referral rate to audiology services, findings in those referred, age at first hearing aid fitting in a given year in that locality and retrospective audit of children with sensorineural loss. The last two will enable the service to be assessed in terms of the UK National Deaf Children's Society targets. For a retrospective audit of cohort of children, the children must be at least 6 years old in order to audit those not detected until the definitive screen at school entry (see below). Audit at this age allows determination of the 15–20 per cent with early onset progressive losses who may have had normal hearing in the first 8–12 months. With a prevalence of 1/1000 births the cohort has to be at least 100 000 births if statistical analysis is to be useful.

SCREENING AT SCHOOL ENTRY

Goal

The goal is to detect middle ear dysfunction, unilateral deafness and acquired or progressive hearing loss in order to minimize the effects upon education.

Procedure

Headphone audiometry in school using sound-excluding audiocups delivering pure tones at 0.5, 1, 2 and 4 kHz at 20–25 dB. Failures are retested once, and second failures are referred for full audiometry. Tympanometry is not used for screening as it is too sensitive and is not a measure of hearing.

Testing children's hearing

Accurate hearing assessment can be achieved even in very young children providing the environment is child orientated and the testers experienced in handling children. As hearing loss affects language development, testing children's hearing always includes testing hearing for speech and making an evaluation of expressive language and comprehension. In children with other disabilities it is occasionally necessary to undertake auditory evoked potential tests to verify behavioural thresholds, but the information thus obtained can be of limited benefit in terms of frequencies testable and the relationship between cochlear function and hearing in children with disabilities.

The best results are obtained in multidisciplinary paediatric assessment centres in which the environment and organization are child orientated. The atmosphere should be relaxed and friendly if the child's performance is to be optimal. The decor and facilities of the waiting area are important for relaxing the child and mother before the interview, and for providing an opportunity for informal observation of the child. The test room should be at least 4 metres square (16 square metres) with a minimum of visual distractions, including visible apparatus. The ambient noise level must be less than 30 dBA for testing in soundfield. At least half an hour is required for preliminary assessment, and more than one session may be required as children become tired and attention is lost. For this reason it is sometimes wiser to leave the history and examination until hearing levels have been established.

BEHAVIOURAL AND OBJECTIVE HEARING ASSESSMENT UNDER 6 MONTHS

With the advent of neonatal screening and increased awareness of congenital hearing impairment in parents and primary care it is necessary to evaluate the hearing of infants fully so that amplification may begin. Otoacoustic emissions demonstrate normal hearing, but give no indication of the severity of any loss. Brainstem auditory evoked potentials elicited in the standard manner give the threshold at 3–6 kHz only, and even then the normality of the central nervous system has to be assumed. Although most congenital hearing loss is high frequency, in a small proportion the loss affects the low frequencies only. Full frequency brainstem auditory evoked responses can be obtained using notched noise, but this is not available on most clinical systems and takes much longer to perform, so that sedation would be required. The soft ear canal of neonates can produce artefactual tympanograms if a high (660 Hz) probe tone is not used.

It is therefore essential that behavioural methods are used to substantiate hearing loss detected by objective measures before amplification is begun. Infants do respond behaviourally to sound from birth, and this is the basis of the auditory response cradle. Observations include stilling, altered respiration, eye widening, eye turning, blinking, head turning, opening the mouth or chewing, wriggling the toes and moving the arms. These responses are to sounds presented within 10 cm of and in the plane of the ear, and are inconsistent. The startle response defines the infant's response to loud sound. Best results are obtained to broad band familiar noises.

Because behavioural responses are inconsistent at this age and objective tests give limited information, these test results must be substantiated by the observations of parents and peripatetic teachers visiting the home. Some of these infants who appear congenitally deaf by all the methods so far described will have delayed auditory maturation and respond normally to sound by the age of 1 year. The limitations of hearing assessment in the first 6 months of life must be explained to the parents, along with the benefits of early amplification. Any child suspected of hearing loss during this period must be followed up until a full distraction test or visual reinforcement audiometry is possible.

THE DISTRACTION TEST (7–17 MONTHS)

The technique described here is a formalized method of behavioural orientation audiometry (BOA) in which there is no conditioning, and is a modification of that first developed in Manchester, England by the Ewings. Best results are obtained by a pair of testers who are used to working together. The infant is supported forward on the mother's knee. The first tester ensures that the infant is able to track a moving object visually with full head turns in each direction in order to detect preferred head turning. This tester then raises the

level of attention and awareness using toys. When the child is alert the activity is plateaued and the tester behind the infant presents the signal at a distance of 1 metre, in the plane of the ear and at an angle of 45°. If no response is obtained at 25–30 dBA, the signal is presented again at an increased intensity or at a decreased distance. Care must be taken to avoid visual clues (e.g. shadows), auditory clues (squeaking shoes or rustling clothes), olfactory and tactile clues. Tactile clues with voice test arise from exhaled air and are avoided by the use of a screen. Parents give tactile clues by the manner in which they support the baby. If no response is obtained the responsiveness of the baby is checked by gently touching or blowing upon the child's ear. After each response the signal intensity used to elicit that response is measured using a sound level meter. The units are dBA, which is a scale weighted for testing in soundfield.

Signals used for distraction testing

1. High frequency rattle (8–10 kHz)
2. Sibilant letter 'S' (4–6 kHz)
3. G chime bar (1.6 kHz)
4. Voice, low frequency hum, or C chime bar (250–500 Hz)
5. Warble tones or narrow bands of noise (to avoid standing waves) at 0.5, 1, 2 and 4 kHz
6. 90–100 dBA drum beat or shout to elicit the auropalpebral reflex if no other response has been obtained
7. Broad band sounds such as a cup and spoon, musical box, squeakers and rattles are used when there is no response to conventional sounds in order to support the more formal observations

Observed responses

Head turn and localization of the signal. Eye turn is sometimes used when head turn is inhibited. Observations that include stilling, altered respiration, eye widening, blinking, opening the mouth or chewing, wriggling the toes, and moving the arms may be the only responses obtained in handicapped children, and should be interpreted with extreme caution. The distraction test thus performed can give an accurate assessment of hearing in soundfield at 500–8000 Hz. Normal hearing children with normal development respond to levels of 25–30 dBA. Differences between the ears can be detected but some children with monaural deafness such as that due to atresia will correctly identify the side on which the sound is presented, even at low intensities. False turns can be obtained in visually aware, otherwise normal, hearing impaired children. As already mentioned, up to 30 per cent can pass a screening distraction test, and even in the best clinic environment turns may be obtained in the absence of hearing. The results of the distraction test are therefore interpreted in the light of speech development. By 7 months tuneful babble should be present, and by the first birthday recognizable words should be heard in an otherwise normal child. Children with visual impairment, developmental delay or communication disorders such as autism may not respond to the distraction test in spite of normal hearing. If any of these scenarios is suspected behavioural observations may need to be confirmed by evoked response testing, but visual reinforcement audiometry should be attempted first.

VISUAL REINFORCEMENT AUDIOMETRY (7–30 MONTHS)

Visual reinforcement audiometry (VRA) differs from the distraction test by virtue of structured conditioning of the head-turning response. This test requires a sound proof room with speakers and audiometer. Above or below each speaker is a reinforcing toy that lights up (sometimes with moving parts) when the child turns to the sound. The child sits on the carer's lap facing either a tester or a mechanical toy. The child's attention is directed forward and a sound stimulus presented via the speaker situated in front of the child at an angle of 30° from the midline. To condition the child the sound is initially presented at suprathreshold levels (around 60–70 dBA) with the visual reinforcement activated. Once the child is turning to every presentation of sound plus reinforcing light the sound stimulus is presented alone. When the child turns to the speaker the reinforcing light is activated, keeping the sound stimulus on. The child's attention is then redirected forward and the procedure repeated until thresholds are obtained.

The signals are warble tones or narrow bands of noise, at 500–4000 Hz, to avoid standing waves in the soundfield. Normal hearing children respond at 20–25 dBA and hearing impaired children at 5–25 dBA above their true threshold. Very young children do not always respond to warble tones, and some children with communication disorders do not respond to unfamiliar sounds. In such cases taped theme tunes from television, emergency vehicle sirens, and other stimuli may be presented. An automated screening version of VRA is available using sounds similar to those of the distraction test. One of the advantages of VRA is that it can be undertaken by one tester, although it is useful to have a second observer or occupier.

COOPERATIVE TEST (18–30 MONTHS)

For most children there is a stage when responses to the distraction test and VRA are inhibited and they have not yet reached the maturity required for performance testing. At this stage a test of language comprehension may be all that is possible. The child is requested to hand toy items using fixed choice of mother, teddy, sister, another adult or into a box. Alternatively, the question 'where are your shoes/eyes/nose?' may be asked. This is a suprathreshold test, the levels required being more than 10 dBSL (sensation level) in the speech frequency range. Normal children respond at levels of 40 dBA.

PERFORMANCE TEST (2½–5 YEARS)

From a developmental age of 2½ years it is possible to condition a child to perform a simple action in response to a given signal. This can be the word 'go', a sibilant 'S' or warble tones. Seated opposite the child the examiner draws the child's attention to the source of the sound. A loud (70 dBA) sound is introduced with visual clues and the child's hand guided into the required action, for example dropping bricks into a box. This is repeated until the child is automatically performing the task without guidance. The visual clue is then removed and correct responses to stimuli encouraged. The sound stimuli are then decreased in intensity until threshold is obtained for frequencies 250–4000 Hz. The procedure may then be repeated for bone-conducted tones. As the attention span is short a large selection of 'games' is required. Children may not repond at threshold to 8000 Hz as the sound is unfamiliar. Low frequencies such as 250 Hz can only be undertaken in adequately silent rooms.

SPEECH DISCRIMINATION TESTS

2–5 years

Speech discrimination testing is undertaken on *all* children in order to verify the soundfield audiogram and to identify any language delay or disorder in the presence of normal hearing. Miniature toy items are used, which the child is first asked to name, then identify with lip-reading available, and finally without lip-reading, gradually decreasing the intensity until the minimum level for full discrimination of known items is achieved. Words may be presented from the front using a screen, or from each side, keeping the child's attention on the toys placed on the table in front of the child. There are a number of toy sets, all of which contain items with common phonemes such as 'cup' and 'duck' or 'shoe' and 'spoon'. Commonly used sets include the *McCormick toy discrimination test*, consisting of cup, duck, shoe, spoon, house, cow, horse, fork, plate, plane, lamb and man. The *Kendal toy test* contains cup, duck, shoe, spoon, house, mouse, plate, gate, string, brick, fish, dish and a number of 'distractors' such as a glove. The *E2L toy test* is specifically designed for children whose second language is English and live in cities. It includes cup, duck, bus, brush, car, bath, shoe, spoon, egg, bed, sweet and key. If the criterion used is the level for 100 per cent correct, this is likely to be 20 dBA above the warble tone threshold, if 50 per cent correct it should match the warble tone threshold as for any speech or pure tone comparison. Normal hearing children should achieve 100 per cent correct at 30 dBA. Children with mild to moderate conductive impairment commonly require 45–55 dBA for discrimination.

5–6 years

At this age children are reluctant to point to toys and picture cards are used instead with similar instructions. The *Manchester picture cards* have a fixed choice of four items/cards, and the *Manchester junior word lists for pictures* have a fixed choice of six items/sheet. Each card or page has only one test word and the scoring is as for conventional speech audiometry.

7–10 years

At this age speech discrimination can be performed in soundfield or with earphones in the same manner as for adults except that the word lists consist of items familiar to children. The *Manchester junior word lists* are commonly used. In the USA toy, picture and taped word material uses spondees familiar to children such as 'hotdog' and 'cowboy'. When using earphones the non-test ear is masked.

EXPRESSIVE SPEECH AND LANGUAGE

Expressive speech is an invaluable guide to the child's hearing status during the period critical for language acquisition. A relaxed environment and interesting toys will encourage the child to talk sufficiently for a general impression of speech development to be obtained. Failure to acquire age-appropriate speech is the only way in which many hearing impaired children may present. Children with primary speech or communication disorders, or both, commonly present to ENT and audiology clinics for hearing assessment. The pos-sibility of speech delay or disorder should be considered in every child presenting for hearing assessment. Any child suspected of delayed or deviant speech or of a communication disorder should be formally assessed by a speech and language therapist. All children with sensorineural hearing impairment need to have speech and language assessed, and therapy if required, from a specialist speech and language therapist for the hearing impaired.

IMPEDANCE TESTING

Adult techniques of impedance studies are applicable to children, but in small children machines capable of obtaining a tympanogram rapidly are easier to use as the time available for the test is often limited. For preschool children a tympanogram alone is all that is usually required as the task is to ascertain the presence or absence of chronic secretory otitis media in children in whom a hearing loss is suspected. *The tympanogram is not a hearing test, it is a means of ascertaining the cause not the presence of a hearing loss.* The hearing loss associated with secretory otitis media can be anything from 0 to 55 dB. If the hearing loss is more than this it cannot be due to secretory otitis media alone. In neonates and very young children 660 Hz, not 220 Hz, is required for accurate audiometry. In general terms, the more rapid the tympanogram the more likely it is to give a flat pattern of secretory otitis media. The test can be oversensitive.

Stapedius reflexes are used in children to assess middle ear function, as a measure of recruitment when fitting hearing aids, and as supporting evidence in the interpretation of behavioural hearing assessment. The rapid reflexes obtained from ipsilateral probes should be viewed with extreme caution, especially below the age of 9 months. Transcranial transmission of these suprathreshold stimuli may be sufficient to elicit a reflex from the contralateral ear, especially at 500 Hz, which may also cause an artefact with an ipisilateral 600 Hz probe tone.

OTOACOUSTIC EMISSIONS

The principals of this test have been described in Chapter 4. Both distortion products and click evoked otoacoustic emissions are used to test children's hearing. One advantage of their use in children is that the only cooperation required is for the child to keep still and very quiet for the 2–5 minutes required for the test. This is best achieved in a sleeping baby. As the ear probe is less invasive than electrodes required for electric responses, the baby is less likely to wake up, and parents find the test less distressing. Small children will accept a probe similar to an impedance probe, when electrode placement would not be acceptable. The other advantage is that all frequencies are tested, unlike brainstem auditory evoked responses. Responses can be obtained with tympanostomy tubes in place, and under anaesthetic or sedation. The disadvantages are that the test

- is very sensitive and only demonstrates the presence of normal hearing (better than 30 dB)
- gives no indication of the severity of any hearing impairment
- cannot be recorded in the presence of secretory otitis media (although this is not always the case)
- requires the child to be completely quiet without noisy breathing or sucking.

AUDITORY EVOKED POTENTIAL TESTS

The principals of this procedure have been described in Chapter 4. Brainstem auditory evoked potentials (BAEPs) are the method of choice as they are easier to perform in terms of time and the effect of sleep or sedation. The best traces are obtained when the child is asleep. The procedure is applicable to children providing the latencies of the waves are corrected for maturity and potentials are interrupted in the light of the integrity of the nervous system. Extremely premature babies, sick babies, and those with central nervous system abnormalities, including damage from meningitis, may have absent evoked potentials in the presence of normal hearing. It is often precisely these infants in which objective tests are required, as behavioural responses are also poor. Delayed auditory maturation can cause absence of behavioural responses and evoked potentials to sound, and these tests should therefore be supported by otoacoustic emissions. Placement of electrodes is possible in sleeping infants below the age of 4 months, but in children older than this sedation or anaesthesia will be required.

Sedation is undertaken as a day case under paediatric care. Thresholds are obtained by performing a latency–intensity function, following the waves down from a point at which they are clearly visible to where they are just identifiable and reproducible. Each level should be reproducible for two traces. Latency–intensity functions are steep in recruiting hearing impairment (cochlear pathology) and in other conditions such as hypoxia. BAEPs only give high frequency information and will therefore miss low frequency losses and may overemphasize the degree of deafness when used for hearing aid fitting. Other frequencies may be tested using

notched noise, but this requires special equipment and a much longer test time, so there may not be time to complete the test before the child awakes.

Maturation of BAEPs affects latency and amplitude. Latencies attain childhood values at the end of the first year of life. When testing neonates and infants a 20 ms recording window is required, rather than the 10 ms window usually used for this procedure. The change in latency with postconceptual age is curvilinear, with the greatest changes occurring in the first 3 months. Although wave I is delayed in infants below this age, it is the interpeak latency of waves I–V that shows the greatest maturational change as myelination progresses. In the neonatal period the I:V amplitude ratio is variable, with wave I often being greater than wave V. The amplitude of wave I is enhanced by horizontal montage (mastoid/mastoid). The stability and reliability of the brainstem potentials in infants is poor because of incursion of slow wave EEG activity and fluctuating levels of motor activity. Because of changes with maturity and variability of the potential, abnormal results should always be repeated after an interval before interpretation is undertaken.

Cortical auditory evoked potentials are undertaken in cooperative older children to establish hearing thresholds, as for adults. They are also subject to maturational changes and can be extremely variable.

Transtympanic electrocochleography ECoG is a better indicator of the threshold of hearing than any other auditory evoked potential and is not affected by maturation. As anaesthesia is required it is best combined with other procedures such as myringotomy and high resolution CT of the temporal bone (see Chapter 6). This combination of procedures is the best way of demonstrating complete absence of hearing in young children, together with establishing a cause. This is of great advantage in subsequent management.

CENTRAL AUDITORY PROCESSING TESTS

Cortical deafness is suspected when the pure tone thresholds are much better than the hearing for speech. Central auditory processing disorders are suspected when hearing is worse in noisy situations, such as the classroom, than it is in quiet. Testing children for central auditory disorders is difficult as the spread of normality is considerable, and standardization difficult. Tests of speech discrimination in noise, competing speech, and degraded speech have been used. The easiest to standardize is the *masking level differences*, which is a less demanding test in terms of time per test. Tests of auditory memory, sequencing and processing are part of the test battery used by clinical and educational psychologists when assessing children with suspected disorders of auditory processing.

HEARING TESTING IN CHILDREN WITH OTHER HANDICAPS

Hearing assessment is required for all children undergoing the process of 'statementing', described below, for special educational needs as even minor hearing problems can have a major effect upon the language development and behaviour of children with other disabilities. When testing handicapped children, allowance must be made for any motor difficulties and developmental delay. The tests used are those appropriate to the developmental rather than chronological age of the child. Impedance tests are always undertaken because of the high prevalence of chronic secretory otitis media in this population. Electrical evoked responses must be interpreted in the light of the functioning of the central nervous system. Otoacoustic emissions can be very useful in this population providing middle ear function is normal. Hearing assessments in this population can be difficult, and may require the joint expertise of paediatrician and audiologist.

History, examination and investigation

HISTORY

Details of *gestational, perinatal, previous, family* and *developmental history* are required and this is most efficiently ascertained by questionnaire. The name of the school or nursery is required. The facts to be elicited are outlined in Table 10.3 and may be taken in stages. The parent's estimation of the child's hearing status is correct in around 70 per cent of cases, and details of *duration, fluctuation* and *progression* are elicited. Leading questions may be necessary for *vertigo, imbalance* and *tinnitus* as the child does not have the vocabulary to describe the symptoms nor realize their relevance to hearing. Children do not complain about tinnitus or vertigo until their body image is fully developed. Both symptoms are more common in childhood than is often recognized, and the tinnitus is one reason that children cannot fall asleep at night without a tape to listen to. The *social* and *educational history* are important in determining cause, prognosis and defining parents' expectations. The developmental history is taken

Table 10.3 Factors to be elicited in the history

Gestation	Duration of pregnancy, any complication e.g. infections
Perinatal	Birth weight, jaundice, anoxia, infection, trauma, birth defects
Past history	Infections, age at first attack of otitis media, serious illnesses
Present history	Current hearing status, duration of impairment, fluctuations, progress, tinnitus, vertigo, accompanying symptoms
General health	Atopy, other disabilities, mobility
Speech and language	Age of first word, age of joining into sentences, vocabulary, current status of communication
Vision	Any visual defect, strabismus etc
Development	Age of sitting, standing, walking, blowing, sucking, feeding difficulties
Family history	Deafness, tinnitus, vertigo, eye, thyroid, diabetes, neurological disorder, renal disease
Educational and social history	Name of school, how child functions at school academically, socially and in communication, peer interaction, parental expectations, family dynamics

with particular reference to postural control and the *development of speech and language.*

EXAMINATION

The examination begins with observation of the child interacting with the parents in the waiting area. Once in the consulting room the child may need a little time to adjust to the surroundings, but rapidly becomes restless if too long is spent on the history. The hearing level is then established, and while thresholds for speech and pure tone are being established the child's overall developmental status will become apparent. The ears are then examined using pneumatic otoscopy if possible. The rest of the otorhinolaryngology system is examined with special attention to the speech apparatus. The eyes are examined for colour, vision, eye movements and epicanthic folds, and a general examination undertaken if appropriate. The examination and history may have to be spread over several visits if the cooperation of the child is to be maintained. Priority is given to establishing the hearing level and middle ear status. Family audiograms are undertaken if sensorineural loss is present.

INVESTIGATIONS OF AETIOLOGY

Selective investigations of children with sensorineural hearing impairment enables aetiology to be established, and provides information that improves management. The most important investigations are *ophthalmology, developmental assessment* and *speech and language evaluation*. Many children with hearing loss also have some abnormality of the eyes such as strabismus, refractive errors, retinopathy or corneal opacity. The detection and correction of visual impairment is crucial to the management of the hearing impaired child as habilitation depends upon visual input for lip-reading or sign language. Likewise it is essential not only to monitor the progress in speech development, but also to detect any speech and language disorder, as this will confound the effect of any hearing impairment. The investigations undertaken are related to the age of the child and some will need to be repeated at intervals.

- 0–6 months: viral studies for intrauterine infection, chromosomes, renal ultrasound (oto-brachio-renal syndrome)
- 0–18 months: urinalysis for mucopolysaccharidosis
- 0–3 years: high resolution CT of the temporal bone for congenital malformation or cholesteatoma; urinalysis for casts, red blood cells and protein (Alport syndrome); ophthalmology, developmental and speech assessment
- 3–6 years: ECG for Jervell and Lange–Neilson syndrome (long QT, syncopal attacks); EEG if epilepsy, central deafness or ataxia suspected
- 6–9 years: ophthalmology for heredodegenerative retinitis pigmentosa; urinalysis for casts and red blood cells; high resolution CT of the temporal bone; EEG for neurological syndromes presenting at 6 years; serology for syphilis; biochemistry for thyroid and renal function; full blood count and ESR for Cogan syndrome and sickle-cell trait; autoimmune profile; vestibular assessment

Vestibular testing can be undertaken from the age of 6 years, but requires some adaptation of the adult approach (see Chapter 5) because of immaturity of eye movement control and variable attention. Smooth pursuit may be needed to achieve calibration. Smooth pursuit is somewhat irregular as this system is not mature until the age of 18 years. Rotation tests can be used from infancy, sitting the infant on the parent's lap. Caloric and rotation responses can only be reliably recorded with eyes open in the dark, as fixation is very good at this age and there are excessive random movements behind closed lids. The child must con-

stantly be talked through the procedure and appropriate mental alerting is vital. Vestibular assessment is useful in diagnosis (e.g. Usher syndrome, labyrinthitis, secondary hydrops), in planning therapy and in providing informed recreational and vocational counselling for school leavers.

Management

PREVENTION

Prevention may be considered as minimizing disability from and decreasing the prevalence of the impairment. Disability is minimized by detection before 1 year and effective, appropriate intervention. Prevalence is reduced primarily by immunization. If diagnosis is on target, genetic counselling will enable parents with a high risk of recurrence (recessive and dominant disorders) to plan their families accordingly.

SURGERY

Surgical management for chronic secretory otitis media, cholesteatoma, congenital stapes fixation and related conditions is discussed elsewhere in this volume. The role of surgical management of hearing loss in children depends upon the type and extent of any hearing loss and the presence of other disorders such as developmental or speech delay. Surgical management is therefore considered in the context of the whole child and may exist in tandem with other approaches such as medical treatment and hearing aids. It is important that hearing is assessed before and after surgery.

MEDICATION

Medical management is aimed at alleviating Eustachian tube dysfunction, allergic rhinitis and sometimes at improving cochlear function. Treatments include low-dose antibiotics as a prophylactic, antihistamines, decongestants, topical steroids and betahistine. Wax may be treated with syringing, aural toilet or ceruminolytics. Control of allergic rhinitis and infection in the postnasal space can be effective in the management of fluctuating conductive hearing loss.

PSYCHOLOGICAL MANAGEMENT AND COUNSELLING

Psychological management and counselling begins with diagnosis. Permanent hearing impairment is bad news and needs to be imparted with care. This should be followed up with both parents being given the opportunity to discuss their concerns and a full and detailed explanation of the possible causes, the prognosis and possible management options. There is a statutory duty upon the doctor making the diagnosis to inform the parents of local and national voluntary bodies, such as the UK National Deaf Children's Society, and to inform the education authority. For children statemented for special education needs the education authority has a statutory obligation to inform social services of the needs of the child.

Parents pass through a period of bereavement expressed as the stages of mourning: shock, denial, anger, guilt, acceptance and constructive action. The parents need to be supported and counselled through these stages if management is to be successful. It is not appropriate to take impressions for hearing aids while the parents are still in a stage of shock or denial as hearing aid fitting in this period will be unsuccessful. The stage of anger is prolonged and bitter if diagnosis has been delayed. The parents will also blame themselves for late diagnosis in spite of the fact that it is responsibility of the professionals. Early diagnosis enables the parents to pass through the stages of denial, anger and guilt as quickly as possible, and this facilitates good hearing aid use. The parents will pass through additional stages of bereavement at each stage of the child's life: starting school, the child's realization that hearing loss is permanent, transferring to secondary education, choosing a career and school leaving. The child also passes through bereavement at similar times, particularly around the age of 8 years when the realization comes that they will still need hearing aids as adults, as teenagers when they cannot conform with their peers and again at school leaving when the difficulties of being hearing impaired in a hearing world are fully realized. Psychological problems are extremely common in hearing impaired children and their families. A *specialist child and adolescent psychiatry for the hearing impaired programme* is available at only one UK National Centre at Springfield Hospital in Tooting, London. The need for this type of help can be minimized by early diagnosis and management sensitive to the psychological and communication needs of the child and family. The availability of a hearing impaired adult role model is also useful.

EDUCATION

The psychological management of the hearing impaired child and their family is shared with the child's peripatetic or unit advisory teacher for the hearing impaired. The teacher is effectively the key worker and will bear the day-to-day counselling load. Without this support, management of hearing impaired in children is unlikely to succeed.

In the UK there is no statutory duty for an education authority to provide for children under the age of 2 years, or to provide for children in the preschool period unless a formal statement of specified special educational needs has been prepared and accepted by the education authority. Most education authorities do, however, provide extensive input during the preschool years as this period is critical for language acquisition and enables the child to reach their potential. Without shared care between education and health at this stage, the child is unlikely to acquire language, even if the hearing aids are adequate. Indeed, constant feedback from the teachers of hearing responses in the home environment contribute significantly to the hearing aid prescription. The UK Education Act of 1981 Section 1 advocates the education of children with special needs in mainstream classes whenever possible. Section 4 of the Act gives parents the right to information upon which placement of their child is determined. They can provide their own statement and appeal to the Secretary of State if they disagree with the provision. The formal statement will give an indication of the communication system that is thought most appropriate to the child's needs and, similarly, the type of education: mainstream, partially hearing unit or school for the deaf.

Doctors are required to give medical input to the educational statement and this takes the form of a description of the child's impairment and handicap and likely requirements for amplification and speech therapy, both of which are provided free by the health authority. The final document is a formal statement of need to which the parents and the education authority have to agree and upon which provision is based. The procedure of preparing a statement usually begins at the age of 2 years or as soon thereafter that an impairment likely to affect educational progress is recognized.

Advisory teachers for the hearing impaired monitor children in school even if a formal statement of need has not been prepared or accepted and their hearing loss is unilateral, mild or otherwise unsuitable for a hearing aid. They will make recommendations on seating, note takers or additional help such as non-teaching aids.

SPECIALIST SPEECH AND LANGUAGE THERAPY

Specialist speech and language therapy for the hearing impaired complements the auditory training and language training given by the advisory teachers. More detailed language assessments are undertaken and the possibility of communication disorders explored. Work is also undertaken on the child's sound production system. Speech therapy is ongoing until after school leaving as many of these children never attain speech understandable to strangers.

HEARING AIDS FOR CHILDREN

The principles of hearing aid provision are the same as those for adults given in Chapter 8. The fitting of hearing aids is undertaken as soon as hearing loss severe enough to affect speech acquisition or education is diagnosed, the UK National Deaf Children's Society target being within 4 weeks of diagnosis. The majority of children are fitted with postaural hearing aids from the NHS or a commercial range. Almost all children are fitted with two hearing aids. Occasionally, as children grow up they reject the second aid, and this is usually because the discrimination for speech is much worse in one ear than the other. Factors taken into consideration when prescribing are power as determined by the severity of impairment; output limiting or compression for tolerance of loud sound; the need for direct input to the instrument from radio microphones et cetera; frequency response to conform to the configuration of the impairment; and acoustic feedback suppression.

Earmoulds pose a challenge as the external auditory canal is small and a small pinna results in the microphone of the hearing aid being close to the output, generating acoustic feedback. Impression technique is crucial, as is the skill with which the earmould is manufactured. Growing canals require new earmoulds at frequent intervals. Wax, even in small quantities, will cause feedback and detract from the accuracy of the impression.

Some children will require bone conduction instruments, in-the-ear aids, body-worn hearing aids or bone-anchored hearing aids.

The suitability of the prescription is assessed by measuring the hearing thresholds with the hearing aids worn at the prescribed settings. This requires a soundfield system capable of delivering warble tones. The response technique will be determined by the developmental stage of the child. In children over the age of 5 years it is possible to perform insertion gain estimations to aid prescription.

Children reject hearing aids that are not powerful enough, too powerful, faulty or have feedback. Once hearing aids have been fitted for the first time it takes the child months of listening before recognizing sounds around them and a year or more before producing words. This is a difficult time for the parents as little result is seen for the effort involved.

Funding for hearing aids, particularly the expensive commercial hearing aids required by children, is always problematic, not made any easier by the high rate of loss and breakage of hearing aids worn continuously by small children.

Radio systems are used in school in order to improve the signal to noise ratio by delivering speech to the ear which has been picked up by a radio microphone worn by the teacher. The child wears a radio receiver that either drives a body-worn hearing aid, an electromagnetic neck loop or a direct input system to a postaural hearing aid.

BONE-ANCHORED HEARING AIDS

(See Chapter 8).

COCHLEAR IMPLANTS (SEE CHAPTER 9)

A *cochlear implant* should be considered when the aided thresholds with the best hearing aids available still fall outside the speech range of intensity and frequency. They are also considered when speech fails to develop despite early and appropriate amplification. Cochlear implants are of great benefit in those children who progressively lose their hearing during childhood or have acquired profound hearing loss. CT tomography and magnetic resonance imaging is required to ensure that the cochlea is patent and the auditory nerve present. Of children referred to cochlear implant programmes only one-half are eventually implanted. Some of those referred are found not to require an implant as the residual hearing is adequate and lack of progress has been the result of poor local management. This illustrates the difficulties posed by amplification in children and the need for centres specializing in the amplification needs of children. A cochlear implant programme requires a great commitment in time after the implant for parents and professionals alike, as the child learns to recognize and use the new sounds. Considerable teaching and speech therapy input is required for many years, and this may be beyond the resources of the referring locality team. Ability to complete the habilitation programme is a significant factor in choosing implantation. Cochlear implants are most effective in children born deaf if they are undertaken well before the age of 7 years. The presence of chronic secretory otitis media increases the complication rate for this procedure.

Prognosis

Chronic secretory otitis media is a self-limiting condition that always resolves with time if there is no underlying cause such as Down's syndrome or cleft palate. Sensorineural hearing loss does not recover and is progressive in at least 15 per cent by the age of 5 years and as many again by 16 years. The psychological sequelae of childhood hearing impairment are great, particularly in those who have had no access to language for the first decade. This is an argument for the early introduction of total communication using speech, sign, gesture and lipreading. Child abuse is more common in handicapped than normal children, and of those with handicaps it is most common in those with hearing impairment. Early intervention maximizes the chance of developing good speech and language, but this is a struggle for hearing impaired children and their families. Restricted language development hampers education and may prevent access to the national curriculum. Most hearing impaired school leavers will go on to further education, and all have access to social workers for the deaf and help from disablement resettlement officers.

With the advent of better hearing aids, earlier identification and cochlear implants when required, the prognosis for hearing impaired children is better than ever before.

Suggested reading

Bennett MJ, Wade HK. Computerised hearing test for neonates. *Hearing Aid Journal* 1981; **10**:52–3.

Bess FH. The minimally hearing impaired child. *Ear and Hearing* 1985; **6**:43–7.

Bhattacharya J, Bennett MJ, Tucker SM. Longterm follow-up of newborns tested with the auditory response cradle. *Archives of Diseases of Childhood* 1984; **59**:4–11.

Butler J. *Child health surveillance in primary care: a critical review*. London: HMSO, 1989.

Das VK. Aetiology of bilateral sensorineural deafness in children. *Scandanavian Audiology Supplement* 1988; **30**:43–52.

Davis AC, Sancho J. Screening for hearing impairment in children; a review of current practice with special reference to the screening of babies from special care baby units for severe/profound hearing impairment. In:

Gerber SE, Mencher GT eds. *Human communication disorders: a worldwide perspective*. Washington DC: Galludet University Press, 1987.

Downs MP, Sterrit GM. A guide to newborn and infant screening programmes. *Archives of Otolaryngology* 1967; **85**:15–22.

Ewing IR. Screening tests and guidance clinics for babies and young children. In: Ewing AWG. *Educational guidance of the deaf child*. Manchester: Manchester University Press, 1957.

Fortnum H, Farnsworth A, Davis A. The feasibility of evoked otoacoustic emissions as an inpatient hearing check after meningitis. *British Journal of Audiology* 1993; **27**:227–32.

Galambos R, Hicks G, Wilson M. Hearing loss in graduates of a tertiary intensive care nursery. *Ear and Hearing* 1982; **3**:87–90.

Haggard MP, Hughes EG. *Screening children's hearing – a review of the literature and the impact of otitis media*. London: HMSO, 1991.

Hall, DMB, *Health for all children: a programme for child health surveillance, 3rd ed*. Oxford: Oxford University Press, 1996.

Hunter MH, Kimm L, Cafarelli Dees D, Kennedy CR, Thornton ARD. Feasibility of otoacoustic emission detection followed by ABR as a universal neonatal screening test for hearing impairment. *British Journal of Audiology* 1994; **28**:47–51.

Johnson MJ, Maxon AB, White KR, Vohr BR. Operating a hospital based universal newborn hearing screening program using transient evoked otoacoustic emissions. *Seminars in Hearing* 1993; **14**:46–56.

Kemp DT, Ryan S. The use of transient evoked otoacoustic emissions in neonatal hearing screening programs. *Seminars in Hearing* 1993; **14**:30–45.

Kennedt CR, Kimm L, Cafarelli Dees D, Evans PIP, Hunter M, Lenton S, Thornton RD. Otoacoustic emissions and auditory brainstem responses in the newborn. *Archives of Diseases in Childhood* 1991; **66**:1124–9.

Last J. *A dictionary of epidemiology*. Oxford: Oxford University Press, 1983.

Markides A. Age of fitting hearing aids and speech intelligibility. *British Journal of Audiology* 1986; **20**:165–8.

Martin JAM, Bentzen O, Colley JRT, *et al.* Childhood deafness in the European Community. *Scandanavian Audiology* 1981; **10**:165–74.

Maxon AB, White KR, Vohr BR, Behrens TR. Using transient evoked otoacoustic emissions for neonatal hearing screening. *British Journal of Audiology* 1993; **27**:149–53.

Newton VE, Rowson VJ. Progressive sensorineural hearing loss in childhood. *British Journal of Audiology* 1988; **22**:287–95.

Peckham CS, Sheridan M, Butler NR. School attainments of seven year old children with hearing difficulties. *Developmental Medicine and Child Neurology* 1972; **14**:592–602.

Quality standards in paediatric audiology: part 1. London: NDCS, 1994.

Simmons FB, Russ FN. Automated newborn hearing screening: the crib-o-gram. *Archives of Otolaryngology* 1974; **11**:1–7.

Sorensen JR, Levy HL, Mangione TW, Sepe SJ. Parental response to repeat testing of infants with false positive results in a newborn screening program. *Paediatrics* 1984; **73**:183–7.

Stevens JC, Webb HD, Hutchinson J, Connell J, Smith MF, Buffin JT. Click evoked otoacoustic emissions compared with brainstem electrical response. *Archives of Diseases of Childhood* 1989; **64**:1105–11.

Stevens JC, Webb HD, Smith MF, Buffin JT, Ruddy HA. A comparison of otoacoustic emissions and brainstem electric response audiometry in the normal newborns and babies admitted to a special care baby unit. *Clinical Physics and Psychological Measurements* 1987; **8**:95–104.

Tucker SM, Bhattacharya J. Screening of hearing impairment in the newborn using the auditory response cradle. *Archives of Diseases of Childhood* 1992; **67**:911–9.

Watkin PM, Baldwin M, McEnery G. Neonatal at risk screening and the identification of deafness. *Archives of Diseases in Childhood* 1991; **66**:1130–5.

White KR, Vohr BR, Behrens TR. Universal newborn infant hearing screening using transient evoked otoacoustic emissions: results of the Rhode Island hearing assessment project. *Seminars in Hearing* 1993; **14**:18–29.

Section B

Tinnitus

CHAPTER 11

Incidence, classification and models of tinnitus

JONATHAN HAZELL

Introduction

The traditional view that tinnitus is a degenerative disorder of the cochlea caused by damaged hair cells has led to a philosophy that nothing much can be done to alter it, and patients can only be helped to cope with the situation or learn to live with it. This model reflects the concept of hearing as something that is centred in the ear, and ignores the complex areas of central auditory processing and perception which are characteristically omitted from the curriculum of otologists and audiologists alike. Although our knowledge of auditory processing is far from complete, enough is known to explain the basic mechanisms for the emergence and persistence of tinnitus, and also to describe quite accurately the mechanism of distress caused by tinnitus. Even a superficial understanding of these mechanisms makes it obvious how tinnitus must be treated. However, those with strong beliefs about the concept of tinnitus being purely an inner ear disorder frequently find the change of belief and understanding difficult to make.

Definitions of tinnitus

Tinnitus has been defined as the conscious experience of a sound that originates in the head of the owner.[1] Most authorities have qualified this statement by adding 'in the absence of any acoustic electrical or other external stimulation'. From a management point of view it is best to confine tinnitus to that of phantom auditory sensation[2,3] for which no acoustical generator can be identified. This places tinnitus securely within the neural aspects of the auditory system from the cochlea up to the auditory cortex, and excludes the experience of sounds generated by mechanical processes within the head or body, which are best described as somatosounds.[4] Although the processing of auditory information resulting in tinnitus and that of somatosounds may have some similarities in terms of neurophysiology and management, it is important to distinguish between them. Somatosounds have different psychoacoustical properties (e.g. masking by external tones) and may in many cases be amenable to surgical correction or medical treatment.

In all cases tinnitus refers to the subjective description of what the patient hears. It is a perception occurring at or just below the auditory cortex, and it is not a description of abnormalities that may or may not be present in the auditory periphery. Each perception of tinnitus, like any other auditory perception, is subject to considerable subcortical processing, signal detection and pattern matching, which has a profound effect on any focus or source that may be responsible for the origin and emergence of tinnitus.[2,5]. Therefore, in each and every case the central auditory system plays a vital and critical role in the experience of tinnitus. Moreover parts of the brain not involved in audition at all (e.g. the limbic system and prefrontal cortex) play a primary role in the development of tinnitus distress, which is the main reason for patients presenting with tinnitus. The traditional concept, therefore, that tinnitus is due to hair cells 'lying down' in the cochlea is unhelpful, misleading and counterproductive when it comes to devising an effective means for eradicating tinnitus perception based on a scientific model.

Classification

Having identified, in broad outline, what tinnitus is, it is clearly unhelpful to classify tinnitus in any of the traditional ways, for example into peripheral or central, or even by identifiable pathology. Although otological pathology (e.g. otosclerosis, Menière's disease) may play a part in tinnitus emergence and its natural history, it is equally possible for these pathologies to be present without any tinnitus perception whatever. The best approach is to divide the subject into somatosounds and phantom auditory perception (true tinnitus) (Fig 11.1). Somatosounds may be further subdivided into cochlear (spontaneous otoacoustic emissions) and extracochlear (vascular, respiratory, muscular or joint crepitus). Neurophysiological tinnitus, or phantom perception, may arise from a source or trigger (tinnitus related neural activity – TRNA) in the cochlea, brainstem or at higher levels; however, with few exceptions, we are currently unable to identify the source clinically. In each case tinnitus may be facilitated and sustained by the addition of a conductive hearing loss. The fact that the surgical correction of such a conductive loss may result in any change in the tinnitus underlines the mechanism whereby tinnitus in this case is a true phantom perception simply made more audible by the exclusion of external environmental sounds.

Auditory imagery[6] is the persistent perception of music and singing, commonly hymn tunes and jingles, which may with time become broken up into annoying snatches, a few musical bars in length. This condition should not be confused with the hallucination of psychotic disorders such as schizophrenia (which nevertheless is a phantom perception), and occurs in older people, who often have a hearing loss. It seems to be due to 'leakage' of auditory memory into perceptual areas in the central auditory system.

It should be noted that tinnitus and somatosounds may be part of everyone's normal experience. Transient tinnitus associated with feeling a blockage in the ear is universal and physiological, as is the ability to hear one's heart beating or sounds of Eustachian tube function or swallowing. People frequently describe 'the sound of silence'.[7] Occasionally these experiences can cause distress if they are thought to reflect pathological processes or disease.

Non-organic tinnitus can occur in individuals seeking compensation for industrial or accident claims.

Incidence and epidemiology

Tinnitus was described in the Egyptian papyri (6000 BC) and has clearly been with us a long time. The ability to detect tinnitus rises to 94 per cent in individuals with normal hearing placed in a soundproof room for up to 5 minutes.[7] The sounds perceived by such individuals are identical to those perceived by

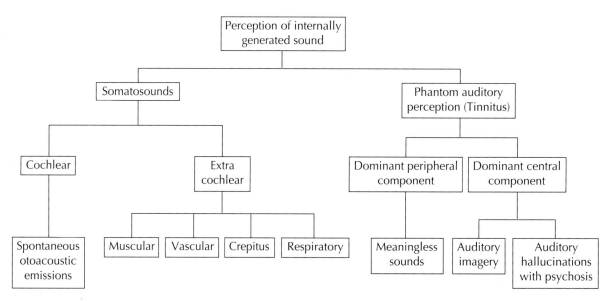

Fig 11.1 A new classification of tinnitus taking into account the Jastreboff[2] neurophysiological model.

individuals complaining of tinnitus distress. The mechanism by which tinnitus emerges in an extremely silent environment is of importance in its proper management. The National Study of Hearing (Institute of Hearing Research UK) showed that 10 per cent of adults have at some time experienced tinnitus for more than 5 minutes and apart from immediately after noise exposure, and 4 per cent have tinnitus causing moderate or severe annoyance.[8] In addition, 4 per cent of adults have tinnitus causing sleep disturbance and 0.5 per cent have tinnitus causing a severe effect on their ability to lead a normal life. Seven per cent of adults have at some time reported tinnitus during a visit to their family doctor. There is no sex difference, but a slightly increased incidence of reported left-sided tinnitus to right-sided tinnitus. This is not due to differences in noise exposure and is consistent with the epidemiological data on left-sided hearing being worse than right-sided.

Tinnitus and hearing loss

The increased incidence of tinnitus with age reflects the effects of ageing throughout the auditory system, but also worsening hearing. The Jastreboff model of tinnitus[2] stresses the importance of the 'straining to hear' phenomenon as a cause of tinnitus with increased hearing loss. Likewise, noise exposure is associated with tinnitus in only 23 per cent of patients, but this does indicate a twofold increased risk of developing tinnitus over a population not exposed to noise. It is not true to say that whatever caused the hearing loss probably caused the tinnitus too, although it may be responsible for its initial emergence. In many cases the traditional approach of identifying a high frequency sensory hearing loss and indicating this as 'the cause of the tinnitus' is inappropriate and unproven. Often the hearing loss has been present without change for a long time before the emergence of tinnitus. Even in the most severely hearing impaired population there is a very significant group who experience no tinnitus at all. In a study of 800 patients being assessed for cochlear implantation, 27 per cent had experienced no tinnitus whatever at anytime. Only 30 per cent had experienced distressing tinnitus.[9] In the Nottingham study of hearing (tier A data), 39 per cent of a group who said that they could not hear at all had no experience of tinnitus. Clearly, extreme hair cell destruction in the cochlea is frequently associated with the absence of tinnitus perception, and one must look elsewhere for a mechanism to account for its emergence and persistence.

Tinnitus in children

Tinnitus is present in 56 per cent of hearing impaired children although it is mostly intermittent. In a study by Graham and Butler[10] tinnitus was present in 66 per cent of 100 partially hearing children and 29 per cent of 66 deaf children. Again the tinnitus was mostly intermittent. It is quite common for clinicians not to ask of children whether they experience tinnitus and some authorities have actually counselled against it. Nevertheless, studies of adults with prolonged distressing tinnitus often reveal that this started in childhood, and that great unhappiness was experienced during this period. Equally, the experience of childhood tinnitus can be associated with the belief that 'everyone must have it'. Retraining therapy is highly effective in treating tinnitus in children because of the higher levels of plasticity in central auditory pathways.

Models of tinnitus mechanisms

The model of tinnitus that will be presented here is based on the Jastreboff model.[2] The introduction of this model has resulted in the design of a new therapeutic approach, which for the first time has resulted in prolonged absence of tinnitus perception. It also explains many of the conundrums that have haunted tinnitus research for so long. Traditional models have been strongly centred on cochlea function, largely because clinicians and auditory physiologists were strongly focused on this part of the hearing mechanism. In the case of clinicians, their ability to focus attention elsewhere was constrained by their training, which did not include a knowledge of central auditory mechanisms or understanding of the neural processing of perceptual information. Cochlear models of tinnitus were also encouraged by strong reports from tinnitus patients that their experience of internally generated sound emanated from the ear. In many cases patients are able to point to the part of the ear from which they think the sound is coming.

Such forceful reporting unhappily generated a naive belief in professionals that tinnitus was indeed a condition of the inner ear, and this accounts for the direction of clinical and research effort, which has been heavily focused on looking for abnormalities of cochlea function and treating the ear with drugs and other therapeutic approaches in an attempt to effect a cure. The reason why most approaches have been ineffective is because tinnitus is not a phenomenon confined to the inner ear.

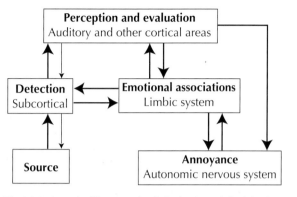

Fig 11.2 Jastreboff[2] neurophysiological model of tinnitus.

In the Jastreboff model tinnitus is primarily a subcortical perception, and results from the processing of weak neural activity in the periphery. It is important to think of 'tinnitus related neural activity' (TRNA) occurring, for the most part, near the periphery of the system, undergoing considerable processing in subcortical auditory pathways and finally being perceived at a conscious level as sound. The psychoacoustical qualities, such as the loudness and perceived frequency content of tinnitus, will depend on the strength and patterns of electrical activity arriving at the cortex of the temporal lobe of the brain after subcortical signal detection and pattern matching has occurred. TRNA will have undergone a similar process of signal detection, categorization and pattern matching as the neural activity generated by the external sounds detected by the cochlea (Fig 11.2).

Evidence for tinnitus related neural activity

With a normal cochlea and in the absence of external sound the normal subject is likely to describe the experience of silence. In the auditory nerve in silence there is random neural activity.[11] Disturbance of this random activity occurs when a sound is applied to the ear, which induces a synchrony of firing of nerve fibres of the appropriate characteristic frequency. Therefore anything that may alter this random activity may result in TRNA, which is ultimately perceived as tinnitus. The patterns of TRNA are usually very faint compared with those generated by external sounds. Nevertheless, in complete silence these very weak signals can easily be detected as discreet sounds in certain situations. Furthermore, discordant damage between outer and inner hair cells is able to

produce abnormalities of auditory nerve patterning, resulting in further TRNA.[3] TRNA could be further enhanced by efferent activity controlling the functioning of outer hair cells.[12] Very small differences in efferent function between tinnitus and non-tinnitus patients can be observed in the contralateral suppression of otoacoustic emissions.[13] In all cases the changes that can be measured are less than 1 dB and can in no way compare with the intensity of tinnitus that is experienced by sufferers. The high incidence of tinnitus in patients who have normal audiograms[14] suggests that cochlear abnormalities are not the most important factor in the generation of distressing tinnitus.

There has been a general failure of attempts to identify peripheral abnormalities that consistently relate to tinnitus, and consequently we do not find any asymmetry in the brainstem auditory evoked potentials except in grouped data. Tinnitus is not derived from a spontaneous otoacoustic emission except in rare circumstances,[15] and it cannot be detected in auditory nerve random activity.

Auditory processing – its importance in the generation and perception of tinnitus

THE COCHLEA

The main role of the cochlea is to transform sound energy into electrical patterns in the auditory nerve. In this form it is available for analysis by higher levels in the brain. The cochlea also performs a frequency analysis, extracting the individual frequencies that are present in any complex sound. Outer hair cell activity, apart from increasing sensitivity to very small sounds, also improves the frequency discrimination of the basilar membrane, particularly at low intensities of sound.[16] Patterns of electrical activity in the auditory nerve exactly reflect the patterns of acoustic activity in the external ear canal (see Chapters 2 and 4). The information transmitted from the cochlea by the auditory nerve is the 'raw data' of hearing. All the frequencies present in the acoustic environment are represented there, without the possibility of identifying any specific external acoustic message. In humans there is limited possibility for the ear to change the attentional focus of hearing. This is in contradistinction to vision, in which movement of the eye can concentrate a single item of visual interest onto the sensitive fovea to the exclusion of other images within the visual environment. With hearing, although the

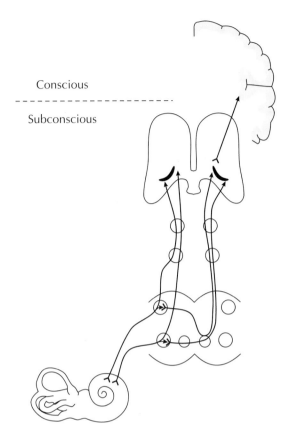

Fig 11.3 Auditory pathways: cochlea to auditory cortex.

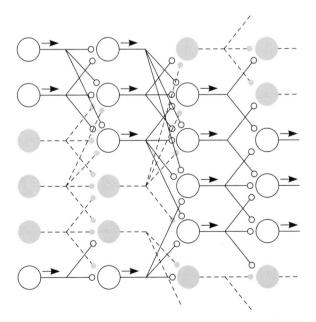

Fig 11.4 Neuronal networks involved in subcortical processing. Hatched cells are inactive. Neurons working in concert are able to act as filters in subcortical signal detection and pattern matching.[17]

pinna and head movement play a role, the main focusing of sensory attention has to be performed by central auditory processing.

SUBCORTICAL AUDITORY PATHWAYS

These pathways are often depicted as electric cables (Fig 11.3) joining the cochlea to the cortex, but this model is inaccurate. In reality a dense network of interconnecting neurons exists (Fig 11.4), which plays a vital role in detecting signals and categorizing information in an hierarchical fashion.[5,17] In the brainstem and midbrain, phase and loudness data from both ears allow precise localization of sound. As the auditory signals pass centrally, categorization of information proceeds in an increasingly complex manner so that different frequencies can be grouped according to their origin and type, for example speech, environmental sounds, warning signals and new information. Indeed, new patterns of information are always dealt with as a priority as their importance has not already been established.

There are many examples of this subcortical and subconscious signal detection at work. We are all familiar with the experience of hearing the sound of our first name being mentioned in a nearby conversation at a noisy party. In this situation, first, only the bearer of the name will detect the sound and second, no other part of the sentence in which it occurs will be audible. We know we are being talked about but we do not know what is being said about us. In this situation subcortical neuronal networks are working as a complex filter or pattern recognition mechanism below our level of conscious awareness to alert us to signals that have special importance, even if our attention is diverted elsewhere, or in some instances, even if we are asleep. The experience of mothers waking to the sound their baby makes just before it begins to cry while father sleeps on is well known to many of us. In each case a process of learning or special programming of neuronal networks has to occur to allow the identification of complex and prolonged auditory stimuli. The same process of auditory learning distinguishes the conductor of an orchestra, who is able to hear each instrument individually, from the 'tone deaf' member of the audience for whom the music is simply a wash of sound.

Perception of sound

Sound perception occurs some 200–300 ms after electrical signals leave the cochlea (Fig 11.3). Perception involves activity in other areas of the brain, but it is convenient to think of this as being the time and place of perception for the purpose of this model. When we go to sleep at night cortical activity is greatly suppressed and this is why perception of all sensory modalities (hearing, vision, touch, smell etc) is suspended. Nevertheless, during sleep and anaesthesia, activity at lower levels in the auditory system (from cochlea to inferior colliculus) are unchanged. In the rare condition of bilateral temporal lobe stroke there is total deafness (and no perception of tinnitus either) despite the fact that structures lower down in the auditory system continue to function normally. Quite clearly perception of sound occurs only after neural patterns reach the cortical perceptual areas and only after extensive subcortical processing of auditory information has occurred.

The auditory attentional focus

Auditory perception is further characterized by an attentional focus. It is only possible to have one focus of auditory attention at any one time. A constant process of prioritization or rank-ordering of auditory information takes place, the item of greatest importance occupying the attentional focus to the exclusion of other environmental sounds. Once our attention moves from one auditory item to another, the previous perception is suppressed; in most cases we simply cannot hear it. This strategy makes for the most effective processing of information such as language, but it does mean that we have great difficulty in performing two auditory tasks at the same time. All of these aspects of normal central processing of auditory information have a very direct bearing on the clinical presentation of tinnitus.

The evolution of pattern matching strategies in the auditory system

It is unlikely that such complex neuronal networks capable of the detection of long utterances and able to extract these from a background of considerable noise were developed to enable us to detect people talking about us at a cocktail party. In nature, a hostile environment and the constant threat of many predators demands first and foremost the ability to detect their presence. Successful predators make very little sound and their signals must be extracted from a background of natural sounds

that may be of considerable intensity. Moreover, the sound of a snake slithering through the grass must be distinguished from similar sounds such as the wind in the grass. The ability to do this results in the survival of the animal with the best attributes for escaping the snake. These include the possession of highly developed signal detection and pattern matching mechanisms in the auditory subconscious. These neural processes and the ability to detect very small signals that threaten us in the presence of high levels of background noise rapidly develop under the influence of natural selection.[18] Humans might be seen as the end product of this selection process.

Significance of sound and its emotional content

When faced with any signal that could indicate a warning, whether it be a threat to life or simply something that might have a mild negative influence on day-to-day living, it is important that an emotional message is conveyed with it. Indeed, no learning process is complete without its emotional label. In a survival reflex there is very strong and immediate stimulation of the limbic system, the centre of emotion and learning in the brain, which includes important structures such as the hippocampus, cingulate gyrus and connections with the reticular formation in the brainstem. There are at least two million connections between subcortical neuronal networks in the auditory system concerned with signal detection and the limbic system (Fig 11.5). Strong emotional response can be obtained when life-threatening signals are first detected, even before there is a cortical awareness. In this situation cortical evaluation of danger would be too slow. In the case of the sound of the snake, extreme anxiety or fear would bring about instant flight or freezing of movement to avoid attack. In the case of a threatened mongoose, anger would be produced in order to prepare for combat with the snake. It is important to realize that all of these extremely powerful emotions evoking an invariate and irresistible response are brought about by structures outside the auditory system, and may be initiated by the very weakest auditory signal.

Even in very primitive organisms with the simplest central nervous systems, changes in homeostasis, that is to say variations in the environment in terms of temperature change, increases in the amount of light, et cetera, produce specific activity in the reticular formation. The sensation that we experience in an analogous situation might be

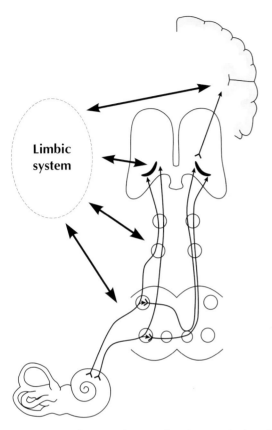

Fig 11.5 Auditory pathways showing cortical and sub-cortical connections with the limbic system.

described as annoyance or ill ease, the object of which is to make us react so as attempt to restore the status quo in our environment.

PHOBIAS AND FEARS

In a so-called civilized environment the exposure to predators of a life-threatening kind is an uncommon occurrence. However, the same neurophysiological processes continue to set up reflex responses in susceptible and vulnerable individuals. These are exhibited by various kinds of phobic response to benign objects such as the house spider. In this case a small visual stimulus from a harmless creature (the house spider) evokes a very powerful unpleasant emotional response because of early learning, for example finding a spider in your bed or bath when young. Other well known phobias include a dislike of small spaces, open spaces, lifts, flying, heights, et cetera. The mechanism is very similar to the survival response in that there is an immediate and invariate unpleasant emotional feeling, often fear or anxiety, and there is also stimulation of the

autonomic nervous system with appropriate symptoms such as sweating, palpitations and nausea. A characteristic of all these phobic responses is that they do not easily habituate, unlike the presence of other stimuli that are without significant meaning for which habituation is usually rapid and complete. Think of the universal experience of annoyance created by a newly purchased refrigerator. Habituation to this sound takes on average about 2–3 weeks as every refrigerator salesman knows.

MOOD STATE AND THE SURVIVAL REFLEX

Anxious animals tend to react much more strongly to potential danger, but those in a depressed mood state (e.g. after injury or illness) need to be even more aware of the presence of predators. A broken limb may restrict mobility and require an awareness of the presence of snakes when they are twice as far away. Fluctuations in mood state therefore result in a non-specific 'widening' of subcortical filters to increase threat detection potential. We are all aware of the feeling of walking down a dark street in the middle of the night in a foreign city when every footstep or sound echoes a hundred times louder in our ears than would be the case if we were out shopping in our own town centre on a Saturday afternoon. The connections between the limbic system and signal detection mechanisms in all sensory modalities is two directional. Detection of a threat signal triggers an appropriate emotion, and changes in emotional state change the sensitivity and specificity of this signal detection mechanism.[18,19]

Tinnitus emergence and persistence

EMERGENCE OF TINNITUS

For tinnitus to grow into any kind of a clinical problem it has to be detected for a first time. In fact the emergence of tinnitus is an extremely common phenomenon, much commoner than tinnitus of clinical importance. Present day social life dictates a high incidence of 'disco tinnitus', which nearly always disappears within a day or so, often after a few hours. Significant temporary changes occur in the cochlea after such noise exposure. These changes are reflected in auditory nerve patterning, which is perceived as high frequency whistles and

(a)

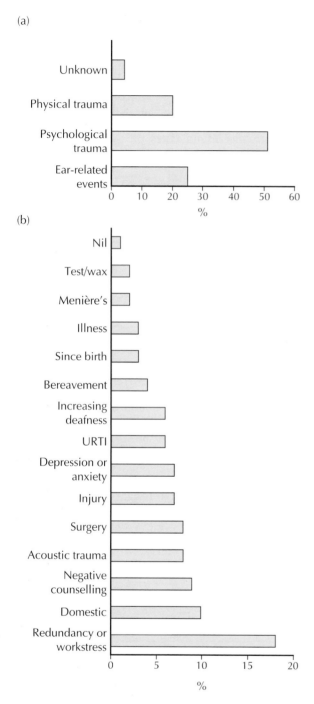

(b)

though some hair cell damage may have occurred, tinnitus rarely persists. Contrast this experience with a particular episode associated with very loud noise, enough to cause pain in the ear, when a very clear conviction develops that the ear has been damaged, because of the presence of pain. This is always the occasion when tinnitus persists, becomes louder and intrusive, and becomes associated with unpleasant emotional responses.

Another example of tinnitus emergence, which is almost universal, is described in the classic experiment by Heller and Bergman.[7] Eighty normally hearing individuals were placed one by one in a soundproof room for less than 5 minutes at a time and asked to record their auditory experiences. Ninety-three per cent described a high frequency hiss, ringing, hissing and pulses identical to those described by patients with clinically significant tinnitus. Again tinnitus disappeared after the experience. Nearly all of us can try the Heller and Bergman experiment every time we retire for bed at night to the quiet of a bedroom with closed, often double-glazed windows by which we have managed to exclude most environmental sound. This is quite different from the noise of nature in a nest or burrow. It is often in this silent environment at night, or on waking in the morning, when tinnitus emerges and is first experienced.

TRIGGERS TO TINNITUS EMERGENCE

During a recent study of 100 consecutive patients presenting with severe persistent tinnitus, it was found that over 80 per cent had triggers of emergence that could be classified as reflecting changes in mood state (Fig 11.6). These included bereavement, job loss, retirement, unrelated injury or accident, episodes of clinically significant depression or anxiety and as domestic and work stress. In only relatively few cases was there an easily identifiable cochlear or 'ear' trigger such as Menière's syndrome or a verifiable incident of acoustic trauma. The mechanism for tinnitus emergence here can be seen as the opening of central auditory filters allowing the perception of previously inaudible TRNA.

PERSISTENCE OF TINNITUS

Persistence of tinnitus and its associated emotional response is the reason for patient complaint. Temporary short duration tinnitus not associated with anxiety or depression rarely prompts a need for professional help.

Persistent tinnitus has been shown to be associated with the development of negative beliefs about

Fig 11.6 (a) Trigger factors in the emergence of tinnitus (100 consecutive cases). (b) A more detailed breakdown of the same data. URTI, upper respiratory tract infection.

hisses by the individual. The experience of disco tinnitus has (unfortunately) very little meaning for the individual. Everybody gets tinnitus after going to a disco, it is associated with having a good time. Even

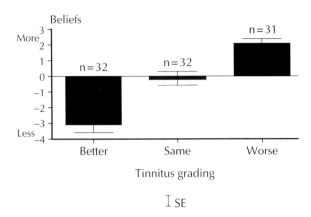

Fig 11.7 Changes in negative beliefs (see Table 11.1). Patients getting better show a reduction in negative beliefs about tinnitus over a 6-month period. Changes in beliefs also occur with worsening tinnitus.

Table 11.1 Common negative beliefs* acquired by patients with tinnitus distress

Tinnitus will get worse
Tinnitus will go on for ever
Tinnitus is a physical disease
There is no treatment for tinnitus
I will be deprived of sleep because of tinnitus
Tinnitus will make me go deaf
Tinnitus will make me go mad/I will not be able to stand it
Tinnitus is caused by a tumour
Tinnitus means I will have a stroke
My ability to cope will be severely reduced
My family life and social life will suffer greatly
It is an intrusion into my right to remain silent

*Such beliefs are frequently reinforced by negative counselling.

what tinnitus means.[20] Moreover, the number of negative beliefs held by the individual directly relate to the severity of the tinnitus and its natural progression (getting better, worse or staying the same) (Fig 11.7). Therefore, those patients in whom tinnitus was worsening showed an increase in the number of negative beliefs and those in whom it was naturally habituating showed a decrease. Although this does not prove that the beliefs themselves were responsible for the change of tinnitus perception, it is consistent with that hypothesis. As will be seen later, one of the most effective therapies focuses on changing these inappropriate beliefs about the meaning of tinnitus.

Inappropriate beliefs about tinnitus

For the past 5 years we have been monitoring and recording patient beliefs and fears about what their tinnitus means (Table 11.1). There is a highly consistent short list, on which the worries about tinnitus getting worse, persisting for all time and being incurable are the most important. On this basis, fears that tinnitus may be associated with ensuing deafness or other intracranial disease create very understandable distress in the individual. The effect that the tinnitus may have on the individual's life in terms of their sleep, enjoyment of recreational activity and life quality generally are also of extreme importance (see below). Many patients with severe tinnitus distress have been exposed to negative counselling, which has helped to reinforce

beliefs about the serious effects that tinnitus may have.

ENHANCEMENT OF NEGATIVE BELIEFS ABOUT TINNITUS

A careful history will often reveal that the patient experienced tinnitus emergence on several occasions sometime before tinnitus became permanent and started to produce feelings of distress. The feelings of distress are generally related to the development of negative ideas about tinnitus (Table 11.1) and it is understandable that at this stage patients immediately begin a search for help. It is unfortunate that health-care professionals usually respond to a patient's complaint of tinnitus with the short homily that 'there is nothing that can be done about tinnitus', 'you need to go away and learn to live with it', 'you could have an operation but this could render you totally deaf', 'I am very sorry but there is no known cure for this condition' et cetera. This has been the conventional wisdom and teaching for nearly 100 years. If the patient exhibits extreme distress that might be classified as psychological disturbance, a referral for a psychological or psychiatric appointment may be made, and in the meantime scans may be done 'in order to exclude a tumour'. Although many of these actions may be well intended, they do nothing to allay the patient's anxieties about the meaning of their tinnitus, and it is usually during this period of negative reinforcement that the tinnitus become louder and the emotional responses generated become far stronger. We have documented thousands of case histories in which this is the exact sequence of events.

Also the exhibition of interventionist, unproven and empirical therapies ('take these tablets and come back in 3 weeks') further reinforces the concept that no effective treatment is available.

It must be stressed, from a neurophysiological point of view that all of these powerful perceptions that the patient has are entirely real and are represented by high levels of neuronal activity at the auditory cortex.[21] They also reflect the presence of TRNA, which in most cases has been present for a long time before emergence, and conscious awareness occurs. Once tinnitus perception is identified with a potential life threat or even a life quality threat, there is a compelling need to monitor its progress on a minute-to-minute basis. Constant monitoring of tinnitus, either by diary keeping or simply to obtain reassurance that it is not getting any worse, acts as a training and reinforcement programme to assure that tinnitus perception persists and may indeed become stronger.

Emotional response to tinnitus and distress mechanisms

The neurophysiological interaction of the limbic system (and prefrontal cortex) with the auditory subcortex is a two-pronged process (Fig 11.1). Whereas alterations in mood state may be responsible for the emergence of tinnitus, it is common experience that distressing tinnitus frequently results in alterations in mood, usually anxiety and depression. This occurs more commonly when mood swings predate tinnitus onset. These and other emotions become involved in a complex interaction with the tinnitus. Anxiety symptoms (worrying about it, fear, panic) may mingle with anger symptoms (ranging from irritation to eruptions of violent behaviour). The general clinical picture is one of anxiety symptoms mixed with irritation and annoyance, giving an overall feeling of distress. These powerful emotions, elicited by the tinnitus itself, are what militate against its habituation. In addition to emotions resulting directly from tinnitus, other feelings indirectly associated with tinnitus play an important part in its persistence. These usually centre around anger at the dismissive way in which health-care professionals make it clear that they have no interest in the condition. Patients often feel guilty if they have submitted to treatment that they feel may have made things worse, or they may consider themselves responsible for noise exposure or the application of ineffective home remedies.

In a study of 54 patients with unilateral deafness and severe tinnitus, we found that 41 per cent had failed otosurgery (an otherwise very rare cause of unilateral deafness). The cause of their distress was strongly related to anger about the surgeon and guilt about submitting to the procedure.[22] Behavioural therapy focused on these emotional issues was very beneficial in reducing tinnitus perception and annoyance.

Hyperacusis

Many patients complain of hyperacusis either with or without tinnitus. Sixty per cent of patients in our tinnitus clinic also complained of hyperacusis and some 80 per cent show abnormally low levels of

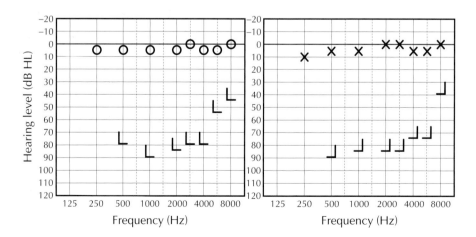

Fig 11.8 Loudness discomfort levels in a typical phobic tinnitus patient. Hyperacusis is most marked around the perceived tinnitus frequency. Hyperacusis improves with retraining therapy.

loudness discomfort to pure tones particularly around the perceived pitch of the tinnitus. The Jastreboff model[2] predicts that inappropriate setting of auditory filters giving tinnitus perception may also facilitate the enhanced detection of external sounds that sound similar. If a phobic response to tinnitus exists, this may trigger aversive emotional reactions to sounds similar to the tinnitus coming from the environment. If there are strongly held beliefs that noise damage to the ear has occurred, inappropriate beliefs can develop about the damaging properties of normal levels of environmental noise, even though they were previous well tolerated. Hyperacusis (and phonophobia) frequently develops around the perceived pitch of the tinnitus (Fig 11.8). Hyperacusis (measured by persistent and repeatable measures of reduced loudness discomfort to pure tones) may also be generalized across other frequencies, and usually affects the contralateral ear indicating that a central mechanism is involved. It is important to differentiate this sensitivity to external sounds, which is properly referred to as hyperacusis, from the cochlear abnormality of recruitment. Hyperacusis is reversible by behavioural therapy and sound therapy,[23] and indicates an enhanced gain in subcortical auditory processing.

References

1. McFadden D. *Tinnitus: facts, theories, and treatments.* Washington DC: National Academy Press, 1982:1–150.
2. Jastreboff PJ. Phantom auditory perception (tinnitus): mechanisms of generation and perception. *Neuroscience Research* 1990; **8**:221–54.
3. Jastreboff PJ, Brennan JF, Coleman JK, Sasaki CT. Phantom auditory sensation in rats: an animal model for tinnitus. *Behavioral Neuroscience* 1988; **102**:811–22.
4. Hazell JW. Tinnitus. II: Surgical management of conditions associated with tinnitus and somatosounds. *Journal of Otolaryngology* 1990; **19**:6–10.
5. Goldman-Rakic PS. Topography of cognition: parallel distributed networks in primate association cortex. *Annual Review of Neuroscience* 1988: **11**:137–56.
6. Goodwin PE. Tinnitus and auditory imagery. *American Journal of Otology* 1980; **2**:5–9.
7. Heller MF, Bergman M. Tinnitus in normally hearing persons. *Annals of Otology* 1953; **62**:73–83.
8. Coles RRA. Epidemiology of tinnitus: (1) prevalence. *Journal of Laryngology and Otology Supplement* 1984; **9**:7–15.
9. Hazell JWP, Mckinney CJ, Aleksy W. Mechanisms of tinnitus in profound deafness. *Annals of Otology, Rhinology and Laryngology Supplement* 1995; **166**:418–20.
10. Graham JM, Butler J. Tinnitus in children. *Journal of Laryngology and Otology Supplement* 1984; **9**:236–41.
11. Moller AR. Pathophysiology of tinnitus. *Annals of Otology, Rhinology and Laryngology* 1984; **93**:39–44.
12. Hazell JWP. A cochlear model for tinnitus. In: Feldmann H ed. *Proceedings of the Third International Tinnitus Seminar, Munster, GDR.* Karlsruhe: Harsch Verlag, 1987:121–8.
13. Graham RL, Hazell JWP. Contralateral suppression of transient evoked otoacoustic emissions: intra-individual variability in tinnitus and normal subjects. *British Journal of Audiology* 1994; **28**:235–47.
14. Hazell JWP, Wood SM, Cooper HR, *et al.* A clinical study of tinnitus maskers. *British Journal of Audiology* 1985; **19**:65–146.
15. Penner MJ, Coles RRA. Indications for aspirin as a palliative for tinnitus caused by SOAEs: a case study. *British Journal of Audiology* 1992; **26**:91–6.
16. Zenner HP, Plinkert PK. A.C. and D.C. motility of mammalian auditory sensory cells – a new concept in hearing physiology. *Otolaryngologia Polska* 1992; **46**:333–49.
17. Pribram KH. *Languages of the brain – experimental paradoxes and principles in neurophysiology.* Englewood Cliffs, NJ: Prentice Hall, 1971:1–432.
18. Hazell JWP. Models of tinnitus. Generation, perception, clinical implications. In: Vernon J, Moller A eds. *Mechanisms of tinnitus.* Boston: Allyn and Bacon, 1995:57–72.
19. Hazell JWP. Support for a neurophysiological model of tinnitus: research data and clinical experience. In: Reich G, Vernon J eds. *Proceedings of the Fifth International Tinnitus Seminar.* Portland, OR: American Tinnitus Association, 1996:51–7.
20. Mckinney CJ, Hazell JWP. Retraining therapy can abolish perception of tinnitus [abstract]. *Paper presented 22nd Int. Congress of Audiology: Halifax July 4–8.* 1994:151.
21. Lockwood AH, Salvi RJ, Coad ML, *et al.* Neural correlates of subjective tinnitus as identified by positron emission tomography (PET) of cerebral blood flow. *Proceedings of the Association for Research in Otolaryngology 19th midwinter research meeting, Florida, USA Feb 4–8.* 1996.
22. Hazell JWP, von Schoenberg LJ, Meerton LJ, Sheldrake JB Tinnitus and the unilateral dead ear. In: Aran JM, Dauman R eds. *Proceedings of the Fourth International Tinnitus Seminar, 1991 Aug 27–30; Bordeaux.* Amsterdam: Kugler Publications, 1992:261–4.
23. Hazell JWP, Sheldrake JB. Hyperacusis and tinnitus. In: Aran JM, Dauman R eds. *Proceedings of the Fourth International Tinnitus Seminar, 1991 Aug 27–30; Bordeaux.* Amsterdam: Kugler Publications, 1992:245–8.

CHAPTER 12

Assessment and psycho-acoustical aspects of tinnitus

JONATHAN HAZELL

Introduction

Once there is an understanding of the complex neurophysiology that is involved in the generation of tinnitus and tinnitus distress, it can be readily appreciated that a simple approach for assessment based on audiometric testing is unlikely to give useful information or bring consistent results. We have established that tinnitus is a perception, the result of pattern matching events near the auditory cortex that strongly reflect previous subcortical processing of tinnitus related neural activity (TRNA), and that it is highly dependent on input from the limbic system and also the prefrontal cortex. In addition, the distress caused by tinnitus, which is the essential part of tinnitus complaint, cannot be assessed by auditory testing. That is why measurements of loudness matching and masking or suppression measurements have no statistical relationship to the overall severity of the tinnitus.[1]

The tinnitus clinic

Problem tinnitus cannot be dealt with satisfactorily in a routine ENT clinic, although those simply needing reassurance may be, provided the clinicians have a good understanding of the neurophysiogical model. For problem patients there must be a mechanism for referral to a specialist tinnitus clinic in which a realistic length of time can be allocated to each patient. The tinnitus clinic takes place on a monthly, weekly or daily basis according to need

and demand, but it must be a formal part of the organization of each regional service. An average of 45 minutes must be allocated to the assessment of each new patient, a much longer time than is needed for the assessment of routine ENT problems. A team needs to be assembled and must include an interested and committed ENT surgeon or audiological physician, who takes the first consultation with the patient. An audiologist or audiological technician with skills in tinnitus testing, fitting of appropriate instruments and initial counselling works in close proximity with the physician or surgeon running the tinnitus clinic. The follow-up sessions of retraining therapy in the UK are most commonly undertaken by a hearing therapist, but other disciplines are also variously involved, depending on departmental structure. In addition to this core team, it is highly desirable to have immediate access to a clinical psychologist with a special interest in tinnitus, and also a medical colleague in psychiatry. The close interaction of the team members is more important than their actual numbers but there must be at least two, one medical and one non-medical. The role of the audiological physician or ENT surgeon is to diagnose or exclude otological disease, organize appropriate investigations, take a proper tinnitus history and perform the first in a series of directive medical counselling sessions with the patient. The role of the non-medical therapists is to organize a programme of retraining; to introduce the patient to any instruments, such as white noise generators or hearing aids; to make sure that their use is understood and to outline a programme for their use; and to undertake further periods of directive counselling, relaxation training therapy, et cetera as appropriate in the period between medical counselling and assessment sessions. The therapist must also be prepared to perform measurements to determine the level of habituation that has occurred as the programme proceeds.

TINNITUS CLINIC ENVIRONMENT

It is obvious that this must be a quiet and unhurried environment in which confidentiality is ensured and the patient has time and opportunity to talk about their symptoms. Many will have experienced disinterest and dismissive attitudes. The first job of a committed tinnitus clinic is to make it clear to the patient that this approach has changed, and that there are many positive things that can be done to help the patient's symptoms.

Descriptions of tinnitus

The perceived psychoacoustical properties of the tinnitus and its location simply reflect the difficulties of central perceptive mechanisms in interpreting new and unusual patterns arriving from the auditory periphery. Difficulties are always experienced in interpreting new signals from a new location especially if it be inside the head, a place previously only associated with silence.

Minute changes in pitch, location and loudness are often perceived as a new turn in pathological events, and it is vital that the patient understands the relative unimportance of these perceptual changes. Most commonly tinnitus is perceived as a high frequency hiss or whistle, something approaching a pure tone, which may be surrounded by a narrow band of noise. Pulsatile elements are commonly described (in about 12 per cent of patients). They do not necessarily indicate the presence of somatosounds, although they may suggest the 'imprint' of vascular activity transmitted through the cochlear fluids. The reported position of tinnitus is highly dependent on cortical evaluation. The process of externalization of perception,[2] by which we create a virtual reality of the world around us, results in the accurate placement of the origin of sights, sounds and tactile information within our immediate environment. No coordinates pre-exist for placing the experience of internally generated sound, and for this reason many patients will initially describe tinnitus as a sound coming from outside. They frequently open windows, prise up floorboards and generally search high and low for the source of an external sound.

'Hummers'

For some people the belief that tinnitus is an external sound is so powerful that they remain permanently convinced that the sound is generated by some external source (e.g. gas pipes under the ground or overhead electric lines). These patients have sometimes been referred to as 'hummers'. Although this group merges with the hyperacusis group, in whom there is a highly increased sensitivity to some disturbing sound in the environment, the majority of 'hummers' describe sounds that cannot be detected by others, even with the most sensitive listening apparatus. Many of them also have a hearing loss. However, complaints of environmental noise causing distress should be treated sensitively. The individual's perception that the sound is external is complete reality to them, and is often reinforced by strong emotions, enhanced by years of legal battles against utility companies. The fact that sounds may only be heard near the home results from an automatic process of subcortical monitoring and enhancement of TRNA in the environment in which the annoying sound is expected. Logic says it cannot be detected elsewhere. Understanding of tinnitus mechanisms and the phenomenon of externalization of perception helps those who are really looking for relief from their noise. For those who can never come to terms with the idea that they are experiencing tinnitus, and for those who are having to deal with the reality of environmental noise that they have come to dislike, a masking approach is permissible for symptom relief, although this will not result in habituation. Inoffensive background sound should be created in the bedroom (such as a large electric fan). The ability to hear 'hums' in the presence of ear plugs or masking sounds, confirms their internal origin.

Perceived location, description and course of tinnitus

In the majority of patients, tinnitus is finally identified as coming from one or other or both ears or from within the head. Unilateral tinnitus commonly becomes bilateral when it persists. Up to 40 different sound locations have been identified by a single patient. This simply indicates the ability of central processing mechanisms to identify TRNA coming from more than one site. It is important to chart the overall duration and temporal fluctuations of tinnitus, particularly with respect to psychological triggers. Fluctuation and periods of remission should be viewed as evidence of the beginning of habituation rather than a reinforcement phenomenon. The subjective loudness of tinnitus is perhaps the most changing phenomenon to record, and bears least statistical relationship to any other variable. In general, the more annoying the tinnitus is the louder it is perceived, but some patients with extremely phobic responses may be extremely troubled by tinnitus that is barely audible. Tinnitus is masked by a variety of environmental sounds, but the masking effect does not follow any parameters of psychoacoustical masking. In many patients extremely distressing tinnitus will only be heard in the absence of daytime environmental noise. The fact that it is troublesome only in the evening during periods of quiet recreational activity and at night does not negate its importance. Many patients will discover by themselves that tinnitus can be masked or made less intrusive by the use of radios, television sets, music and household equipment such as fans and loudly ticking clocks. The therapeutic significance of this will be discussed later.

Hyperacusis

Sixty per cent of patients with significant tinnitus also experience discomfort from environmental noise. In 40 per cent of these patients this hyperacusis to normal environmental sounds predated the onset of tinnitus indicating an increased sensitivity, increase of central auditory gain, or the development of a behaviourally based annoyance response to certain sounds because of their meaning. Reported experience of environmental hyperacusis is often supported by reduced loudness discomfort levels on audiometry. In many cases hyperacusis will trigger increased tinnitus. When these sounds indicate a threat or territorial intrusion, the focusing of auditory filters results in enhancement of TRNA and louder tinnitus at the same time. Questioning of the patient should cover these points.

Effects of tinnitus on patient's life

It is important to assess the effects of tinnitus as a complaint. Three separate and non-dependent categories are concentration (at work), quiet recreational activity and sleep. These functions may be variably and separately affected. Sleep disturbance is very common with tinnitus onset, but often habituates early. Persistent insomnia is a separate issue that

often requires specialized management by a psychologist. If sleep disturbance has existed before tinnitus onset, then sleep is most likely to be affected. Elements that need separate assessment are difficulty in getting off to sleep, difficulty in getting back to sleep on waking, and early morning waking (which itself maybe a sign of coexistent depressive illness). For many patients the loss of the ability to be completely silent is the hardest part to bear. Tinnitus interferes with quiet recreational activities such as reading, painting and sewing. Whether the recreation is able to move the attentional focus away from the tinnitus, or whether the tinnitus intrudes so strongly as to make the recreation impossible should be noted. If concentration at work is affected, then serious worries may develop about sick leave, unemployment, loss of income and inability to support the family et cetera. Many patients have a tendency to 'what if' and produce fantastic scenarios in their minds that are far removed from reality. These anxieties and worries may be the main preoccupations rather than the tinnitus itself, and must be uncovered by gentle questioning.

Interaction of tinnitus with mood state

The Jastreboff model[3] indicates the importance of limbic activity both in terms of cause and effect (see Fig 11.1). Pre-existing anxiety and depression may re-emerge in the presence of persistent tinnitus and become the most important clinical entity. Tinnitus may persist as a barometer of the emotional state. In patients with very clear emotional triggers, continued family or work stress may result in predictable fluctuations in tinnitus caused by a non-specific opening and closing of subcortical filters monitoring environmental threats. We have usefully identified a very small group of patients as 'flag wavers'. These patients need to use their tinnitus (in itself not very important or significant) as a means of identifying a mountain of abject misery and despair that lies buried just beneath the surface of an otherwise calm exterior. Life problems may be long-standing and insoluble, but the tinnitus is a respectable symptom that may be presented to the unwitting otologist in circumstances of extreme despair.

Communication disorder

Many tinnitus patients presume that it is the tinnitus that makes it difficult for them to hear, for instance in a noisy environment. The perception is that tinnitus masks hearing. In almost all such cases there will be a degree of high frequency hearing loss reducing directional hearing in noise. The patient's ability to hear in noise does not improve as their tinnitus reduces (for instance in the process of tinnitus retraining therapy). Enlightenment about tinnitus mechanisms is important in order to ensure understanding of these relationships and compliance with treatment. In some patients, however, the hearing difficulty relates to a lack of concentration engendered by an extremely intrusive and distressing tinnitus, and here other evidence of failure of attentional focus will be found on questioning. In patients with completely normal audiograms and extreme difficulty in hearing noise, particularly if this symptom predates the tinnitus, it is important to question for other evidence of 'obscure auditory dysfunction' (OAD) syndrome, another manifestation of central auditory processing dysfunction.[4] Specific tests and strategies for management exist for this condition, and it is important to have a member of the tinnitus team equipped to deal with the diagnosis and therapy required for OAD.

Habituation assessment

The percentage of waking hours in which the patient is aware of tinnitus over a 2- to 3-month period should be recorded at the beginning when the tinnitus started, from the history, and at the present moment. The same assessment should be made for the percentage of waking hours during which tinnitus distress or annoyance exists; it will nearly always be less than the first measurement. These figures may seem to be rather arbitrary, but they do indicate the general direction, that habituation of perception (the first value) or habituation of reaction (the second value) are already to some extent taking place. The fact that the annoyance figure is different from the awareness figure indicates two separate mechanisms: one by which tinnitus is perceived as an auditory sensation and the other by which unpleasant emotional effects are generated (outside the auditory system). This helps to support and reinforce the importance of the Jastreboff model[3] to the patient.

Questionnaire data

Pitch, loudness, time scale, aggravating factors and other subjective parameters of tinnitus may be most easily recorded on an analogue scale, either by history taking or by the patient on their own. Such measurements are extremely useful to log the progress of the patient's tinnitus and identify different aspects of it. The fact that such measurements are highly non-linear is of less consequence, as it is the direction of progress that counts.

BELIEFS, FEARS AND MEANINGS

The questionnaire should contain a list of negative beliefs about tinnitus commonly expressed by sufferers (Table 11.1). Whereas patients with mild tinnitus annoyance may not have developed any of these beliefs, those with very powerful anxieties or phobias about their tinnitus will often hold many or all of these beliefs from time to time. It is vital to identify these negative beliefs in the very phobic tinnitus patient, because reversal of this phobic or survival-style response will not be possible without removal of the inappropriate beliefs associated with it.

PREDISPOSING OR TRIGGER FACTORS

In our experience trigger factors most commonly have a psychological or stress content, rather than something otological, and it is most important to document these. Even in cases of noise exposure or painful ear syringing there is a powerful belief generated that irreparable damage is being done to the ear, although in most cases this has been found not to be so. It is the generation of the fear, rather than the physical action of water or sound on the eardrum, that is of importance here.

If tinnitus is associated with the sudden onset of deafness or increasing deafness, two factors are important. First, there is a change of patterning of auditory nerve resting discharge potentials, which may be quite subtle, but nevertheless is identified as a 'new' signal. Second, there may be an increase in 'straining to hear phenomena' causing an increase in central auditory gain. These are not inevitable occurrences, and in the majority of cases of sudden or increased hearing loss there is no associated tinnitus perception. If the hearing loss or associated balance disturbance causes undue alarm, tinnitus emergence and persistence may be mediated through connections with the limbic system.

Traditional triggers (appropriately sought in the diagnosis of a sensorineural hearing impairment such as family history or ototoxic drugs) have little relevance to the tinnitus. Despite this, it is important to investigate the hearing loss properly at the same time as taking an intelligent history of the tinnitus.

Clinical examination

Any tests or examinations that are indicated on the basis of identifiable pathology must be dealt with in a proper and conventional manner. This is one reason for the presence of a competent otologist in the tinnitus clinic. In addition to routine examination, auscultation of the neck, head and ears should be made if somatosounds are suspected, and gentle jugular compression for pulsatile tinnitus is useful in the diagnosis of jugular outflow syndrome (e.g. in benign intracranial hypertension).[5]

Blood tests

There are no haematological investigations that are directly relevant to tinnitus, but a deafness 'screen' is indicated to check for anaemia, abnormal serology, thyroid function, abnormal lipids, vitamin B12, blood sugar and zinc levels. Ten years of continuous monitoring of these factors has not revealed a single patient with tinnitus alone who showed any abnormality.

Acoustic neuroma exclusion

Enormous, and sometimes unnecessary resources are poured into the diagnostic procedures required for acoustic neuroma exclusion. Whereas 10 per cent of all acoustic neuromas begin with a symptom of unilateral tinnitus only, in the UK this amounts to probably less than 40 cases a year with this presentation. We perform brainstem auditory evoked potentials (BAEPs), with caloric testing as a primary screen, although one must be aware that many such tinnitus patients are hyperacusic to 80 dB clicks presented during BAEP testing and that BAEP is much less sensitive to small tumours. MRI (preferably with gadolinium enhancement) should be used as audiologically indicated. Proper counselling is needed, especially for hyperacusic patients, about MRI noise (provide earplugs) and the fact that they will be locked in a small tube for 45 minutes or so (many phobic tinnitus patients are also claustrophobic). Patients waiting for MRI should not be told that there is a possibility of a tumour if this is their main worry. However, once a normal examination is completed this reassurance can be of great therapeutic value. Neuroma investigation without alarming the tinnitus patient is an art that should be acquired.

Audiometric testing

Auditory thresholds to the lowest limit of the audiometer should be tested at all frequencies, including half octaves. Loudness discomfort levels (LDLs) should be recorded between 250 Hz and 8 kHz with the instructions 'please indicate when the sound I am making starts to become uncomfortably loud'. The presentation tone should be increased in 5 dB steps, starting well below the predicted LDL and with the ear likely to have the better dynamic range. Pure tone and LDL measurements together give a good picture of the dynamic range of the ear, and frequently show contraction in dynamic range caused by a widening of central auditory filters around specific frequencies, most often the tinnitus frequency. Initial assessment of LDLs will avoid causing the patient distress by presenting tones above the LDL (e.g. when testing for reflexes). Sometimes extremely reduced LDLs, even as low as 30–40 dB, are seen in patients with normal hearing and hyperacusis (see Fig 11.8). These are real and repeatable measurements and should be done first in the test battery. They of course preclude the measurement of stapedius reflexes. LDLs should be measured throughout treatment, and improvement in hyperacusis and tinnitus will often be mirrored by higher values for LDL.

Pitch match frequency

These tests are only an approximation of the perceived pitch of the tinnitus by the patient. Sometimes they are extremely inaccurate because of the difficulty of comparing an external sine wave with an internal signal that is far from a simple sound and has not undergone normal categorization by central processing. A simple adaptive technique with a standard fixed frequency audiometer that uses tones around 10–20 dB sound level ensures that the patient understands the meaning of the word pitch or frequency and is not thinking in terms of loudness. Approximate measurements of perceived tinnitus frequency are useful in supporting the Jastreboff model[3] to the patient, and occasionally for diagnostic purposes (e.g. low frequency tinnitus in endolymphatic hydrops).

Tinnitus loudness matching

Tinnitus loudness matching is almost always a meaningless exercise.[6] Many attempts have been made to overcome the problem of increased sensitivity to noise around the tinnitus frequency. Comparing tinnitus loudness with a tone at another frequency at which the dynamic range is normal and different formulae have been proposed[7] but none of these measurements have been found helpful in evaluating or dealing with tinnitus distress.

Minimal masking level

To find the minimal masking level a signal, either pure tone, narrow band or broad band of noise, is used to make a measurement of the point at which tinnitus is masked or suppressed.[8] This is really suppression rather than psychoacoustical masking and the term tinnitus masking should be abandoned, although historical precedent may make this difficult. The masking or suppression level (MML) may be indicated in audiometric terms (i.e. in hearing level) or as a sensation level (i.e. the level of masking sound above threshold required to mask or suppress the tinnitus).

MML does not indicate who can be helped by white noise generators ('maskers'). It does indicate how well central auditory processing can identify TRNA in the presence of noise, and how well developed and focused the auditory filters are on the TRNA. In our study,[6] changes in tinnitus were matched by changes in MML; patients improving with behavioural training showed a decrease in MML. Changes in MML were very small, mostly less than 5 dB, and were only observable as a statistical change in group data. Loudness measurement did not change. MML measurements were not in themselves predictors of those patients who would improve with therapy. In many cases repeated measurements of MML result in emergence of the tinnitus even with an intensity of masking noise that previously suppressed it (temporal decay of masking[9]). This identifies the enhancement of TRNA detection by subcortical signal processing.

Residual inhibition

In some cases tinnitus can be suppressed by sounds applied to the ear or ears for a test period (generally 60 seconds at 10 dB above the MML), using wide band noise.[10] This is found in some 40 per cent of tinnitus patients, suppression lasting usually for seconds or minutes, but rarely for longer periods. It is unlikely that there is any disturbance of cochlea function. The changes observed in residual inhibition testing can be explained by the Jastreboff model[3] in terms of changes in central auditory filters. The test has been shown to have no value as a predictor for the results of tinnitus therapy,[1] and is at present simply viewed as an interesting phenomenon without clinical significance. Very often the performance of a simple pure tone audiogram is enough to provoke temporary suppression of tinnitus. The mechanism may be related to some extent to attentional phenomena at a cortical level.

Otoacoustic emissions

The measurements of transient otoacoustic emissions and distortion products may be helpful in understanding early cochlear pathology before any abnormality in the audiogram appears. In most cases such changes reflect normal ageing effects. They may be seen as part of a trigger mechanism according to the discordant damage theory proposed by Jastreboff.[3] In some cases of tinnitus there may be abnormalities of cochlea efferent control that may influence tinnitus related activity. The effect of contralateral suppression of transient otoacoustic emissions in tinnitus patients was found to be much more variable than in normal individuals and also to be generally a smaller effect with a loss of non-linear components.[11]

References

1. Hazell JWP, Wood SM, Cooper HR, *et al.* A clinical study of tinnitus maskers. *British Journal of Audiology* 1985; **19**:65–146.
2. Bekesy G. von. *Sensory inhibition.* Princeton: Princeton University Press, 1967:220–6.
3. Jastreboff PJ. Phantom auditory perception (tinnitus): mechanisms of generation and perception. *Neuroscience Research* 1990; **8**:221–54.
4. Higson JM, Haggard MP, Field DL. Validation of parameters for assessing Obscure Auditory Dysfunction – robustness of determinants of OAD status across samples and test methods. *British Journal of Audiology* 1994; **28**:27–39.
5. Sismanis A, Smoker WR. Pulsatile tinnitus: recent advances in diagnosis. *Laryngoscope* 1994; **104**:681–8.
6. Jastreboff PJ, Hazell JWP, Graham RL. Neurophysiological model of tinnitus: dependence of the minimal masking level on treatment outcome. *Hearing Research* 1994; **80**:216–32.
7. Jakes SC, Hallam RS, Chambers CC, Hinchcliffe R. Matched and self-reported loudness of tinnitus: methods and sources of error. *Audiology* 1986; **25**:92–100.

8. Feldmann H. Homolateral and contralateral masking of tinnitus by noisebands and by pure tones. *Audiology (Basel)* 1971; **10**:138–44.

9. Coles RRA, Baskill JL, Sheldrake JB. Measurement and management of tinnitus. Part I. Measurement. *Journal of Laryngology and Otology* 1984; **98**:1171–6.

10. Vernon JA, Meikle MB. Tinnitus masking: unresolved problems. *Ciba Foundation Symposium* 1981; **85**:239–62.

11. Graham RL, Hazell JWP. Contralateral suppression of transient evoked otoacoustic emissions: intra-individual variability in tinnitus and normal subjects. *British Journal of Audiology* 1994; **28**:235–47.

CHAPTER 13

Management of tinnitus

JONATHAN HAZELL

Introduction

Well over 90 per cent of patients presenting in our tinnitus clinic will not have an identifiable pathology amenable to conventional otological treatment. The advent of tinnitus retraining based on the Jastreboff model[1] has meant for the first time that there is a structured approach that can effect permanent eradication of tinnitus distress in many patients without the need for further treatment. This relatively new approach will be dealt with first. In addition, the issue of somatosounds and tinnitus as a symptom of another surgical or medical condition will be considered separately. Finally, a critique will be made of current approaches to tinnitus management that I no longer consider appropriate.

Tinnitus retraining therapy

The basic principle underlying tinnitus retraining therapy (TRT) is that persistence of tinnitus, and the distress it causes, is due to changes that occur in central auditory processing involving signal detection and pattern recognition. There is an enhancement of internally generated signals, referred to here as tinnitus related neural activity (TRNA), resulting in the continued perception of tinnitus (see above). If tinnitus distress or annoyance is present, this is generated in extra-auditory centres, principally the limbic system, but also involves the reticular formation in the brainstem and the autonomic nervous system. TRT is a behaviourally based approach aimed at altering plasticity in the neuronal networks involved with central processing, and effecting permanent changes in auditory filters and

pattern recognition involved in the detection and enhancement of TRNA. When the trigger or cause of TRNA is a cochlea-related event such as discordant damage to cochlear hair cells, no attempt is made to repair this damage, which is not possible at present. Despite the undoubted diversity of triggers, sources or causes of emergence of TRNA the tinnitus retraining approach is applicable in every case of persistent distressing tinnitus, whatever its cause.

HABITUATION OF REACTION AND PERCEPTION

By effecting changes in central auditory processing and areas of association, we are able first to remove the distressing emotions associated with tinnitus (habituation of reaction) and second, to reduce and finally remove the perception of persistent tinnitus (habituation of perception). If the otologist or audiological physician feels somewhat daunted at the prospect of being faced with activities that seem more appropriate for a psychologist or psychiatrist, they should not give up at this point. Otological and audiological expertise are essential to the success of this technique, and are needed for diagnosis and treatment of related disorders. However, at least one member of the team must be capable of applying these behavioural techniques.

ROLE OF THE OTOLOGIST OR AUDIOLOGIST – MEDICAL COUNSELLING

The first consultation should last at least 1 hour and may combine the diagnostic interview with the start of directive counselling.

DIAGNOSIS AND PATHOLOGY

The first duty of the otologist or audiological physician is to identify and treat any pathology that may be present. Absent pathology presents the opportunity for strong reassurance about the absence of damage; this has a powerful therapeutic effect. When there is a hearing loss, it is important to stress the knowledge that hair cell loss occurs normally, and that deafness is commonly associated with *no* tinnitus. If pathology is identified, then a programme for its medical or surgical management will be put to the patient. TRT will be given either alongside or after the treatment of such pathology, to cope with any residual tinnitus that may persist, such as after middle ear surgery or after treatment for endolymphatic hydrops.[3]

EXPLANATION OF HEARING MECHANISM

The preliminary explanation of how our hearing mechanism works should be given by the otologist. It is very difficult to present tinnitus as a disorder of central auditory processing, unless both the otologist and the patient have a working knowledge of how the central auditory systems actually performs. It is precisely because of the absence of this knowledge that little progress has been made in managing tinnitus in the past.

The otologist will have no problem in presenting the mechanism of the cochlea and hair cell function; however, outer hair cells should be presented not in terms of their damaged members that cannot be repaired, but as a model for a weak source of energy that contributes to TRNA. It can be stressed that TRNA is a natural sound, part of nature, something that has been present throughout the patient's life, before tinnitus was first perceived. Diagrams of the peripheral and central nervous system are of an enormous help in this crucial first exercise in directive counselling. A section of the brain indicates clearly the junction between white matter and grey matter which can be viewed as the point where perception of any sound (including tinnitus) occurs.

Patients, if untutored, continue to believe that tinnitus pathology must be confined to the place where perception is localized, rather than understanding that perception may be imperfect (see above – externalization of perception). The concept of end organ and auditory cortex separated by central pathways involved in signal processing is crucial to the understanding that the patient (and doctor) needs to take part in a retraining programme.

The function of the subcortical pathways can be demonstrated using diagrams (Figs 11.2, 11.3, 11.4 and 11.5). Patients can be shown that the pathways consist of neuronal networks containing millions of nerve cells and interconnecting neurons capable of complex acts of signal detection and pattern recognition. They are not simple electric cables connecting ear to brain. Much signal detection is subconscious, like the ability to respond to the sound of your first name, or a mother waking to the sound of her baby moving in the night. The auditory nerve contains patterns of electrical activity that are very similar to the patterns of sound frequencies in the environment. No categorization of these different frequencies into specific signals has been made. It is like a jigsaw puzzle with all the pieces contained mixed up in their box. The gradual characterization of bits of this jigsaw into 'sky' 'trees' 'people' 'background' and 'foreground' occurs in a progressive manner as they pass up the subconscious pathways towards the cortex. In just such a way the auditory system is categorizing groups of different frequencies into those identified as being part of speech, part of environmental sounds, warning signals, new signals et cetera. The categorization process gives particular emphasis to new signals or those that have previously been identified as warnings.

It is useful to describe to the patient the historical basis by which such neuronal networks developed with the passage of time as a means for identifying predators in a previously hostile environment. Signals emitted by predators are customarily weak, but must be detected by the prey with unerring certainty, and in addition should produce a strong emotional response, usually fear, but also anger, if combat is envisaged. These mechanisms involve signal detection at a subconscious level and strong stimulation of the limbic and autonomic nervous systems even before full conscious awareness of any such signal is received. This survival reflex has many rules, the most important of which is that it should not habituate throughout the life of its owner.

In a so-called civilized environment generally devoid of traditional animal predators, phobias and aversive reactions nevertheless commonly occur, and by a similar mechanism. In each phobic situation (lifts, heights, flying) there is a belief, sometimes irrational but always strongly held, that the individual's security will be compromised by the encounter.

IDEA OF TINNITUS AS A THREAT

In cases of severe tinnitus distress it is easy to identify the process by which tinnitus has acquired threatening status. In almost all cases one or more of the beliefs on the 'threat list' (Table 11.1) are held strongly by the individual. It may be helpful to let the patient know the extremely close relationship between the number of negative beliefs and the state of tinnitus, for example whether it is getting better or worse or staying the same. Those patients with mild tinnitus exhibiting annoyance, or possible anxiety about things getting worse, but being able to cope with the situation quite well at present may well not have developed any negative feeling about their tinnitus. Those with severe tinnitus, however, are easily identifable as having a strong phobic reaction to their tinnitus.

EMERGENCE AND PERSISTENCE OF TINNITUS

It is important to stress the difference between the emergence of tinnitus which is an almost universal event, and its persistence. Describe to the patient the experience of normal individuals in a sound-proof room, the Heller and Bergman experiment.[3] Stress that TRNA is a very weak signal, which so far we have been unable to detect in patients but that after central processing it may result in a strong and powerful perception with associated unpleasant emotional stimulation (the limbic system). In general we try and avoid the word psychological, although this concept is often suggested by the patient. Emergence of tinnitus is common in those exposed to noise, for example disco tinnitus, but in most people this disappears as it is associated with a pleasant experience. It is only when noise exposure is accompanied by pain and a belief that damage has occurred that persistence of tinnitus becomes likely. The distressed tinnitus patient will have persistent tinnitus even though this may be intermittent. The task of the otologist is to show that this is not due to any peripheral pathology but to inappropriate settings of the central auditory filters, as already described. The good news here is that these can be 'reprogrammed' so that perception of TRNA eventually ceases.

FIT THE MODEL TO THE PATIENT'S EXPERIENCE

Examine the counselling the patient has already had; was it appropriate? Was it excessively negative? Was the negative counselling associated with an enhancement of tinnitus perception or reaction? What triggers were associated with the onset of tinnitus? Did these have a psychological element? Has the tinnitus fluctuated with stress? If this has been the case, then the influence of the limbic system can be indicated to the patient with appropriate anatomical and functional charts.

OUTLINE OF TINNITUS RETRAINING PROGRAMME

It is important to introduce the therapist (audiologist, hearing therapist or psychologist) who will be taking on the patient's longer term management session by session. Follow-up appointments with the medical specialist are vital to assess the patient's progress and to retain and develop confidence in their new beliefs about tinnitus. The physician also needs to learn from these encounters whether the initial 'directive counselling' approach has been successful, or whether it requires modification. The patient should be asked to specify what helped in the explanation and what did not.

At the first session decisions will be made about the appropriateness of different 'noise or sound therapies' – either white noise generators or hearing aids. In addition, the importance of further directive counselling is stressed. If the patient has acquired a major phobic response to tinnitus, it will be clear to the therapist and the patient that it will take some time to achieve a reversal of the situation. Although it should be stressed that there is no quick fix for tinnitus, it should also be indicated that the long-term results are excellent and maintained. It should be explained that there is a reduction of the emotional response (habituation of reaction) during which time the perception may remain virtually unaltered. Further retraining then results in the gradual disappearance of tinnitus perceptions as the auditory filters concerned with detection of TRNA gradually close (habituation of perception).

In practical terms it is worth having a team meeting, which need not last more than about 5 minutes, after the patient's history and initial investigations, to decide on the initial strategy. Consistency of approach and training is essential if the patient is to change strongly held beliefs about the negative properties of tinnitus.

TINNITUS RETRAINING THERAPY – ROLE OF TINNITUS THERAPIST

Here we introduce a new professional, the tinnitus therapist. This role may be taken on by anyone with aptitude and knowledge appropriate to carry out behavioural retraining therapy. In the UK this is commonly performed with great expertise by hearing therapists whose work normally entails counselling and instruction of hearing impaired patients, the teaching of lip-reading skills and the use of environmental aids. The otologist or audiological physician must work in close rapport with the tinnitus therapist. The four elements of retraining therapy are

- instrumentation or sound therapy
- directive counselling
- reduction of autonomic arousal
- treating of coexisting or resultant emotional disturbance

Instrumentation

Since Saltzmann and Ersner identified the beneficial effect of hearing aids on tinnitus, it has been clear that sound therapy of one type or another can greatly influence tinnitus perception.[4] In the 1970s Vernon promoted the concept of 'tinnitus masking'.[5,6] Tinnitus masking is a misleading term and should properly be called tinnitus suppression by sound. It has none of the properties of psychoacoustical masking of one sound by another. Although so-called tinnitus masking provided symptomatic relief for about 30 per cent of patients,[7] many patients did not benefit, or found the masking sounds intolerable. The retraining approach using the Jastreboff model[3] requires that tinnitus should not be masked. In trying to promote habituation of any signal it is essential that the signal remains detectable by the central nervous system. We are now using retraining approaches on patients who have been successfully masking their tinnitus for the past 20 years, but on removal of the masking sound experience no improvement in the loudness or annoyance of the tinnitus. With retraining, during which the tinnitus remains audible, it is possible to proceed to complete habituation of tinnitus perception. In retraining therapy instruments or noise generators have a completely different, secondary, role compared with the masking approach.

REDUCED CONTRAST OF THE TINNITUS SIGNAL

All sensory modalities respond strongly to contrasting information. We are inclined to reduce levels of background noise, particularly at night. Many tinnitus patients admit to a lifetime of seeking extreme silence because of a behavioural preference for the absence of auditory intrusion. This degree of silence is an abnormal environment in nature. It facilitates the performance of the

Heller and Bergman experiment,[3] and makes emergence of tinnitus almost inevitable. Because TRNA is such a small signal, very low levels of environmental noise introduced into the bedroom or living room can greatly reduce the contrast between tinnitus signal and background activity in the auditory system. This makes it much easier for the attentional focus to switch off the tinnitus and onto other things of greater importance.

INCREASE IN PLASTICITY IN SUBCORTICAL PATHWAYS

Once it is accepted that the process of habituation involves the resetting of neuronal networks concerned with signal detection, then increased activity in these network helps promote their reconfiguration. We have used low levels of broad band noise for, generally, up to 6 hours a day over a period of 6–9 months. In the past these instruments have been referred to 'maskers', but now they are designated white noise generators in order to avoid confusion about their role in tinnitus retraining. The level at which the noise generator should be set is between the threshold of hearing the instrument and a small distance below the point at which masking of the tinnitus occurs. The intensity of the sound must be at or below its comfortable listening level (Fig 13.1). The effectiveness of wide band noise therapy in increasing plasticity in these neuronal networks is negated once one moves into the area of tinnitus suppression ('masking' in old terminology) as has been shown by our long-term patients who had been using previously advised masking therapy.

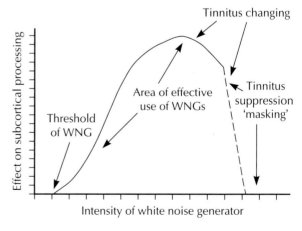

Fig 13.1 Curve showing approximate relationships between intensity of white noise therapy and effectiveness in inducing habituation. 'Masking' or suppression of tinnitus is contraindicated. WNG, white noise generator.

CHANGING ATTENTIONAL FOCUS

In some patients the presence of a soothing mean-ingless sound in the ear under their own personal control helps to attract the auditory attentional focus from the tinnitus. This can constitute a train-ing experience whereby for increasing periods tin-nitus ceases to occupy the perceptional attentional focus. In the early stages of extreme tinnitus distress tinnitus may occupy the attentional focus for up to 100 per cent of the waking hours, so any movement away from this situation is seen as a move towards habituation.

THE USE OF HEARING AIDS

Hearing aids are fitted to all patients experiencing hearing impairment, and to some patients with high frequency sensory losses in whom difficulties in hearing noise may or may not have been identi-fied. Hearing aid fitting techniques must be of an extremely high quality in order to help the tinnitus patient. Over-amplification of low frequency sounds by ear canal occlusion or inappropriate hearing aid selection can make tinnitus worse. In the majority of patients in whom postaural aids are used, open moulds or extremely well vented moulds are necessary, and careful introduction of amplification is needed particularly when there is coexisting hyperacusis. About 10 per cent of patients will experience a total suppression of their tinnitus with hearing aids. During these periods, although the patients may be very happy with the results, the process of habituation of perception cannot progress. It is therefore important to have periods of the day when hearing aids are not worn and the behavioural exercises of retraining therapy can be applied to habituate tinnitus perception. The selection of instruments is made according to Table 13.1. Combination instruments, which include white noise generators combined with hearing aids are used much less frequently now

than in the masking–suppression days, but are occasionally indicated and helpful if additional reduction of contrast is needed for tinnitus that is not ameliorated by hearing aid use alone.

Directive counselling

Directive counselling is the major role of the tinni-tus therapist. The work done in the initial medical counselling session has to be reinforced. Patients' inappropriate beliefs and fears about their tinnitus must be challenged, and explanations for the patients' experiences must be given in terms of the neurophysiological model. This model is of neces-sity quite complicated, and even with supplemen-tary reading material it cannot be completely understood in a single session. The main aims of directive counselling are as follows:

- to identify the patient's wrongly held beliefs and negative emotional associations regarding tinni-tus
- to increase understanding of central hearing mechanisms
- to challenge the negative beliefs and fears, sub-stituting a benign model of tinnitus unrelated to ear damage; to work on the effects of previous negative counselling
- to encourage the patient to recognize and under-stand the differences between emotional reac-tion to tinnitus and perception of tinnitus
- to reinforce the new belief that tinnitus is a dis-order of central processing that can be fixed
- to remove the concept of tinnitus as a threat
- to remember that strongly held beliefs, phobic responses and survival-style reflexes take time to change
- to teach the use of distraction techniques and thought blocking to shift awareness from the tin-nitus, for early symptom control.

The acquisition of conventional counselling skills can be very helpful; they are also useful in protect-ing the therapist from emotional overload from these patients. However, conventional counselling involves the principle of allowing the patient to talk and so focuses on listening to sometimes quite long and extended dialogue from the patient. This does have a part to play in TRT, and it also allows the therapist to acquire knowledge about symptoma-tology and natural history of tinnitus from first-hand experience. However, it does not bring about retraining and resetting of neuronal networks. Directive counselling requires the teaching of new ideas and beliefs, and in this case the therapist or counsellor will do very much more of the talking.

Table 13.1 Hearing aids and white noise generators in retraining therapy

Degree of hearing impairment	Instrumentation
Normal hearing +/– some HF loss	Noise generators
Significant hearing loss	Hearing aids +/– noise generator

Many of the symptoms experienced by the patient relate to autonomic symptoms such as palpitations, sweating, feelings of anxiety, stomach and bowels disturbance, neckache and headache. Classic relaxation techniques, taught either by the therapist or with the help of the psychology or physiotherapy department, are of great benefit. Because the autonomic system feeds back into the auditory pathways (Fig 11.2), reduction of autonomic tone in many patients results in a reduction in tinnitus loudness and accompanying distress. Relaxation techniques are also very helpful, promoting the onset of sleep if this is disturbed. Sleep disturbance is a separate entity and, as has been said, affects a high proportion of patients with tinnitus, particularly in the early stages when tinnitus is threatening and intrusive. In some patients there will be a long history of sleep disturbance, and specialist help will be needed from a psychologist. Older patients who have been on hypnotics for long periods should not have their medication altered, at least until the retraining programme is well on the way and the patient is confident about controlling the emotional responses to their tinnitus.

Tinnitus and insomnia

The management of insomnia in tinnitus is a large subject and many behavioural management strategies exist.

Sleep education about different sleep stages and the functions and effects of sleep is important. Many patients have very rigid and inappropriate beliefs about the effects of not sleeping on their life and health.

Sleep hygiene: exercise should be avoided near bedtime; late afternoon and early evening is best. Fit people definitely sleep better, and snacks and fluid intake should be limited. Caffeine should be avoided and alcohol is a poor hypnotic as it disturbs the sleep pattern. The environment must be comfortable in terms of the bed and the room temperature.

It is important that the patient establishes an optimal sleep pattern. They should go to bed when they feel sleepy rather than by habit, and should put lights out immediately on retiring. If sleep does not come within 20 minutes they should sit in another room until they are sleepy again; the bedroom should not be thought of as a place of torment (lying awake all night listening to tinnitus). Napping during the day should be avoided and the alarm should be set for the same time everyday. No attempt should be made to try and recover sleep to compensate for previous bad nights.

Relaxation is important; the patient should try to wind down mentally and physically during the second part of the evening. No work or other activity should be done for about an hour and a half before bedtime and then a relaxation routine should be practised when in bed such as concentrating on breathing, tensing and relaxing muscles and becoming gradually calmer. A prescribed relaxation technique should be used at other times in the day too.

Intrusive thoughts must be dealt with. The patient should try and focus on the concept that sleep will come when it is ready, and that relaxing in bed is almost as good as sleep. They should not try too hard to go to sleep, but should use thought-blocking techniques such as repetition of a semantically neutral word (e.g. the- the- the- the) subvocally.

The patient should do a mind dump, that is, sit for 20 minutes in the evening with a pencil and paper reflecting on the day, its objectives and achievements and reallocating time to deal with these thoughts on a subsequent day. They should not be taken to bed. This session should be used as a means of dividing daytime and evening time activities.

Treatment of coexisting or resultant emotional disturbance

If there is very long history of anxiety or depression, this may require new or renewed analysis and management by an appropriate professional, either a psychiatrist or a psychologist. During retraining therapy as far as possible it is best to avoid drug therapy, but a short course of antidepressants can be very valuable if patients are so depressed that they have extreme sleep disturbance and are also unable to concentrate on the cognitive aspects of the TRT. Experience will indicate how much of this emotional disturbance can be dealt with in the audiology department, but the lines of communication with the psychology and psychiatric department must be maintained open at all times for referral of patients, and for dealing with acute emergencies. Very occasionally tinnitus patients can be identified as a suicide risk, and in this case a psychiatric consultation must be made urgently.[8] Occasionally this may be a definite indication for admission to an ENT ward. Admission can result in a resolution of the acute crisis quite rapidly by taking the patient out of their previous highly stressful environment.

Desensitization programme for hyperacusis

In patients in whom hyperacusis is an important part of the tinnitus, or exists in the absence of tinnitus, a slightly different approach is required. The mechanism is very similar, and there is frequently the establishment of phobic or aversive responses to external sounds, usually based on the belief that these sounds will damage the ear. Hyperacusis to normal environmental sounds is a common precursor of tinnitus.[9] Desensitization therapy is aimed at closing auditory filters inappropriately set to enhance external sounds. In patients in whom tinnitus is also present the frequency contents of poorly tolerated environmental sounds is often similar to that of the perceived pitch of the tinnitus. The mechanism is one of increased central auditory gain. Audiometric testing frequently shows a normal hearing threshold with greatly reduced dynamic range and loudness discomfort levels. The approach to desensitization follows that of tinnitus, but instrumentation plays a more important part. In most patients the fitting of binaural white noise generators used for a minimum of 6 hours a day at a comfortable listening level produces immediate symptomatic relief. The volume should be increased to a point at which it 'interferes' with the uncomfortable sounds. It is essential to withdraw the use of earmuffs and earplugs, which are commonly used even in normal sounds situations and are most counterproductive. Excluding environmental sounds from the ear simply increases central auditory gain and makes hyperacusis worse. This does *not* mean that normal hearing conservation practice should be avoided, for example when shooting, in discos or in industry.

Directive counselling techniques are essential, and are frequently effective even in the absence of noise generators. Education about the exact mechanism of hyperacusis, the realization that normal environmental sounds will not damage the ears even though these sounds appear to be painful and the knowledge that this mechanism can be completely reversed by appropriate retraining must be heavily pressed on the patient. The gradual reintroduction of the patient back to their normal environment is planned, and as confidence is gained, patients are able to return to work and social activity that was previously precluded by the distress caused by environmental noise. After a period of 6–9 months the noise generators are gradually withdrawn as a normal dynamic range of hearing returns. The patient's progress should be charted by loudness discomfort levels, which in most cases will map the progress made in learning to deal again with normal levels of environmental sound.

Follow-up appointments and expectations

Habituation of reaction and reduction in the emotional distress caused by tinnitus usually begins to occur after the initial consultation in which tinnitus diagnosis, prognosis and management are discussed. In the first 6 months tinnitus perception is likely to remain much unchanged, that is, the loudness will be the same, but the periods of non-awareness will lengthen and the tendency to monitor or look for tinnitus will be reduced. A realistic aim in the average case of severe tinnitus distress is to achieve total habituation of reaction after 2 years of TRT.

The question of what a good result means in this situation depends on the patient's interpretation. At the beginning of treatment they cannot understand how it is possible to hear tinnitus without having extreme distress. Once the responses of the limbic system have been habituated, a different attitude evolves about what is acceptable and what is not acceptable in terms of still being able to hear tinnitus. However, those patients who persist with the programme will experience varying degrees of perceptual habituation, measured in increasing periods of non-awareness, or an overall significant reduction in tinnitus loudness, or both.

Retraining therapy can abolish tinnitus perception

In a recent study[10] of 149 patients with an average duration of tinnitus of 11 years who were getting consistently worse up to the point of entry into the retraining therapy programme, 19.6 per cent achieved eradication of perception of their tinnitus for periods of up to 11 days after 18 months. Ninety-six per cent of this group had worthwhile improvement, particularly in their emotional response to the tinnitus. Studies that include patients who are not so profoundly distressed tend to show much better results in terms of habituation of perception (i.e. the inability to hear tinnitus even when it is listened for).

In general our patients are seen by the otologist or audiological physician at the initial consultation, 4–6 months later and then at 6-monthly intervals until the patient declares that no further management is required. The tinnitus therapist will have between three and six 1-hour sessions in the first 6-month period, the number of sessions relating to the speed at which the patient is able to absorb the ideas, concepts and training that is involved in this programme. Usually some 8–12 sessions with various members of the team are required over an 18-month period.

Somatosounds

Once the neurophysiological mechanism of tinnitus perception is understood, it becomes clear why there is no surgical solution for it. However, surgery is sometimes indicated for somatosounds, although it is definitely contraindicated for tinnitus (phantom auditory perception). Otosurgery when tinnitus is a presenting or an important symptom needs careful planning and appropriate counselling of the patient to avoid exacerbation of the tinnitus. The term somatosound refers to any internally generated sound perceived by the patient for which there is an acoustic correlate. It can often be detected by an external observer. It obeys the rules of psycho-acoustical masking.

PULSATILE SOMATOSOUNDS

Venous hums

Venous hums can be abolished by light venous pressure and are caused by turbulent flow through the jugular bulb. They may be altered by neck movement or posture; the sounds are unilateral and the pulse synchronous. It may be possible to detect a pulse either by a stethoscope or intrameatal microphone. It is important to excluded benign intracranial hypertension.[11]

Arterial loops (auditory nerve compression syndrome)

This condition has had a somewhat chequered history. Initial enthusiasm led to over diagnosis of this condition and an increase of inappropriate neurosurgery to correct it.[12] CT or MRI angiography may detect a kinked artery within the internal auditory canal in patients in whom there is pulsatile tinnitus, often with fluctuating hearing loss and

vestibular symptoms. Separation of the artery by the introduction of a small piece of silastic sheeting has been reported as producing symptomatic relief, but there have also been reports of labyrinthine failure due to arterial spasms and even facial paralysis.

Carotid transmissions

All cases of pulsatile tinnitus should be examined for the presence of carotid bruits, or systolic heart murmurs, or both, which may be transmitted to the ear via the carotid circulation. In carotid stenosis appropriate arterial surgery will often abolish the perception of the somatosound. Dialogue between the otologist and vascular surgeon is essential to weigh up the surgical indications based on the risk of hemiplegia and the distress caused by the somatosound.

NON-PULSATILE SOMATOSOUNDS

Patulous Eustachian tube syndrome

In this condition the Eustachian tube becomes widely patent and does not close automatically after opening. Distressing symptoms of autophony for nasal respiration and vocalization can produce extreme distress. There may be feelings of ear fullness, vestibular symptoms and sensorineural hearing loss.[13] The symptoms may emerge after weight loss, because of the loss of peritubal fat, and weight gain may result in improvement of symptoms. The symptoms are often abolished by lying down (venous engorgement of submucosal vessels). Diagnosis may be made by the introduction of mildly irritant powder such as talc through a Eustachian catheter (if these skills are still retained). In severe cases it is justified to apply Eustachian diathermy, most easily achieved with a urological diathermy probe which is malleable and can be passed easily through the nose to the opening of the Eustachian tube.[14] Secretory otitis media develops in 10–15 per cent of patients so treated, and these patients will require middle ear ventilation. Most are happy to exchange this inconvenience for the extreme distress caused by patulous tube syndrome. The injection of Teflon paste into the Eustachian cushions and silver nitrate application are less effective.

Palatal myoclonus

In palatal myoclonus the patient hears an irregular clicking sound coming from one or other or both ears caused by myoclonic contractions in tensor or levator palati muscles, or both. The sound is created by the opening snap of the Eustachian tube as the wet surfaces part. The clicks may regularly be heard by others in a quiet environment, and in children can even be loud enough to keep siblings or guests awake at night. Myoclonic contractions of the palate, and sometimes of other suprahyoid muscles in the neck, can be seen synchronously with the acoustic click. Some patients also have facial tick or titubation, and the neurological mechanism is probably similar. We have experienced some success in suppressing myoclonic contraction with masking techniques.[15] If the hyperactive muscle reflex can be blocked for a period, permanent relief can sometimes be achieved. As all somatosounds are real acoustic events they follow the rules of acoustic masking. In some cases the injection of botulinum toxin into the soft palate has been effective, but this must be repeated every 2–3 months.[16]

Tensor tympani syndrome

Tensor tympani syndrome is an important and common condition in which increased tension in the tensor tympani muscle produces a fluttering low frequency sound in the ear, and was first described by Klockhoff.[13] In many cases the sound is also 'felt', as if there is a fluttering insect in the bottom of the ear canal. Indeed the tympanic membrane is being moved rapidly by the fibrillation of this middle ear muscle. A classic rapid fluctuation of impedance recordings may be identifiable. In most cases reassurance about this mechanism is all that is needed, but occasionally patients can be helped by section of the tensor tympani muscle behind the neck of the malleus.

The management of tinnitus in surgical diseases

MENIÈRE'S DISEASE

Medical and surgical treatment for Menière's disease may result in the improvement of tinnitus in these cases.[2] In the majority of patients vertigo and hearing loss are a much more severe problems, but, particularly in those patients who no longer have vertigo but may be profoundly deaf, tinnitus can be very troublesome. The tinnitus of Menière's syndrome responds particularly well to sound therapy with white noise and surgical strategies should be aimed at preserving residual hearing for this reason among others. Saccus decompression and drainage operation and vestibular nerve

section are to be preferred to labyrinthectomy, which makes the ear inaccessible to any kind of sound therapy either by hearing aids, noise generators or even cochlear implants.

OTOSCLEROSIS

Many patients with advanced otosclerosis and severe tinnitus have been refused surgery because of the fears of making tinnitus worse. The mechanism of tinnitus in most cases of conductive hearing loss is an enhancement of internally generated sounds as a result of the 'earplug' effect and also the 'straining to hear phenomenon'. The few reported series of otosclerosis surgery in which tinnitus has been recorded show excellent results with respect to the tinnitus.[13] Provided that appropriate directive counselling is initiated before surgery, the surgeon has much less to fear about postoperative tinnitus even in the unfortunate event of a sensorineural hearing loss after surgery. It is nevertheless important to counsel the patient that tinnitus may be worse temporarily after failed surgery, but that in such a situation tinnitus is quite amenable to retraining therapy.

TYMPANIC MEMBRANE PERFORATION

In patients with distressing tinnitus it is well worthwhile performing a patch test with a small piece of sterile tissue paper in the clinic before deciding on a tympanoplasty. Not only will this identify what component of the conductive hearing loss is due to the hole in the eardrum and what is due to ossicular dysfunction, but it will also indicate any improvement in tinnitus that the patient may expect postoperatively. Audiometry should be performed before and after the patch test, and an improvement in tinnitus may be experienced even though there is little closure of the air–bone gap.

ABLATIVE SURGERY

Some of the worst tinnitus in a unilateral hearing loss comes from failed otosurgery.[17] It is sad that there are still otosurgeons who have advised acoustic nerve section as a means of curing intractable tinnitus. This indicates a lack of understanding of the neurophysiological mechanisms of tinnitus, and a conviction, often strongly reinforced by the patient, that the problem is situated in the cochlea and nowhere else. Again the need to preserve residual hearing either for the purpose of acoustic or electrical stimulation is paramount. In most cases TRNA is coming not only from the cochlea or auditory nerve but also from neuronal sources in the brainstem due to increased central auditory gain. Cutting the acoustic nerve is not effective as it is peripheral to the generator, and can also result in an electrically active stump neuroma. Review the poor results of auditory nerve section in tinnitus in different pathologies.[18,19]

Medical treatments

There is naturally a strong tendency to search for a medical quick fix for tinnitus. The neurophysiological model makes it clear such a search is unlikely to be rewarded, but this does not mean that drugs do not play a part in the alleviation of symptoms in some patients, in the aggravation of tinnitus in others and in occasional rare patients they abolish the underlying trigger or source.

SPECIFIC DISEASE-ORIENTATED APPROACHES TO TINNITUS AND SOMATOSOUNDS

Anaemia

Occasionally, anaemia is responsible for pulsatile somatosounds due to increased blood flow. Severe anaemia may also result in reduced oxygenation of parts of the brain, including the auditory system. Appropriate treatment of anaemia under specialist medical care may produce an improvement, but self-administration of drugs is inadvisable and is useless when the body has adequate supply of these substances.

Migraine

Tinnitus can occur in association with migraine, often as part of the aura. Patients who have suffered from migraine in the past, who experience classic migraine symptoms or in whom there is a family history can be given the opportunity to try migraine therapy, particularly with beta-blockers and serotonin antagonists.

Waking tinnitus

It is very common to experience tinnitus on waking, either in the morning or after a 'catnap'. All sensory systems, including hearing, are put on alert at the moment of waking and the environment is scanned for threat. This accounts for the enhanced detection at this time. A very small group of patients have been shown to have increased tinnitus because of low blood sugar at these times. A simple trial of dextrose (any proprietary brand drink) will identify whether the tinnitus is in this category.

Thyroid dysfunction

Low thyroid function may result in hearing impairment and occasional tinnitus, which may be corrected by appropriate thyroid replacement hormone. An overactive thyroid may also produce a wide variety of symptoms, including tinnitus, and clinical and haematological diagnosis is necessary for proper management.

Diabetes and insulin

Diabetics may well experience tinnitus if their diabetes is not well controlled. This may be mediated by stress mechanisms rather than directly by changes in levels of blood sugar. There is no evidence that diabetes itself is responsible for hearing loss or tinnitus. As diabetes is common many people with diabetes may also have tinnitus that is unconnected.

Zinc therapy

Zinc therapy has been promoted in the past for the treatment of tinnitus on a totally empirical basis. It is an essential element, and low zinc levels may be associated with otherwise unexplained sensory hearing loss. We have measured zinc blood levels in our patients for nearly 10 years and have not identified a single patient whose tinnitus has benefited from zinc therapy.

Hypertension

There is no real agreement over hypertension as a factor in tinnitus emergence or persistence. Increased blood pressure is very common in older people, who are also more likely to experience tinnitus. It is most likely that these two conditions commonly coexist. Occasionally, tinnitus will improve once blood pressure is controlled, but in most cases it is unrelated either to the condition or its treatment.

Spontaneous otoacoustic emissions

In very rare cases tinnitus or (more appropriately) somatosounds may be associated with an otoacoustic emission (see Chapter 4), and this can be identified by spectral analysis of the cochlea. Sometimes the emission and the perception can be abolished by aspirin.[20]

Diet

Enormous time and effort is spent, particularly by patient-support groups, in identifying elements in the diet and the environment that may be 'responsible for tinnitus'. There is no evidence that tinnitus, as described in the neurophysiological model, has any allergic element. Nevertheless people whose life quality is already reduced subject themselves to rigorous diets, finally removing the last elements of enjoyment in their otherwise miserable existence.

Caffeine and other cerebral stimulants may exacerbate tinnitus and should be tested for on an individual basis. Alcohol variously produces an improvement in tinnitus, an exacerbation or has no effect whatever. Some patients experience such relief that alcoholism may develop.

Xanax (alprazolam)

This powerful benzodiazepine tranquillizer, Xanax, has been advocated specifically for the treatment of tinnitus in the USA. A double-blind trial showed a measurable improvement in reducing tinnitus.[21] Xanax is a powerful anxiolytic drug. The problem of dependency even after medium-term treatment with this drug has been well documented, and occasioned some law suits. We do not recommend it as a therapy in any situation because of this.

Prozac (fluoxetine)

Prozac is a relatively new antidepressant, hailed as a miracle drug, which is also being promoted for tinnitus. Again, tinnitus patients frequently develop high dependency or have significant side effects from this drug and we do not recommend it.

TREATMENT OF EFFECTS

Anxiety

In the short term there is no doubt that some benzodiazapine drugs like valium can do much to reduce severe anxiety and panic, which might be quite disabling. Behavioural techniques, however, such as relaxation therapy and thought blocking are much to be preferred than tranquillizers, which often cause dependency in the long term. In the tinnitus clinic the introduction of tinnitus retraining therapy can effectively compliment the withdrawal of benzodiazapine tranquillizer in many patients.

Depression

Many patients with tinnitus have coexisting or pre-existing depression. Appropriate antidepressant therapy can be extremely valuable in the short term, and a relatively safe antidepressant such as amitriptylene or prothiadine, preferably taken at night, may be indicated for a restricted period of a few months. Slow withdrawal is recommended.

TREATMENT OF THE SYMPTOM (TINNITUS)

There is no drug that will abolish tinnitus permanently but some do have temporary effect. These are found particularly in the group of drugs used in epilepsy, which act as membrane stabilizers and reduce the overactivity of neural tissue.

Lidocaine (lignocaine)

Lidocaine (lignocaine) is one of the few drugs that works in a high proportion (about 60 per cent) of patients, but only when given by intravenous administration.[22] Tinnitus is usually abolished for a period of a few minutes or so, but occasionally for longer periods. Profound changes in neural transmission are experienced throughout the central nervous system and there are other side effects on organs such as the heart and liver so that continuous administration has not been possible. Oral analogues such as tocainide have been tried in the past but have severe side effects thus precluding their use.

Carbamazepine

Carbamazepine is the drug that has had the longest running success as a 'tinnitus suppressor'. It has been used in dosage of 100 mg/day up to 200 mg three times a day.[23] Despite its widespread use there are very few patients who will admit to any meaningful therapeutic effect in the long term. We no longer prescribe it.

Clonazepam

Clonazepam is also used in the treatment of epilepsy and is related to valium. Drug dependency occurs if taken longer for a month and strict medical supervision is essential.

Furosemide

Furosemide has been advocated by some authorities especially in the USA. It is a diuretic that in high doses can actually cause cochlear damage. Recent research has shown that furosemide may block neurotransmitters in the central nervous system as well as affecting the stria vascularis.

Control trials have failed to show any benefit to tinnitus patients.

Nimodipine

Nimodipine interferes with calcium channels and has been shown to abolish tinnitus in animals. A trial conducted in humans showed that there was some short-term response, but it is certainly not a panacea.

Ginkgo biloba

The extract of *Ginkgo biloba* has been widely promoted in Europe for the treatment of tinnitus. It comes from the Chinese maidenhair tree. Controlled trials have been controversial and we have no patients who have benefited in the long term. Interestingly, animal studies show that tinnitus can be influenced (Jastreboff PJ personal communication).

DRUG THERAPIES AND THE FUTURE

The neurophysiological model shows the important part that is played by extra-auditory systems in the brain, particularly the limbic system and the autonomic nervous system. This explains the failure of any one therapeutic agent or interventionist procedure in helping the patient. Moreover, when strong phobic responses to tinnitus are generated the patient will continue to 'search' for TRNA within the auditory system. Short-term intervention with drugs is unlikely to have any long-term effect on tinnitus without the concurrent application of appropriate behavioural retraining. This does not, however, negate the importance of searching for ways of using combined therapy and also of influencing TRNA in the periphery when this becomes possible. All future research on tinnitus should take account of what is now known of its neurophysiology and avoid using a naive and simplistic model of ear dysfunction.

PROPHYLAXIS

There are many factors within and outside the auditory system that can be responsible for triggering tinnitus emergence. In the absence of a tinnitus trigger persistence of tinnitus and its distress will not occur. It is therefore important to promote the avoidance of auditory damage from noise, drugs and other ototoxic events as a means of avoiding tinnitus. In addition, it is important to indicate the part that inappropriate absence of environmental noise

plays. Indeed, silence can be dangerous for patients who have a tendency to high levels of sensory gain or sensory hypersensitivity. Environments that are totally free from sound are not common in nature or in a natural state, and their acquisition during the process of civilization in the form of the hermetically sealed and silenced bedroom or living accommodation is to some extent responsible for the levels of tinnitus emergence that occur in the population. The development of tinnitus distress is dependent in large part on the negative beliefs and 'bad press' that have been attached to the word 'tinnitus'. Proper education about tinnitus and its natural appearance as a part of audition in various circumstances will do much to avoid the development of severe phobic and aversive reactions to it. Advisory services provided by primary health care and available by telephone must be developed to give the right advice at a stage when tinnitus is a new experience without sinister meaning.

Cultural differences with respect to treatment

Several authorities have noticed the absence of certain cultural or ethnic groups in their clinics complaining of tinnitus. The neurophysiological model helps to explain this phenomenon. In village life in the Indian subcontinent for instance, there is a strong cultural belief that the experience of tinnitus means that the gods are speaking to you. In such an instance it is unlikely that powerful negative beliefs associated with unpleasant emotions will develop. The effect of tinnitus, and also the ease with which retraining approaches may be applied, depends on many aspects of culture and background, for example the expressive emotions, the feeling about the authority of the medical profession, the ability to follow orders and the basic level of background scientific knowledge. In applying retraining therapy it is important to remember these cultural differences and to behave appropriately. Avoid analogies to natural selection or evolution if these beliefs conflict with the individual's religious upbringing.

Conclusion

The traditional model of tinnitus as a cochlear pathology has been responsible for the lack of progress in treating this condition over the past 100 years. Tinnitus retraining therapy can now remove the emotional reaction to tinnitus and its perception. This process involves a habituation of reaction in the first instance, with a reduced emotional response and gradually decreasing distress with the reversal of negative beliefs about the tinnitus, which otherwise might lead to a phobic or aversive response to it. This process is followed by habituation of perception, in which there are increased periods of non-awareness of tinnitus, in its perceived loudness, and eventually by the disappearance of tinnitus from auditory experience.

References

1. Jastreboff PJ. Phantom auditory perception (tinnitus): mechanisms of generation and perception. *Neuroscience Research* 1990; **8**:221–54.
2. Ryan RM, Hazell JWP. Ménière's disease: are investigations of any value? A retrospective study. *Journal of Audiological Medicine* 1995; **3**:160–70.
3. Heller MF, Bergman M. Tinnitus in normally hearing persons. *Annals of Otology* 1953; **62**:73–83.
4. Saltzman M, Ersner MS. A hearing aid for the relief of tinnitus aurium. *Laryngoscope* 1947: **57**:358–66.
5. Vernon J. Attempts to relieve tinnitus. *Journal of the American Audiology Society* 1977; **2**:124–31.
6. Schleuning AJ, Johnson RM, Vernon JA. Evaluation of a tinnitus masking program: a follow-up study of 598 patients. *Ear Hearing* 1980; **1**:71–4.
7. Hazell JWP, Wood S. Tinnitus masking – a significant contribution to tinnitus management. *British Journal of Audiology* 1981; **15**:223–30.
8. Lewis JE, Stephens SD, McKenna L. Tinnitus and suicide. *Clinical Otolaryngology* 1994; **19**:50–4.
9. Hazell JWP, Sheldrake JB. Hyperacusis and tinnitus. In: Aran JM, Dauman R eds. *Proceedings of the Fourth International Tinnitus Seminar: 1991 Aug 27–30; Bordeaux.* Amsterdam: Kugler Publications, 1992:245–8.
10. Sheldrake JB, Jastreboff PJ. Hazell JWP. Perspectives for the total elimination of tinnitus perception. In: Reich G, Vernon J eds. *Proceedings of the Fifth International Tinnitus Seminar.* Portland, OR: American Tinnitus Association, 1996:531–6.
11. Meador KJ, Swift TR. Tinnitus from intracranial hypertension. *Neurology* 1984; **34**:1258–61.
12. Moller MB, Moller AR, Jannetta PJ, Jho HD. Vascular decompression surgery for severe tinnitus: selection criteria and results. *Laryngoscope* 1993; **103**:421–7.
13. Hazell JW. Tinnitus. II: Surgical management of conditions associated with tinnitus and somatosounds. *Journal of Otolaryngology* 1990; **19**:6–10.
14. Robinson PJ, Hazell JWP. Patulous Eustachian tube syndrome: the relationship with sensorineural hearing loss. Treatment with Eustachian tube diathermy. *Journal of Laryngology and Otology* 1989; **103**:739–42.
15. East CA, Hazell JW. The suppression of palatal (or intra-tympanic) myoclonus by tinnitus masking devices. A preliminary report. *Journal of Laryngology and Otology* 1987; **101**:1230–4.
16. Saeed SR, Brookes GB. The use of clostridium botulinum toxin in palatal myoclonus. A preliminary report. *Journal of Laryngology and Otology* 1993; **107**:208–10.
17. Hazell JWP, von Schoenberg LJ, Meerton LJ, Sheldrake JB . Tinnitus and the unilateral dead ear. In: Aran JM, Dauman R eds. *Proceedings of the Fourth International Tinnitus Seminar: 1991 Aug 27–30; Bordeaux.* Amsterdam: Kugler Publications, 1992:261–4.
18. Baguley DM, Moffat DA, Hardy DG. What is the effect of translabyrinthine acoustic schwannoma removal upon tinnitus? *Journal of Laryngology and Otology* 1992; **106**:329–31.
19. Parving A, Tos M, Thomsen J, Moller H, Buchwald C. Some aspects of life quality after surgery for acoustic neuroma. *Archives of Otolaryngology – Head and Neck Surgery* 1992; **118**:1061–4.
20. Penner MJ, Coles RRA. Indications for aspirin as a palliative for tinnitus caused by SOAEs: a case study. *British Journal of Audiology* 1992; **26**:91–6.
21. Johnson RM, Brummett R, Schleuning A. Use of alprazolam for relief of tinnitus. A double-blind study. *Archives of Otolaryngology – Head and Neck Surgery* 1993; **119**:842–5.
22. den Hartigh J, Hilders CG, Schoemaker RC, Hulshof JH, Cohen AF, Vermeij P. Tinnitus suppression by intravenous lidocaine in relation to its plasma concentration. *Clinical Pharmacology and Therapeutics* 1993; **54**:415–20.
23. Murai K, Tyler RS, Harker LA, Stouffer JL. Review of pharmacologic treatment of tinnitus. *American Journal of Otology* 1992; **13**:454–64.

Section C

Disorders of balance

CHAPTER 14

Disorders of balance – assessment and psychological aspects

LINDA M LUXON

Extent of the problem

Disorders of balance span conditions giving rise to dysequilibrium, vertigo, vague giddiness or dizziness, unsteadiness or ataxia and falls. In the UK Roydhouse[1] reported that 30 per cent of the population have consulted a doctor for giddiness by the age of 65 years, whereas annually 5 out of every 1000 patients consult their general practitioner because of symptoms that are classified as vertigo and a further 10 in every 1000 are seen for symptoms of dizziness or giddiness.[2] Moreover, after head injury and whiplash injury, vestibular symptoms are one of the most likely sequelae to prevent rapid return to work,[3] whereas falls are recognized as one of the most important health problems of the elderly and represent the commonest cause of accidental death in those over 75 years old.[4] Other important sequelae of balance disorders include psychiatric morbidity, particularly anxiety, depression and phobias,[5] which limit social and occupational activities in one-third of hospital referrals and lead to early retirement and chronic invalidism in 18 per cent.

Dizzy patients frequently present in cardiological, neurological, geriatric, general medical and ENT clinics and thus individual specialities may develop a strategy for evaluating symptoms of dysequilibrium in their own particular area of expertise, but may either overlook the many causes of dizziness arising in other systems, or refer the patient to a different specialist, often after expensive and inappropriate investigations such as MRI scanning or angiography. Such an approach is unsatisfactory for the patient, who may wait months for a diagnosis and appropriate management, and is economically wasteful for the patient, who is likely to lose their job, and for any health-care system, which shoulders the cost of repeated referrals with no satisfactory outcome. Therefore, the need to develop a systematic, efficient and formal assessment strategy for the diagnosis of the symptom complex of dizziness or vertigo and dysequilibrium is paramount in order to provide appropriate management and rehabilitation.

Humans have developed a sophisticated mechanism for maintaining balance, which relies upon visual, vestibular and proprioceptive input. The sensory inputs are integrated and modulated with activity from other neurological centres within the central nervous system (Fig 14.1). Considering the complexity of balance, it is not surprising that pathology in a wide variety of systems may give rise to symptoms of dysequilibrium (Fig 14.2).

It is well established that minor pathology in the vestibular system may lead to major disability and handicap if left unmanaged (Fig 14.3),[7–9] and the importance of disability and handicap, rather than pathology alone, in management strategies has become recognized.

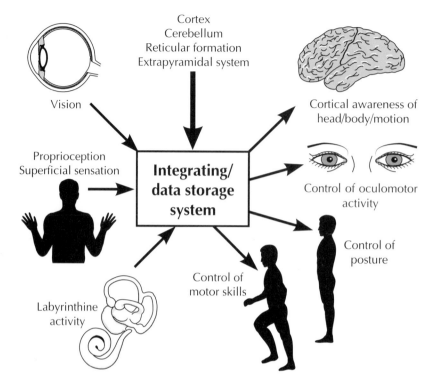

Fig 14.1 Mechanisms subserve balance in humans. (Reproduced from Savundra and Luxon[5] with permission.)

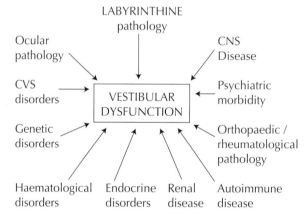

Fig 14.2 The variety of disorders that can give rise to vestibular dysfunction. CNS, central nervous system; CVS, central vestibular system.

WHO schema for disablements

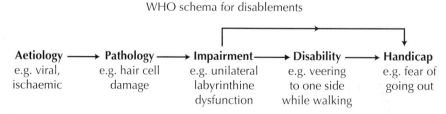

Fig 14.3 The progression of pathology to handicap following the World Health Organization Scheme for Disablement. (Reproduced from Luxon[6] with permission.)

Assessment

Good management relies upon accurate diagnosis. A single pathology may frequently be identified, but certain generalizations deserve mention. Some pathologies may give rise to symptoms as a result of involvement of more than one site, for example cardiovascular disease may give rise to an ischaemic labyrinthitis or ischaemic events in the brainstem or cerebellum, or both, or a combination of all three. Second, patients who suffer a peripheral labyrinthine event, such as labyrinthitis, may make an excellent initial recovery, but after either psychological (e.g. redundancy, bereavement, divorce) or physical stress (e.g trauma or intercurrent illness) may 'decompensate' and suffer a recurrence of symptoms (Fig 14.4). Third, in the elderly population dysequilibrium may be consequent upon the interaction of a multiplicity of pathologies, for example there may be visual impairment due to cataracts, proprioceptive impairment due to arthritis and vestibular impairment due to vascular disease. Although individually each of these impairments may be trivial, together they give rise to a significant balance problem,[10] which is commonly termed 'the multisensory dizziness syndrome'. It should also be borne in mind that age-related neuronal loss in the older patient makes the integration and modulation of information required for balance less efficient, such that compensation for vestibular or visual or proprioceptive defects is less efficient.

Clinical assessment, as in all medical conditions, is based on a detailed clinical history and examination, which allow appropriate investigations to define the correct diagnosis from a differential list. I would advocate a standard assessment strategy for all symptoms of dysequilibrium in order to optimize the likelihood of achieving the correct diagnosis.

CLINICAL HISTORY

A full general medical history should be taken with special reference to the cardiovascular and neurological systems. In addition, certain specific aspects of the dizziness or imbalance should be sought.

Character of symptoms

'Vertigo' is defined as an illusion of movement and is a key feature of disordered vestibular function. 'Dizziness' is a lay term and is usually taken to mean non-specific light-headedness, faintness or giddiness, and is common in many general medical disorders, such as cardiovascular disease, anaemia,

NATURAL HISTORY OF PERIPHERAL
VESTIBULAR PATHOLOGY

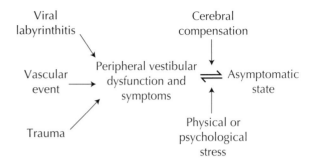

Fig 14.4 The reversible nature of vestibular compensation and decompensation in peripheral vestibular pathology. (Reproduced from Luxon[6] with permission.)

gastrointestinal disease and endocrine and neurological disorders. Although in clinical terms a distinction between dizziness and vertigo is of value, frequently a patient frightened by new and unphysiological symptoms may experience profound difficulties in expressing their symptomatology, such that a clear distinction between dizziness and vertigo cannot be made. Hyperventilation, because of anxiety induced by vertigo, can induce lightheadedness and complicate the description (see below).

Moreover, not infrequently patients report bizarre complaints, such as 'my brain is sloshing around inside my skull', 'I feel like I am a goldfish in a bowl, watching my life go by' and symptoms of visual vertigo, for example a dislike of walking on highly patterned carpet, watching football matches on television, ironing striped material, or watching type move on the computer or VDU. Not surprisingly, for the inexperienced clinician such symptoms may be dismissed as psychological and the underlying balance disorder not recognized.

Classically, vertigo of peripheral labyrinthine origin occurs as acute, unprecipitated, short-lived episodes of rotational movement of the world (objective vertigo) or of the patient themselves (subjective vertigo). Frequently, there is accompanying nausea and vomiting, more rarely diarrhoea. The patient becomes pale and sweats profusely. Vertigo of central neurological origin is more insidious in onset and constant in nature, with the patient commonly complaining that they feel they are walking on a moving surface or that they are swaying or rocking.

A history of falls requires the evaluation of risk factors such as drug intake, neurological conditions, cognitive function, general medical disorders and environmental factors, including uneven or slippery surfaces, poor lighting or an unfamiliar environment. Potentially treatable predisposing factors leading to falls can, thus, be identified and corrected. A patient who suffers a single uncomplicated fall with no sequelae may be reassured and discharged, but recurrent falls with or without injury require careful assessment (Fig 14.5) and, in

particular, a detailed evaluation of balance (Chapter 5). As Downton[11] highlights in her excellent monograph on falls, it is valuable to consider 'Why did this particular person fall at this particular time in this particular place?' For any particular fall, there is a *liability* to fall factor and *opportunity* to fall factor.

A complaint of unsteadiness or 'weakness' of the legs, the legs 'not moving properly' or 'not going in the right place', unaccompanied by any symptoms of dizziness or vertigo, requires neurological investigation specifically to exclude cerebellar and brainstem disease, associated with ataxia, and proprioceptive loss, associated with neuropathy.

Time course of dysequilibrium

The time course of the overall illness, together with the duration of individual 'episodes' should be considered (Fig 14.6). It is important to define whether the symptoms are constant, or whether episodes are erratic or occur in 'clusters', with relapses and remissions. Attacks of acute, rotational vertigo that are of less than 1 minute's duration and occur in clusters are most commonly associated with benign

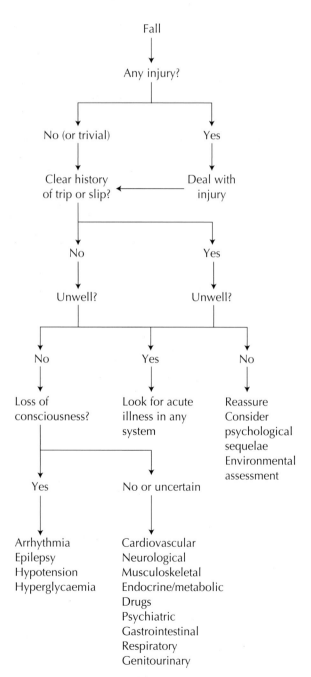

Fig 14.5 The management of falls. (Reproduced from Downton[11] with permission.)

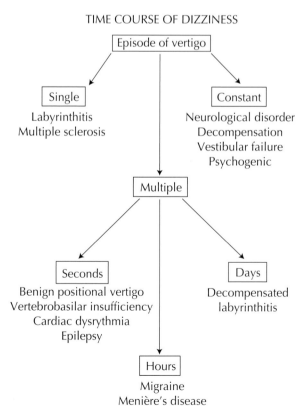

Fig 14.6 Time course of vertigo in different vestibular disorders.

positional vertigo of paroxysmal type, which is particularly common after head injury, in association with vascular disease and in the older age group. The periods of freedom from episodes may last many weeks or months. Particularly in the elderly, such attacks are frequently ascribed to vertebrobasilar ischaemia, but in the absence of any concomitant neurological symptoms or signs, this diagnosis is unlikely to be correct.[12]

Vertigo of several hour's duration is commonly associated with acute peripheral labyrinthine events, such as viral or ischaemic labyrinthitis. Such pathology may or may not be associated with cochlear symptoms. Recurrent acute symptoms of vertigo, with hearing loss and tinnitus, form the characteristic triad of Menière's disease. However, this diagnosis is frequently made rather casually and it is important that strict criteria are followed if the diagnosis is to be correct (Chapter 38). Pressure and fullness in the ear is a frequent accompanying symptom with acute attacks of Menière's disease, although it does not form part of the classic triad.

In patients with recurrent episodes of acute vertigo, more usually unassociated with cochlear symptoms, migraine is a diagnosis that should be considered and it is, therefore, prudent to enquire specifically about headaches. It should be recalled that vestibular symptoms associated with migraine may occur with or without headache, although a clear family history or past history, or both, of migraine should be established if this diagnosis is to be considered.

After an acute labyrinthitis, symptomatic recovery occurs over a period of several weeks, as a result of a variety of mechanisms, which are collectively known as cerebral compensation (Chapter 15). The crucial role of vision, somatosensory inputs and the cerebellum in the recovery of animals and humans after labyrinthine destruction has been well documented. The commonest cause of chronic vertigo is failure of compensation, or intermittent decompensation, after an acute labyrinthitis (Fig 14.7). A variety of factors may prevent compensation (Fig 14.8) and the clinician should specifically seek to identify the presence of any such factors and institute appropriate therapy if possible.

(a)

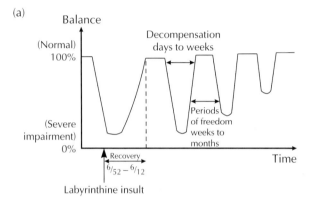

(b)

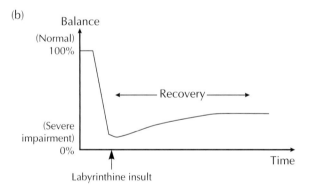

(c)

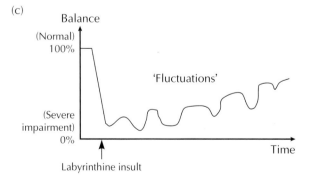

Fig 14.7 (a) The clinical presentation of symptomatic recovery after an acute labyrinthine episode with intermittent decompensation. (b) and (c) Two clinical presentations of failure of compensation after an acute labyrinthine event. (Reproduced from Luxon[6] with permission.)

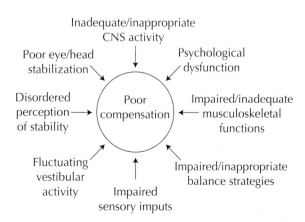

Fig 14.8 Factors predisposing to failure of compensation.[13]

Chronic persistent vertigo may, more rarely, be the result of central neurological disease, such as multiple sclerosis, spinocerebellar degenerations or vascular disease, but associated neurological symptoms or signs (particularly eye movement abnormalities) are the rule. Bilateral vestibular failure may also manifest with chronic dysequilibrium, which is usually accompanied by 'bobbing oscillopsia'.

Associated symptoms

Pathology within the VIIIth nerve and labyrinth may involve vestibular and auditory elements, which lie in close anatomical proximity. Thus, in any patient with disorientation, it is wise to enquire specifically about hearing loss or tinnitus, or both, particularly as a slowly progressive hearing loss may pass unobserved, or the elderly patient may assume that the hearing loss is due to ageing and unrelated to the primary complaint of dysequilibrium (Fig 14.9).

Pathology involving the vestibular pathways within the central nervous system rarely manifests as isolated dysequilibrium and is almost always associated with other specific neurological complaints. It is, therefore, advisable to enquire specifically about brainstem symptoms such as hemiparesis, hemianaesthesia, ataxia, facial weakness or numbness, dysarthria and eye movement difficulties. A full general medical history should be sought with specific enquiry about each bodily

Table 14.1 Factors precipitating vertigo

Head movement
Critical head position
Body movement
Eye movements
Motion
Movement of visual field
Movement of objects in visual field
Exertion
Fear or panic
Hyperventilation
Stress

system to identify any relevant symptoms, such as polyuria, excess malaise, angina, dysrythmia and leg pain on walking.

Precipitating factors

Precipitating factors for the patient's symptoms (Table 14.1) should be identified, as these may indicate possible aetiologies: for example, dizziness on standing from lying may indicate postural hypotension; dizziness on tipping the head backwards may indicate benign positional vertigo; dizziness due to strong visual targets such as a striped carpet may indicate peripheral vestibular pathology; and oscillopsia and unsteadiness on walking may indicate vestibular failure.

Drug history

The importance of a detailed drug history cannot be overemphasized (Table 14.2), as many drugs give rise to dizziness as a side effect and the ototoxic effect of the aminoglycoside antibiotics should be borne in mind particularly, as failure to evaluate renal function and trough and peak serum drug levels regularly may have serious medicolegal consequences, quite apart from devastating balance sequelae for the patient recovering from a life-threatening illness.

CLINICAL EXAMINATION

A full general medical examination is essential, with particular evaluation of the fundi, visual fields, visual acuity and general neurological, cardiovascular and peripheral vascular systems.

On the basis of a comprehensive history and a thorough examination (Fig 14.10), the possibility of a number of neurological and general medical disorders will be raised such that appropriate specific

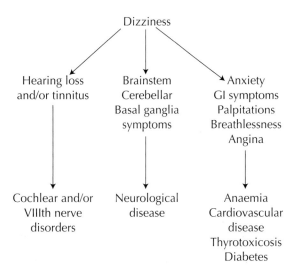

Fig 14.9 The diagnostic value of eliciting associated symptoms in the differential diagnosis of vertigo. GI, gastrointestinal.

Table 14.2 Drugs causing dizziness or vertigo

Psychotropic drugs	
Antidepressants	Tricylics, tetracyclics, MAOIs
Tranquillizers	Phenothiazines, benzodiazepines
Anticonvulsants	Phenobarbitone, phenytoin, carbamazepine
Analgesics	Paracetamol, acetylsalicylate, non-steroidal anti-inflammatory drugs, opiates
Anaesthetics	Nitrous oxide, halothane
Cardiovascular drugs	
Antihypertensives	Diuretics (thiazides and loop), beta-blockers, captopril, calcium channel blockers, methyldopa, hydralazine
Anti-arrhythmic	Verapamil, amiodarone, di-isopyramide, mexiletine, flecanide
Anti-angina	Glyceryl trinitrate, isosorbide dinitrate, nifedipine, verapamil
Antimicrobials	Aminoglycosides, minocycline, isoniazid, rifampicin, chloroquine, erythromycin
Anti-allergic drugs	Chlorpheniramine, cyproheptadine, ephedrine, promethazine
Hormone replacement or substitute	Hypoglycaemics, corticosteroids, HRT
Chemotherapeutic agents	Cis-platinum, busulphan, vinblastine

HRT, hormone replacement therapy; MAOIs, monoamine oxidase inhibitors.

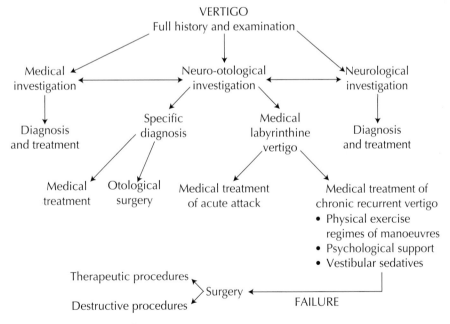

Fig 14.10 The management of vertigo.

investigations may be undertaken. There will then be a significant group of patients with neuro-otological symptoms, that is, vestibular and auditory complaints, in whom further vestibular investigation (Chapter 5) is indicated. Inevitably, there is some interrelationship between the three main subgroups of disorders that give rise to vertigo, for example diffuse vascular disease may manifest as angina, a cerebrovascular accident and thus labyrinthine dysfunction, which causes ischaemic labyrinthitis with or without vertebrobasilar insufficiency.

The specific clinical examination of vestibular pathology includes

- an examination of the external ear and tympanic membrane, together with clinical tests of auditory acuity and tuning fork tests
- an assessment of vestibulo-ocular function
- an assessment of vestibulospinal function.

A basic understanding of vestibular physiology (Chapter 2) is essential for the understanding of a detailed vestibular examination and vestibular test procedures, but for the purposes of understanding the neuro-otological examination certain points will be re-emphasized. Under normal circumstances, resting activity generated by each of the paired vestibular receptors is equal and maintains gaze, body and head position and the perception of normal balance. Any head movement brings about an alteration in neural activity, such that the input from one labyrinth is increased, whereas the input on the opposite side is decreased. This asymmetry of information is 'monitored' within the central nervous system, allowing perception of a head movement and forming the neurophysiological basis of the vestibulo-ocular and vestibulospinal reflexes. Thus, a head movement to the right induces a compensatory eye movement to the left, as a result of vestibular activity, and, if this eye movement is sufficiently great, neurological mechanisms produce a rapid eye movement (saccade) in the opposite direction, giving rise to the sawtooth eye movement known as spontaneous nystagmus. In normal physiological situations, turning rapidly on the spot or swivelling in a secretary's chair will bring about nystagmus, whereas in the pathological situation, damage to vestibular receptors or pathways on one side brings about an asymmetry of neural activity and, thus, the perception of motion (i.e. vertigo) and pathological nystagmus.

Otological examination

In all patients with episodic vertigo, active chronic middle ear disease with labyrinthine erosion must be excluded and any obvious otological abnormality noted and evaluated in the context of the clinical history and other signs. The presence of an auditory deficit, as judged by tuning fork tests or whispered voice tests, may suggest labyrinthine or VIIIth nerve pathology, but audiometry should be the definitive test to exclude such disorders.

VESTIBULO-OCULAR EXAMINATION

Eye movements

An assessment of spontaneous nystagmus is of paramount importance in the evaluation of the vestibular system. This is described in Chapters 3

and 5. Rapid eye movements (saccades) should be assessed by asking the patient to fixate a target subtending an angle of 20–30° to the right and left of the midposition of gaze to assess horizontal saccades and 30° up and down to assess vertical saccades. Delayed initiation, inaccuracy of fixation or slow velocity of the saccades may all indicate neurological disese and will impair the vestibular nystagmic response because of impairment of the fast phases of nystagmus. Slow *smooth pursuit* eye movements are intimately involved with the mechanism, which brings about suppression of vestibular nystagmus by optic fixation (see below). Thus, smooth pursuit should be assessed clinically by asking the patient to follow a target moving in the horizontal and vertical planes and assessing 'smoothness' of the eye movement. Asymmetrically deranged pursuit almost always indicates neurological pathology, but symmetrically disordered pursuit may be pathological (i.e. neurologically induced) or may be associated with psychotropic drugs (anticonvulsants, tranquillizers, antidepressants), fatigue and old age.

Spontaneous nystagmus

A detailed assessment of the presence and type of spontaneous nystagmus provides invaluable information about vestibular pathology (see Chapters 3 and 5).

The patient should be asked to gaze at a target (approximately half a metre in front of their eyes) and then deviate their gaze to the target held 30° to the right, left, up and down. Deviation of the eyes to a greater angle may result in physiological end-point nystagmus, which should not be confused with pathological nystagmus.

As noted above, a paralytic peripheral vestibular lesion (one arising in the labyrinth) gives rise to spontaneous nystagmus, which is directed (i.e. the direction of the fast phases) in the opposite direction to the affected labyrinth. Irritative lesions cause nystagmus with the quick component towards the disordered ear. Horizontal nystagmus of peripheral (i.e. labyrinthine or VIIIth nerve) origin obeys Alexander's Law, which states that the nystagmus is always in one direction, irrespective of the direction of gaze, and that the intensity of the nystagmus is greatest when the eyes are deviated in the direction of the fast phase (Fig 14.11). Nystagmus is described as first degree (when it beats in the same direction as gaze deviation); second degree (when it beats in a particular direction with the eyes held in the midposition of gaze) or third degree (when it beats in the opposite direction to the direction of gaze, e.g. to the right when the eyes are deviated to the left). Bidirectional, or direction changing, nystagmus (e.g.

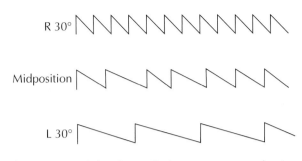

Fig 14.11 Peripheral vestibular nystagmus obeying Alexander's Law.

Table 14.3 Characteristics of spontaneous vestibular nystagmus

	Peripheral type	Central type
Duration	Temporary	Permanent
Direction	Unilateral	May be multidirectional
Character	Sawtooth Always conjugate	May be pendular May be dysconjugate
Effect of removal of optic fixation	Enhances	Unchanged or inhibited

first degree nystagmus to the right on looking to the right and first degree nystagmus to the left on looking to the left); vertical nystagmus (i.e. upbeat nystagmus or downbeat nystagmus, or both) and dysconjugate nystagmus (differing nystagmic response in each eye) arise only from central nervous system disease, and imply need for further neurological investigation (Table 14.3).

Under normal circumstances, the nystagmus generated by a peripheral labyrinthine stimulus, be it pathological or physiological, may be suppressed by visual fixation upon a target. Thus, in attempting to differentiate peripheral horizontal nystagmus from central horizontal nystagmus, it is of value to assess the effect upon any observed nystagmus of visual fixation upon a target (Fig 14.12). In the presence of an intact central nervous system, when a subject fixates, any observable nystagmus will be much less obvious than when fixation is removed. This suppression of vestibular nystagmus is not observed in cases of neurological origin (see Chapters 3 and 5).

Positional nystagmus

The presence of positional nystagmus is a most valuable and frequently overlooked clinical sign, which should be sought in every dizzy patient by performing a brisk Hallpike manoeuvre (Fig 14.13). It is important to explain the manoeuvre to the patient, particularly the possibility of the development of acute vertigo. The patient sits near the end of a flat examination couch. The head is held firmly between the examiner's hand and turned 30°or 40° to the right or left. The patient is then carried rapidly backwards, so that the head is extended on the neck over the edge of the couch and the eyes are carefully observed. If positional nystagmus develops, it is observed until it disappears or for 2–3 minutes, after which it may be assumed that the nystagmus is persistent. The patient is then

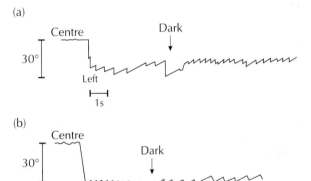

Fig 14.12 Vestibular nystagmus. (a) Central disease – after the removal of optic fixation nystagmus decreases. (b) Peripheral disease – after the removal of optic fixation nystagmus increases.

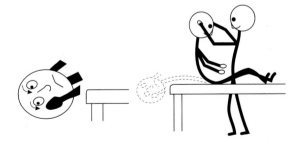

Fig 14.13 The techniques of performing the Hallpike manoeuvre to test for the presence of positional nystagmus.

returned to the upright position and the eyes carefully observed for any reversal of positional nystagmus. The procedure is then repeated with the head turned in the opposite direction.

Table 14.4 Characteristics of positional nystagmus

	Benign paroxysmal type	Central type
Latent period	2–20 seconds	None
Adaption	Disappears in 50 seconds	Persists
Fatiguability	Disappears on repetition	Persists
Vertigo	Always present	Typically absent
Direction of nystagmus	To undermost ear	Variable
Incidence	Relatively common	Relatively uncommon

In broad clinical terms, the positional nystagmus that may develop can be divided into two main types, as outlined in Table 14.4. It should be emphasized that there are a number of patients with positional nystagmus that does not fit neatly into either category and demonstrates features of benign positional nystagmus and central positional nystagmus. These patients should be further investigated neurologically.

If the positional nystagmus is of peripheral labyrinthine origin, there is a latent period of up to 30 seconds; severe vertigo develops in association with rotatory nystagmus directed towards the undermost ear and during this period the patient may be distressed and feel nauseated. Symptoms and signs then gradually adapt and if the procedure is repeated in the same direction, it is frequently observed that the nystagmus fatigues, that is, becomes less marked on repeated testing. Care must be taken to carry out the procedure correctly on the first attempt, as it is possible that this will be the only occasion on which the clinical signs will be elicited. The importance of this procedure was originally emphasized by Harrison and Ozsahinoglu[14] who found central nervous system pathology in 38 per cent of patients with persistent positional nystagmus compared with only 4 per cent of patients with benign paroxysmal positional nystagmus. Moreover, benign positional vertigo of paroxysmal type can be treated effectively in a large proportion of patients, using one of the particle repositioning procedures (Chapter 5) or, rarely, by operation (Chapter 38).

Optokinetic nystagmus

The clinical assessment of optokinetic nystagmus, which is a reflex oscillation of the eyes in response to movement of the visual surround (e.g. as seen in train passengers watching objects moving rapidly past the window), is of importance in balance disorders, as the pathways subserving this response pass through the vestibular nuclei. Clinically, the response may be elicited using a hand-held striped

Table 14.5 Optokinetic nystagmus

Anatomical site	Normal (%)	Abnormal (%)
Brainstem	41	59
Cerebellum	28	72
Basal ganglia	43	57
Parietal lobe	26	74
Labyrinth	99	1

n = 614 (Reproduced from Yee *et al.*[5] with permission.)

drum or a piece of striped material, which is moved to the right and left, and up and down in front of the patient's eyes. The examiner observes any asymmetry in the nystagmic response to right and left or in the vertical plane. The importance of this test is that in patients with peripheral vestibular pathology abnormalities in optokinetic nystagmus are not observed, except in the acute phase of a peripheral labyrinthine disorder, when spontaneous nystagmus is present and may contaminate the optokinetic response. However, in neurological disease giving rise to dysequilibrium, optokinetic abnormalities are seen in 57–74 per cent of patients depending on the precise site of the lesion (Table 14.5).

VESTIBULOSPINAL ASSESSMENT

Vestibulospinal function cannot be assessed directly, and clinical examinations of 'balance' are non-specific and insensitive compared with tests of vestibulo-ocular function, but they may provide an indication of the extent of a patient's diability. The *Romberg test* is performed by asking the patient to stand in the upright position with feet together, arms by the side, head straight forward and eyes closed. A tendency to sway to one side usually suggests peripheral vestibular pathology, whereas an inability to stand with the feet together is more characteristic of cerebellar ataxia. However, it must be emphasized that the Romberg test was originally designed for use in assessing posterior column loss in tabes dorsalis and is influenced by a variety of sensory and motor disorders. Thus, it is non-specific for vestibular disease. In anxious patients there is frequently a tendency to fall backwards, like a wooden soldier, and this is indicative of a non-organic component to their symptoms. Nonetheless, it should be emphasized that this is almost always observed in the presence of an underlying abnormality, which is elucidated on full investigation.

Unterberger testing

Unterberger testing involves the patient marching up and down on the spot, with their eyes closed and their hands clasped at arms length in front of them. Normal patients show less tendency to deviate to the right or left than patients with peripheral or central vestibular disorders. However, the value of this test is questionable in view of the multiplicity of factors that influence the response.

Gait testing

Gait testing is assessed by asking the patient to walk towards a fixed point in a normal manner with the eyes closed. Again, a tendency to veer in one direction is most commonly the result of an ipsilateral peripheral vestibular disturbance, but may on occasions be observed with cerebellar disease. The latter diagnosis is commonly associated with a broad-based ataxic gait. A variety of other gait disorders that are associated with balance disorders may be observed, for example the slow shuffling parkinsonian gait, the high-stepping foot-dropping gait of posterior column loss or peripheral neuropathy and the bizarre, non-organic gait that is frequently observed in patients with vestibular disorders, in whom a diagnosis has not been made and psychological overlay is prominent.

A detailed clinical history and examination, as outlined, allows most disorders of balance to be diagnosed. Specific diagnoses such as Menière's disease, benign positional vertigo and acoustic neuroma, for which specific medical or surgical treatments are available (Fig 14.10), will be defined. In addition, there is a significant proportion of 'dizzy' patients (approximately one-third in hospital practice), in whom chronic vertigo is the result of poor compensation for a previous 'labyrinthitis'. Vestibular rehabilitation (Chapter 15) is required in this group. Vertigo attributable to neurological disease occurs in approximately 10 per cent of 'dizzy' patients referred to specialist balance clinics, but it

should be emphasized that a detailed eye movement assessment will, with experience, allow identification of virtually all such patients.

Psychological aspects

The management of chronic vertigo is detailed in Chapter 15 but the psychological aspects of vestibular pathology are worthy of specific consideration, although they are often overlooked and poorly understood. The relationship between physical disease and psychiatric disorders is well recognized and 13 per cent of neurological outpatients have been reported to suffer primary psychiatric disease, although the prevalence of psychatric dysfunction in patients with hearing loss is lower.[16] In patients with persistent dizziness, psychiatric disorders have been demonstrated to be the second most common cause of symptoms, occurring in 10–25 per cent of patients.[10,17–19] Conversely, complaints of dizziness and feelings of loss of balance are extremely common in psychiatric patients, especially those with panic and other anxiety disorders, such as agoraphobia.

In a study in a geriatric dizziness clinic (>60 years of age), Sloane et al.[20] found that primary psychiatric disease was present in only 3 per cent of patients, but psychiatric factors were contributory in 24.5 per cent. A more detailed study of patients with demonstrable vestibular disease,[21] identified that one-third of those presenting to a specialist neuro-otological clinic recovered totally over 3–5 years, whereas a further one-third experienced some improvement. The remainder, however, reported no improvement or a worsening of symptoms. Interestingly, the degree of vestibular impairment as judged by vestibular tests was not correlated to symptomatic outcome or psychiatric morbidity. Residual vestibular symptoms, however, were directly related to psychiatric morbidity, which in turn correlated with measures of anxiety, perceived stress and previous psychiatric illness. It is of note that other otological conditions do not show the same prevalence of psychiatric dysfunction. Clark et al.[16] compared patients with vestibular disorders with those with confirmed hearing loss and found that, although between 20 per cent and 40 per cent of patients with vestibular disorders suffered from panic disorder or panic attacks, none of the hearing loss patients had panic disorder and only 7 per cent suffered panic attacks.

A variety of studies have shown that the commonest psychiatric disorders associated with symptoms of dysequilibrium are panic disorder, generalized anxiety disorder, phobic anxiety disorder and depression. More specific syndromes such as 'space' phobia[22] and the 'motorist's disorientation syndrome'[23] have also been described in patients with peripheral and central vestibular disorders.

Anger, fear and mild depression are common responses to chronic physical illness and may provide the stimulus for active participation in rehabilitation programmes, but, depending on the patient's psychological make-up and environmental factors, severe psychological illness may supervene. The complex interaction of vertigo with associated physical and psychological factors is shown in Figure 14.14.

Hyperventilation is commonly associated with anxiety and may cause dizziness as a result of cerebral ischaemia. It has been cited as the cause of dizziness in as many as 25 per cent of dizzy patients.[10] The common features of hyperventilation include dyspnoea, chest pain and light-headedness, together with specific symptoms of sighing, yawning and excess use of the chest wall and accessory muscles of respiration, which may serve as pointers to the diagnosis. Typically, hypocapnia in muscle tissue leads to cramps and may manifest as carpopedal spasm. The psychiatric manifestations include anxiety, panic attacks, unreal feelings and depersonalization. To make the diagnosis a provocation test is recommended. The patient is instructed to describe how they feel during the test, and the precise purpose of the test should be explained. They are asked to take 30–40 deep breaths per minute, following the breathing pattern of the examiner. This should be continued for 4 or 5 minutes or until dizziness supervenes. The patient may or may not report similarities to their own symptoms. Symptoms may be brought under control by rebreathing from a paper bag. This test

should not be carried out in patients with ischaemic heart disease, anaemia, cerebrovascular disease or chronic obstructive airway disease.

For the clinician supervising the diagnosis and care of patients with dizziness and dysequilibrium, the ability to identify the main psychiatric disorders common in balance disorders is of value. In *generalized anxiety disorders*, the primary symptoms are anxiety, including non-specific apprehension, and constant motor activity (e.g. fidgeting, trembling) with an inability to relax and autonomic overactivity (including tachycardia, tachypnoea and dry mouth), occurring most days for a period of at least several weeks. Dizziness occurs in 63 per cent of patients with this condition and is the fourth most common symptom next to palpitations, head and muscle aches and sweating.[24] Importantly, these symptoms are also common in primary vestibular pathology and, thus, vestibular investigations are essential, if clear evidence of vestibular disease is to be defined.

Panic disorder is common in patients with balance dysfunction and is characterized by recurrent attacks of severe anxiety, which are not particularly restricted to any single situation. Somatic features include dizziness, palpitations, chest pain and feelings of unreality, whereas psychological sequelae include fear of dying or going mad. Usually there are several attacks within 1 month and in between the attacks the patient is free from symptoms of anxiety, unlike generalized anxiety disorder.

Phobic anxiety disorders are characterized by anxiety provoked by a certain well defined situation and such situations are characteristically avoided or endured with dread. Reassurance is unhelpful in relieving the anxiety and there is frequently coexistent depression. Patients with vestibular disorder may develop, in particular, agoraphobia or social phobia as a result of fear of an attack of dizziness or becoming incapacitated in a public or social situation. In an attempt to avoid provoking attacks, particularly in public, patients tend to impose restrictions on their activity and lifestyle, which generate feelings of helplessness and frustration and reinforce the phobia. The effects on the patient's life and environment (work, home and social activities) is marked, and severely affected patients may become housebound and intensely depressed.

Depression is more commonly recognized by most clinicians and is characterized by a depressed mood with feelings of worthlessness, pessimism and tearfulness, which is associated with persistent physical and mental fatigue, after even trivial effort, and a complete loss of interest in and enjoyment of life. Frequently, patients complain of poor attention

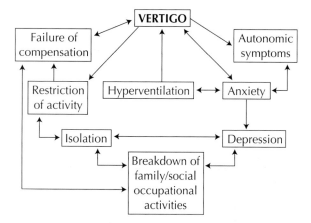

Fig 14.14 The interaction of physical and psychological factors associated with vertigo.

and concentration and marked slowing down in all activities. This may be more easily distinguishable from vestibular disease than the anxiety disorders, as the spectrum of clinical symptoms is different and dizziness is not a major feature.

The first step in identifying the need for psychiatric intervention relies upon the clinician's awareness of the relationship between psychological and vestibular disease. Self-rating questionnaires, such as the Hospital Anxiety and Depression Scale, the Beck Depression Inventory, the Fear Questionnaire (which detects phobic anxiety and avoidance behaviour) and the General Health Questionnaire are of value in identifying psychiatric dysfunction, as part of an overall clinical assessment. Patients may feel that psychiatric referral indicates that their symptoms are 'less real' than those exhibited by patients with an organic disease and it is, therefore, very important to convey to the patient that psychological sequelae are 'normal' and common in association with vestibular pathology and that the clinician understands the difficulties they are confronting psychologically and in terms of vestibular pathology. The clinician should be aware of the substantial body of literature that supports the view that an effective treatment package for chronic dysequilibrium addresses the physical and the psychiatric components of the disorder.[25] Importantly, the patient should come to realize that active participation in the management of their treatment, including the psychological symptoms, is helpful in the recovery process. Appropriate psychological treatment should be organized and this may take the form of behavioural psychotherapy, for those with avoidance behaviour and panic attacks,[26] or counselling or drug therapy for depression.

Cognitive behavoural therapy is a goal-orientated, practical technique aimed at examining the perceptions of the patient regarding their illness, which may be negative, false or wrongly attributed, and modifying the behaviour by substituting it with more appropriate coping strategies. Anecdotal evidence suggests these techniques are of particular value in vestibular pathology, but a controlled study has not yet been reported.

Antidepressants are of particular value in patients with depression and vestibular disease, but there is no place in the long-term treatment of anxiety disorders for addictive benzodiazepines. Moreover, the use of temazepam as night sedation can be avoided by the use of a sedative antidepressant. Any psychological drug therapy must be rationalized to avoid dangerous drug interactions or interactions that may give rise to dizziness. Many patients are fearful of taking such drugs, and reassurance and explanation are therefore necessary.

Antidepressants in general take 7–21 days to bring about improvement of symptoms and patients should be aware of this delay in response.

In conclusion, balance disorders are common and may be encountered by a variety of specialists. Although rarely life-threatening, they may be associated with significant morbidity. Psychological sequelae may be particularly troublesome, leading to significant handicap. A rational, systematic diagnostic strategy enables rapid diagnosis in the majority of cases, such that appropriate management may be started, allowing significant social, occupational and economic benefits to accrue.

References

1. Roydhouse N. Vertigo and its treatment. *Drugs* 1974; **7**:297–309.
2. Royal College of General Practitioners and Office of Population Census and Surveys (RCGP/OPCS). *Morbidity statistics from general practice.* London: HMSO, 1986.
3. Luxon LM. Post-traumatic vertigo. In: Baloh RW, Halmagyi M eds. *Handbook of vestibular disorders.* New York: Oxford University Press, 1996.
4. Downton JH. Falls in the elderly – epidemiology, classification and causes. *Journal of Audiological Medicine* 1994; **3**:iii–xiii.
5. Savundra P, Luxon LM. The physiology of equilibrium and its application to the dizzy patient. In: Kerr AG ed. *Scott-Brown's diseases of the ear, nose and throat, 6th ed.* London: Butterworths, 1996. [Wright D ed. Basic sciences, **1**.]
6. Luxon LM. Vestibular compensation. In: Luxon LM, Davies RA eds. *A handbook of vestibular rehabilitation.* London: Whurr, 1997:17–29.
7. Jacobsen GP, Newman CW. The development of the dizziness handicap inventory. *Archives of Otolaryngology – Head and Neck Surgery* 1990; **116**:424–7.
8. Yardley L. *Vertigo and dizziness.* London: Routledge, 1994.
9. Sheperd NT, Smith-Wheelock M, Telian SA, Raj A. Vestibular and balance rehabilitation therapy. *Annals of Otology, Rhinology and Laryngology* 1993; **102**:198–204.
10. Drachman DB, Hart CW. An approach to the dizzy patient. *Neurology* 1972; **22**:323–34.
11. Downton JH. *Falls in the elderly.* London: Edward Arnold, 1992.
12. Luxon LM. Signs and symptoms of vertebrobasilar insufficiency. In: Hofferberth B ed. *Vascular brainstem diseases.* Basel: Karger, 1990.
13. Shumway-Cook A, Horak FB. Rehabilitation strategies for patients with vestibular deficits. *Neurology Clinics of North America* 1990; **8**:441–57.
14. Harrison MS, Ozsahinoglu C. Positional vertigo. *Archives of Otolaryngology* 1975; **101**:675–8.
15. Yee RD, Baloh RW, Honrubia V, Jenkins HA. Pathophysiology of optokinetic nystagmus. In: Honrubia V,

Brazier M eds. *Nystagmus and vertigo: clinical approaches to the patient with dizziness.* New York: Academic Press, 1982:251–75.

16. Clark DB, Hirsch BE, Smith MG, Furman JMR, Jacob RG. Panic in otolaryngology patients presenting with dizziness or hearing loss. *American Journal of Psychiatry* 1994; **151**:1223–5.

17. Nedzelski JM, Barber HO, McIlmoyl L. Diagnoses in a dizziness unit. *Journal of Otolaryngology* 1986; **15**:101–4.

18. Herr RD, Zun L, Matthews JJ. A directed approach to the dizzy patient. *Annals of Emergency Medicine* 1989; **18**:664–72.

19. Kroenke K, Lucas CA, Rosenberg ML, *et al.* Causes of persistent dizziness. *Annals of Internal Medicine* 1992; **117**:898–904.

20. Sloane PD, Hartman M, Mitchell CM. Pyschological factors associated with chronic dizziness in patients aged 60 and older. *Journal of Americal Geriatric Society* 1994; **42**:847–52.

21. Eagger S, Luxon LM, Davies RA, Coehlo A, Ron MA. Psychiatric morbidity in patients with peripheral vestibular disorder: a clinical and neuro-otological study. *Journal of Neurology, Neurosurgery and Psychiatry* 1992; **55**:383–7.

22. Marks IM. Space 'phobia': a pseudo-agoraphobic syndrome. *Journal of Neurology, Neurosurgery and Psychiatry* 1981; **44**:387–91.

23. Page NGR, Gresty MA. Motorist's vestibular disorientation syndrome. *Journal of Neurology, Neurosurgery and Psychiatry* 1985; **48**:729–35.

24. Noyes R, Clancy J, Hoenk PR, Slymen DJ. The prognosis of anxiety neurosis. *Archives of General Psychiatry* 1980; **37**:173–8.

25. Yardley L, Luxon LM. Treating dizziness with vestibular rehabilitation. *British Medical Journal* 1994; **308**:1252–3.

26. Davidson AD. Behavioural psychotherapy. In: Luxon LM, Davies RA eds. *A handbook of vestibular rehabilitation.* London: Whurr, 1997:74–9.

CHAPTER 15

Rehabilitation and management of balance and vestibular disorders

LINDA M LUXON

Introduction

Disorders of balance may arise as a result of visual, priorioceptive or vestibular pathology or as a result of the inability of the central nervous system to integrate and modulate this information appropriately (Fig 14.1). Pathologies in many different bodily systems, including cardiovascular, endocrine, musculoskeletal, neurological, renal, haematological and psychological disorders, may cause dysfunction of the mechanisms for balance and lead to chronic symptoms with significant disability and handicap.

A detailed history and general medical and neurological examination will allow the identification of the majority of non-labryinthine disorders that may give rise to balance disorders and allows the otologist to refer these patients to the appropriate specialist. The aim of this chapter is to consider the management of chronic vertigo and unsteadiness, which is most commonly associated with uncompensated peripheral vestibular lesions and, more rarely, with central neurological disorders.

Vertigo and dysequilibrium associated with an acute unilateral vestibular lesion normally improve over a period of 6–12 weeks as a result of a number of processes that are collectively known as cerebral compensation. These processes can be subdivided into two main physiological categories: habituation or adaptive responses and sensory substitution.

Habituation or adaptive responses allow the central nervous system to 'adjust' to changes in labyrinthine signals as a result of repetitive stimulation and thus render the patient asymptomatic. Similar processes occur in acrobats, ice skaters and ballet dancers, who perform repetitive rotational movements but do not become dizzy because the brain 'adapts' to the repetitive signals.

In sensory substitution the central nervous system 'relies' more heavily on, for example, vision and proprioception, than vestibular input, and thus readjusts the inputs controlling perfect balance in the face of a deficit in the vestibular system.

These two different mechanisms of recovery do not always occur spontaneously and patients may be left with persistent symptoms after an acute vestibular episode such as viral labyrinthitis. Continuing symptoms may be constantly present or may occur as intermittent episodes of dizziness, frequently triggered by a coincidental illness such as influenza, or a psychological upset such as redundancy, divorce or bereavement (Fig 14.4). The symptoms may be mild and merely described as a 'nuisance', or they may be severe enough to lead to loss of employment and disruption of social activities.

The various mechanisms encompassed in the term cerebral compensation are dependent upon brainstem, cerebellar and cortical structures in addition to the sensory inputs – vision, proprioception and vestibular input – required for balance.[1] The causes of failure of compensation or intermittent decompensation are not clear, but cerebellar damage, impairment of prioprioception, visual impairment and psychological disorders have all been cited as possible contributing factors.[2] Compensation processes cannot be effective in the presence of ongoing or intermittent pathology within the labyrinth, as may occur in such conditions as Menière's disease and failed or incomplete destructive surgical procedures. There is also some evidence to suggest that drugs with an effect on the central nervous system may delay vestibular compensation.[3]

Vestibular rehabilitation

Vestibular rehabilitation refers to a structured programme of treatment aimed at expediting and enhancing vestibular compensation and rendering the dizzy patient asymptomatic (Table 15.1), such that they may return to full occupational and social activities.

As noted in Chapter 14, a systematic diagnostic strategy for balance disorders allows general medical, neurological and otological balance disorders to be differentiated and appropriate management to be set in place (Fig 14.10). Vestibular rehabilitation is of particular value in the remaining group of patients with chronic vestibular symptoms, which are most commonly attributable to unilateral labyrinthine pathology, but may be associated, more rarely, with VIIIth nerve, bilateral labyrinthine and central vestibular pathology.

Patients with chronic vertigo due to unilateral vestibular disorders fall into two main categories: those with specific conditions for which there is a recognized treatment regime, such as Menière's disease, benign positional vertigo of paroxysmal

Table 15.1 Rehabilitation programme

1. Investigation and diagnosis
2. Explanation
3. Rehabilitation plan:
   Correction of remedial problems
   General fitness programme
   Physical exercise programme
   Psychological assessment
   Medication
   Realistic goals
      family
      social
      occupational
4. Monitoring, feedback and follow-up
5. Discharge

type and acoustic neuroma, and those in whom, although there is test evidence of peripheral labyrinthine dysfunction, a specific aetiological condition may defy diagnosis. In addition, it should be recalled that standard vestibular tests (caloric and rotation testing) assess only horizontal semicircular canal function and thus vestibular pathology in the vertical canals or the otolith organs may be overlooked in a symptomatic patient in whom standard tests are normal.

GENERAL REHABILITATION PLAN

A number of practical points are of importance in the development of an individual rehabilitation programme for a specific patient.[4] An initial assessment should be undertaken to identify factors that may compromise the rehabilitation effort (Fig 14.8). A patient in poor physical condition is unable to take part in an active exercise-based rehabilitation programme; therefore it is important to encourage patients to participate in a general fitness programme, which may begin slowly but gradually builds up fitness levels (Table 15.2).

The treatment of musculoskeletal disorders such as arthritis is of importance and retraining in appropriate stance and gait strategies is required. Proprioception and visual inputs should be assessed to allow appropriate remediation of defects, for example cataract removal, appropriate optical correction and optimal management of joint inflammation. Inappropriate perception of stability has been observed in elderly people with dizziness and disequilibrium and this may be improved by making the patient aware of the disordered perception and introducing retraining using biofeedback (posturographic self-monitoring).

Rehabilitation of patients with peripheral vestibular pathology is aimed at alleviating acute symptoms and then introducing a regime based on physical exercises to enhance inadequate compensation. Animal experiments showing that visual and

Table 15.2 Physical exercise regimes and manoeuvres relevant to rehabilitation

General fitness programme
Systematic exercise programme e.g.
   Cawthorne–Cooksey
'Customized' exercise programme
Specific therapies
   Brandt–Daroff exercises
   Semont manoeuvre
   Epley manoeuvre

proprioceptive stimulation promote recovery of balance in animals subjected to a unilateral vestibular neurectomy provide the scientific basis for this approach. If psychological symptoms (anxiety, depression, phobic symptoms) have developed, psychological support may be required. Thus, the basic principles of vestibular rehabilitation may be called to mind by the three Ps:

- pharmacological treatment
- physical exercise regimes (Table 15.2)
- psychological intervention

PHARMACOLOGICAL INTERVENTION

Anti-emetics, such as prochlorperazine by buccal absorption, intramuscular injection or by suppository, followed by a vestibular sedative such as cinnarizine are of value in the management of acute vertigo. However, in the management of chronic labyrinthine symptoms, such drugs may suppress vestibular activity within the central nervous system, which is crucial for the development of compensation. Thus, a vestibular sedative may be used in very symptomatic patients to enable physical exercise regimes to be introduced, but should be withdrawn as soon as possible and, in general, has no place in the long-term management of chronic balance disorders.

PHYSICAL EXERCISE REGIMES

Cawthorne–Cooksey exercises

Physiotherapy for patients with peripheral vestibular disorders was first introduced by Cawthorne and Cooksey in the mid 1940s.[5,6] They recognized the tendency for patients suffering from vestibular damage as a result of head injury to drift into chronic invalidism and designed a series of graduated exercises (Table 15.3) aimed at encouraging head and eye movements that provoked dizziness in a systematic manner, recognizing that a patient recovered more rapidly using these techniques. The Cawthorne–Cooksey exercises were performed in various positions and at various speeds depending on the severity of the patient's symptomatology. The patients were required to perform the exercises with the eyes open and closed, in order to promote compensation using vestibular and proprioceptive mechanisms. The importance of psychological aspects of vestibular disorders was recognized and daily group sessions for patients undertaking the Cawthorne–Cooksey exercises were recommended to encourage the more hesitant patients and identify

malingerers. Moreover, it was also recommended that patients should be encouraged to encounter noisy and crowded environments, from which the majority of patients with vestibular disorders tend to shy.

Subsequently, it has become clear that it is important to emphasize to the patient that the exercise regime is not an endurance test and that a gentle, systematic, consistent approach is more effective than infrequent bursts of aggressive exercise, which merely precipitate troublesome vertigo associated with nausea and vomiting and deter the patient from wishing to persevere with the exercises.

Table 15.3 Cawthorne–Cooksey exercises

A. RESTING
Only one exercise at a time should be carried out and this exercise should be continued until any unpleasant symptom ceases. Only then should the next exercise be started.
1. *Eye movements* – at first slow, then quick
   up and down
   from side to side
   focusing on finger moving from 3 feet to 1 foot away from face
2. *Head movements* – at first slow, then quick.
   Later with eyes closed
   bending forwards and backwards
   turning from side to side

B. SITTING
1. and 2. as above
3. shoulder shrugging and circling
4. bending forwards and picking up objects from the ground

C. STANDING
1. as A1 and 2 and B3
2. changing from sitting to standing position with eyes open and shut
3. throwing a small ball from hand to hand (above eye level)
4. throwing a ball from hand to hand under knees
5. change from sitting to standing and turning round in between

D. MOVING ABOUT
1. circle round centre person who will throw a large ball and to whom it will be returned
2. walk across room with eyes open and then closed
3. walk up and down slope with eyes open and then closed
4. walk up and down steps with eyes open and then closed
5. any game involving stooping or stretching and aiming such as skittles, bowls or basketball

Early studies assessing symptomatic response[7] showed that approximately 80 per cent of patients with vestibular disorders responded favourably to the Cawthorne–Cooksey regime, and the importance of 'emotional stress' was noted. Norré[8] extended the original work of Cawthorne and Cooksey by defining vertigo-provoking manoeuvres and devising an objective measure of the patient's functional response. Patients were asked to score the intensity, type and duration of vertigo produced by each of the test manoeuvres (rapidly performed and each position held for 120 seconds before returning to the resting position). Subsequent workers[9] have also emphasized the importance of objective post-therapy outcome measures.

Customized exercises

Early work on the physical exercise regimes concentrated on progression through a fixed system of exercises aimed at presenting a full range of visual and vestibular stimuli in all planes of space. However, recent programmes of physical exercise regimes have concentrated on a 'customized' set of exercises developed for each individual patient, as outlined initially by Norré and Beckers[10] and, more recently, by Shepard *et al.*[11] and Herdman.[12]

These workers emphasize pre-rehabilitation assessment of vestibular deficits and of posture, gait and balance disorders, in order to identify the best stimuli to induce compensation, that is, 'customized' exercises based on the patient's functional difficulties. Patients are instructed to work at the limit of their ability and are involved in an overall rehabilitation programme, including a general fitness programme, with specific goals aimed at reintegrating them into normal social and occupational activities (Table 15.1). Like the Cawthorne–Cooksey exercises, these customized programmes are instructed initially by a physiotherapist, after which a 'home programme' of exercises two or three times a day is encouraged, with review by the clinician or physiotherapist based on the patient's need and progress. A telephone helpline is of value to ensure patient compliance and provide readily available assistance and encouragement for patients who are uncertain about the exercise regime or are anxious about symptoms precipitated by the exercises.

Recent work has suggested a role for physical exercise regimes in all forms of disorientation, regardless of diagnosis.[11,13] In addition, there is some evidence that there may be a critical time period within which significant functional improvement and an ability to return to the workforce may be achieved, although Shepard *et al.*[11] did not identify duration of symptoms or age as negative prognostic factors for recovery. Financial compensation, however, has been identified as a negative factor, as have head injury and severe postural control abnormalities, as judged by posturography.

PSYCHOLOGICAL SUPPORT

Significant psychological benefits accrue from a structured vestibular rehabilitation programme, as a detailed explanation of the regime is required in order for patients to comply with the instructions. This necessitates an understanding of dizziness and, thus, allays fears of sinister pathology. In addition, patients are encouraged to cope actively with their symptoms rather than avoid them,[13] and this reassures the patient by placing them in control of their symptoms.

Many patients with vestibular disorders experience bizarre symptoms, such as feeling 'spaced out' and sensing that their brain is 'disconnected' from their skull. They are embarrassed to report such symptoms and this may be compounded by the inexperienced clinician, who dismisses their complaints as 'in the mind' rather than identifying the underlying vestibular abnormality. Moreover, such symptoms may reinforce the patient's view that there is sinister neurological pathology, which is being overlooked by their medical advisers, or, equally importantly, confirms in their mind that they are 'going mad'. Poor management of this situation must be avoided, and it is encumbent on clinicians dealing with patients with vestibular disorders to be aware of the bizarre symptomatology with which such patients may present.

The development of psychological symptoms in patients with dysequilibrium is well documented[14] and in particular panic attacks, anxiety disorders and depression have been noted. Recent work has suggested that active management of these symptoms, particularly behavioural therapy, is of considerable value in correcting avoidance behaviour and bringing about more rapid recovery of vestibular symptoms in these psychologically disturbed patients.[15,16] Although there is no controlled study to assess the value of early counselling in patients with peripheral vestibular disorders, the negative outcome in patients with psychological symptoms is well documented. It is, therefore, suggested that a detailed and appropriate explanation of the patient's symptoms early in the natural history of the disorder may alleviate long-term psychological sequelae and therefore improve the ultimate outcome. Hyperventilation has been discussed in the previous chapter.

Although uncompensated, unilateral peripheral vestibular disorders are the commonest cause of persistent dysequilibrium, bilateral vestibular hypofunction, benign paroxysmal positional vertigo and central vestibular symptoms should be considered in the context of vestibular rehabilitation.

BILATERAL VESTIBULAR HYPOFUNCTION

Patients with bilateral vestibular failure may benefit from intensive physical exercise regimes,[17] with the expectation of better recovery in the presence of residual vestibular function. Patients may also be helped by such simple measures as wearing thick rubber soles, to reduce oscillopsia associated with walking and the use of a walking stick to provide additional proprioceptive input through the upper limb. They should be advised to avoid specific situations in which they may be in danger, for example swimming alone, especially under water, and standing on the edge of railway platforms and the edge of cliffs. Vestibular sedatives should be avoided to maximize the input of any residual vestibular function in these patients.

BENIGN PAROXYSMAL POSITIONAL VERTIGO

The consideration of vestibular rehabilitation is incomplete without discussion of the new methods of managing benign paroxysmal positional vertigo, which is a common cause of chronic vertigo after head injury, in association with vascular disease and in a variety of otological conditions, most importantly viral labyrinthitis. The diagnosis is made on the basis of the characteristic rotational nystagmus, which develops after a latent period and adapts and fatigues on performing the Hallpike manoeuvres (Chapters 3 and 14).

Cupulolithiasis, in which debris from the otolith organ become attached to the cupula of the posterior semicircular canal, was the pathophysiological mechanism (Fig 15.1) that was first proposed to explain this condition. When the patient assumed a critical head position, usually with the neck extended and the head turned to right or left, it was postulated that a burst of neuronal activity arising from the crista of the posterior semicircular canal would result from the 'heavy' cupula, which had become hypersensitive to the effect of gravity in the critical head position. However, more recent work has led to the theory of canalithiasis, which better explains all the characteristic features of benign positional nystagmus.[19] This theory proposes that debris of calcium carbonate crystals forms in the most dependent portion of the posterior canal and, when a critical head position is assumed, the debris moves in an ampullofugal direction, thus having a 'plunger' effect within the narrow posterior semicircular canal. This causes movement of the cupula in an ampullofugal direction, with a brief paroxysm of vertigo and nystagmus as a result.

This new hypothesis of the pathophysiological mechansim of benign positional vertigo of paroxysmal type has rationalized the development of new management techniques. Cawthorne–Cooksey exercises were previously used in the treatment of this condition, but were considerably less effective than in the management of peripheral vestibular disorders, with evidence of abnormalities of horizontal semicircular canal function. In 1980, Brandt and Daroff[20] reported complete relief of symptoms in 66 out of 67 patients with benign positional vertigo as a result of precipitating head positions 'on a repeated and serial basis' (Fig 15.2). On the basis of the canalithiasis model, it seems likely that these manoeuvres cleared the debris from the most dependent part of the posterior semicircular canal into the utricle, where it is presumed that it disperses or becomes attached to the lining and can, therefore, no longer interfere with semicircular canal dynamics.

More recently, details of single positional manoeuvres[21,22] have been published that rely on the anatomical configuration of the posterior semicircular canal and the ability to move the head in such a way as to allow the offending debris in the posterior canal to migrate, by gravitation, via the common crus into the utricle (Fig 15.3). Epley[22] has advised the use of mastoid vibration to ensure that, at each stage of the manoeuvre, all the debris is transferred to the most dependent part of the canal.

The patient is instructed to avoid lying flat for at least 2 days after the manoeuvre is performed, to prevent the debris re-entering the posterior canal orifice. Most workers have recommended that the manoeuvre be repeated at least twice, particularly if the patient continues to be symptomatic after the initial treatment. There are rare reports of patients becoming acutely vertiginous while the repositioning procedure is being performed, and it has been suggested that this is the result of debris becoming obstructed in the posterior semicircular canal. Patients may require sedation and antiemetics and immediate 'reversal' of the positions adopted during the particle repositioning procedure, together with mastoid vibration, to 'clear' the canal.

Approximately 10–20 per cent of patient suffer a relapse or are not cured by the initial manoeuvre, and typically this recurrence is relieved by repeating the procedure. Pretreatment sedation is not

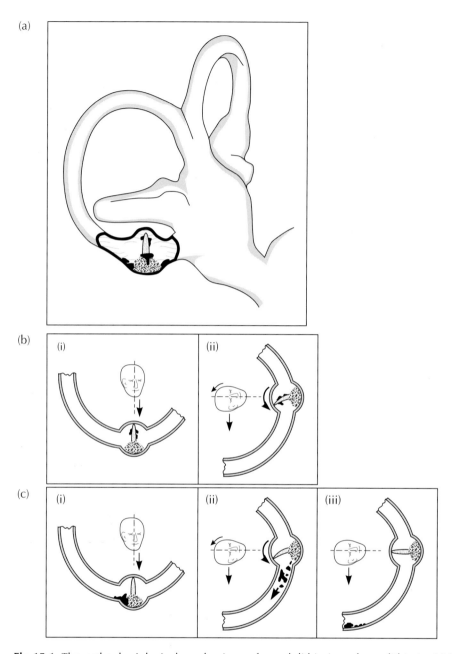

Fig 15.1 The pathophysiological mechanisms of cupulolithiasis and canalithiasis. (a) The cupula in the ampulla of the posterior semicricular canal, with debris attached to and surrounding the cupula. (b) The effect of gravity on the cupula and debris as proposed by the theory of cupulolithiasis. (c) The effect of gravity on the cupula and debris as proposed by the theory of canalithiasis. (Reproduced from Brandt and Steddin[18] with permission.)

required, except for the most anxious of patients. After the procedure some 10–20 per cent of patients are reported to feel a persistent unsteadiness or disorientation, or both, which may last for up to 1 week. In a small percentage of patients, it would appear that the particle repositioning procedure may not be effective and, in intractable cases, plugging of the posterior semicircular canal or section of the posterior ampullary nerve may be considered (Chapter 38).

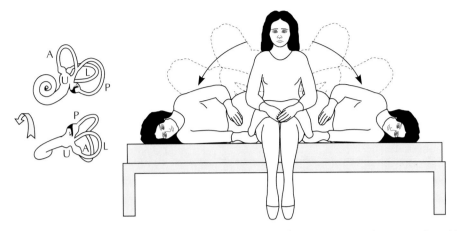

Fig 15.2 Brandt–Daroff exercises. A, anterior; L, lateral; P, posterior; U, utricle. (Reproduced from Brandt and Daroff[20] with permission.)

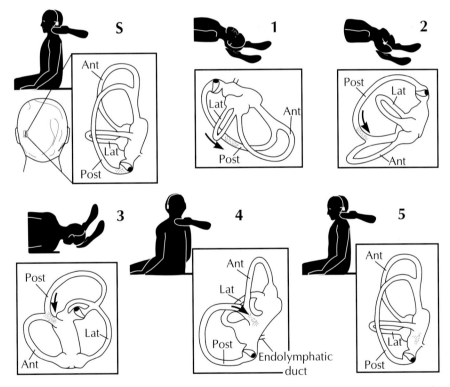

Fig 15.3 The particle repositioning procedure for canalithiasis of left posterior semicircular canal as described by Epley. (Reproduced from Epley[22] with permission.)

CHRONIC CENTRAL VESTIBULAR SYMPTOMS

The management of central vestibular dysfunction remains poorly understood and empirical in approach. Neurological disorders associated with vertical nystagmus, such as multiple sclerosis, brain-stem strokes and the Arnold–Chiari malformation, may give rise to persistent oscillopsia with dysequilibrium and marked nausea. Such symptoms are extremely distressing and, indeed, to the inexperienced clinician may appear out of proportion to the clinical signs. In this situation clonazepam, titrating the dose against sedative side effects, may be of value, as may baclofen, limiting the dose to avoid the side effect of muscular weakness in this instance.

In patients with pathology involving the brainstem or cerebellum, or both, there may be evidence of central vestibular dysfunction, with bidirectional direction changing or dysconjugate horizontal nystagmus and derangements of eye movements, including dysmetric saccades and disordered pursuit and optokinetic responses. In these cases, a trial of cinnarizine should be attempted, although the success rate is low. Additionally, carbamazepine or clonazepam have been reported to be of value in individual cases. In those patients who have a sense of instability and falls, which are frequently associated with basal ganglia disorders and cerebellar disease, physiotherapy to teach alternative gait strategies may prove invaluable in enabling them to regain a sense of confidence and improve their stability.

VESTIBULAR REHABILITATION AND SURGERY

Two conditions associated with chronic or recurrent vertigo that require early surgical intervention are chronic suppurative otitis media, with cholesteatoma (erosive middle ear disease) and, much more rarely, the possibility of a perilymph fistula (see Chapter 38).

In Ménière's disease active intermittent labyrinthine activity may, rarely, justify a destructive operation (Chapter 38). It cannot be overemphasized that before any destructive vestibular surgery sophisticated vestibular investigations must confirm the abnormal diseased side, and the possibility of bilateral disease must also be considered. The cardinal points to emphasize are

- a destructive operation can only offer benefit for changing erratic, intermittent, activity – it cannot help the problems of vestibular deficit
- rehabilitation is effective only for fixed deficits with an unchanging (or very slowly changing) vestibular state; it is of no use in the presence of active disease causing irregular intermittent vestibular stimuli
- all possible factors that may prevent adequate compensation should be considered and any possible remediation attempted before destructive surgery
- vestibular compensation is less effective and slower in older subjects and those with neurological disease
- there is no reason to believe that compensation for a total vestibular failure will be more rapid or more effective than for a partial vestibular loss

Conclusion

Aggressive, early vestibular rehabilitation based on specific physical exercise regimes and supported by appropriate psychological management is the cornerstone of rapid and efficient vestibular recovery for chronic peripheral vestibular disorders. Such a regime is highly effective in unilateral and bilateral vestibular dysfunction of peripheral type. The treatment of choice for benign positional vertigo of paroxysmal type is a particle-liberating manoeuvre of the type described by Epley[22] and Semont *et al.*[21] Surgical measures for treating causes of vertigo are discussed in Chapter 38.

References

1. Lacour M, Xerri C. Vestibular compensation: new perspectives. In: Flohr H, Precht W eds. *Lesion-induced neuronal plasticity in sensorimotor systems.* Berlin: Springer–Verlag, 1984:240–53.
2. Luxon LM. Vestibular compensation. In: Luxon LM, Davies RA eds. *A handbook of vestibular rehabilitation.* London: Whurr, 1996.
3. Zee DS. The management of patients with vestibular disorders. In: Barber HO, Sharpe JA eds. *Vestibular disorders.* Chicago: Year Book Medical Publishers, 1988:254–74.
4. Shumway-Cook A, Horak FB. Rehabilitation strategies for patients with vestibular deficits. *Neurology Clinics of North America* 1990; **8**:441–57.
5. Cawthorne TE. Vestibular injuries. *Proceedings of the Royal Society of Medicine* 1945; **39**:270–3.
6. Cooksey FS. Rehabilitation of vestibular injuries. *Proceedings of the Royal Society of Medicine* 1945; **39**:273–8.
7. Dix MR, Rehabilitation of vertigo. In: Dix MR, Hood JD eds. *Vertigo.* Chichester: Wiley and Sons, 1984:23–39.
8. Norré ME. Rationale of rehabilitation treatment for vertigo. *American Journal of Otolaryngology* 1987; **8**:31–5.
9. Sheprad NT, Telian SA, Smith-Wheelock M. Habituation and balance retraining therapy: a retrospective review. *Neurologic Clinics* 1990; **8**:459–75.
10. Norré ME, Beckers A. Benign paroxysmal positional vertigo in the elderly, treatment by habituation exercises. *Journal of American Geriatric Society* 1988; **36**:425–9.
11. Shepard NT, Telian SA, Smith-Wheelock M, Raj A. Vestibular and balance rehabilitation therapy. *Annals of Otology, Rhinology and Laryngology* 1993; **102**:198–204.
12. Herdman SJ. *Vestibular rehabilitation.* Philadelphia: FA Davis, 1994.
13. Yardley L, Luxon LM. Treating dizziness with vestibular rehabilitation. *British Medical Journal* 1994; **308**:1252–3.

14. Eagger S, Luxon LM, Davies RA, Coehlo A, Ron MA. Psychiatric morbidity in patients with peripheral vestibular disorder: a clinical and neuro-otological study. *Journal of Neurology, Neurosurgery and Psychiatry* 1992; **55**:383–7.

15. Laczko-Schroeder T. Psychological aspects. In: Luxon LM, Davies RA eds. *A handbook of vestibular rehabilitation*. London: Whurr, 1996.

16. Davidson A. Behavioural psychotherapy. In: Luxon LM, Davies RA eds. *A handbook of vestibular rehabilitation*. London: Whurr, 1996.

17. Takemori S, Ida M, Umezu H. Vestibular training after sudden loss of vestibular function. *ORL Journal of Otorhinolaryngology and Related Specialties* 1985; **47**:76–83.

18. Brandt T, Steddin S. Current view of the mechanism of benign paroxysmal positioning vertigo: cupulolithiasis or canalolithiasis? *Journal of Vestibular Research* 1993; **3**:373–82.

19. Baloh RW. Benign positional vertigo. In: Baloh RW, Halmagyi M eds. *Handbook of neuro-otology/ vestibular system*. New York: Oxford University Press, 1996.

20. Brandt T, Daroff RB. Physical therapy for benign paroxysmal positional vertigo. *Archives of Otolaryngology* 1980; **106**:484–5.

21. Semont A, Freyss G, Vitte E. Curing BPPV with a liberatory manoeuvre. *Advances in Otorhinolaryngology* 1988; **42**:290–3.

22. Epley JM. The canalith repositioning procedure: for treatment of benign paroxysmal positional vertigo. *Otolaryngology – Head and Neck Surgery* 1992; **107**:399–404.

Facial nerve paralysis

CHAPTER 16

Tests of facial nerve function

DAVID A MOFFAT

Introduction

Clinical testing of facial nerve function is an essential part of otological practice. An accurate and detailed knowledge of the motor and sensory anatomical pathways of the facial nerve and the physiological functions that it subserves is a vital prerequisite to this and to the development of clinical acumen in the management of facial palsy.

Anatomy of the facial nerve

The facial nerve is the nerve of the second branchial arch, which explains its complex and intimate relationships with the middle ear cleft and the ossicular chain (see Chapter 1). The nerve possesses a motor and a sensory root, the latter called the *nervus intermedius*. The two roots appear at the lower border of the pons just lateral to the recess between the olive and the inferior cerebellar peduncle, the motor part being the more medial. The vestibulocochlear nerve lies immediately to the lateral side of the sensory root.

The motor fibres supply the muscles of facial expression, scalp and auricle, the buccinator, platysma, stapedius and stylohyoid muscles and the posterior belly of the digastric muscle. The sensory root conveys taste fibres via the chorda tympani nerve for the anterior two-thirds of the tongue, and, from the palatine and greater petrosal nerves, the fibres of taste from the soft palate.

The sensory root also conveys secretomotor preganglionic parasympathetic fibres for submandibular and sublingual salivary glands, for the lachrymal gland and for the glands of the nasal and palatine mucosa. In addition, some evidence suggests that there may be cutaneous sensory fibres from a small area of the external ear, accounting for the distribution of the vesication in herpes zoster oticus.

The motor fibres have their cell bodies in the facial nucleus, which is in the reticular formation of the lower part of the pons. It is situated behind the dorsal nucleus of the trapezoid body and ventrimedial to the nucleus of the spinal tract of the trigeminal nerve. The nucleus receives pyramidal fibres from the contralateral motor cortex and a smaller number from the homolateral side (Fig 16.1). In addition, some of the efferent fibres of the facial nerve take origin from the *superior salivatory nucleus*, which lies in the reticular formation, dorsilateral to the caudal end of the motor nucleus. It represents the general visceral efferent column, and it sends its fibres to join the sensory root, by which they are ultimately distributed through the chorda tympani to the submandibular and sublingual salivary glands. Fibres from the spinal tract of the trigeminal nerve and fibres from the corpus trapezoideum play upon the facial nucleus. The motor fibres sweep around the nucleus of the VIth cranial nerve and emerge from the brainstem at the lower border of the pons between the olive and the inferior cerebellar peduncle (Fig 16.2). Crossing the cerebellopontine angle in a lateral and forward direction, the nerve is closely related to the two divisions of the auditory nerve, the nervus intermedius and posteriorly the anterior inferior cerebellar artery. The nerve enters the temporal bone through the porus acousticus and internal auditory canal together with the cochlear nerve, the nervus intermedius and the internal auditory artery and veins, all these structures being ensheathed in a prolongation of the subarachnoid space with its meninges (Fig 16.3).

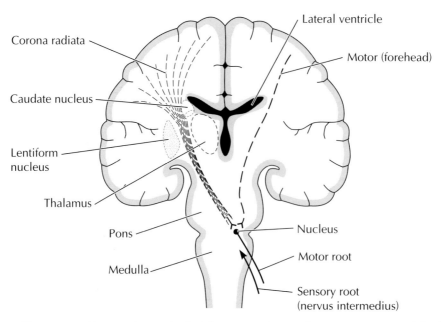

Fig 16.1 The source of innervation to the facial nerve nucleus in the pontine portion of the brainstem derives from the contralateral hemisphere, which supplies all of the nucleus, and from the ipsilateral hemisphere, which supplies that portion of the nucleus that supplies the forehead. The sensory root of the facial nerve enters the brainstem separate from the main trunk as the nervus intermedius.

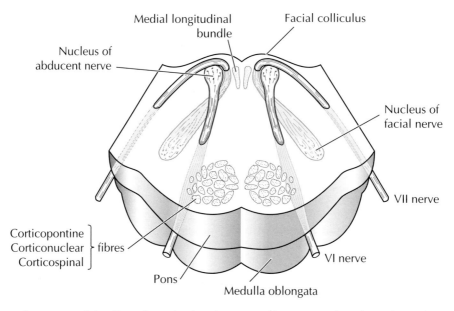

Fig 16.2 The course of the fibres from the facial nerve nucleus is not directly to the surface of the brainstem but by a tortuous route that turns around the nucleus of the VIth (abducent) nerve nucleus in the floor of the fourth ventricle.

(a)

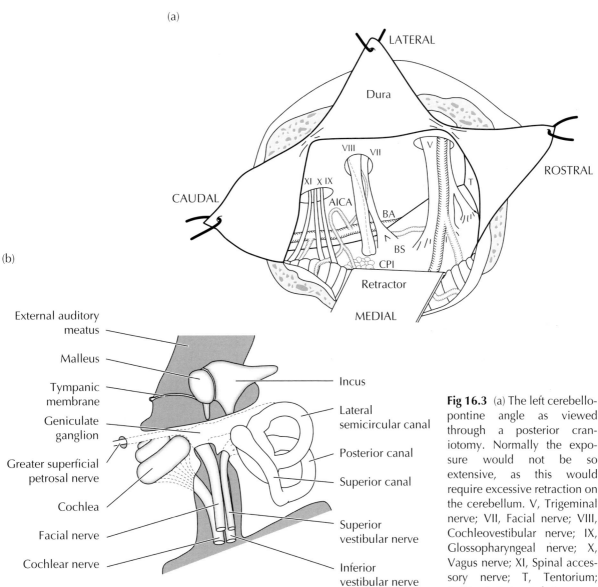

(b)

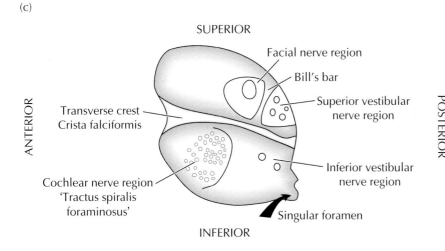

(c)

Fig 16.3 (a) The left cerebello-pontine angle as viewed through a posterior craniotomy. Normally the exposure would not be so extensive, as this would require excessive retraction on the cerebellum. V, Trigeminal nerve; VII, Facial nerve; VIII, Cochleovestibular nerve; IX, Glossopharyngeal nerve; X, Vagus nerve; XI, Spinal accessory nerve; T, Tentorium; AICA, Anterior inferior cerebellar artery; BA, Basilar artery; BS, Brainstem; CPI, Choroid plexus. (b) A diagrammatic view of the floor of right middle cranial fossa with the internal auditory meatus opened to show the disposition of the nerves. In reality the cochlear and vestibular nerves have joined to form a single large bundle by the time they enter the cerebellopontine angle. (c) A view of the apex of the right internal auditory meatus as seen from the cerebellopontine angle with the contents of the canal removed.

At the fundus or lateral extremity of the internal auditory canal the nerve continues, with the nervus intermedius, into the bony Fallopian canal, which runs laterally above the vestibule (the labyrinthine portion of the facial nerve), separated from the middle cranial fossa by a thin layer of bone. Upon reaching the medial wall of the epitympanic recess, it bends sharply backwards above the promontory and arches downwards in the medial wall of the aditus to the tympanic antrum. The point at which it bends sharply backwards is the first genu, at which point it manifests a reddish ganglioform swelling, the geniculate ganglion. In some cases the bony roof of the canal is absent, so that the ganglion is directly related to the dura mater.

From the geniculate ganglion the nerve runs posteriorly and slightly inferiorly in the medial wall of the tympanum. Here the bony Fallopian canal forms a cylindrical ridge familiar to otologists as the tympanic course of the nerve, lying slightly inferior to the horizontal semicircular canal and superior to the oval window and promontory. The anterior limit of this section of the nerve is marked by the processus cochleariformis with its emerging tensor tympani tendon, a valuable landmark (Fig 16.4).

In the bony floor of the aditus the nerve makes a gradual bend, the second genu, turning inferiorly 1 or 2 mm behind the pyramid to the commencement of the vertical or mastoid segment. This descending

(a)

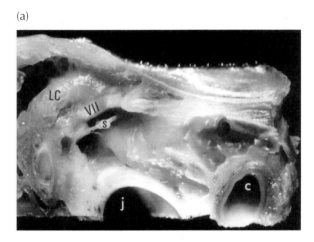

(b)

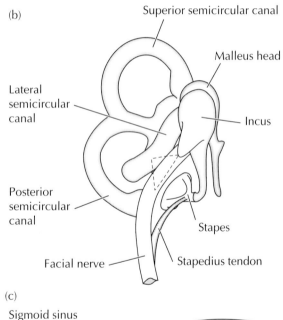

(c)

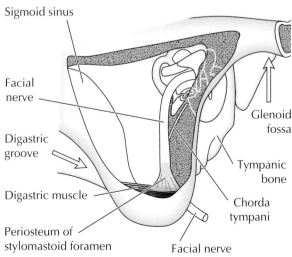

Fig 16.4 (a) A longitudinal section of the right temporal bone viewed from a lateral aspect. The section has passed through the incudostapedial joint and the facial nerve can be seen above the stapes (S) with the processus cochlearformis anterior and the tensor tympani running along the roof of the Eustachian tube, above the internal carotid artery (C). The jugular bulb (J) lies in the floor of the middle ear. Superior and posterior to the facial nerve is the dome of the lateral semicircular canal (LC). Posterior to this is the mastoid antrum. The descending portion of the facial nerve has just been uncapped by the sectioning posterior and a little inferior to the pyramid and the stapedius tendon. (b) The relationship between the short process of the incus, the lateral semicircular canal and the second turn of the facial nerve as it becomes the descending portion. The dimensions of the sides of the triangle adjacent to the right angle are of the order of 1.5 mm. (c) The descending portion of the facial nerve in a cortical mastoid cavity with a posterior tympanotomy.

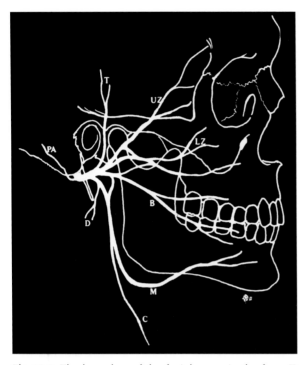

Fig 16.5 The branches of the facial nerve in the face. T, Temporal; UZ, Upper zygomatic; LZ, Lower zygomatic; B, Buccal; M, Mandibular; C, Cervical; PA, Postauricular.

portion of the facial nerve runs directly inferior to the stylomastoid foramen and is surrounded by the mastoid air cells. It is rarely less than 2 cm from the outer mastoid surface in the adult.

On emerging from the stylomastoid foramen, the facial nerve runs forwards in the substance of the parotid salivary gland, crosses the styloid process, the retromandibular vein and the external carotid artery, and divides behind the vertical ramus of the mandible into five main branches, the *pes anserinus*, comprising, from above downwards, temporal, zygomatic, buccal, mandibular and cervical (Fig 16.5). These supply the muscles of facial expression.

The sensory nucleus of the facial nerve is the upper part of the nucleus of the tractus solitarius in the medulla oblongata. The sensory root or nervus intermedius contains efferent preganglionic parasympathetic nerve fibres originating in the superior salivatory nucleus. At the geniculate ganglion these fibres mingle with those of the motor nerve trunk. Those destined to innervate the submandibular and sublingual glands continue in the facial nerve as far as the chorda tympani. They finally arrive at the submandibular ganglion by way of the chorda tympani and the lingual nerve. Parasympathetic motor fibres supplying the lachrymal gland leave the geniculate ganglion in the

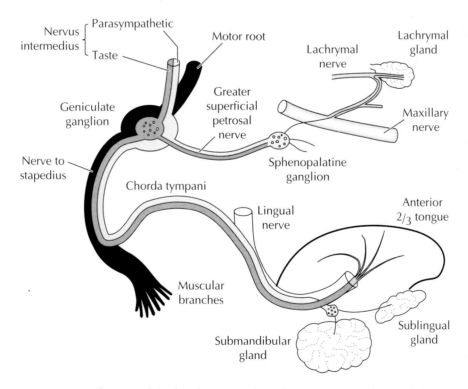

Fig 16.6 Composite diagram of the facial nerve: its branches, constituent fibres and distribution.

greater superficial petrosal nerve and reach their destination by way of the vidian nerve, the maxillary nerve and its zygomatic branch. The secreto-motor fibres for the nasal mucosa leave the facial nerve by the same route. The taste fibres from the anterior two-thirds of the tongue travel in the lingual nerve and then join the facial nerve by way of the chorda tympani. After ascending in the facial nerve, the taste fibres have their cell bodies in the geniculate ganglion. From the palate taste fibres first follow the palatine nerves, and then pass through the sphenopalatine ganglion, vidian nerve and greater superficial petrosal nerve to reach the geniculate ganglion. The central axons of all these taste neurons continue in the nervus intermedius to the brainstem. Their final destination is the tractus solitarius.

BRANCHES OF THE FACIAL NERVE

From proximal to distal the branches of the facial nerve are as follows (Fig 16.6). First, the *greater superficial petrosal nerve*, which comes off at the geniculate ganglion. Second, the *nerve to stapedius*, which arises from the facial nerve opposite the pyramidal eminence on the posterior wall of the mesotympanum. It passes forwards through a small canal to reach the stapedius muscle. Third, the *chorda tympani nerve* arises from the facial nerve usually 6 mm from the stylomastoid foramen, but the distance is variable and it may be anywhere from 1 to 2 mm below the nerve to stapedius to the stylomastoid foramen. Furthermore, the chorda tympani may emanate from the front, lateral, or posterior aspect of the nerve trunk. These variables can create difficulties in operations on the nerve if the chorda is used as a landmark for the main trunk. Fourth, the *posterior auricular nerve* supplying the occipitofrontalis and external auricular muscles, the *digastric branch* to the posterior belly of the digastric muscle and the *stylohyoid branch* to the stylohyoid muscle all arise close to the stylomastoid foramen. Fifth, the final fanwise branching of the facial nerve has five main branches:

- *temporal branches* supply the intrinsic muscles on the lateral surface of the auricle, the anterior and superior auricle muscles, the frontal belly of the occipitofrontalis, the orbicularis oculi and the corrugator
- *zygomatic branches* supply the orbicularis oculi muscle
- *buccal branches* supply the procerus, zygomaticus major and levator labii superioris; they also supply levator anguli oris, zygomaticus minor, levator labii superioris, alaeque nasi and the small muscles of the nose

- the *mandibular branch* supplies depressor anguli oris, depressor labii inferioris, mentalis orbicularis oris and risorius
- the *cervical branch* supplies the platysma muscle.

Clinical testing of facial nerve function

The first thing the clinician should do is to observe the patient's face at rest and during movement while talking and with emotion looking for asymmetry, hemifacial spasm and facial tics. Close observation of blinking at rest is very important because delay in blinking may be the earliest manifestation of a facial palsy.

THE BLINK TEST

The patient is asked to stare at the examiner who then suddenly taps the patient on the glabella with their forefinger. The ensuing blink is then studied and a delay in blinking on one side may be noted due to facial weakness.

TESTING FACIAL MOVEMENT

The temporal branches are tested by asking the patient to wrinkle the forehead and elevate the eyebrows. The zygomatic branches are assessed by asking the patient to screw up the eyes, the buccal by wrinkling the nose, the mandibular by showing the teeth and blowing out the cheeks and the cervical by grimacing.

In an attempt to reduce interobserver variability in the assessment of the degree of facial weakness, a standardized, internationally acceptable system for reporting recovery of facial function after injury to the facial nerve has been established (Table 16.1).[1]

An illustration of the six grades of facial function on the House–Brackmann grading system can be seen in Figure 16.7.

The first diagnostic decision involves the recognition that the paralysis is due to a lower motor neuron lesion. This is not always as straightforward as it may seem. Indicators of an upper motor neuron lesion would be associated central nervous system abnormalities and sparing of the forehead, but lower motor neuron palsies may be seen in which only the lower face is affected, and the distinction can then sometimes be difficult.

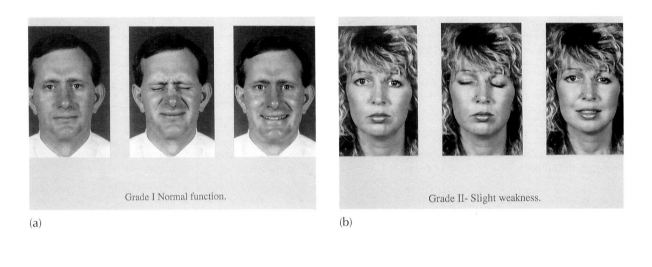

(a)

Grade I Normal function.

(b)

Grade II- Slight weakness.

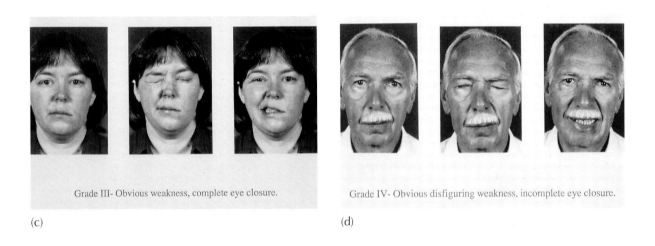

(c)

Grade III- Obvious weakness, complete eye closure.

(d)

Grade IV- Obvious disfiguring weakness, incomplete eye closure.

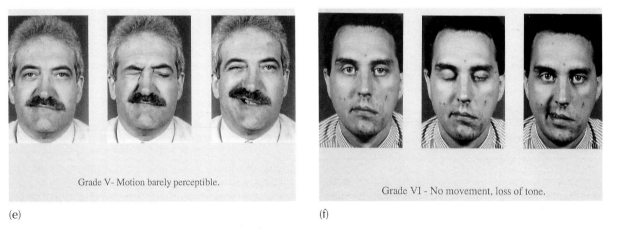

(e)

Grade V- Motion barely perceptible.

(f)

Grade VI - No movement, loss of tone.

Fig 16.7 (a)–(f) Typical examples of the six House–Brackmann grades of facial nerve paralysis. Grade I is normal and grade VI is a complete flaccid paralysis. These figures should be viewed in conjunction with Table 16.1.

Table 16.1 Classification system for reporting results of recovery from facial paralysis

Degree of injury	Grade	Definition
Normal	I	Normal symmetrical function in all areas
Mild dysfunction (barely noticeable)	II	Slight weakness noticeable only on close inspection. Complete eye closure with minimal effort. Slight asymmetry of smile with maximal effort. Synkinesis barely noticeable, contracture, or spasm absent
Moderate dysfunction (obvious difference)	III	Obvious weakness, but not disfiguring. May not be able to lift eyebrow. Complete eye closure and strong but asymmetrical mouth movement with maximal effort. Obvious, but not disfiguring synkinesis, mass movement or spasm
Moderately severe dysfunction	IV	Obvious disfiguring weakness. Inability to lift brow. Incomplete eye closure and asymmetry of mouth with maximal effort. Severe synkinesis, mass movement, spasm
Severe dysfunction	V	Motion barely perceptible. Incomplete eye closure, slight movement of corner of mouth. Synkinesis, contracture, spasm usually absent
Total paralysis	VI	No movement, loss of tone, no synkinesis, contracture or spasm

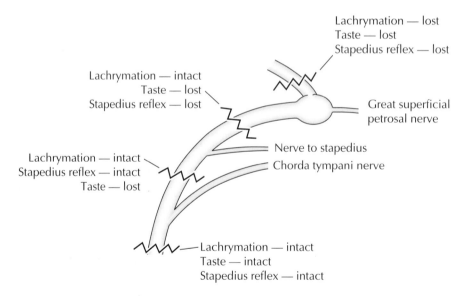

Fig 16.8 Results of topognostic testing in the presence of lesions to the facial nerve at different sites.

Topognostic testing

Topognostic testing is sometimes helpful in determining the site of a facial nerve injury (Fig 16.8) and requires the foregoing anatomical knowledge of its branches.

In a nuclear lesion in the pons, only the motor functions of the nerve will be affected, with no disturbance of taste or lachrymation or salivation or loss of the stapedial reflex. There may be involvement of other brainstem structures, such as the nucleus of the VIth nerve.

A lesion in the cerebellopontine angle, within the internal auditory canal, within the intralabyrinthine segment or at the geniculate ganglion will impair lachrymation, the stapedial reflex and taste and salivation on the same side.

If the lesion is between the geniculate ganglion and the nerve to stapedius, lachrymation will be intact but the stapedius reflex and taste on the anterior two-thirds of the tongue (and salivation) will be lost on the ipsilateral side.

If the lesion is between the nerve to stapedius and the chorda tympani nerve, lachrymation and the stapedius reflex will be intact but taste on the anterior two-thirds of the tongue on the ipsilateral side will be impaired.

In a lesion below the level of the chorda tympani there will be a pure motor deficit, with intact lachrymation, stapedial reflex, taste and salivation.

The Schirmer test, the stapedial reflex test and testing taste are recommended by some authors as a means of preoperative localization of the site of a VIIth nerve injury, but electrogustometry and submandibular gland flow testing are of less diagnostic value.[2]

SCHIRMER TEST

The technique for the Schirmer test is as follows. Two strips of paper are folded and placed in the lower conjunctival fornix for 5 minutes. Lambert and Brackmann[3] describe an abnormal Schirmer test as being a decrease of lachrymation of 75 per cent or more on the affected side as measured by the amount of paper soaked by tears on each side, or a bilateral decrease in lachrymation (less than 10 mm for both sides at 5 minutes). The latter may be due to the fact that unilateral injury to the geniculate ganglion can paradoxically cause a bilateral reduction in lachrymation.

STAPEDIAL REFLEX TESTING

Stapedial reflex testing is accomplished at the time of impedance testing, and should be part of comprehensive audiometrical evaluation indicated for all patients with facial nerve weakness after head trauma. If the stapedial reflex is absent in the face of normal hearing, then the site of lesion is likely to be between the geniculate ganglion and the stapedius muscle. If the reflex is present, then the site of the lesion is distal to the stapedius muscle.

TESTING TASTE

Taste testing kits include four bottles containing solutions that are concentrated sweet, salt, sour and bitter. The patient is asked to protrude the tongue and it is gently rubbed with a cotton bud soaked in the solution being tested along the lateral margin in the anterior two-thirds towards the tip. It is important to ensure that that the patient does not retract the tongue into the mouth because the taste receptors inside the mouth will render the result invalid. The patient is then asked to rinse out the mouth with water and the second modality is introduced. The results of the responses to all four flavours are recorded and compared with the other side.

Electrogustometry is an electrical method of testing taste. A small current is applied to the lateral border of the protruded tongue in its anterior two-thirds via a metal rod angulated at its tip. The current is slowly increased in a stepwise fashion until the patient perceives a metallic taste. A normal threshold is about 1 mA and this may be raised to 4 mA if the chorda tympani is involved. The threshold on the test side is then compared with the contralateral side.

Electrogustometry can also be used as a test of greater superficial petrosal nerve integrity, by applying the same stimulus to the taste buds of the palate.

SUBMANDIBULAR GLAND FLOW

Submandibular gland activity can be compared on the two sides by sialometry. Under local anaesthetic polythene tubes are passed into Wharton's ducts after probing with a stylet. Salivation is provoked by a stimulus of 6 per cent citric acid on the anterior part of the tongue. The measurement of the number of drops of saliva from each side during 1 minute, or until the total flow reaches, say, 25 drops.

Electrodiagnosis and the severity of the lesion

The question that is of paramount importance to the otolaryngologist is which facial nerve palsy will recover and which will not. In the past 2 decades, this question has led to the development of electrical tests to determine the status of the facial nerve and predict its potential for recovery. The electrical tests that offer the most useful information are the maximal stimulation test and electroneuronography. These are tests of nerve conductivity and can demonstrate evidence of degeneration as early as 3 days after the onset of the paralysis. The nerve is stimulated through the skin with an electrode.

MINIMAL EXCITABILITY TEST

This test determines the minimal current necessary to stimulate muscle movement when applied to a branch of the facial nerve. The Hilger nerve stimulator was designed for use in this test. A comparison is made between the normal and abnormal sides, and a difference of 3.5 mA or greater between the two sides is thought to be significant and an indicator for surgical decompression of the facial nerve.[4]

MAXIMAL STIMULATION TEST

The maximal stimulation test (MST) was first described by May *et al.*[5] in 1971 and represents an evolution of the minimal excitability test. The MST also utilizes the Hilger nerve stimulator at the highest setting tolerated by the patient, usually 5 mA or greater. The response of the involved side is compared with the normal side and evaluated as an equal response, a reduced response or an absent response. Degeneration of the nerve is inferred from total loss of nerve excitability. Neurapraxia does not raise the threshold, whereas partial degeneration raises the threshold above that of the contralateral side. May *et al.*[5] found this test to be more accurate in predicting facial nerve outcome after injury. Interestingly, the MST is of no value for the first 72 hours after injury. Normal values are obtained during this period, even in facial nerves that have been completely transected. This means that nerve conduction tests may show evidence of degeneration as early as 3 days after the onset of the paralysis and the longer after that time that the normal threshold is maintained, the more likely it is that the lesion has caused only a neurapraxia. Frequent testing, even daily, will allow recognition of continuing degeneration by a progressively rising threshold.

ELECTRONEURONOGRAPHY

Electroneuronography (ENoG) was described by Esslen[6] and popularized by Fisch.[7] ENoG records the actual compound action potential of the facial nerve after stimulation. May *et al.*[8] have used the term 'evoked electromyography' or EEMG, which is probably more accurate, because it is the compound action potentials of muscle fibres that are measured. The stimulating electrode is placed on the skin over the stylomastoid foramen and a supramaximal stimulation is applied to ensure that all functioning nerve fibres are stimulated. The recording electrode is placed in the region of the nasolabial fold, which has been shown to be the optimal site for this electrode.[9] The stimulus is gradually increased in magnitude until there is no further increase in the amplitude of the response. Again, the normal side is compared with the abnormal side. The amplitude loss on the involved side is directly proportional to the degree of degeneration taking place in the nerve. Therefore, if the amplitude of the affected side is 25 per cent of the normal side, a 75 per cent degeneration has occurred in the abnormal facial nerve. May[10] recommended surgery when the amplitude of the affected side was 25 per cent of the normal side. Esslen[6] has shown, however, that the majority of patients with less than 90 per cent degeneration will have complete recovery of facial nerve function, prompting the majority of authors to advocate the figure of 10 per cent or less amplitude of the affected side compared with the normal as a more appropriate indicator for surgical decompression. Fisch[11,12] has recommended surgical intervention within 3 weeks in patients in whom traumatic injury has resulted in 90 per cent amplitude reduction by ENoG testing within 6 days of the injury. Current recommendations are for operative exploration as soon as the patient's condition permits in cases of immediate paralysis with greater than 90 per cent degeneration.

Like the MST, ENoG is not useful for at least 72 hours after injury, and most authors advocate that testing begin on the third or fourth day after the trauma.

STRENGTH–DURATION CURVES

Strength–duration curves (SD curves) are obtained by plotting the current intensity of a stimulus delivered to the muscle against the time required to excite. They are not used as frequently as previously. The current is generated by a constant output muscle stimulator, which delivers an impulse of rectangular form, selectable between 0 and 5 mA. The threshold value of the current is plotted along the ordinate, and the duration of the stimulus in milliseconds logarithmically along the abscissa. The threshold for an indefinitely long stimulus is called rheobase, and the time needed for a stimulus of twice the rheobase is called chronaxie. In degeneration the rheobase becomes increasingly ineffective below 100 ms, and the curve is displaced to the right, becoming kinked if degeneration is partial. Strength–duration curves do not begin to show abnormalities until degeneration reaches and involves the motor end-plate in the muscles, which may take as long as 2 or 3 weeks. Improvement in the curve may precede recovery of voluntary movement in the muscles.

ELECTROMYOGRAPHY

Measurement of the electrical activity in muscle is useful to demonstrate the survival of motor units, implying preservation of some intact nerve fibres; the presence of fibrillation potentials, indicating denervation; and an indication of recovery before it is clinically apparent. As evidence of denervation does not become manifest for 2 weeks after the onset of the paralysis, its value is for assessing prognosis in those patients whose nerve degeneration has already been shown by nerve conduction studies.

At rest, normal muscle shows no electrical activity. On the insertion of a needle electrode, normal muscle responds to the stimulus with a brief shower of normal insertion action potentials. Denervated muscle may demonstrate abnormal insertion fibrillation potentials. On voluntary contraction of normal muscle fibres, normal motor unit potentials appear, building up to what is called normal interference pattern. Lesions that affect the motor neuron to the point of denervation of muscle result in a reduction of motor unit activity, revealed electromyographically by failure of the motor unit potentials, on maximal volition, to form a normal interference pattern.

Degeneration of a lower motor neuron is followed in about 2 weeks by spontaneous activity in the muscle supplied, detected as fibrillation potentials.

The electrical potentials detected by the needle electrode are, after amplification, transmitted to a loudspeaker, measured on a meter, and displayed on an oscilloscope screen for observation and photography or printout. An individual motor unit potential is usually diphasic with a duration of 3–10 ms and an amplitude between $100\,\mu V$ and $2\,\mu V$. The complete interference pattern, resulting from asynchrony of motor firing, is characterized by a completely disturbed baseline on the screen audible as a low rumbling from the loudspeaker. Fibrillation potentials produce a repetitive clicking noise and appear as small diphasic potentials of 1–2 ms duration and amplitudes less than $100\,\mu V$.

Complete degeneration cannot be shown by electromyography (EMG) until about 2 weeks after the onset, and often longer. Insertion fibrillation potentials may appear by the sixth day, but sustained fibrillation comes much later. The presence of some motor unit potentials in response to voluntary efforts indicates that some nerve fibres are intact. Increasing signs of spontaneous motor unit activity, in the absence of voluntary efforts at contraction, are unfavourable features with regard to denervation.

Electromyography can demonstrate the earliest signs of recovery. First fibrillation ceases, and then polyphasic motor unit potentials appear, which may precede the return of facial movement by up to 12 weeks. They are explained by dispersion of the neural stimulus, temporally because of variation in the conduction rates of the regenerating fibres, and spatially because the regenerating fibres branch to supply more muscle fibres each. Their appearance is sought while the patient attempts voluntary contraction, and they indicate the continuity of some fibres, and that regeneration is under way. If the wasted muscle becomes converted to scar tissue, as it will after 18–24 months, fibrillation potentials disappear, and the electrical output becomes silent.

Electromyography is not helpful in the evaluation of facial paralysis of recent onset. It does not demonstrate denervation potentials until 8–10 days after denervation has occurred.[6] All electrical testing is therefore limited by the fact that it cannot provide an indication of the status of the facial nerve in the immediate postinjury state.

References

1. House JW, Brackmann DE. Facial nerve grading system. *Otolaryngology – Head and Neck Surgery* 1985; **93**:146–7.
2. Hough JVD, McGee M. Otological trauma. In: Paparella MM, Shumrick DA, Gluckman JL, Meyerhoff WL eds. *Otolaryngology*. London: WB Saunders, 1991:1137–60.
3. Lambert PR, Brackmann DE. Facial paralysis in longitudinal temporal bone factures: a review of 26 cases. *Laryngoscope* 1984; **94**:1022–6.
4. Alford BR, Jerger JF, Coats AC, *et al.* Neurodiagnostic studies in facial paralysis. *Annals of Otology, Rhinology and Laryngology* 1970; **79**:227–33.
5. May M, Harvey JE, Marovitz WF, *et al.* The prognostic accuracy of the maximal stimulation test compared with that of the nerve excitability test in Bell's palsy. *Laryngoscope* 1971; **81**:931–8.
6. Esslen E. Electromyography and electroneurography. In: *Proceedings of the Third International Symposium on Facial Nerve Surgery, 9–12 Aug. 1976, Zurich, Switzerland*. Amsterdam: Kugler Medical, 1977:93–100.
7. Fisch U. Surgery for Bell's palsy. *Archives of Otolaryngology* 1981; **107**:1–11.
8. May M, Blumenthal F, Taylor FH. Bell's palsy: surgery based upon prognostic indicators and results. *Laryngoscope* 1981; **91**:2092–103.
9. Gutnick HN, Kelleher MJ, Prass RL. A model of waveform reliability in facial nerve electroneurography. *Otolaryngology – Head and Neck Surgery* 1990; **103**:344–50.
10. May M. Facial nerve paralysis. In: Paparella MM, Shumrick DA eds. *Otolaryngology, 2nd ed.* London: WB Saunders, 1980:1680–704.
11. Fisch U. Facial paralysis in fractures of the petrous bone. *Laryngoscope* 1974; **84**:2141–54.
12. Fisch U. Management of intratemporal facial nerve injuries. *Journal of Laryngology and Otology* 1980; **94**:129–34.

CHAPTER 17

Causes and management of facial paralysis

BARRY SCHAITKIN AND MARK MAY

Paralysis of the facial nerve may result from a wide variety of insults. This chapter is based on Mark May's approach to diagnosis and management, based on experiences evaluating more than 3000 patients with facial paralysis.

Anatomy of the facial nerve

The detailed anatomy of the facial nerve is described by Moffat in the preceding chapter.

Neuropathophysiology

Approximately 70 per cent of the 10 000 or so fibres in the facial nerve are myelinated motor axons to the facial muscles,[1] and the nature of facial dysfunction depends on which of these fibres is injured and to what degree. The system we use to classify facial nerve injury focuses on the potential for spontaneous return of facial function and is based on systems described by Sunderland[2] and House and Brackmann.[3]

FIRST-DEGREE AND SECOND-DEGREE INJURY AND RECOVERY

First-degree or second-degree injury to the facial nerve involves compression of the nerve and typically occurs with viral inflammatory disorders such as Bell's palsy and herpes zoster cephalicus. In a Sunderland first-degree injury to the nerve, there is no evident change in morphology when the nerve is examined histopathologically. With second-degree injury there is some loss of axons, but the endoneurial tubes remain intact.

A first-degree injury to the facial nerve is usually followed by a House–Brackmann (HB) grade I (complete) spontaneous recovery of facial muscle function beginning 1–3 weeks after nerve injury. After a second-degree injury, the axons grow into intact endoneurial tubes at the rate of about 1 mm/day, and clinical recovery of facial nerve function starts between 3 weeks and 2 months after injury. Spontaneous recovery of nerve function after a second-degree injury is usually House–Brackmann grade II (fair), with some noticeable abnormality in facial muscle movement due to faulty regeneration of nerve fibres.

THIRD-DEGREE INJURY AND RECOVERY

With third-degree injury to the facial nerve, more severe or sustained compression causes loss of myelin tubes, so that as new axons grow peripherally from the site of injury they may come to innervate a quite different facial muscle than originally. Thus when clinical recovery of facial muscle function begins (2–4 months after facial nerve injury), motor impulses from the injured portion of the nerve might cause abnormal contraction of completely different facial muscles than normally. Infectious processes such as suppurative acute otitis media or chronic otitis media with cholesteatoma and slow-growing benign neoplasms may cause second-degree or third-degree injury to the facial nerve.

Spontaneous recovery after a third-degree injury is moderate (HB grade III, obviously incomplete) to poor (HB grade IV, significant deformity) and is usually marked by complications.

SEVERE INJURY AND RECOVERY

Fourth-degree and fifth-degree injuries to the facial nerve typically occur as a result of surgical transection or trauma from a rapidly growing neoplasm.

A fourth-degree injury to the facial nerve involves not only all of the changes in the nerve characteristic of the first three degrees of injury (compression) but also disruption of the perineurium. With a fourth-degree injury, when axons start to grow towards the periphery they are blocked by scar tissue. Not only is recovery of facial nerve function delayed (clinical signs of recovery do not appear until 4–18 months after nerve injury), but recovery is usually grade V (poor). With House–Brackmann grade V recovery, complications of faulty regeneration are not as noticeable as with House–Brackmann grade III or IV recovery, but the overall result is worse because the patient has marked weakness of facial muscles on the involved side, so that facial expression is noticeably abnormal.

Fifth-degree injury to the facial nerve (transection) is followed by scarring that prevents regrowth of axons. There is thus no spontaneous recovery of facial function, and results are categorized as House–Brackmann grade VI (none). Recovery from facial paralysis is summarized in Table 16.1.

COMPLICATIONS OF NERVE REGENERATION

When facial nerve fibres regenerate, the spacing between the nodes of Ranvier changes and the myelin that covers the axon is thinner than the myelin covering normal axons. In addition, axons regenerating from one cell body may split and cross axons from another cell body. The result is that facial muscles innervated by regenerated axons may exhibit hypokinesis, hyperkinesis, or synkinesis.

Hypokinesis might occur as a result of too few regenerated fibres innervating a muscle or regenerated fibres from different branches 'competing' to innervate the muscle.

Synkinesis, or inappropriate movement of a muscle, is manifest in a tic or involuntary twitch. Synkinesis occurs when regenerating nerve fibres from one branch of the facial nerve innervate muscles originally activated by another branch of the nerve.

Hyperkinesis or spasm of facial muscles may occur by a mechanism called ephaptic transmission, in which depolarization of a nerve fibre at the site of injury excites firing of adjacent neurons.[4,5]

On the other hand, free intermingling of regenerating facial nerve fibres with fibres from other nerves might also account for the occasional instance in which surgical repair of a facial nerve injury gives results superior to those expected from the severity of the injury.

Diagnosis of facial paralysis

Facial paralysis is challenging to diagnose and treat because in most cases the paralysis is idiopathic[6] but a long list of potentially treatable causes must be excluded before this diagnosis is reached. The goal of diagnosis is to arrive at a prognosis and treatment plan, thus answering the patient's three major questions: 'What caused the paralysis?' 'When can recovery be expected?' and 'What can be done to speed recovery?'

HISTORY AND PHYSICAL EXAMINATION

In most cases, the results of a thorough history and physical examination will narrow the diagnoses needing further consideration as possible causes of facial paralysis.

Time-course of paralysis

A history of recent injury, especially involving the head and neck, should lead the examiner to investigate trauma as the cause for facial paralysis in a patient of any age. Presence of facial paralysis at birth indicates that the differential diagnosis must also include an inherited or developmental disorder.

Bell's palsy is characterized by peripheral facial weakness that progresses to maximal loss of function by 3 weeks after onset. Such an onset may also be seen when a neoplasm involves the facial nerve, but with Bell's palsy the paralysis begins to resolve within 6 months of onset.

Other conditions affecting the facial nerve may cause incomplete or complete, sudden or delayed onset of facial paralysis.

Recurrence of facial paralysis on the same side was noted in 4 per cent of patients with Bell's palsy in our series, but it was present in 17 per cent of those found to have a neoplasm involving the facial nerve. Therefore, ipsilateral recurrence of paralysis in patients with Bell's palsy should prompt further evaluation for a neoplasm. A history of malignancy is additional grounds for suspecting a neoplasm as the cause of paralysis.

Contralateral recurrence of facial paralysis occurred in 8 per cent of those with Bell's palsy in our series, and alternating recurrent facial paralysis is characteristic of Melkersson–Rosenthal syndrome. However, contralateral recurrence is rare with other disorders of the facial nerve.

In a small proportion of cases in our series, facial paralysis occurred bilaterally. The most common cause was Guillain–Barré syndrome. Other causes included Bell's palsy, leukaemia, sarcoidosis, skull fracture, Moebius syndrome, rabies, Lyme disease and infectious mononucleosis.

Physical findings

A number of conditions causing facial paralysis can be diagnosed by certain findings on the physical examination.

More than 50 per cent of patients in our series complained of pain with facial paralysis. Pain over the mastoid or pre-auricular area is typical of Bell's palsy. If pain is severe, the examiner should look for vesicles on the pinna and in the ear canal or on the face or neck, signalling herpes zoster cephalicus. The palate should also be examined.

Bruising or other signs of injury over the affected segment of facial nerve point to trauma as a likely cause of paralysis. A red chorda tympani nerve or vascular flaring in the posterosuperior aspect of the tympanomeatal area, which can be seen by otoscopy, is characteristic of Bell's palsy. Otoscopy may also reveal signs of acute or chronic otitis media that may have affected the facial nerve.

If examination of the head and neck, including the mouth and pharynx, reveals a mass or tests of cranial nerve function show abnormalities in other cranial nerves, a neoplasm could be causing facial paralysis. However, function of other cranial nerves may also be affected by Bell's palsy (associated with hyperacusis, dizziness, loss of lachrymation and altered taste) or herpes zoster cephalicus (sensory distribution of cranial nerves V, VII, X and XI and the cervical plexus).

If examination of the eyes reveals intranuclear ophthalmoplegia, multiple sclerosis is a possible diagnosis. Ptosis and weakness of laryngeal and facial muscles suggests that further evaluation for myasthenia gravis is indicated.

TESTS OF FACIAL NERVE FUNCTION

Tests of facial nerve function have been described in Chapter 16.

Diagnostic categories of facial paralysis

Broad diagnostic categories for facial paralysis may be listed as congenital (including inherited and developmental disorders), infectious (including Bell's palsy), neoplastic and traumatic (including iatrogenic injury during surgery).

CONGENITAL FACIAL PARALYSIS

Facial paralysis present at birth may be traumatic or developmental in origin. It has been estimated that between 0.8 and 1.8 per 1000 infants are born with facial paralysis, and in each case, diagnosing the cause accurately and early is important to help the family manage this crisis well.

Birth trauma

The literature suggests that in the majority of cases when a child is born with facial paralysis, the condition is due to trauma during delivery (Fig 17.1).[7–9]

Birth trauma is more likely when the labour has been prolonged or difficult, or both, as typified by the birth of a large infant to a primiparous mother. The use of forceps during delivery has been associated with facial nerve palsy in the newborn. However, facial paralysis due to birth trauma typically involves the entire distribution of the facial nerve,[7,9,10] so the difficult birth itself rather than forceps specifically may be implicated in these cases. For example, Parmalee[11] suggested that pressure of the mother's sacrum on the infant's facial nerve could lead to paralysis.

When a newborn presents with facial nerve paralysis, the evaluation for a traumatic cause should include searching for signs of temporal bone or facial injury such as haematoma or laceration, haemotympanum, or ecchymosis over the mastoid. The facial nerve is not likely to be transected by birth trauma, so a first-, second- or third-degree injury with corresponding spontaneous recovery of House–Brackmann grade I, II or III would be expected in most cases. Some evidence of hyperkinesis or synkinesis may become evident later in the child's life if the facial nerve has suffered a third-degree injury. The fact that such injury is not often found supports the likelihood that most congenital cases are probably inherited.[12]

If there is a possibility that facial paralysis in a newborn is traumatic, electrophysiological testing may be performed. When paralysis is due to an inherited or developmental condition, there will be

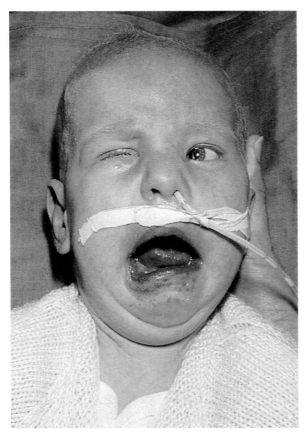

Fig 17.1 A baby born by forceps delivery with a left facial nerve paralysis.

no response on electromyography (EMG), that is, EMG responses will be abnormal in such a newborn and there will be no change with serial testing, in contrast to the progressive decline in amplitudes of compound action potentials that occurs after traumatic facial nerve injury.

Computed tomography may be performed to evaluate bony structures such as the Fallopian canal, which may be poorly developed or non-existent, and other temporal bone structures, checking that there are no concealed fractures.

Any child who presents with facial palsy should also undergo brainstem auditory evoked potential testing to determine whether a hearing loss is present (abnormal amplitudes of waves I and V and abnormal interwave latency).[13]

In the rare cases when a diagnosis of birth trauma has been made but the infant fails to recover some function, surgical intervention might be considered if complete facial paralysis was documented at birth; EMG shows complete loss of facial nerve function by 3–5 days after birth; the infant still has facial paralysis and no electrical activity at 5 weeks of age; physical examination reveals evidence of

temporal bone trauma; or a fracture is evident on radiological images.

Inherited or developmental causes of facial paralysis

Abnormalities in craniofacial structures such as the ear, palate, maxillary structures or other cranial nerves usually accompany facial nerve paralysis caused by an inherited or developmental condition.[14] For example, an abnormality in the course of the facial nerve is often accompanied by a malformed incus or stapes, because the facial nerve develops within the second pharyngeal arch while the external and middle ears are forming from the first external groove and internal pouch. In these cases, the facial nerve may present as a mound over the stapes footplate or the promontory,[15] putting it at risk of avulsion during stapedectomy.[16]

Even normal facial nerves have quite variable courses, as described by Proctor and Nager.[17] For example, in the temporal bone the facial nerve may course with the chorda tympani nerve, so that the two structures appear intraoperatively as an enlarged chorda tympani nerve. In other cases, the nerve may be enlarged in the temporal segment because it contains motor fibres. Alternatively, the facial nerve may be represented by a fibrous strand.

The results of a thorough history and physical examination are often sufficient to determine that congenital facial palsy is due to an inherited or developmental disorder rather than to birth trauma. If the abnormalities present do not seem to fit an established syndrome, a dysmorphologist may be consulted. Such a consultation may also help to determine what other organ systems should be evaluated.

Inherited disorders

Myotonic dystrophy and Albers–Schoenberg disease are the two types of facial paralysis that may be inherited.

Myotonic dystrophy is inherited as an autosomal dominant disorder. It is characterized by progressive muscle wasting and variable degrees of mental impairment. Facial muscle weakness is usually among the first symptoms noted as it is often present at birth.

Albers–Schoenberg disease follows an autosomal recessive pattern of inheritance or may appear as a new mutation. With this disorder of bone metabolism, bone density increases and primary bone resorption decreases. Osteopetrosis of bony canals for cranial nerves causes compression of the nerves, resulting in blindness, deafness and facial paralysis when the IIIrd, VIIIth, and VIIth cranial nerves, respectively, are affected.

Developmental abnormalities

Poor facial muscle function may be part of four congenital syndromes: Moebius syndrome, CHARGE syndrome, OAV syndrome and asymmetric crying facies.

Moebius syndrome involves abnormalities in many cranial nerves. Typically, unilateral or bilateral facial paralysis and a VIth cranial nerve palsy are present, and function of cranial nerves III, IV, V, VIII, X and XII may also be abnormal. The lower face may be less affected than the upper face, but about one-half of children with this disorder also have malformed extremities or lack the pectoralis muscle. When facial palsy is bilateral, the diagnosis of facial nerve paralysis may be delayed. Although the cause of Moebius syndrome is unknown, its clinical presentation can be identical to that seen with teratogens such as thalidomide, and agenesis of the facial nucleus, nerve or musculature has been implicated.[18]

About 43 per cent of children with the symptom complex of *c*olobomata, *h*eart defects, *a*tresia choanae, *r*etarded growth, *g*enital hypoplasia and *e*ar anomalies (CHARGE syndrome) have facial nerve dysfunction. Some children with CHARGE syndrome also have anomalies that meet the criteria for Moebius syndrome.[19]

Oculo-auriculo-vertebral syndrome (OAV) is characterized by abnormal formation of first and second branchial arch derivatives on one side that becomes more pronounced as facial growth progresses. Unilateral hypoplasia of bone and soft tissues typically involves the maxilla, mandible and ear, causing microstomia and microtia. Facial nerve weakness is usually only one of a number of central nervous system abnormalities in OAV syndrome. However, facial weakness is present in nearly all of the 10 per cent of children with OAV syndrome who also have epibulbar dermoids and vertebral anomalies (Goldenhar syndrome).

Asymmetric crying facies is one of the more common congenital conditions affecting the facial nerve. Also known as congenital unilateral lower lip palsy (CULLP) or hypoplasia of the depressor anguli oris muscle, asymmetric crying facies of itself causes no particular functional deficit. This condition may, however, signal the presence of other defects or abnormalities, including cardiac defects, which may be severe, in about 10 per cent of cases.

INFECTIOUS CAUSES OF FACIAL PARALYSIS

Infectious causes of VIIth cranial nerve dysfunction include Bell's palsy, herpes zoster cephalicus, Lyme disease, acute or chronic otitis media and malignant otitis externa.

Bell's palsy

Bell's palsy, an acute peripheral facial paralysis due to a viral inflammatory process, is self-limiting, non-progressive and not life-threatening. Bell's palsy is the most prevalent disorder associated with facial paralysis, accounting for between 15 and 40 cases per 100 000 population.[20–22] Furthermore, Bell's palsy can cause the patient significant distress.

In one series of patients with Bell's palsy, 14 per cent had a positive family history for the disorder. The majority of these patients (60 per cent) had experienced a viral prodrome. One-half had pain around the ear or changes in taste, nearly one-half (40 per cent) had facial numbness, and one-fifth had numbness of the tongue. Twelve per cent of these patients experienced a recurrence of Bell's palsy.[23]

In another study, involving more than 1000 patients with Bell's palsy seen over a 15-year period, complete recovery of facial nerve function occurred in 71 per cent and recovery with barely noticeable deficits occurred in 13 per cent; only 4 per cent had severe sequelae of Bell's palsy.[22] All patients in this study experienced some improvement in facial nerve function, beginning 3 weeks after onset of paralysis, with earlier return of function being correlated with better prognosis for the final grade of recovery.

As long as the palsy is first evaluated within 14 days of onset and remains incomplete patients can be given an appointment to return in 3–6 weeks for further evaluation. However, they should be told to check daily for progression and to return sooner if the palsy worsens. Daily home evaluation of facial movement should be performed by the patient standing in front of a mirror or having a family member observe the effects of the patient raising the eyebrows, squeezing the eyes closed, wrinkling the nose, attempting to whistle, blowing out the cheeks and grinning so as to show their teeth. The patient with an incomplete palsy should begin to recover in 6 weeks.

Herpes zoster cephalicus

Herpes zoster cephalicus (herpes zoster oticus or Ramsay Hunt syndrome) has been reported to account for between 3 per cent and 12 per cent of cases of facial paralysis.[24] The onset of this condition is rapid and characterized by pain and the appearance of vesicles in the ear canal, pinna and on the face, in addition to facial nerve paralysis. If the infection involves the VIIIth cranial nerve, hearing loss and vertigo may also occur. Antibody

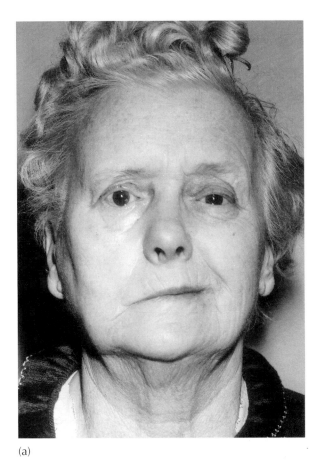

(a)

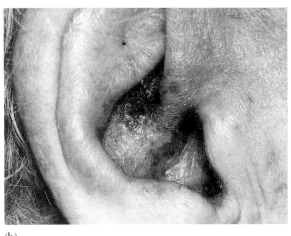

(b)

Fig 17.2 (a) An elderly lady with a complete right sided facial nerve palsy. Note the drooping eyelid, the loss of the nasolabial fold and the asymmetry of the lips at rest. (b) The right auricle shows the crusting overlying the vesicles of a typical herpetic lesion.

titres or complement fixation studies may be used to confirm the diagnosis.

Between 30 per cent and 50 per cent of patients with herpes zoster cephalicus have persistent weakness of facial muscles after the episode, giving it a worse prognosis then Bell's palsy (Fig 17.2).

Medical management of Bell's palsy and herpes zoster cephalicus

The use of steroids in Bell's palsy has been extensively reported.[18] Like the use of steroids in many conditions, their use in this condition has been more empiric then proven. Using stratified patient groups, May demonstrated in 1976 that outcome remains unaffected by steroid therapy.[25] However, prospective randomized trials using a larger dose of steroids did demonstrate some improvement in treatment groups although this was not statistically significant.[26] This was presented best in an overview by Stankiewicz in 1987.[27] He reviewed prospective and retrospective studies and reported the following: 'the use of steroids prevents crocodile tearing (autonomic synkinesis) and *may* prevent denerva-

tion, prevent or lessen synkinesis, prevent progression of incomplete to complete paralysis, and may help hasten recovery.' In his conclusions he stated 'only a few studies indicate that steroid therapy is not beneficial, and these studies have statistical deficiencies.' However, the definitive study to prove the statistical value of steroids has not yet been done. For those who choose to use steroids the dose as recommended by Adour for adults is a daily total of 1 mg/kg body weight in divided doses morning and evening. If the palsy is incomplete by the fifth day the dosage can be tapered to zero during the next 5 days. If there is a question about the severity or the progression of severity during the first 5 days, he recommends the full dosage for 10 days and then tapering over the next 5 days.

Acyclovir is an antiviral drug indicated in the treatment of herpes viral infections in immunocompromised hosts. It is poorly absorbed from the gastrointestinal tract, which led Dickins *et al.*[28] to give acyclovir intravenously 10 mg/kg every 8 hours over a 7-day hospitalized period in 1987. This preliminary study suggested improved outcome in patients treated soon after the onset of their facial paralysis. These results although promising are still waiting for a definitive double-blind controlled study to show improvement superior to the natural history of this disorder.

Lyme disease

Lyme disease, caused by a tick-borne spirochaete, has been found worldwide and in some study populations was the leading cause of facial paralysis in children.[29] About three-quarters of patients have a red skin lesion apparent at the site of the tick inoculation and most have rash, headache, stiff neck, arthralgia and fatigue. Facial paralysis is usually associated with a bite in the head or neck[29,30] and may be more common in children because they are more likely to be inoculated in this region. Unilateral and bilateral facial paralysis may occur in up to 11 per cent of patients with Lyme disease but Clark et al.[31] noted 99 per cent had spontaneous recovery, confirming that operative intervention is not indicated.

A diagnosis of Lyme disease may be confirmed by enzyme-linked immunosorbent assay (ELISA) detection of immunoglobulin G and immunoglobulin M antibody to the spirochaete, and in one study serologic evidence of Lyme disease was found in 20 per cent of those whose facial paralysis had been diagnosed as Bell's palsy.[32]

Treatment is the use of tetracycline or a macrolide antibiotics for 3–4 weeks.

Autoimmune deficiency syndrome (AIDS)

Individuals infected with the human immunodeficiency virus may develop facial paralysis as a result of herpes zoster oticus,[23] progressive multifocal leucoencephalopathy,[34] or neoplasm.[35]

Suppurative otitis media and externa

Facial paralysis may complicate acute or chronic suppurative otitis media or malignant otitis externa.

Paralysis of the facial nerve occurs with acute otitis media due to compression of the nerve as inflammation spreads through congenital dehiscences or along neural or vascular structures.[36] The facial nerve palsy is usually relieved with treatment of the acute otitis media, including wide myringotomy to drain the middle ear effusion and obtain a specimen of exudate for culture, followed by administration of appropriate antibiotic drugs.

Chronic otitis media can lead to the formation of a cholesteatoma or granulation tissue that then compresses the facial nerve and causes facial paralysis. Facial nerve function usually recovers well after surgical excision of the abnormal tissue and decompression of the facial nerve proximal and distal to the site of lesion.

Facial nerve paralysis as a consequence of malignant otitis externa is most likely to develop in patients with diabetes mellitus or who are immunocompromised. Infection in the ear canal is typically due to *Pseudomonas* and is characterized by severe ear pain and drainage from the canal. On otoscopy, granulation tissue is usually found at the bony–cartilaginous junction in the ear canal. Malignant otitis externa should be treated by intravenous antibiotics.

NEOPLASMS AFFECTING THE FACIAL NERVE

Facial nerve paralysis may be caused by a tumour on or near the nerve anywhere along its course from the brainstem to the facial muscles.

Tumours of the facial nerve

The most frequent benign lesion of the facial nerve is a schwannoma. In our experience about one-half of facial neuromas are located in the cerebellopontine angle or internal auditory canal and the other half involve the temporal bone portion of the facial nerve or chorda tympani nerve (Fig 17.3).

Vascular lesions such as meningiomas, angiomas and intraosseous haemangiomas are the next most frequent cause of facial paralysis, caused by a benign lesion on the facial nerve. Most such tumours are located outside the nerve itself, at or proximal to the geniculate ganglion and, unlike schwannomas, can be resected with preservation of residual facial nerve function.

In our experience, the malignant tumours most often affecting the facial nerve are adenoid cystic or mucoepidermoid carcinomas, usually located in the parotid gland. A small number of these tumours have manifested occultly. Pathologic diagnosis of the facial paralysis was made at the time of surgery with no palpable parotid mass.

Acoustic neuromas

Excision of an acoustic neuroma puts the facial nerve at risk, although anatomical preservation of the facial nerve has been reported in more than 90 per cent of cases.[37,38] In one study, 98 per cent of patients with good facial nerve function at discharge from the hospital after resection of an acoustic neuroma recovered an acceptable degree of facial nerve function compared with only 77 per cent of patients who had poor function at the time of discharge.[38]

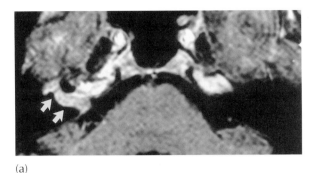

(a)

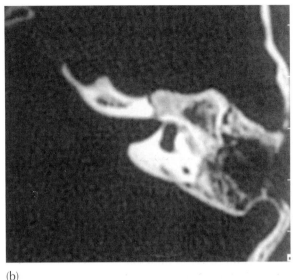

(b)

Fig 17.3 (a) Fast spin echo T2-weighted MRI scan showing a tumour of the facial nerve in the internal auditory meatus. The shape of the lesion suggests that it was expanding the Fallopian canal at the level of the geniculate ganglion. The tumour was an adenocarcinoma. The patient had had a 'benign' parotid tumour removed some 20 years previously. (b) Axial and (c) coronal CT scans of an 8-year-old girl with a 2-year history of a conductive deafness and a facial palsy, which had been labelled as a Bell's palsy. Before the palsy she had had 1 year of facial twitching. A white swelling was easily visible behind and bulging the tympanic membrane. The scans show a large mass of new bone formation surrounding the geniculate ganglion. At surgery via a combined mastoid and middle cranial fossa approach an odontogenic cyst was removed and the tympanic membrane grafted.

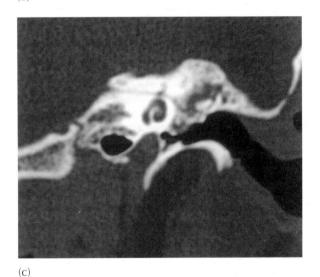

(c)

TRAUMATIC FACIAL PARALYSIS

One cause of trauma to the facial nerve is disruption during surgery for resection of a parotid tumour or with the drill during chronic ear surgery. Temporal bone fractures and facial wounds are other causes of traumatic facial nerve injury.

Iatrogenic injury

The facial nerve most often suffers iatrogenic injury during resection of a tumour, either on the facial nerve itself or in tissues close to the facial nerve, such as an acoustic neuroma.

Iatrogenic injury to the facial nerve during otological surgery occurs most often at the level of the second genu in the mastoid and is more frequent when the facial nerve has an aberrant course or the course is altered by disease. Neurophysiological monitoring may help to locate facial nerve tissue, although it cannot protect the facial nerve from injury.[39,40]

Parotid gland surgery is another frequent cause of iatrogenic injury to the facial nerve.

When the facial nerve is known to have been disrupted, it is best repaired in the same operation, ideally by direct anastomosis of the cut ends. In some situations this cannot be accomplished without tension on the anastomosis, so placement of a nerve graft is indicated. Nerve grafting can restore facial nerve function in a high proportion of cases; however, in patients who have paralysis before the operation, the results of nerve grafting are less reliable.[41,42]

If facial paralysis occurs soon after surgery but the facial nerve was intact at the completion of surgery (as confirmed by proximal stimulation of the facial nerve), the patient can be allowed to recover from the effects of anaesthesia and surgery. However, if nerve continuity was not confirmed at the end of surgery, the patient should be monitored by serial electrophysiological testing. Complete paralysis with lack of electrical response by the fifth postoperative day indicates that re-exploration of the facial nerve may be necessary. However, if paralysis is incomplete and electrical testing shows some facial nerve function or facial nerve function begins to return within 3 weeks postoperatively, the prognosis is good for satisfactory spontaneous return of facial nerve function.

Temporal bone fractures

Patients who may have suffered a temporal bone fracture should be evaluated for injury to the facial nerve as early as possible. Physical examination should include a determination of tonus in facial muscles and the adequacy of eye closure. Electrical testing of facial nerve function should be performed, and CT scans should be examined for signs of fracture. This subject is explored in greater detail in Chapter 16.

Facial wounds

A wound affecting the extracranial facial nerve should be explored as early as possible, and no more than 3 days after injury. After this time, the distal neural bundle will begin to degenerate.

If the wound is clean, the facial nerve should be repaired by primary anastomosis, if this is possible without putting tension on the anastomosis. Otherwise, an interposition graft should be placed. If the wound is contaminated, the facial nerve should not be repaired immediately because grafts placed in contaminated wounds have a relatively high rate of failure. Instead, the ends of the facial nerve should be tagged and the wound left to heal by secondary intention. The facial nerve should then be repaired as soon as possible up to 3 weeks after the injury.

IDIOPATHIC FACIAL NERVE PARALYSIS

Idiopathic facial nerve paralysis occurs with Melkersson–Rosenthal syndrome and Kawasaki disease.

Melkersson–Rosenthal syndrome is a rare disease with familial tendencies but no identified pattern of inheritance.[43] It consists of facial motor dysfunction, episodic or progressive facial oedema and fissured tongue. The facial paralysis in individuals with Melkersson–Rosenthal disease may be partial or complete, unilateral or bilateral. Often the paralysis precedes other signs by months to years. Histological examination of oedematous tissue has revealed the presence of non-caseating granulomas.[44,45] The facial paralysis usually resolves spontaneously, but complete decompression of the facial nerve has been recommended for patients who have multiple recurrences of Melkersson–Rosenthal syndrome.[46]

Symptoms of Kawasaki disease include high fever, cervical adenitis, erythema of the oral mucosa, injection of the conjunctiva, upper and lower extremity oedema and desquamation of the palms of the hands and soles of the feet. Some patients with Kawasaki disease also have peripheral neuropathy, frequently facial paralysis, which typically resolves completely along with other symptoms.[47]

General management of facial nerve paralysis

Because most patients with facial paralysis will recover spontaneously, clinicians frequently approach this problem with no particular urgency. However, occasionally a patient is seen with a facial paralysis that has an underlying life-threatening disorder; others may spend their lives as facial cripples because treatment was not offered until the death of the facial nerve was established by electrical tests. This section of the chapter develops management plans for patients with facial paralysis. It is essential when embarking on these plans to provide the patient and the family with a realistic assessment of the expected degree of recovery and the therapeutic options that are available. Certain families may benefit from contact with appropriate support groups or psychological counselling.

MEDICAL TREATMENT OF THE PARALYSED EYELID

Most patients with facial paralysis require some type of initial medical programme to prevent extension of orbital problems into corneal ulceration. The specific programme used depends on multiple factors: the age of the patient, the cause of the paralysis, the degree of the paralysis and the likelihood of recovery of eyelid function. When looking at the eye one wants to note the position of the lower eyelid, the position of the lachrymal puncta, the wideness of the scleral exposure and the presence of the BAD syndrome, that is, absence of Bell's phenomenon, corneal anaesthesia and dry eye. Tear secretion can be measured by the Schirmer test.

After thorough evaluation the majority of patients will require the addition of a lubricant. Our programme is replacement with an artificial tear solution every 1–2 hours during the day and an ointment at bedtime. The majority of over-the-counter products are well tolerated and helpful for most patients. However, there are certain patients who are intolerant of the preservatives used in many artificial tear solutions. For these patients we recommend switching to a preservative-free preparation. This seems to be much less irritating and gets rid of the dissatisfaction for patients with a sensitivity. In addition, there are more viscous preservative-free solutions that can be used for the patient who has a wide eye and finds that the artificial tears do not give long-term relief. For these patients we have found that the use of Ocucoat PF (Storz Ophthalmics, St. Louis, Missouri, USA) provides a very high level of lubrication without sacrificing visual acuity.

Protection in addition to medication may be needed in some patients, especially at night. Cellophane wrap using cellophane as an occlusive dressing with lubricating ointment at the periphery has been used for a long time. Patients generally prefer a moisture chamber (Pro-Optics, Palatine, Illinois, USA), which is available from a variety of sources. The use of tape can be quite helpful for patients with a paralytic eyelid. Adhesive tape cut in the shape of a half moon and applied to the upper lid can provide some closure, and a lower lid ectropion can be supported with a very fine strip of tape taken out to the lateral canthal region. The use of spectacles, especially sun glasses in the open, provides additional security and some patients benefit from side panels to the spectacle frame to reduce the chance of irritation from wind or dust further.

This series of medical treatments will make the majority of patients comfortable regardless of their clinical situation.

SURGICAL MANAGEMENT OF THE PARALYTIC EYELID

The traditional surgical management of the paralytic eye has been tarsorrhaphy. This generally provided satisfactory protection, but at the cost of function and cosmesis. Reanimating the upper eyelid by placement of a gold weight or a wire spring has been found to be a more attractive option. Our mainstay is the use of the gold weight prosthesis. This is the easiest technique and provides good results for the majority of patients. Weight size is determined preoperatively by taping various weights to the central upper lid margin. Gravity and relaxation of the levator palpebral muscle allows for lid closure. The weights most commonly employed are 0.9 and 1.1 g. Children do well with smaller weights. The technique of insertion is as described by Jobe and Levine and modified by May.[48]

Conjunctival anaesthesia is achieved with a topical anaesthetic and a scleral shield is placed to protect the cornea. One per cent lidocaine (lignocaine) 1:100 000 adrenaline is injected into the tarsal supratarsal fold region. Under loop magnification a 1 cm incision centred just medial to the midpupillary line is made using a razor blade knife. Subcutaneous tissues, orbicularis oris and levator aponeurosis are divided straight down from skin incision until the tarsal plate is reached. Haemostasis is maintained with judicious use of bipolar cautery. The pocket is extended to 3 mm above the lash line. Each weight is approximately 1 mm thick, 5 mm high and 10 mm long. Three holes are provided in the weight to allow for suture fixation to the deeper tissues. An 8-0 monofilament suture is used to attach the lowest hole to the soft tissue lateral to the tarsus. The upper two fixation holes are sewn to the tissue overlying the orbital septum. The weight is placed medial to the midpupillary line and 3 mm above the lash line to provide maximal closure and minimize the cosmetic deformity. Soft tissues are closed with a 7-0 absorbable suture and the skin is closed with a 6-0 plain gut suture (Fig 17.4).

Some patients' eye problems are not amenable to gold weight placement. These patients in general have a greater degree of lagophthalmos. Trial weight placement in the consulting room may show that a weight heavy enough to provide closure is too heavy for the levator and causes a significant ptosis, which is unacceptable for vision. These patients have been successfully managed with a palpebral spring (Fig 17.5), which is fashioned and tried in the consulting room preoperatively. The spring is formed of 0.25 mm orthodontic wire using orthodontic pliers. Anaesthesia is as for gold weight placement. The tarsal supratarsal fold is incised as above and a second anaesthetized area of the lateral orbital rim is created and carried down to the level of the periosteum. The wire is adjusted on the table to conform to the patient's orbital profile. A 19-gauge spinal needle is gently curved and passed between the two incisions lateral to the tarsus. The upper lid is everted to be sure that the conjunctiva has not been violated. The obsturator of the needle

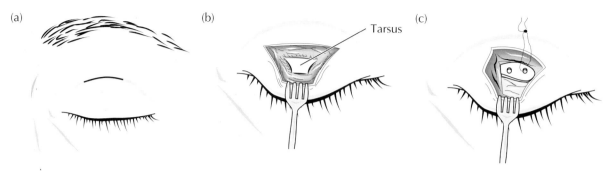

Fig 17.4 Implantation technique for gold weights. (a) An incision is made in the supratarsal crease centred just medial to the midpupillary line. (b) Dissection is carried down to the tarsus within 3 mm of the lash line. (c) The gold weight is stabilized with a three-hole suture technique.

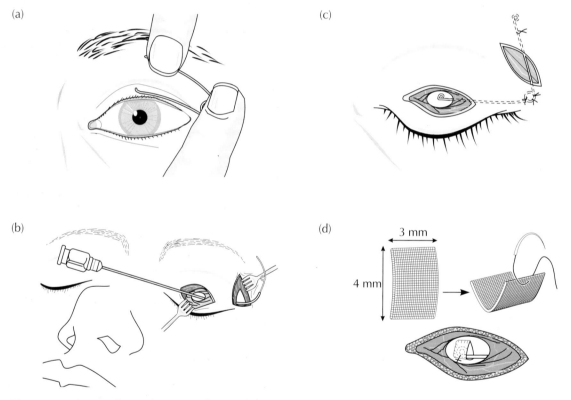

Fig 17.5 Technique for implantation of an eyelid spring. (a) The spring is moulded to achieve proper closure. (b) The two incisions are fashioned to allow for passage of the spring through an intravenous catheter. (c) The ends of the spring are curved and the spring is fixed by a suture. (d) Dacron 'booties' are placed over the end of the spring to reduce the risk of extrusion.

is removed and the spring is passed into position. Two 5-0 permanent sutures fix the fulcrum of the spring to the periosteum. The upper rim of the spring is looped distally and placed in a soft-tissue pocket. The palpebral rim is designed to extend medial to the pupil. It is looped at its distal rim away from the lash line. The corneal shield is removed

and eyelid function is checked and final adjustments made. The distal loop of the palpebral rim is covered in a Dacron sleeve sewn in place with an 8-0 monofilament suture. Soft tissue closure is as for gold weight.

Because the upper eyelid excursion is 10 times that of the lower lid, it receives the majority of the surgical focus. However, lower eyelid procedures are available to counteract the loss of normal lower lid tone and the loss of the 0.5–1.0 mm elevation contribution of the lower lid.

Lower lid extropion can be improved by a number of lateral tightening procedures. These can also improve the position of the lachrymal puncta. The implantation of auricular cartilage into the lower eyelid provides better positioning of the lid margin, bringing it well up to the normal position of the limbus.[49] Cartilage implantation is useful in the young patient with poor lid position who otherwise has excellent eyelid skin tone.

SURGICAL MANAGEMENT OF FACIAL NERVE PARALYSIS

Indication for surgery

Ongoing studies continue to look at the indications for facial nerve surgical decompression. The benefits of decompression for Bell's palsy or herpes zoster cephalicus have yet to be convincingly shown. Surgical decompression of acute suppurative otitis media, necrotizing external otitis, or facial paralysis occurring after iatrogenic or an external temporal bone fracture must be individualized on a patient by patient basis.[12,50] When facial paralysis occurs as a result of an ongoing process such as the case of chronic suppurative otitis media with or without cholesteatoma, surgery is the only thing that can be offered to eradicate the primary disease process. Surgery has the best chance of success if one intervenes before evidence of electrical denervation. Surgical intervention should also be undertaken in patients who have a nerve transection, a facial nerve tumour or a facial nerve infiltrated by tumour.

Marsh and Coker[51] noted that most evidence points to the meatal segment of the facial nerve as the site at which nerve entrapment is likely to occur. Because we know that 84 per cent of patients with Bell's palsy will spontaneously recover to a House–Brackmann grade I or II result, it is the remaining 16 per cent who we are trying to identify as candidates to improve their long-term outcome.[22] Marsh and Coker[51] set the following criteria for a prospective trial to assess the role of decompression: acceptable anaesthetic risk, age less than 60 years, EMG results greater than 90 per cent of normal and no evidence of neurapraxia deblocking on EMG.

The majority of surgeons performing surgical decompression use a middle fossa approach.[52] However, we prefer to decompress the facial nerve through a transmastoid supralabyrinthine approach (Fig 17.6).

The transmastoid approach to the facial nerve begins as with many otological procedures with a simple mastoidectomy. The anterior exposure is quite important and the cells leading into the route of the zygoma must be opened. The upper edge of the incus and the bony prominence of the horizontal semicircular canal must be seen.

Using the posterior tip of the incus above and the digastric ridge near the mastoid tip, the surgeon identifies the facial nerve as in any mastoid procedure. The bony facial canal is thinned using a diamond burr with copious irrigation. The surgeon encounters the nerve as a white shiny structure with vascular markings on its surface. When the surgeon requires exposure to the tympanic portion of the facial nerve the facial recess is opened. In patients without hearing in the ear a translabyrinthine approach is quite appropriate; however, for most patients this is not the situation. Instead we disarticulate the incus by gently separating the incudostapedial and malleoincudal joints. The short process of the incus is rotated based on its attachment in the fossa incudus down towards the middle ear. This allows for exposure of the proximal tympanic, geniculate and distal labyrinthine segments of the facial nerve. With this dissection complete the incus can be rotated towards the mastoid so that the midtympanic portion of the facial nerve can be dissected without fear of transmitting vibration from the incus to the stapes. The surgeon decompresses the nerve by slitting the nerve sheath. Bleeding should not be treated with bipolar cautery, instead gentle tamponade with absorbable materials is preferred. This approach can be performed with a fairly minimal risk to hearing.[53]

Management of traumatic facial nerve injuries

After Bells's palsy, facial trauma is the next most frequent cause of facial paralysis. The treatment of choice for these injuries depends on the age of the patient, cause of the injury, the location of the injury, the status of hearing and the length of time since the paralysis occurred.

Temporal bone fractures

Patients with a facial paralysis after head trauma can be followed expectantly without the need for surgery, and a favourable spontaneous recovery can be expected in patients who have a delayed onset even with loss of electrical response. Patients with a sudden complete onset, loss of electrical response, a history of major head trauma, a profound sensorineural hearing loss and radiological evidence of transverse fracture through the Fallopian canal

(a)

(b)

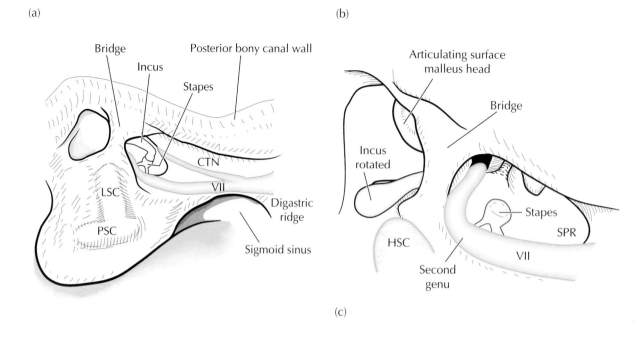

(c)

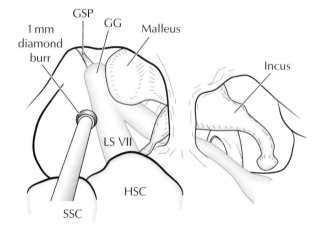

Fig 17.6 Transmastoid supralabyrinthine approach to the facial nerve and geniculate ganglion in the right ear. (a) A wide mastoidectomy is performed and the facial recess opened. CTN, chorda tympani nerve; LSC, lateral semicircular canal; PSC, posterior semicircular canal. (b) The incus is disarticulated and rotated, and the facial nerve is exposed in the horizontal segment. HSC, horizontal semicircular canal; SPR, suprapyramidal recess. (c) The dissection is continued and the geniculate ganglion and the intralabyrinthine portion of the nerve are exposed and decompressed. GG, geniculated ganglion; GSP, great superficial petrosal; LS, labyrinthine segment; SSC, superior semicircular canal.

should be considered surgical candidates. In a recent study we found that 30 per cent of patients with these criteria had severe facial nerve injury and at surgery facial nerve disruption required nerve repair.[53] We approach patients with hearing through the submiddle fossa transmastoid approach, and in those with severe hearing loss we use a translabyrinthine approach. Most authors still use a middle fossa approach as first proposed by Fisch[54] and later by Glasscock.[40]

Once the surgeon has exposed the nerve through whatever approach he or she feels is most appropriate, treatment of these patients requires evaluation of the nerve injury. If the fragments have been displaced onto the nerve creating a crush injury and haematoma, decompression may be all that is nec-

essary. However, in many of the patients who meet the above criteria the nerve must be freshened proximally and distally and an interposition graft placed. Within the temporal bone because of lack of movement in this area no sutures are required. The earliest possible intervention allows for ease of surgery and the best possible outcome for nerve repair. Patients treated with nerve repair 2 years on and even 1 year on never achieve the results of patients operated on within 6 months.

Injury occurring during surgery

Otolaryngology has a dictum that the sun should never set on facial paralysis that follows otological surgery. In the majority of patients we recommend that the surgeon does wait a day or longer before re-exploration. This additional time allows for the family and the patient to be consulted and more importantly allows the surgeon to regain his composure and use his best skills or allows time to call in colleagues with those skills to provide the best final outcome. Equally importantly, it allows for assessment of the circumstances of the injury, which may preclude the need for reoperation.

Otological surgery

At the conclusion of otological surgery the facial nerve should be stimulated proximally with the nerve stimulator. If good stimulation occurs the surgeon and the patient can expect spontaneous recovery. If at the conclusion of the procedure the surgeon is unsure of the status of the nerve, serial electrical tests can be performed. If nerve excitability is lost by the fifth postoperative day, re-exploration may be appropriate. However, what appeared to be a total paralysis in the recovery room may prove to be incomplete paralysis when the effects of local and general anaesthesia dissipate fully. The prognosis for favourable outcome is improved when response to electrical stimulation is maintained beyond 10 days and voluntary motor unit action potentials persist or return.

Parotid gland surgery

When performing parotid gland surgery the same caveats apply. If at the conclusion of the case proximal stimulation of the facial nerve provides brisk facial movement, the surgeon can be reassured that the nerve is in continuity. Recovery would be expected within 4–6 months of surgery even if complete paralysis is seen immediately postoperatively. The result will depend on the degree of nerve injury when the nerve is intact so that a House–Brackmann grade III recovery can occur in these circumstances although a grade I or II recovery is more common. On the other hand, if the nerve does not respond to electrical stimulation, the surgeon should reinspect the nerve from proximal to distal to make sure nerve disruption has not occurred.

FACIAL REANIMATION

Facial reanimation is approached in a hierarchical fashion from the simplest to the most complicated techniques. These techniques are designed to address the circumstances of the injury and to allow for the best possible recovery. This will be illustrated by some case examples.

Case number 1 – a young man presents with a facial laceration and immediate facial weakness of the upper division of the facial nerve.

In this patient all would agree that re-establishing facial nerve continuity provides the best possible outcome. When the patient is stable the nerve should be explored, preferably within the first 3 days to allow for distal stimulation. The nerve ends must then be assessed and freshened. If the wound is a grossly contaminated one, then we recommend coming back and doing the nerve repair at a separate sitting. The temptation is to reapproximate the facial nerve, but if infection were to occur one would not know that the nerve repair had not survived until the window for obtaining the best possible results had been lost.

On the other hand, if it is a clean wound there is no reason not to go ahead and perform nerve repair at the initial procedure. The main point to stress is that the nerve repair must be tension free. If this can be performed with gentle mobilization extratemporally or within the temporal bone, then the nerve should be brought together in a tension-free fashion. However, what frequently seems to happen is that the more the nerve is freed up the more it seems to shorten and the more the blood supply to the nerve is jeopardized. In our experience the results were as good or better when a free graft was introduced as when the nerve was rerouted. The choice of donor nerve depends on the length of nerve needed. The cervical cutaneous nerve provides up to 9 cm of nerve graft and the sural nerve can be used when longer grafts are required. The segment of nerve used should be longer than the gap to be bridged to provide tension-free closure. Freshened ends under the microscope allow for good grafting using a 10-0 monofilament suture. A fascicular anastomosis is used at this institution although reports of a variety of repair techniques have been espoused. Recently the idea of using autogenous axially aligned free-style skeletal muscle has been proposed. Early work with this technique suggested that it might be an alternative to the sacrifice of a sensory nerve, and it may be less technically difficult to perform.[55]

The above principles are also applied in the resection of tumours affecting the facial nerve, regardless of whether they are primary facial nerve tumours that invade the facial nerve. The best possible results occur when proximal and distal facial nerves can be reconstructed.[41] This includes the treatment of acoustic neuromas. In the patient whose facial nerve is resected during excision of acoustic neuroma, a direct VII–VII facial nerve to facial nerve anastomosis usually requiring an interposition nerve graft provides results superior to any other reanimation technique. The length of graft has not been shown to be a deterrent to a favourable outcome. However, patients who exhibit a facial paralysis preoperatively do not fair well with nerve interposition grafting.[42]

The use of facial nerve monitors particularly in acoustic surgery has been shown to have a positive outcome, especially in larger tumours[56] and many physicians use facial nerve monitors routinely in otological and extratemporal facial nerve surgery. We follow more closely the practice of Roland and Meyerhoff[57] and do not use monitors except in unusual cases with greatly distorted anatomy or in acoustic tumour surgery.

Case number 2 – a 15-year-old who developed a unilateral hearing loss and was found to have an acoustic tumour. He underwent excision of a 4 cm acoustic tumour with facial nerve disruption of essentially no proximal facial stump at the brainstem. He awoke with a total facial paralysis and was referred after an initial healing period of 3 weeks.

In patients in whom the facial nerve is not available proximally our choice is a XII–VII jump graft for reconstitution of the facial nerve.[58] Since the initial publication, evaluation of the graft results shows that superb outcomes occur only in patients treated within the first 6 months. Good results can be achieved at 6–12 months and poor results beyond 2 years (Schaitkin B, May M, unpublished data).

It is therefore important for the surgeon to make an attempt to confirm facial nerve continuity at the conclusion of the acoustic procedure to allow for timely referral if the nerve has been disrupted or to allow for the placement of a nerve graft if a proximal stump is available.

Case number 3 – a patient presents to the consulting room with a facial paralysis of 6 months' duration. He was told initially that the diagnosis was Bell's palsy but he has had no recovery. Evaluation in the consulting room shows in addition to the facial paralysis a 4 cm hard fixed parotid mass. A fine needle aspirate is consistent with a malignant process.

After appropriate imaging and discussion with the patient, a strategy for treatment that involves surgery with facial nerve resection should be decided upon. In this particular case the tumour has infiltrated the nerve into its more distal extent. Reanimation of the face that does not allow for distal nerve grafting still offers two main alternatives. In patients who have dermal infiltration requiring a soft-tissue paddle and facial reanimation, a microvascular free flap with the muscle innervated by the proximal facial nerve provides a good outcome.

Alternatively, a temporalis rotation flap can be used to provide reanimation of the lower face with separate eye reanimation for the upper face in patients who do not require a soft tissue skin island. The microvascular procedure takes longer to perform and is more challenging technically. Complication rates are higher for free flaps and their long-term outcome continues to be assessed. It may very well turn out to be the procedure of choice as more experience is gained. The temporalis muscle provides a very easy fast approach. It is a reliable with a very low complication rate although there is a depression in the temporal fossa and a bulge over the zygoma.

FIRST BRANCHIAL CLEFT ANOMALY

The first branchial cleft is intimately associated with the facial nerve.[59] Despite warnings throughout the otolaryngological literature, we still see more patients referred to our practice with facial nerve paralysis after treatment of this lesion then for treatment of the lesion as a whole. This is possibly because illustrations of this surgical problem still leave the surgeon unclear as to the facial nerve relationship. Even in our own paper the illustrations are not as good as intraoperative photographs.

References

1. Van Buskirk C. The seventh nerve complex. *Journal of Comparative Neurology* 1945; **82**:303–33.
2. Sunderland S. *Nerve and nerve injuries, 2nd ed.* London: Churchill Livingstone, 1978.
3. House JW, Brackmann DE. Facial nerve grading system. *Otolaryngology – Head and Neck Surgery* 1985; **93**:146–7.
4. Granit R, Leksell L, Skoglund CR. Fibre interaction in injuried or compressed region of the nerve. *Brain* 1944; **67**:125–40.
5. Kugelberg E, Cobb W. Repetitive discharges in human motor nerve fibres during the post ischaemic state. *Journal of Neurology, Neurosurgery and Psychiatry* 1951; **14**:88–94.
6. Schaitkin B, May M. Evaluation and management of facial nerve disorders. *Current Opinion in Otolaryngology – Head and Neck Surgery* 1993; **1**:79–83.
7. Falko NA, Eriksson E. Facial nerve palsy in the newborn: incidence and outcome. *Plastic and Reconstructive Surgery* 1990; **85**:1–4.
8. Harris LE, Stayura LA, Ramirez-Talavera PF, *et al.* Congenital and acquired abnormalities observed in live born and stillborn neonates. *Mayo Clinic Proceedings* 1975; **50**:85–90.
9. Smith JD, Crumley R, Harker LA. Facial paralysis in the newborn. *Otolaryngology – Head and Neck Surgery* 1981; **89**:1021–4.
10. Hepner WR Jr. Some observations on facial paresis in newborn infant: etiology and incidence. *Pediatrics* 1951; **8**:494–7.

11. Parmelee AH. Molding due to intra-uterine posture: facial paralysis probably due to such molding. *American Journal of Disease in Childhood* 1931; **42**:1155–9

12. May M. Facial paralysis at birth: medicolegal and clinical implications. *American Journal of Otology* 1995; **16**:711–2.

13. Harris JP, Davidson TM, May M, Fria T. Evaluation and treatment of congenital facial paralysis. *Archives of Otolaryngology* 1983; **109**:145–51.

14. Bergstrom L, Baker BB. Syndromes associated with congenital facial paralysis. *Otolaryngology – Head and Neck Surgery* 1981; **89**:336–42.

15. Jahrsdoerfer RA. The facial nerve in congenital middle ear malformations. *Laryngoscope* 1981; **91**:1217–25.

16. Welling DB, Glasscock ME, Gantz BJ. Avulsion of the anomalous facial nerve at stapedectomy. *Laryngoscope* 1992; **102**:729–33.

17. Proctor B, Nager GT. The facial canal: normal anatomy, variations and anomalies. *Annals of Otology, Rhinology and Laryngology* 1982; **91(suppl 93)**:33–61.

18. May M. Facial nerve disorders in the newborn and children. In: May M ed. *The facial nerve.* New York: Thieme Medical, 1986:401–19.

19. Byerly KA, Pauli RM. Cranial nerve abnormalities in CHARGE association. *American Journal of Medical Genetics* 1993; **45**:751–7.

20. Hauser WA, Karnes WE, Annis J, Karland LT. Incidence and prognosis of Bell's palsy in the population of Rochester, Minnesota. *Mayo Clinic Proceedings* 1971; **46**:258–64.

21. Adour KK, Byl FM, Hilsinger RL Jr, Kahn ZM, Sheldon M. The true nature of Bell's palsy: analysis of 1000 consecutive patients. *Laryngoscope* 1978; **88**:787–801.

22. Peitersen E. The natural history of Bell's palsy. *American Journal of Otology* 1982; **4**:107–11.

23. May M, Hardin WB. Facial palsy: interpretation of neurologic findings. *Transactions of the American Academy of Ophthalmology and Otolaryngology* 1977; **84**:710–22.

24. Robillard RB, Hilsinger RL Jr, Adour KK. Ramsay Hunt facial paralysis: clinical analyses of 185 patients. *Otolaryngology – Head and Neck Surgery* 1986; **95**:292–7.

25. May M, Klein SR, Taylor FH. Idiopathic (Bell's) facial palsy: natural history defies steroid or surgical treatment. *Laryngoscope* 1985; **95**:406–9.

26. Wolf SM. Treatment of Bell palsy with prednisolone: a prospective randomised study. *Neurology* 1978; **20**:158–61.

27. Stankiewicz JA. A review of the published data on steroids and idiopathic facial paralysis. *Otolaryngology – Head and Neck Surgery* 1987; **97**:481–6.

28. Dickins JRE, Smith JT, Graham SS. Herpes zoster oticus: treatment with intravenous acyclovir. *Laryngoscope* 1988; **98**:776–9.

29. Christen HJ, Bartlau N, Hanefield F, *et al.* Peripheral facial palsy in childhood – Lyme borreliosis to be suspected unless proven otherwise. *Acta Paediatrica Scandinavia* 1990; **79**:1219–24.

30. Steere AC. Lyme disease. *New England Journal of Medicine* 1989; **321**:586–96.

31. Clark JR, Carlson RD, Sasaki CT, Kimmelman CP, Harrison WG. Facial paralysis in Lyme disease. *Laryngoscope* 1985; **95**:1341–5.

32. Jonsson L, Stiernstedt G, Thomander L. Tick-borne borrelia infection in patients with Bell's palsy. *Archives of Otolaryngology – Head and Neck Surgery* 1987; **113**:303–6.

33. Mishell JH, Applebaum EL. Ramsay Hunt syndrome in a patient with HIV infection. *Otolaryngology – Head and Neck Surgery* 1990; **102**:177–9.

34. Langford-Kuntz A, Reichert P, Pohle HD. Impairment of cranio-facial nerves due to AIDS. *International Journal of Oral and Maxillofacial Surgery* 1988; **17**:227–9.

35. Linstrom CJ, Pincus RL, Leavitt EB, Urbina MC. Otologic neurotologic manifestations of HIV-related disease. *Otolaryngology – Head and Neck Surgery* 1993; **108**:680–7.

36. Tschiassny K. Facial palsy, when complicating a case of acute otitis media, indicative for immediate mastoid operation? *Cincinnati Journal of Medicine* 1944; **25**:262–6.

37. Nadol JB, Chiong CM, Ojeman RG, McKenna MJ, Martuza RL, Montgomery WW. Preservation of hearing and facial nerve function in resection of acoustic neuroma. *Laryngoscope* 1992; **102**:1153–8.

38. Arriaga MA, Luxford WM, Atkins JS, Kwartler JA. Predicting long-term facial nerve outcome after acoustic neuroma surgery. *Otolaryngology – Head and Neck Surgery* 1993; **108**:220–4.

39. Rulon JT, Hallberg OE. Operative injury to the facial nerve. Explanation for its occurrence during operations on the temporal bone and suggestions for its prevention. *Archives of Otolaryngology – Head and Neck Surgery* 1962; **76**:131–9.

40. Glasscock ME. Unusual facial nerve problems. Some thoughts on identifying the nerve within the temporal bone. *Laryngoscope* 1971; **81**:669–83.

41. Luetje C, Whittaker CK. The benefits of VII–VII neuroanastomosis in acoustic tumor surgery. *Laryngoscope* 1991; **101**:1273–5.

42. Stephanian E, Sekhar LN, Janecka IP, Hirsch B. Facial nerve repair by interposition nerve graft: results in 22 patients. *Neurosurgery* 1992; **31**:73–7.

43. Carr RD. Is the Melkersson–Rosenthal syndrome hereditary? *Archives of Dermatology* 1966; **93**:426–7.

44. Levenson M, Ingerman M, Grimes C, Anand KV. Melkersson–Rosenthal syndrome. *Archives of Otolaryngology – Head and Neck Surgery* 1984; **110**:540–2.

45. Woorsaae N, Christensen KC, Schiodt M, Reibel J. Melkersson–Rosenthal syndrome and cheilitis granulomatosa. *Oral Surgery, Oral Medicine and Oral Pathology* 1982; **54**:404–13.

46. Graham MD, Kartush JM. Total facial nerve decompression for recurrent facial paralysis: an update. *Otolaryngology – Head and Neck Surgery* 1989; **101**:442–4.

47. Kleinman MB, Passo MH. Incomplete Kawasaki disease with facial nerve paralysis and coronary artery involvement. *Pediatric Infectious Disease Journal* 1988; **7**:301–2.

48. May M. Gold weight and wire spring implants as alternative to tarsorrhaphy. *Archives of Otolaryngology – Head and Neck Surgery* 1987; **113**:656–60.

49. May M, Hoffman DF, Buerger GF, Soll DB. Management of the paralyzed lower eyelid by implanting auricular cartilage. *Archives of Otolaryngology – Head and Neck Surgery* 1990; **116**:786–8.

50. Maiman DJ, Cusick JF, Anderson AJ, Larson SJ. Nonoperative management of traumatic facial nerve palsy. *Journal of Trauma* 1985; **25**:644–8.

51. Marsh MA, Coker NJ. Surgical decompression of idiopathic facial palsy. *Otolaryngologic Clinics of North America* 1991; **24**:675–89.

52. Gantz B, Gmur A, Fisch U. Intraoperative electromyography in Bell's palsy. *American Journal of Otolaryngology* 1982; **3**:273–8.

53. Ferraresi S. Transmastoid submiddle fossa approach for facial paralysis associated with head trauma. Submitted *Laryngoscope*.

54. Fisch U. Facial paralysis and fracture of petrous bone. *Laryngoscope* 1994; **84**:2141–54.

55. Glasby MA, Sharp JR. New possibilities for facial nerve repair. *Facial Plastic Surgery* 1992; **8**:100–8.

56. Harner SG, Daube JR, Ebersold MJ. Electrophysiologic monitoring of facial nerve during temporal bone surgery. *Laryngoscope* 1986; **96**:65–9.

57. Roland PS, Meyerhoff WL. Intraoperative facial nerve monitoring: what is its appropriate role? [Editorial]. *American Journal of Otology* 1993; **14**:1.

58. May M, Sobol SM, Mester SJ. Hypoglossal–facial nerve interpositional jump graft for facial reanimation without tongue atrophy. *Otolaryngology – Head and Neck Surgery* 1991; **104**:818–25.

59. May M, DAngelo AJ. The facial nerve and the branchial cleft: surgical challenge. *Laryngoscope* 1989; **99**:564–5.

PART III

Congenital ear disease

CHAPTER 18

Congenital abnormalities of the external and middle ear

PIYUSH JANI AND TONY WRIGHT

Congenital malformations of the external and middle ear are of major importance to the patient and a technical challenge for the otologist. Bilateral malformations are associated with a significant hearing loss from birth and as a result there is poor acquisition of speech and language. Patients may be wrongly labelled as mentally retarded and are occasionally condemned to a lifetime of intellectual deprivation and institutionalization. Cosmetic deformities of the external ear in children may result in extensive and painful teasing and consequent long-term psychological trauma.

Congenital malformation of the external ear are often associated with abnormalities of the middle and inner ear. Clinicians must be aware of the possible association of certain abnormalities with others; when one abnormality is found, others must be sought and in so doing one must have a high degree of suspicion for the possibility of bilateral congenital deafness. When planning surgical treatment it is also important to be aware of the possibilities of associated abnormalities, such as an aberrant facial nerve, to avoid surgical misadventure.

Embryology

Basic understanding of embryology is essential to appreciate the presence of associated abnormalities when one anomaly is detected. A summary of the development of the external and middle ears and of the labyrinth is given in Chapter 1. It should be remembered that the labyrinth develops separately from the outer and middle ears and, therefore, although the external and middle ears may be grossly abnormal, the inner ear function may be unaffected. Normal cochlear function will of course enhance the prospect of successful surgical intervention in the hope of establishing useful hearing.

Aetiology

There are many causes of the huge range of craniofacial abnormalities that can be associated with anomalies of the external and middle ears. A full discussion of all these groups is beyond the scope of this chapter and some further reading is given at the end. The congenital abnormalities of the external and middle ear may be classified into seven groups.

- diseases of unknown aetiology
- diseases associated with chromosome abnormality
- diseases associated with Mendelian inheritance
- diseases associated with prenatal infection
- diseases associated with maternal drug abuse
- diseases associated with iatrogenic ototoxicity
- environmental factors

DISEASES OF UNKNOWN AETIOLOGY

Diseases of unknown aetiology include an aberrant facial nerve, anomalies of ossicles, congenital atresia, anomalies of the auricle and ossified stapedius tendon. Some syndromic abnormalities such as Goldenhar, the CHARGE association and the VATER association also have an unknown aetiology.

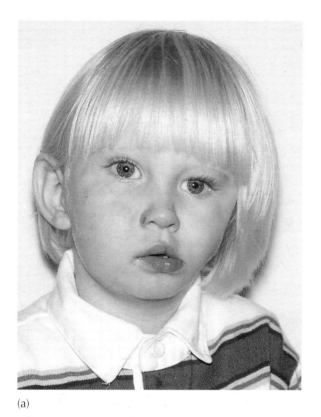
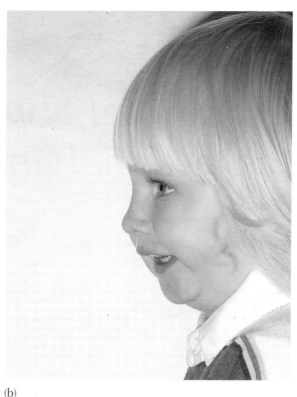

(a)   (b)

Fig 18.1 A young boy with classic Goldenhar syndrome. (a) The left side of the face is clearly underdeveloped on the frontal view and (b) he has long hair to obscure in part the absence of the ear and the facial fissures seen on the left lateral view. (Reproduced with permission of Dr Deirdre Lucas and Dr Kathryn Harrop-Griffiths, consultant audiological physicians at the Nuffield Hearing and Speech Centre at the Royal National Throat Nose and Ear Hospital, London.)

Goldenhar syndrome is, in the main, faulty development of the first and second branchial arches and is frequently called hemifacial microsomia or lateral facial dysplasia as the anomalies are often only found on one side of the face (Fig 18.1). The auricles can be absent, malformed or displaced; the middle ear can be abnormal and the inner ear underdeveloped. There may be hypoplasia of the mandible and maxilla along with macrostomia and cleft palate. Vertebral abnormalities that are present in 50 per cent of children with Goldenhar syndrome include spina bifida, fused vertebrae, additional vertebrae and hemivertebrae.

The CHARGE association comprises colobomata (defects in the iris of the eye from failure of closure of the choroidal fissure), heart disease (commonly Fallot's tetralogy), atresia of the choanae and often oesophagus, retarded growth and development, genital anomalies and ear abnormalities and hearing loss.

The VATER association consists of vertebral anomalies, a ventricular septal defect, anal atresia, tracheo-oesophageal fistula with oesophageal atresia and radial and renal dysplasia. External ear anomalies are common and include an abnormal tympanic membrane.

DISEASES ASSOCIATED WITH CHROMOSOMAL ABNORMALITIES

In recent years many congenital anomalies have been shown to have an underlying major chromosomal abnormality. As the science of genetic mapping advances, the location of more abnormalities will, we presume, be determined and allow a logical classification of the various classes of deformity.

In Turner syndrome (XO) there is an aberration in the sex chromosomes with an absent X chromosome in otherwise phenotypic females. Abnormalities of the external and middle ear include low-set ears, minor abnormalities of the auricle, poorly developed mastoid air cells, abnormalities of the ossicles and Mondini-type deformity of the cochlea in some patients.

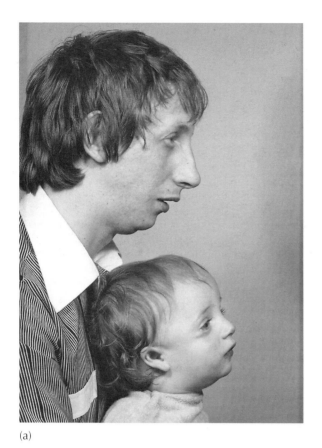

(a)

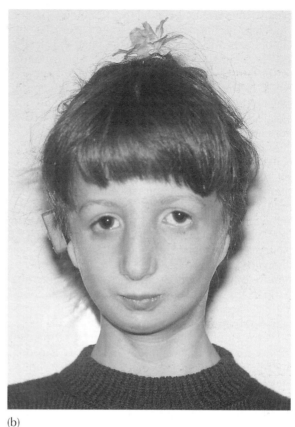

(b)

Fig 18.2 (a) A father and son with Treacher Collins syndrome. The father was not recognized as having a mild expression of this syndrome until his son was born. This child is not severely affected but has, like his father, a hypoplastic mandible. (b) A frontal view of a girl with classic Treacher Collins syndrome. Notice the low-set abnormal ears. On the left side she has been fitted with a bone-anchored hearing aid (see Fig 18.10).

Down syndrome (trisomy 21) is associated with low-set small ears with external canal stenosis. In the middle ear, the ossicles may be bulky with deformed stapes and there is often a wide angle to the second turn of the facial nerve.

In the rather rare Patau syndrome there is an extra chromosome in the 13–15 group. Findings in the external and middle ear include low-set ears, narrow external canals, a thickened handle of the malleus, abnormal incudostapedial joint, deformed stapes, small facial nerve, absent stapedial muscle and persistent stapedial artery. The inner ear is also abnormal. The child has a severe sensorineural hearing loss from birth. These changes are only part of the problem, which is severe and includes microcephaly, severe retardation and a short lifespan.

Trisomy 18 is referred to as Edwards syndrome. Abnormalities in the ear include low-set deformed ears with atretic external auditory canals, deformed malleus and incus, columellar stapes and an abnormal course of the facial nerve.

The general anomalies of the external and middle ear may also be due to abnormalities of chromosome 22 (trisomy) and chromosome 4 (short-arm deletion) but these developmental malformations are rare.

DISEASES WITH MENDELIAN-TYPE INHERITANCE

Diseases with Mendelian-type inheritance include many of the craniofacial abnormalities such as Treacher Collins, Crouzon, Pierre Robin and Apert syndromes, which are usually thought to be inherited in an autosomal dominant pattern. Congenital bony abnormalities such as osteogenesis imperfecta and osteopetrosis also result in abnormal middle ear structures and are also autosomal dominant.

Treacher Collins syndrome is hereditary mandibulofacial dysostosis of the first branchial arch and its derivatives. Hearing loss is common and is usually bilateral and conductive in nature. Abnormalities are frequently seen in the external and middle ears and sometimes in the inner ear. External ear anomalies range from minor abnormalities of the auricle to severe microtia and atresia (Fig 18.2). In the middle ear, the tympanic membrane may be replaced by a bony plate and frequently the ossicles may be malformed. The intratympanic muscles and tendons may be absent. The facial nerve may course directly laterally without a tympanic or mastoid portion.

Crouzon syndrome is a craniofacial dysostosis characterized by premature closure of the cranial vault sutures, maxillary hypoplasia and ocular and aural abnormalities – these give a characteristic 'frog face'. Approximately one-third of these patients have bilateral conductive hearing loss. In the external ear the pinna may be low-set and rotated. There may be stenosis or atresia of the external canal with microtia. Attic fixation of the malleus head is the commonest middle ear abnormality. The tympanic membrane may be absent and stapes may be deformed.

Pierre Robin syndrome is characterized by cleft palate, micrognathia and glossoptosis. It is probably inherited as an autosomal dominant although may occur as a result of intrauterine disease in the first trimester. Abnormalities include low-set cup ears with thickened stapes crura and a small and often dehiscent facial nerve.

Apert syndrome is occasionally an autosomal dominant but often appears to arise spontaneously. The syndrome comprises craniofacial dysostosis, hyperteleorism and proptosis giving a facial appearance not dissimilar to that of Crouzon syndrome, but the presence of syndactyly serves to differentiate the two. External ears are usually normal and the commonest middle ear abnormality is a fixed stapes footplate.

Osteogenesis imperfecta tarda and osteopetrosis are congenital hereditary disorders. Osteogenesis imperfecta is a disorder of the connective tissue caused by a defect in type-I collagen synthesis. Four variants are described and all may have middle ear ossicular abnormalities. The classic combination is blue sclera, fragile bones and deafness due to stapes fixation. This is van der Hoeve's syndrome and appears with progressive hearing impairment, usually in early childhood. Two variants of osteopetrosis have been described and both may be associated with middle ear ossicular abnormalities, persistent stapedial artery and lack of pneumatization of the mastoid antrum and air cells.

The autosomal recessive mode of inheritance is far more common than the dominant mode but there seem to be very few specific examples of deformity of the outer and middle ears that can be reliably ascribed to this form of inheritance.

DISEASES ASSOCIATED WITH PRENATAL INFECTIONS

Congenital rubella syndrome is fortunately decreasing in prevalence in the developed world as a result of increased uptake of preschool vaccination. The syndrome is a result of a maternal viral infection that spreads across the placenta to the fetus. Anomalies in the middle ear include fixation of the malleus head in the attic, abnormal stapes superstructure and fixed footplate. In the inner ear the cochlea is usually abnormal and the patient has severe bilateral mixed hearing loss.

Congenital syphilis is an infection of the fetus caused by *Treponema pallidum* crossing the placenta. Middle ear findings include thickening of the malleus, fusion of the incudomalleolar joint and abnormality of the stapes. Endarteritis obliterans of the otic capsule vessels leads to labyrinthitis that is characterized by endolymphatic hydrops. Audiometric findings include bilateral sensorineural hearing loss, which may have a sudden onset and is severe and profound.

DISEASES ASSOCIATED WITH MATERNAL DRUG ABUSE

The commonest drug abused during pregnancy is alcohol, which may lead to the fetal alcohol syndrome. Although there are major malformations in the central nervous system, cardiovascular system and in the craniofacial region, ear anomalies are comparatively rare and include posteriorly rotated ears, which may be low-set, microtia and a poorly formed concha.

Medications taken during pregnancy that may lead to external and middle ear abnormalities include anticonvulsant drugs, isoretinoin and thalidomide. Anticonvulsant drugs such as phenobarbitone, phenytoin and primidone all have a teratogenic effect. External ear anomalies include prominent, slightly malformed and low-set ears. Middle ear abnormalities include deformed ossicles, absence of the oval and round windows, and an abnormal cochlea and vestibule.

Isotretinoin is a vitamin A derivative that is used for the treatment of severe skin disorders such as cystic acne. It is well known to be teratogenic and can cause serious congenital malformations. The ear may be completely absent (anotia) or there may be a low-set microtia. Rarely the ear may be abnormally enlarged (macrotia) and the pinna may be duplicated. Atresia or stenosis of the external canal is present in approximately 25 per cent of these patients.

In thalidomide toxicity, 20 per cent of those with thalidomide-induced anomalies have anomalies of the external and middle ear. These include deformed or absent pinna, complete or partial atresia of the external auditory canal, deformed tympanic membrane, a fixed malleus and an absent stapes. Inner ear anomalies are also common and include aplasia of the inner ear. Approximately 75 per cent of those with ear anomalies can also be expected to have a moderate to profound sensorineural hearing loss.

DISEASES ASSOCIATED WITH ENVIRONMENTAL FACTORS

Diseases caused by environmental factors include endemic cretinism secondary to low intake of iodine and congenital abnormalities secondary to excessive exposure to radiation. External and middle ear abnormalities may be seen with both these conditions.

Disorders of the external ear

Abnormalities of the external ear may occur in isolation, may be associated with anomalies of the middle and inner ear or may be part of a more widespread syndrome.

ANOTIA

Anotia is the absence of the auricle, which may be replaced by one or two small rudimentary tubercles, or there may be no external evidence of any tissue. The external auditory meatus is usually absent, or is replaced by a blind-ended pit or a sinus. Anotia is a rare abnormality. However, up to one-fifth of children suffering from thalidomide-induced abnormalities exhibit ear deformities and anotia represents over 50 per cent of these.

MICROTIA

Microtia is a smaller than normal auricle, which is usually misshapen (Fig 18.3). It is found in approximately 0.03 per cent of all new born infants. It is associated with atresia or stenosis of the external auditory canal and frequently with ossicular abnormalities. Most of the cases are isolated or sporadic although a familial pattern has been reported. Three groups, graded according to severity, can be recognized:

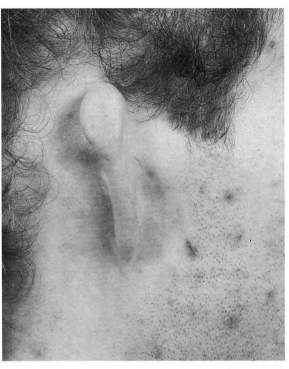

Fig 18.3 A rudimentary grade 2 pinna in a 'non-syndromic' young man. The other ear had been much less severely affected and had been reconstructed. He had good hearing on the reconstructed side and was not interested in further procedures.

- grade 1: malformed pinna, which is small but retains most of the features of a normal auricle
- grade 2: rudimentary pinna consisting of a low, cylindrical bar of tissue that is curved at the cranial end, corresponding to the helix
- grade 3: a more severe deformity in which only a malformed nodule is present and the rest of the pinna is absent (this is close to the classification of anotia and, of course, there is an almost continuous range of deformity that is difficult to classify by a categorical arrangement)

MACROTIA

Macrotia is an auricle that is unduly large while retaining a normal anatomical configuration. The large size may be cosmetically unacceptable and it may be reduced by a wedge excision of the skin and the cartilage. Usually there is no abnormality of function.

POLYOTIA

Polyotia is a very rare abnormality that was first described in 1918 in a child with two well formed auricles facing each other on one side of the head, whereas on the other side there was a normal auricle with two accessory appendages.

SYNOTIA AND MELOTIA

With synotia the auricle is placed posteriorly in the cervical part of the neck. An ear located further forwards on the cheek is referred to melotia.

ANOMALIES OF THE LOBULE

The lobule is the last part of the auricle to develop. It may be enlarged or absent. It is occasionally adherent to the side of the head or it may split because of incomplete union of the first and second arches.

ANOMALIES OF THE HELIX

Anomalies of the helix are of academic and cosmetic interest only and are not associated with abnormal function. A small protuberance seen above the middle of the helix is referred to as Darwin's tubercle (Fig 18.4). In 'cat's ears' the auricle is folded forward and downwards in varying degrees. 'Cup' or telephone ears are unduly hollow. Several eponymous abnormalities are described: Wildermuth ear has an antihelix that is more prominent than the helix; Mozart ear has an enlarged antihelix that is continuous with the helix. Finally, there may be one or more pre-auricular appendages that represent accessory auricles (Fig 18.5). Altman found them in 1.5 per cent of the population. They are usually located in front of the tragus and may be part of a first arch anomaly such as the Treacher Collins syndrome or the Goldenhar syndrome. Each appendage contains elastic cartilage that extends medially. It is therefore insufficient to cut the appendage flush with the skin as the whole of the cartilage needs to be excised taking care not to damage the underlying facial nerve.

ABNORMALITIES OF THE EXTERNAL AUDITORY MEATUS

The external auditory meatus may be

- patent but narrow along its whole length
- patent but stenosed – that is narrowed – at the junction of its cartilaginous and bony part

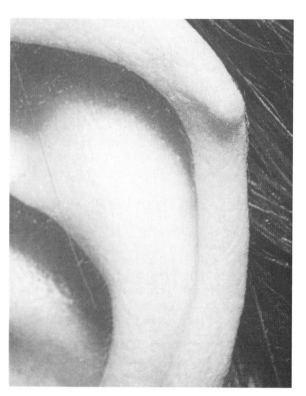

Fig 18.4 A classic Darwin's tubercle.

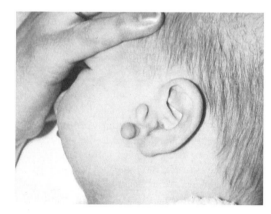

Fig 18.5 Pre-auricular accessory auricles. Unusually, here there are two accessory swellings, both of which had cartilage within them. It is very important to remember that the facial nerve is close to the skin and that removing these swellings is a complex major procedure requiring considerable skill. The child also had Pierre Robin syndrome with micrognathia and a cleft palate as part of the overall pattern.

- atretic – that is closed over – with a membranous or bony (or both) wall across what should have been the canal

Narrowing of the meatus usually does not cause any problems provided that patency is maintained. Regular microsuction may be needed to prevent occlusion by keratin accumulating deep to the narrowed portion.

Meatal stenosis typically occurs at the junction of the bony and cartilaginous canal, where the lumen may be reduced to a pinhole. It is usually unilateral but can be bilateral and familial. There may be other associated abnormalities of the auricle and the middle ear. Meatoplasty may be advised for symptomatic cases.

Congenital atresia is often associated with anomalies of the external and middle ear. It is a relatively common malformation with a frequency of 1–5 in 200 000 live births. Most cases are isolated and sporadic, but a familial pattern has been reported. It results from a failure of the ectodermal cord to canalize and is often associated with abnormalities of the tympanic membrane and the ossicles. It is usually unilateral but may be bilateral (unilateral to bilateral ratio is 4:1) and boys are said to be affected more than girls.

Essentially there is an absence of any bony meatus and a plate of bone exists in place of the tympanic membrane. Frequently there is fusion of the malleus to this atretic plate. The malleoincudal joint may also be fused. The stapes superstructure develops from the second branchial arch and may be normal or deformed, and the footplate (which derives from the labyrinthine capsule) may be fixed. The inner ear is usually healthy. The facial nerve often has an aberrant course and this must be borne in mind if surgery is performed (Fig 18.6).

Congenital meatal atresia is divided into three groups according to severity:

- grade 1 (mild): part of the external canal is present although hypoplastic; the tympanic membrane is present but smaller than normal; the middle ear cavity is usually of a normal size but may be smaller
- grade 2 (moderate): the external canal is completely absent, the tympanic cavity is diminished in size and the ossicles are deformed; the atretic plate is either completely or partially ossified
- grade 3 (severe): the external ear canal is completely absent and the middle ear cavity is markedly smaller or completely absent; the atretic plate is completely ossified

There may be associated abnormalities in the external ear such as deformed pinna, microtia and anotia. Middle ear abnormalities include an abnormal tympanic membrane, replacement of the tympanic membrane by a bony plate, absence of the malleus and incus and fusion of the malleoincudal joint and head of the stapes. In the inner ear there may be abnormalities of the cochlea, vestibule, semicircular canals and the internal auditory meatus.

Congenital abnormalities of the middle ear

TYMPANIC MEMBRANE ABNORMALITIES

The tympanic membrane may be small as in congenital rubella syndrome, it may be distorted as in VATER syndrome or it may be replaced by fibrous tissue. As described above, it may be replaced completely by an atretic bony plate in meatal atresia.

OSSICULAR ABNORMALITIES

Many variations of ossicular abnormalities have been described in all three ossicles. These may be observed alone or with other ear abnormalities such as microtia and atresia, and occasionally they may feature as part of a syndrome.

Abnormalities of the malleus include absence of a part or the whole of the ossicle. The malleus may be fused to the lateral epitympanic wall or anteriorly to the tympanic ring. Occasionally all three ossicles are fused together. More frequently the malleoincudal joint is ossified.

Abnormalities of the incus include absence of the long process or the lenticular process. Rarely the whole ossicle is missing. In addition to union with the malleus, the incus may occasionally be fused to the floor of the aditus.

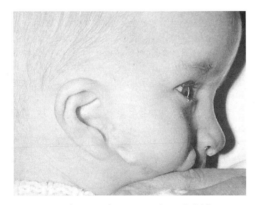

Fig 18.6 External meatal atresia. This child has an external atresia, which is both bony and membranous in extent. There is an associated facial cleft, which can be clearly seen, and a cleft lip, which is more difficult to see because of the restraining hand.

Abnormalities of the stapes include absence of the suprastructure, a decrease in size and a col-umella-type stapes. Occasionally the stapedial tendon is ossified and the stapes head may be fused to the promontory. There may be fixation of the stapes footplate.

Ossicular abnormalities are often associated with abnormalities of the intratympanic muscles. The course of the facial nerve may be aberrant. In cases of a congenitally fixed stapes footplate an abnor-mally patent cochlear aqueduct may be present, which results in a perilymphatic gusher if the foot-plate is removed during stapedectomy.

FACIAL NERVE ABNORMALITIES

It is important to be aware that the facial nerve is much more likely to be abnormal or have an aber-rant course when other congenital external and middle ear abnormalities are present. The major concern in undertaking exploration of a congenital atresia is that in approximately 20 per cent of these patients the facial nerve will have an abnormal course and is therefore liable to surgical damage. To avoid surgical misadventure the surgeon must identify the facial nerve early in the temporal bone exploration. The most constant anatomical course is in the anterior epitympanum where the nerve enters the tympanic cavity. The nerve should be identified at this site early in the dissection and then traced distally, with the surgeon aware of the many possible variations in its course.

There may be a congenital facial palsy, unilateral or bilateral, as seen in the Moebius syndrome. Here there is, classically, a congenital, non-progressive bilateral facial nerve palsy often associated with an abducent (VI) nerve palsy. The syndrome has been broadened to include unilateral palsies and may well be due to focal areas of necrosis in the brain, which have been found in well documented autopsy cases. It is possible that hypoxic episodes during critical periods of development result in selective necrosis of the tegmental nuclei in the brainstem and the facial nerve nucleus.

In the Goldenhar syndrome there is a lower motor neuron facial nerve palsy in about 10–20 per cent of affected children, probably related to bony involvement of the facial nerve in the middle ear and mastoid segment. The nerve is frequently ves-tigial or absent.

The commonest cause of congenital facial palsy has been thought to be trauma during birth when forceps are used to deliver the head of the baby or when other risk factors associated with a difficult delivery are present. This view has recently been challenged by Laing *et al.* (1996) in a study of chil-dren with established non-syndromic, congenital facial palsies. It was found that their births were no more complex than matched controls and the con-clusion was that an intrauterine aetiology was more likely. Thalidomide-induced congenital facial palsy has also been reported.

Congenital dehiscence of the Fallopian canal in the horizontal portion of the facial nerve is a common finding in approximately one-quarter of patients at tympanotomy. The nerve may be dis-placed inferiorly to encroach on the stapes and the oval window. Rarely the nerve lies below the stapes, whose arch is deformed around the nerve. The nerve may be seen to split into two or three branches, which continue separately in the vertical portion. In approximately 15 per cent of temporal bones the descending portion of the facial nerve is displaced laterally and anteriorly. In some cases of congenital atresia, particularly those associated with Treacher Collins syndrome, the nerve may run laterally from the geniculate ganglion and leave the temporal bone immediately. Abnormalities of the tympanic branches of the facial nerve have also been reported. The chorda tympani, the greater superficial petrosal nerve and the lesser superficial petrosal nerve may be absent, poorly developed or have an aberrant course.

ABNORMALITIES OF THE TYMPANIC CAVITY

Vascular abnormalities

Abnormalities of the internal carotid artery are extremely rare. Six cases of anomalous internal carotid artery in the middle ear have been described. It affects girls more than boys and is usually unilateral. Clinical findings include pulsatile tinnitus and a bruit can be heard over the external auditory canal. Examination of the ear shows a red vascular mass in the anteroinferior portion of the tympanum behind an intact tympanic membrane. Usually there are no other associated abnormali-ties. Differential diagnosis includes an aneurysm of the carotid artery and a glomus jugulare tumour. Diagnosis is easily confirmed by a CT scan and a carotid arteriogram or, if the facilities exist, a digital subtraction angiogram using magnetic resonance imaging. No treatment is required if the diagnosis is a carotid artery anomaly, although the problem should be explained in writing as a warning against risks of future intervention.

Aneurysms of the internal carotid artery are rarely seen in the middle ear cavity because they herniate through a defect in the floor of the hypo-tympanum. They present as pulsatile, red smooth masses in the anteroinferior portion of the tympanum, and they also cause pulsatile tinnitus.

Jugular bulb anomalies include a high jugular bulb (Fig 18.7 and Plate section) or a herniation of the bulb into the middle ear cavity through a congenital bony defect in the posteroinferior part of the tympanum. On examination a blue rounded mass is visible arising from the hypotympanum. Occasionally, a diagnosis is made only during a tympanotomy or a myringotomy.

The stapedial artery, which is the artery of the second branchial arch, is sometimes persistent and can be moderately large. It may be a source of troublesome bleeding during a stapedectomy. A large vessel crossing the stapes footplate can make the surgery extremely difficult if not impossible.

Congenital cholesteatoma of the middle ear

Congenital cholesteatoma accounts for approximately 2–3 per cent of all cholesteatomas. It is usually unilateral but may be bilateral. It often appears as a conductive hearing loss. On examination there is a white mass behind an intact tympanic membrane (Fig 18.8 and Plate section). The size varies from a small pearl to a large mass filling the entire middle ear cavity and extending towards the petrous apex. Depending on size, the ossicles may be intact or completely eroded. Congenital cholesteatoma behind an atretic bony plate has been reported. Diagnosis is confirmed by a preoperative CT scan, which also excludes a congenital petrous apex dermoid cyst presenting like the tip of an iceberg in the middle ear.

Congenital perilymph fistula

A congenital perilymph fistula is an abnormal communication between the perilymphatic space of the inner ear and the middle ear cavity. Perilymphatic fluid leaks into the middle ear via this fistula, which is usually located in the region of the oval window. Associated abnormalities of the middle ear and the inner ear are common. Inner ear deformities include a Mondini-type deformity, a wide cochlear aqueduct, an enlarged vestibular aqueduct and a deformity of the fundus of the internal auditory canal. Children with these anomalies present with a fluctuating and progressive sensorineural hearing loss, which is often profound. These symptoms are accompanied by tinnitus, vertigo and occasionally recurrent meningitis. Diagnosis can be confirmed by a CT scan after an intrathecal injection of contrast agent. In those children with recurrent meningitis, the abnormal inner ear and the middle ear cavity must be obliterated together with a blind-pit closure of the external canal.

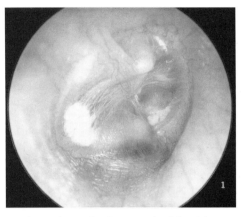

Fig 18.7 An endoscopic photograph of the right tympanic membrane. The patient was an achondroplastic dwarf and had as an incidental finding this high and exposed jugular bulb in the right middle ear.

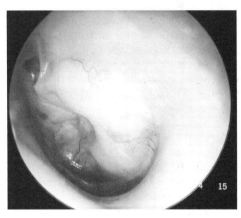

Fig 18.8 An endoscopic photograph of the left tympanic membrane of a 4-year-old child who presented with a unilateral hearing loss detected at routine school screening when headphones rather than free-field testing were used. The intact membrane is bulging with a white mass present in the middle ear. The attic is intact and the mass was soft on palpation with a Jobson–Horne probe.

Management of congenital abnormalities

Correction of severe congenital external and middle ear deformities is a difficult problem. Surgery is technically demanding and there is always a risk of surgical damage to an abnormally placed facial nerve. Results of treatment are variable. The newly fashioned external canal is liable to re-stenose and chronic otorrhoea from the operative cavity is not uncommon. In unilateral cases the improved hearing thresholds – if there are any – do not often match the contralateral normal ear and the patient perceives little benefit. Management of the microtia is difficult.

In bilateral atresia, amplification with bone conduction should be initiated as soon as possible to allow acquisition of speech and language (preferably by the age of 6 months). Correct timing of surgery is important. In the past it was believed that correction of atresia should precede surgery for the microtia. However, this view has been challenged recently and it is now accepted that virgin, unscarred tissue with a good blood supply is essential for the needs of the surgeon performing the reconstruction. Therefore correction of microtia should take place first to be followed by correction of atresia, if necessary, at the age of 5–6 years. Of course surgery should not be contemplated in the presence of an abnormal cochlea with a profound sensorineural hearing loss as there can be no hearing improvement, only the risk of damage.

In unilateral atresia with a normal contralateral ear, surgery of the atresia should be avoided.

CLINICAL ASSESSMENT

A child with severe congenital ear abnormalities should be assessed and managed by a multidisciplinary team comprising a paediatrician, a geneticist, a craniofacial team and an otolaryngologist. A full history is mandatory and must include family history, obstetric history, history of pre-natal and perinatal infections and history of any alcohol and drug abuse together with prenatal medication. A careful systems review must be sought to exclude any systemic abnormalities. During clinical examination congenital atresia will be immediately apparent. Minor anomalies such as pre-auricular tags and pits may indicate other first and second branchial arch abnormalities such as ossicular and facial nerve deformities. Varying degrees of canal atresia may be encountered.

Accurate audiological assessment is important and aims to establish the presence of normal cochlear function and the degree of any conductive hearing loss. Tympanometry may be of some use if the external canal is patent. All children should have brainstem auditory evoked potentials recorded to establish an approximate hearing threshold.

RADIOLOGY

The advent of modern CT scanning has revolutionized the investigation of congenital ear anomalies. Every child should have a scan, which may be helpful in the following areas. In canal atresia the possibility of surgical correction can be assessed on the basis of internal auditory meatal and cochlear anatomy, middle ear cavity aeration, oval window patency and so on. Ossicular abnormalities may be apparent as a source of the conductive hearing loss. An aberrant course of the facial nerve may be apparent. Cochlear dysplasia may be identified.

The various classes of anomaly of the outer and middle ears are discussed in Chapter 6.

SURGICAL CORRECTION OF THE PINNA

Abnormalities of the pinna range from minor abnormalities such as lobule deformities and pre-auricular tags to gross microtia. Minor defects are readily corrected but treatment of microtia is more difficult. It is now widely accepted that microtia surgery should precede surgery to correct the atretic canal as unscarred virgin tissue is critically important to the plastic surgeon.

Various techniques have been devised for correction of microtia. Autogenous grafts are the material of choice. Rib cartilage is harvested and fashioned into the shape of a pinna. The recontoured cartilage is then implanted beneath a skin flap raised in the region of the site of the 'new ear'. The skin flap is encouraged to adhere to the cartilage by scrupulous suction drainage. Subsequently, the implanted pinna is elevated from the scalp and a postauricular fold is created using split skin or a scalp advancement flap. Several surgical stages are required and the results are acceptable when surgery is performed by expert hands.

An alternative method is to use a prosthetic ear made from an alloplastic material such as silastic, which is matched for colour and size to the patient and retained to the side of the head by clip-on attachments to posts on bone-anchored titanium screws (Fig 18.9). The advances in surgical technique over the past decade have now made both approaches to reconstructing the external ear quite acceptable. Operations using rib cartilage entail the creation of chest wall scarring and provide a pinna that will not grow with the child. On the other hand, the silastic prosthesis can be enlarged as the child grows but is never anything more than a prosthesis. It appears that about one-half of the children (or their families) opt for a cartilage reconstruction and one-half for a prosthesis.

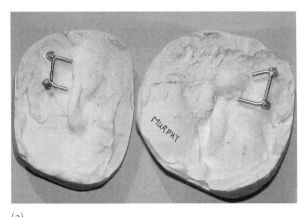

(a)

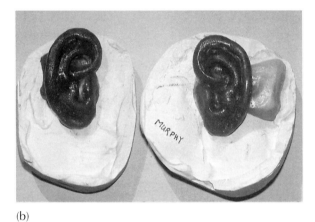

(b)

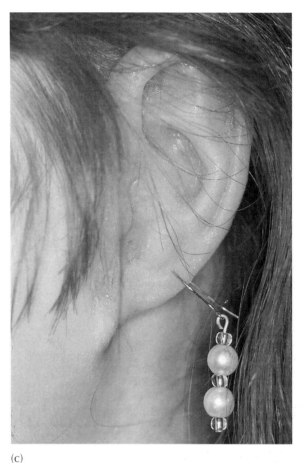

(c)

Fig 18.9 (a) The posts for anchoring the prosthesis modelled on plaster casts of the patient's head to allow for precise planning. (b) Preliminary models are made before final casting in silastic and (c) the completed ear in place and with an earring, which is one of the most common reasons given by girls for wanting 'proper ears'.

SURGERY FOR THE EXTERNAL AUDITORY CANAL

Jahrsdoerfer *et al.* (1992) have devised an excellent preoperative rating scale to assess operability of atresia and the likely outcome of postoperative results. Detailed coronal and axial CT scans are required and certain anatomical factors are assessed and scored (Table 18.1). A perfect score of 10 indicates excellent prospects for a good postoperative result with probable hearing thresholds of approximately 25 dB. Patients who score 5 or less are not considered for surgery. Scores between 6 and 9 are multiplied by a factor of 10 and this gives an approximate percentage of probability for successful outcome.

Table 18.1 Grading system for congenital atresia*

Anatomical feature	Points
Stapes present	2
Oval window open	1
Middle ear space patent	1
Facial nerve course normal	1
Malleus–incus complex present and normal	1
Pneumatized mastoid present	1
Intact incudostapedial joint	1
Patent round window	1
External ear appearance close to normal	1
Total points	10

* Jahrsdoerfer *et al.* 1992

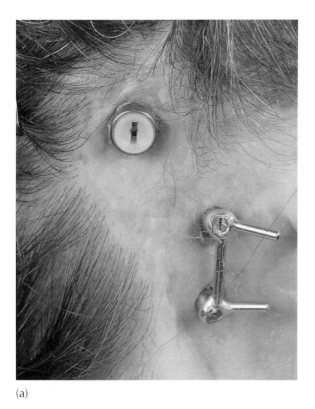

(a)

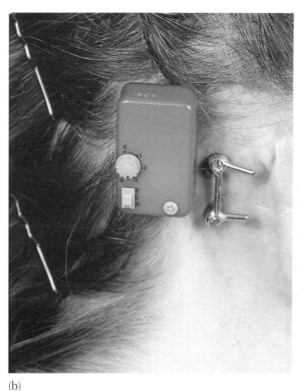

(b)

Fig 18.10 (a) The right ear of a girl with severe Treacher Collins syndrome who has posts for a bone-anchored hearing aid and a prosthetic ear. The modelling for the left ear is shown in Figure 18.9. (b) The bone-anchored hearing aid fitted to the post.

The following cardinal rules should be adhered to before embarking on surgery for congenital atresia.

1. Full audiological and radiological assessment should be performed.
2. The presence of normal internal auditory meatus and cochlear anatomy is essential to any consideration for surgery.
3. Even with normal anatomy of the inner ear, a profound sensorineural hearing loss is a contraindication.
4. Total aplasia (or severe hypoplasia) of the tympanum with very little middle ear air space is a contraindication to surgery. Poorly formed ossicles or an absent stapes will result in a poor outcome.
5. Surgery for microtia should precede correction of atresia.
6. Bilateral atresia should be provided with amplification by the age of 6 months. Surgery for unilateral atresia is unwise.

BONE-ANCHORED APPLIANCES

As mentioned earlier, the results of surgery for congenital atresia are at best mixed. Surgery is technically difficult, with an inherent risk to the facial nerve. The ear canal often re-stenoses and chronic otorrhoea is not uncommon. Any improvement in hearing although audiometrically impressive may not be clinically significant. Postoperative management is often difficult and the child has to attend the specialist clinic at regular intervals. Repeated dressings to the external canal may be required. Surgery for correction of the microtia is complicated, often multistaged and technically difficult.

As a result of these difficulties, many clinicians prefer to use bone-anchored appliances with osseous integrated titanium screws. These can be used to retain bone-anchored hearing aids or a prosthetic ear (Fig 18.10). In selected cases, that is, those with good bone conduction thresholds, there is a high degree of patient satisfaction with fewer complications and a much more favourable postoperative course.

Suggested reading

Altman F. Malformations of the auricle and the external auditory meatus (a critical review). *Archives of Otolaryngology* 1951; **54**:115–39.

Crabtree JA. Congenital atresia: case selection, complications and prevention. *Otolaryngology Clinics of North America* 1982; **15**:755–62.

De La Cruz A, Linthicum FH Jr, Luxford WM. Congenital atresia of the external auditory canal. *Laryngoscope* 1985; **95**:421–7.

Gorlin RJ, Cohen MM, Levin LS. *Syndromes of the head and neck*. Oxford: Oxford University Press, 1990.

Granstrom G, Bergstrom K, Tjellstrom A. Bone anchored hearing aid and bone anchored epithesis for congenital ear malformations. *Otolaryngology – Head and Neck Surgery* 1993; **109**:46–53.

Jahrsdoerfer RA. Congenital atresia of the ear. *Laryngoscope* 1978; **88(Suppl 13)**:1–48.

Jahrsdoerfer RA. The facial nerve in congenital middle ear malformations. *Laryngoscope* 1981; **91**:1217–25.

Jahrsdoerfer RA. Congenital malformations of the ear: an analysis of 94 operations. *Annals of Otology, Rhinology and Laryngology* 1980; **89**:348–52.

Jahrsdoerfer RA, Yeakley JW, Aguilar EA, Cole RR, Gray LC. Grading system for the selection of patients with congenital aural atresia. *American Journal of Otology* 1992; **13**:6–12.

Laing JH, Harrison DH, Jones BM, Laing GJ. Is permanent facial palsy caused by birth trauma? *Archives of Diseases in Childhood* 1996; **74**:56–8.

Sakashita T, Sando I, Kamerer DB. Congenital anomalies of the external and middle ear. In: Bluestone, Stool, Kenna eds. *Paediatric otolaryngology, 3rd edn*. Philadelphia: WB Saunders, 1996:333–70.

CHAPTER 19

Congenital abnormalities of the inner ear

HENRI AM MARRES

Introduction

In Western Europe, the prevalence of early child-hood deafness (average hearing level in the better ear of 25 dB) is estimated to be 1 in 750–1000 births. There is a strong likelihood of a genetic cause in over 50 per cent, whereas in the remainder it is probably possible to attribute the cause to a particular event (i.e. infection) during pregnancy or in the perinatal period, that is, acquired disease (Table 19.1). If hearing impairment is diagnosed in an infant or preschool child, then the following items are of importance when taking a history:

- maternal infection(s)
- use of ototoxic medication during pregnancy or in the postnatal period
- course of delivery
- postnatal infection(s)
- trauma
- family history

Table 19.1 Causes of early childhood (inner ear) hearing loss

Acquired	Prenatal
	Perinatal
	First year postnatal
Inherited	Autosomal dominant
	Autosomal recessive
	X-linked
	Mitochondrial
	Chromosomal

Besides otological and audiometric testing, general physical examination is essential to detect any other anomalies; in some cases it may also be worthwhile to examine the parents and siblings. Ophthalmological and neurological examinations can make valuable contributions to the diagnosis. The younger the child, the more difficult it is to make a diagnosis. However, the earlier the diagnosis, the greater the benefit of adequate hearing rehabilitation to the general development of the child and particularly to their speech and language acquisition.

Acquired hearing loss

RUBELLA (GERMAN MEASLES)

In a large proportion of children with acquired congenital hearing loss, the cause is maternal rubella infection. Estimated rates lie between 10 and 15 per cent. Over the past few decades, the percentage has decreased in the developed world as a result of the introduction of rubella vaccination programmes in the 1970s.

The classic congenital rubella syndrome (CRS) comprises a triad of symptoms: hearing loss, cataracts and cardiac anomalies. The CRS was described for the first time, although incompletely, by Gregg[1] and Swan et al.[2] The infection can have a teratogenous effect at any time during pregnancy, but it is most detrimental in the first trimester. Various studies have shown that the risk of congenital hearing loss as a result of maternal infection is 50 per cent. Maternal infection is characterized by the classic rash, but it can also have a subclinical course and not be recognized. Hearing impairment often appears to be the only symptom when the maternal infection runs a subclinical course.[3] The most reliable indication of maternal infection is an increase in the rubella titre during pregnancy, whereas in a young child a positive rubella titre forms the best indication. The older the child, the greater the chance that primary infection is the cause if the titre is found to be positive. The level of hearing loss is not constant, but the pure tone average is usually poorer than 60 dB. Little is known about the vestibular function in these patients, although various studies have shown that it may be impaired. Audiometry and ophthalmological examination are essential for making the diagnosis. Besides cataracts, the CRS may also include characteristic retinal pigment anomalies, the so-called pepper and salt effect. Tapetoretinal degeneration should also be excluded with the aid of an electro-oculogram and an electroretinogram.

TOXOPLASMOSIS

Congenital toxoplasmosis is diagnosed in 6 out of 1000 newborns. Symptoms of infection are seldom found. The classic serious form of the disease is very rare. Primary infection of the mother during pregnancy holds the greatest risk of symptoms occurring in the offspring. Infection during the first trimester in particular is associated with a high risk of transmission to the infant; symptoms include chorioretinitis, intracerebral calcification, psychomotor disturbances and hydrocephaly or microcephaly. Hearing loss always coincides with several of the abovementioned symptoms and occurs in 10–15 per cent of children with congenital toxoplasmosis. The serological Sabin–Feldman test can be used in the diagnostic work-up, but animal inoculation is essential to make the definitive diagnosis. _Toxoplasma gondii_ is found fairly commonly in cat faeces. Therefore the avoidance or prevention of exposure during pregnancy will reduce the risk of infection in a seronegative expectant mother. Early diagnosis and the subsequent initiation of antimicrobial therapy may help to reduce the level of hearing impairment.[4]

CYTOMEGALOVIRUS

An infection with cytomegalovirus (CMV) nearly always has a subclinical course and for this reason it is impossible to distinguish it as a cause of hearing impairment in retrospective studies. CMV is the most common pathogen in congenital viral infections (up to 2 per cent). Primary maternal infection leads to fetal infection in 20–50 per cent of cases. The outcome may be a spontaneous abortion or cytomegalic inclusion disease: a spectrum of symptoms in the newborn, including microcephaly, periventricular calcifications, chorioretinitis, optic nerve atrophy, sensorineural deafness, cardiac anomalies and growth retardation. It has been estimated that 1 in every 1000 newborns is seriously physically and mentally retarded as a result of congenital CMV infection. So far there is no clear evidence as to whether the time of infection during pregnancy has any influence on the severity of the ensuing anomalies; the transmission of infection can also occur during passage through the birth canal. It is usually possible to detect the virus in the saliva and urine of the newborn infant after about 8–12 weeks using electron microscopy. Sensorineural hearing loss (SNHL) is sometimes the only symptom of congenital CMV infection and it can progress swiftly during the infant's first years.

HERPES SIMPLEX VIRUS

Transplacental infection of the fetus with herpes simplex virus (HSV) type 1 or type 2 is very rare. Transmission of the infection usually occurs during delivery, owing to the presence of the virus in the birth canal. If the mother has herpetic cervicitis, the risk of infection is 40 per cent and there is a preference to perform a caesarian section because infection of the newborn nearly always has a fatal outcome. Hearing impairment as a result of HSV infection has been described, but there is little insight into this aspect of the disease.

CONGENITAL SYPHILIS

Syphilis is caused by _Treponema pallidum_ and can be transmitted _in utero_ via the placenta. This often leads to spontaneous abortion or a stillborn infant. Congenital syphilis, which is rare in western countries, is characterized in the early stages by meningoneuritis and labyrinthitis. Later, between the ages of 10 and 30 years, Hutchinson's triad can be recognized: interstitial keratitis, SNHL and screwdriver teeth. If maternal infection is diagnosed, adequate treatment should be initiated and continued in the newborn. The presence of IgM _Treponema_ antibodies in a newborn's blood, detected using the fluorescent treponomal antibody (FTA-ABS) test, is a good indication of intrauterine infection.

KERNICTERUS

Schmorl[5] introduced the term kernicterus in 1904 on the basis of his histopathological findings at post-mortem in stillborn infants and those who died peri-natally. Kernicterus arises because of rhesus antagonism particularly in premature births, and occasionally it is caused by blood group A and B incompatibility. The incidence of rhesus incompatibility has decreased strongly over the past few decades owing to elective rhesus immunoglobin administration to rhesus-negative mothers who deliver a rhesus-positive infant. Hyperbilirubinaemia of more than 340 mmol/l is considered to be harmful and can lead to kernicterus. Exchange transfusion can form an essential part of treatment for hyper-bilirubinaemia. If left untreated, the consequences of kernicterus can include severe athetoid cerebral palsy, fits and mental retardation. The lesion responsible is localized in the auditory nuclei and in some cases in the auditory nerve. Hair cells are not usually affected, which can be confirmed by means of brain-stem auditory evoked potentials. Retrospective studies have reported that 2.5–17 per cent of hearing loss is caused by hyperbilirubinaemia.[6]

Hereditary hearing loss

Research into the causes of hereditary hearing loss and hereditary deafness was initiated in the second half of the nineteenth century. The first reports of a number of fairly common hereditary syndromes that have hearing loss as one of their characteristic symptoms were published during this period. For example, in 1858 the German ophthalmologist Albrecht von Graefe[7] was the first to describe the occurrence of retinitis pigmentosa and congenital deafness in three affected brothers.

Three years later Liebreich[8] recognized this condition during a study on deaf persons in the Jewish population of Berlin and he drew attention to consanguinity between the parents of the affected individuals. In 1907, Hammerschlag[9] discovered a high frequency of the disorder among the Jewish community in Vienna. This was followed in 1914 by a British description by the Scottish ophthalmologist Charles Usher[10] from Aberdeen. Usher also mentioned the condition in his Bowman Lecture in 1935, which was entitled 'On a few hereditary eye affections'. As a consequence, his name became an eponym for the syndrome, especially in the ophthalmological literature.

Although physicians had known for several centuries that congenital deafness in a young child could also occur in his or her siblings, the first sys-tematic study on the causes of congenital deafness was not conducted until 1853 by Sir William Wilde[11] from Dublin. He recognized heredity as the cause of congenital deafness and also concluded that consanguinity between the parents increased the risk of this disorder. In 1882, Politzer[12] wrote in his text-book on otology on the basis of conclusions from other studies: 'The most frequent causes of congenital deafness are: heredity, including direct transmission from the parents as well as indirect transmission from forefathers and marriage between blood relations'.

It took until the beginning of the twentieth century, however, for Mendel's laws (published in 1865) to be recognized as an explanation for heredity. In the first half of the twentieth century, studies on the causes of deafness were continued on a large scale and several impressively large series including autosomal recessive hereditary deafness, were published in detail. Many of the investigations at that time were devoted to the study of deafness in various types of animal.

Knowledge about the syndromic and non-syndromic forms of hereditary hearing loss has greatly increased, particularly in the second half of this century. The more common syndromes have been described repeatedly and in minute detail, with special attention to the degree of penetrance of the syndrome and the degree of expression of the separate symptoms. On the basis of hereditary, the type of hearing loss and other audiometric characteristics, it has become possible to describe a series of separate non-syndromic hereditary forms of hearing loss. In this period, the first overviews appeared of the many (and ever increasing number of) hereditary syndromes that have deafness as one of the symptoms.

By the 1970s more than 150 (non-)syndromic hereditary forms of hearing loss had been documented, and the number has increased since then to more than 350.[13,14] In a few of these generally autosomal hereditary diseases, gene-linkage studies have very recently led to gene localization.

When hearing loss occurs as an isolated symptom, it can be referred to as non-syndromic hearing loss, whereas if it is associated with other symptoms, these can often be recognized as forming a syndrome. Besides autosomal dominant, autosomal recessive and sex-linked hereditary deafness, there is also mitochondrial hereditary deafness.

AUTOSOMAL DOMINANT HEARING LOSS

Autosomal dominant hearing loss occurs in about 30 per cent of cases with autosomal hereditary

Table 19.2 Several studies of congenital hearing loss

Study	Number in study	Aetiology (%)		
		Hereditary	Acquired	Unknown
Fraser 1964[15]	2355	32	32	36
Huizing 1970[16]	100	20	56	24
Cremers 1976[17]	60	37	38	25
Newton 1985[18]	111	25	32	43
Holten 1985[19]	94	33	41	26
Kankunen 1982[20]	179	55	29	16
Parving 1984[21]	117	48	42	10
Van Rijn 1989[6]	162	38	28	34
These studies together		20–55	27–56	10–43

hearing loss (Table 19.2). In less than one-half of the children with this type of hearing loss, other syndromic features can be recognized. Generally, it is not difficult to make a diagnosis because the familial character of the hearing loss is usually fairly obvious. If hearing loss is found in two or three successive generations, whether or not in association with other features, then there is usually an autosomal dominant pattern of inheritance, especially if the hearing loss has been passed on from father to son. Occasionally, other members of the family will be unaffected. Any syndrome appearing in an isolated patient may be an instance of spontaneous mutation.

Several forms of autosomal dominant hereditary SNHL are described below.

Non-syndromic autosomal dominant hearing loss

On the basis of differences in the time of onset, the rate of progression and the type of audiogram, six types of non-syndromic autosomal dominant SNHL can be recognized (Table 19.3). Actual differentiation will only be possible when gene-linkage studies have been completed.

At present 13 genes have been located that are responsible for a non-syndromic type of hearing impairment. It is striking that these types of hearing loss are milder than the autosomal recessive types of SNHL, probably on the basis of negative marital selection. Chromosome 1p seems to be the most important localization in view of the fact that gene linkage has been accomplished in affected families from various different continents.[22] By investigating several persons within one family (particularly their serial audiograms) it is possible to gain an insight into the rate of progression that can be expected in an individual patient. Vestibular examination seems to be of little value because in various large family studies it hardly made any contribution to interfamily differentiation. However, further examination is warranted if a patient has vestibular complaints or symptoms.

The Waardenburg syndrome

The Waardenburg syndrome was described for the first time as such in the 1940s. At present, two types can be distinguished on the basis of the symptoms present (Table 19.4). Type-II appears to be the more common of the two. The gene responsible for

Table 19.3 Autosomal dominant hearing loss without associated abnormalities

Type of audiogram	Remarks	Gene linkage on chromosome
High-frequency deafness	Slowly progressive at all frequencies	1p
High-frequency deafness	Progressive at high frequencies	7p
Mid-frequency deafness	Most pronounced in mid-frequencies	11q
Low-frequency deafness	Progressive at low and later at high frequencies	5q
High-frequency deafness	Late onset (postlingual) progressive	14q and 6q
High-frequency deafness	Stable hearing loss	13q

Table 19.4 The Waardenburg syndrome

Symptoms	Type I	Type II
Dystopia canthorum	++++	−
White forelock or white eyelashes	++	++
Heterochromia iridis	++	++
SNHL	++	+++
Synophrys	+++	+
Gene location	chromosome 2q	chromosome 3p

++++, always; +++, usually; ++, often; +, sometimes; −, never.

Waardenburg's syndrome type-I has recently been localized on the long arm of chromosome 2. The syndrome shows complete penetrance, but expression is variable. SNHL is a more common feature of type-II than of type-I (60 and 30 per cent, respectively). The characteristic dystopia canthorum in type-I is based on an increased distance between the inner canthi (Fig 19.1). The distance between the outer canthi generally lies within the normal range, but in 10 per cent of patients, actual hypertelorism may be present. A white forelock is present in about 30 per cent of the patients with type-I and type-II and facilitates recognition of the syndrome. A usual feature is heterochromia iridis.

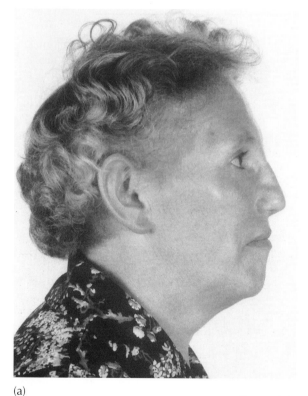

(a)

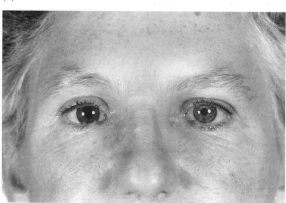

(b)

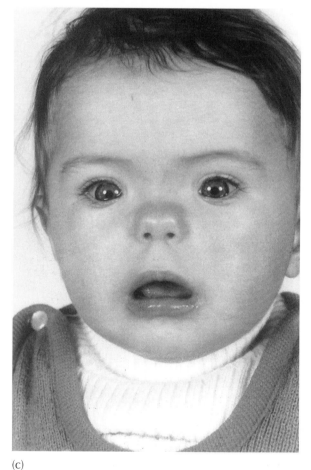

(c)

Fig 19.1 Waardenburg's syndrome type-I (a) the typical profile; (b) heterochromia iridis; and (c) marked dystopia canthorum.

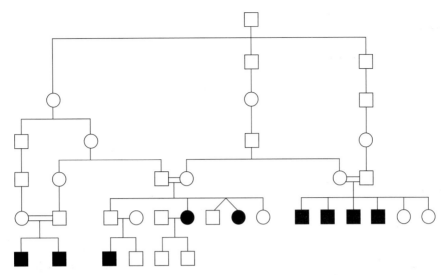

Fig 19.2 Pedigree of family with nine persons with profound SNHL due to autosomal recessive inheritance. Eight of these are offspring of three consanguineous marriages.[23]

AUTOSOMAL RECESSIVE HEARING LOSS

About two-thirds of hereditary hearing loss is caused by an autosomal recessive disorder. These autosomal recessive disorders can be divided into syndromic and non-syndromic types by analogy with the autosomal dominant disorders. Hearing loss is generally more severe than in the autosomal dominant syndromes. Diagnosis is often hindered by the absence of a positive family history. However, if there are siblings with similar symptoms, or if the parents are consanguineous, this will provide support for an autosomal recessive hereditary syndrome as is shown in Figure 19.2. The risk of consanguinity is greater in populations isolated geographically or, for example, by a cultural or religious background.[23]

A syndrome can often be recognized if a patient has several coincidental symptoms. The best known autosomal recessive syndromes are the Usher syndrome and the Pendred syndrome. Hearing loss can also occur as an associated symptom in other syndromes, but the severity of such disorders is based on a completely different area, such as the degree of metabolic disturbance in the Hurler syndrome.

Non-syndromic autosomal recessive hearing loss

So far, 17 genes that are responsible for non-syndromic autosomal recessive hearing loss have been localized. This is probably the most common type of hereditary hearing loss. The incidence is estimated to be 1 in 3000 newborns.

Gene-linkage studies are progressing slowly because it is necessary to perform clinical studies on families that are large enough to have a sufficient number of affected persons. On the basis of the type of audiogram, the time of onset and the rate of progression, different types of this anomaly can be distinguished clinically; the intrafamily variation in expression is low. Unfortunately, it has not been possible to detect carriers on the basis of subclinical symptoms, so genetic counselling of the siblings of an affected person is difficult. The risk that their genetic material is affected is 50 per cent, but the risk of having affected offspring also depends on whether the partner is a carrier of the same gene.

The Usher syndrome

About 6–12 per cent of patients with a hereditary form of hearing loss have the Usher syndrome. Three types of the syndrome can be distinguished; besides retinitis pigmentosa, the level of hearing loss and possible vestibular dysfunction are the most important features (Table 19.5).

Retinitis pigmentosa is present in all three types of the syndrome and in type-I it even causes symptoms at a young age. The first symptom is night blindness, followed by scotoma and eventually by tunnel vision. Patients with the Usher syndrome type-I are the most severely handicapped owing to the early onset of symptoms and the majority need to be cared for at specialized nursing homes.

Table 19.5 The Usher syndrome

	Type I	Type II	Type III
Hearing loss	Profound; all frequencies	Moderate to profound; mainly high frequencies	Progressive
Onset	Congenital	Congenital	First–second decades
Vestibular function	Absent	Normal	Variable
Retinitis pigmentosa	First decade	Second–third decade	Variable
Gene localization	Type IA on 14q Type IB on 11q Type IC on 11p	Type IIA on 1q Type IIB unknown	Type III on 3q

The Pendred syndrome

The hereditary aetiology of this syndrome was not discovered until 1956, 60 years after it was first described by Pendred.[24] Like the Usher syndrome it is one of the more common syndromes. Estimates of the incidence range from 1 to 7.5 per 100 000 newborns. The Pendred syndrome accounts for between 1 and 10 per cent of the hereditary types of hearing loss.

The level of hearing loss is variable and can reach 100 dB. Severe hearing loss sometimes develops within the first 10 years of a patient's life. There may also be vestibular involvement, which is expressed as vestibular hyporeflexia in about 40 per cent of patients. Besides the SNHL, another striking feature is goitre, which occasionally arises in the second or third decade of life (Fig 19.3). Thyroid function is normal in one-half of the patients, but it can also be slightly reduced. This goitre is the result of a thyroid hormone organification defect. The oral perchlorate test can detect a defect in the organic binding of iodine, particularly if potassium iodide is added. Besides audiometric, vestibular and laboratory tests, radiological examination is also essential. In the majority of patients with the Pendred syndrome, a Mondini-like cochlear anomaly can be demonstrated.

Carriers of the gene have a negative perchlorate test and no subclinical audiometric symptoms are present.

X-LINKED HEARING LOSS

The incidence of X-linked hearing loss is low and it is estimated to form 1 per cent of the hereditary types of hearing loss. The symptom usually forms part of a syndrome, such as the Alport syndrome, the Norrie syndrome, the stapes gusher syndrome or the albinism deafness syndrome.[13,14]

MITOCHONDRIAL HEARING LOSS

Our knowledge of a mitochondrial pattern of inheritance is fairly recent and is based on insight obtained into the role of mitochondrial DNA

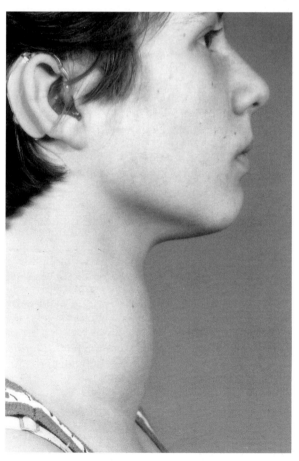

Fig 19.3 Pendred syndrome with marked goitre and SNHL.

(mt-DNA) and nuclear DNA. These two types of DNA can be distinguished by

- exclusive transmission of mt-DNA in the ovum to the offspring, known as maternal inheritance
- a high mutation frequency owing to inadequate repair mechanisms
- the occurrence of heteroplasia, which means that several copies of mt-DNA may exist, but clinical symptoms do not arise until a certain threshold of mutant mt-DNA has been exceeded

Mitochondria play an essential role in metabolism. Therefore, disturbances are expressed most clearly in those with a high metabolic rate, such as striated muscle, the brain, retina and inner ear. Symptoms can be isolated or associated. Late onset is characteristic of syndromes with a mitochondrial pathogenesis. In contrast to the autosomal dominant syndromes, no male to male inheritance can be demonstrated.

So far very few families have been described with isolated hearing loss on the basis of a mitochondrial pattern of inheritance. Very recently this type of hearing loss has been recognized, for example, in association with maternally inherited hypersensitivity to dihydrostreptomycin.[25]

In other mitochondrial syndromes, such as MELAS (mitochondrial encephalomyopathy with lactic acidosis and stroke-like episodes), MERRF (myoclonus epilepsy red ragged fibres), CPO (chronic progressive external ophthalmoplegia) and KSS (Kearns–Sayre syndrome), hearing problems are often the first symptom, whereas the other neurological symptoms do not manifest themselves until about the age of 40 years.

Rehabilitation for genetic deafness

It may often seem to be of little consequence to establish a genetic cause for a patient's deafness, regardless of whether it is an isolated or associated symptom; however, a correct diagnosis is essential for adequate counselling of the patient. Children who are at risk should undergo audiometric tests at the youngest possible age. High-frequency audiometry may help to detect hearing loss at an early stage in development.

As there is no therapy for congenital SNHL, it is better to speak in terms of rehabilitation. The aim of rehabilitation programmes for SNHL is to ensure that the child achieves the optimal level of development with the best possible communication system. From time immemorial, institutes for the deaf have been active in this field. Various schools have emerged aimed at sign language, oral–aural communication (e.g. lip-reading) and so-called total communication in which parts of two abovementioned approaches are applied. The choice of school depends on various factors, such as whether the child has any residual hearing. Even in cases of severe perceptive hearing loss of about 90–100 dB, a powerful hearing aid can be very useful during rehabilitation.

A new development for patients with severe SNHL is cochlear implantation (see Chapter 9). This technique entails opening the cochlea and inserting an array of electrodes connected to a subcutaneous receiver. Via an external microphone and speech processor, sound waves are transmitted to the (usually still well functioning) auditory nerve. Extensive experience has been obtained with postlingually deaf adults and the results are excellent. In prelingually deaf adults, the results are somewhat poorer, but a cochlear implant can make an important contribution to rehabilitation.[26] This is also true to a large extent for patients with an additional visual handicap, for example those with the Usher syndrome. Good results can also be achieved in children, and there appears to be less difference between the results of prelingually and postlingually deaf children because the plasticity of the central auditory system is still intact at this age. A cochlear implant is of great benefit not only to speech perception, but also to speech production, which has a major stigmatizing effect ('speech of the deaf'). Societies for the deaf are following these developments critically, certainly when they concern cochlear implantations in very young children. The medicoethical discussion on this topic has not yet been concluded.

References

1. Gregg N. Congenital cataract following german measles in the mother. *Transactions of the Ophthalmological Society of Australia* 1941; **iii**:35–46
2. Swan C, Tostevin AL, Moore B, Mayo H, Black GHB. Congenital defects in infants following infectious diseases during pregnancy. *Medical Journal of Australia* 1943: **ii**:201.
3. Karmody CS. Subclinical maternal rubella and congenital deafness. *New England Journal of Medicine* 1968; **278**:809–14.
4. McGee T, Wolters C, Stein L, *et al*. Absence of sensorineural hearing loss in treated infants and children with congenital toxoplasmosis. *Otolaryngology – Head and Neck Surgery* 1992; **106**:75–80.
5. Schmorl G. *Pathologisch-Histologischen Untersuchungen*. Leipzig: Vogal, 1904.

6. Van Rijn PM. *Causes of childhood deafness [Thesis].* Nijmegen: University of Nijmegen, 1989.
7. von Graefe A. Vereinzelte Beobachtungen und Bernerkungen. Exceptionelles Verhalten des Gesichtsfeldes bei Pigmentenartung der Netzhaut. *Archiv für Klinische Ophthalmologie* 1858; **4**:250–3.
8. Liebreich R. Abkunft und Ehen unter Blutsverwandten als Grund von Retinitis Pigmentosa. *Deutsche Klinik* 1861; **13**:53–5.
9. Hammerschlag V. Für Kenntnis der Hereditärdegenerativen Taubstummen und ihre differential diagnostiche Bedeutung. *Zeitschrift für Ohrenheilkunde* 1907; **54**:18–36.
10. Usher CH. On the inheritance of retinitis pigmentosa, with notes of cases. *Royal London Ophthalmology Hospital Reports* 1914; **19**:130–236.
11. Wilde WR. *Practical observations on aural surgery and the nature and treatment of diseases of the ear.* London: Churchill, 1853.
12. Politzer A. *Lehrbruch der Ohrenheilkunde, vol 2.* Stuttgart: Enke, 1882.
13. Gorlin RJ, Cohen MM, Levin LS. *Syndromes of the head and neck, 3rd edn.* New York: Oxford University Press, 1990.
14. Gorlin RJ, Toriello HV, Cohen MM. *Hereditary hearing loss and its syndromes.* New York: Oxford University Press, 1995.
15. Fraser GR. A study of causes of deafness amongst 2355 children in special schools. In: Fisch L ed. *Research in deafness in children.* Oxford: Blackwell, 1964:10–3.
16. Huizing EH. Oorzaken van aangeboren slechthorendheid en doofheid. *Proceedings symposium 'Het Slechthorend'.* Amsterdam: 1970:118–32.

17. Cremers CWRJ. *Hereditaire aspectem van vroegkinderlijke doofheid [Thesis].* Nijmegen, The Netherlands: KU Nijmegen; 1976.
18. Newton VE. Aetiology of bilateral sensorineural hearing loss in young children. *Journal of Laryngology and Otology* 1985; **10**:1–57.
19. Holten A, Parving A. Aetiology of hearing disorders in children at the schools for the deaf. *International Journal of Pediatric Otorhinolaryngology* 1985; **10**:229–36.
20. Kankunen A. Preschool children with impaired hearing in Göteborg. *Acta Otolaryngology* 1982; **391**:1–124.
21. Parving A. Aetiological diagnosis in hearing impaired children – clinical value and application of a modern examination programme. *International Journal of Pediatric Otorhinolaryngology* 1984; **7**:29–38.
22. Van Camp G, Coucke P, Kunst H, *et al.* Linkage analysis of progressive hearing loss in five extended families maps the $DFNA_2$ gene to a 1.25-Mb region on chromosome 1p. *Genomics* 1997; **41**:70–4.
23. Marres HAM, Cremers CWRJ. Autosomal recessive nonsyndromal profound childhood deafness in a large pedigree. *Archives of Otolaryngology – Head and Neck Surgery* 1989; **115**:591–5.
24. Draemaker R. Congenital deafness and goitre. *American Journal of Human Genetics* 1956; **8**:253–6.
25. Prezant TR, Agapian JV, Bohlman MC, *et al.* Mitochondrial ribosomal RNA mutation associated with both antibiotic-induced and non-syndromic deafness. *Nature Genetics* 1993; **3**:289–94.
26. Hinderink JB, Mens LHM, Bokx JPL, Van den Broek P. Performance of prelingually and postlingually deaf patients using single-channel or multichannel cochlear implants. *Laryngoscope* 1995; **105**:618–22.

PART IV

Acquired external ear disease

CHAPTER 20

Traumatic disorders of the external ear

ANTHONY F JAHN

Introduction

Despite the exposed location of the auricle and the relatively shallow external ear canal, physical injury to these structures occurs less commonly than might be expected. Several anatomical features protect the outer ear from injury. The auricular framework is elastic cartilage. Unlike hyaline cartilage, this tissue does not normally calcify or ossify. It is therefore easily deflected and difficult to fracture. The auricular cartilage continues into the external ear canal. It is not circumferential, but is interrupted by a gap between the anterior crus of the helix and the tragus. Along the floor of the external canal, the cartilage demonstrates several transverse slits – the fissures of Santorini. These areas of discontinuity further increase the flexibility of the auricular cartilage. The direction of the ear canal is not straight, but has at least two turns. This decreases the likelihood of injury to the tympanic membrane. In other species, such as the cat, the canal is even more tortuous.

Notwithstanding these protective features, the external ear may be damaged by a variety of physical agents. The most important of these are blunt and sharp mechanical trauma and thermal injury.

Blunt injuries of the auricle

Blunt injuries of the auricle usually involve the cartilage-containing pinna portion. The lobule contains fat and fibroconnective tissue only, and offers little resistance to impact. By contrast, the pinna is relatively thin and, despite a degree of flexibility, more easily injured by impacting or shearing forces. The cartilage itself is incompressible and its perichondrium is tightly bound, particularly over the lateral (outer) surfaces.

Seroma of the auricle is a rare condition and comprises a collection of serous fluid in the subperichondrial layer. The seroma forms a fluctuant or tense collection, usually on the lateral surface of the auricle. The area may not be clearly demarcated and is not tender. Its aetiology is either repeated trauma or a single episode, resulting in shearing between the perichondrium and cartilage. An extravasation of serous fluid develops, which may dissect the plane more extensively. I have seen this condition in a retarded child who compulsively rubbed his ear against the mattress for hours at a time. In another case, a man had his ear twisted by his child during boisterous play.

Seromas may be treated initially by sterile aspiration. If the condition recurs, it needs to be evacuated, and the ear bandaged with a compressive dressing. If the seroma is present on medial and lateral surfaces of the auricle, a fracture of the cartilage should be suspected. This is more common with auricular haematomas. If the seroma recurs again, it needs to be surgically opened, the covering perichondrium excised, and the area temporarily oversewn with through-and-through sutures. A bolster pack saturated in antibiotic ointment may be sewn over the area to obliterate the potential dead space.

Haematoma of the auricle also develops after blunt trauma, usually more severe than that which causes a seroma. The classic mechanism for auricular haematoma is a boxing injury. The ear appears

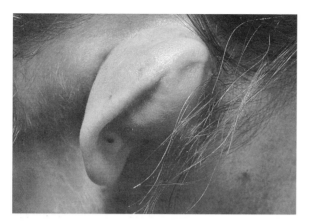

Fig 20.1 Haematoma of the auricle. There is a subperichondrial extravasation of blood along both surfaces of the auricle, suggestive of a fractured cartilage.

bluish and swollen. The swelling is often limited to the lateral surface of the ear, but may involve both surfaces. The swelling is usually in the area over the scaphoid fossa, typically the site of impact, and is limited by the helical rim. The mechanism usually involves traumatic disruption of a perichondrial blood vessel. Blood extravasates into the subperichondrial space, stripping the perichondrium away from the cartilage. If the cartilage is fractured, blood seeps through the fracture line and extends to the subperichondrial plane on the other side (Fig 20.1 and Plate section).

Auricular haematoma may have short-term and long-term consequences. In the short term the condition may lead to chondritis, particularly if the haematoma is drained in a non-sterile fashion. The long-term consequence of an untreated or recurrent auricular haematoma is a deformed ('boxer's') ear. There are three reasons for this: areas of cartilage, deprived of nourishing perichondrium, undergo avascular degeneration; partially resorbed blood and damaged perichondrium form scar tissue; and finally, displaced but viable perichondrium lays down new cartilage, which is no longer part of the original auricular framework. The boxer's ear is therefore often contracted, floppy and deformed in contour (Fig 20.2).

Auricular haematoma is normally sterile unless compounded by a laceration or drainage under substerile conditions. If infected, open drainage and prompt antibiotics must be given to prevent chondritis and significant tissue loss.

Under ordinary circumstances, however, sterile evacuation and application of pressure to prevent reaccumulation is adequate treatment for haematomas. Initially, the blood may be drawn out using a large-bore needle, and the lateral surface of

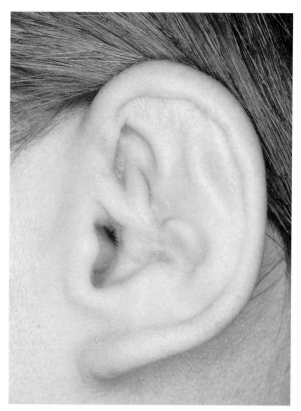

Fig 20.2 Partially deformed auricle, resulting from an untreated haematoma. The contours of the pinna are changed as a result of resorption and redeposition of cartilage.

the auricle packed with Vaseline or Xeroform gauze. This applies the pressure needed to reapproximate the perichondrium to the cartilage. If the haematoma reaccumulates, or blood extravasates on both sides of the auricle as a result of a fractured cartilage, greater pressure needs to be applied after re-evacuation of the blood. Vaseline gauze bolsters can be applied to both sides of the auricle and tied down using through-and-through nylon sutures. Buttons have also been suggested, which allow the sutures to be drawn tight without cutting through. If sutures are placed through the cartilage, oral antibiotics should be given concomitantly.

Sharp trauma of the auricle

Sharp trauma may range from minor lacerations of the pinna or lobule to total avulsion of the auricle. The same basic principles apply to the management of all sharp lacerations, and these are discussed below.

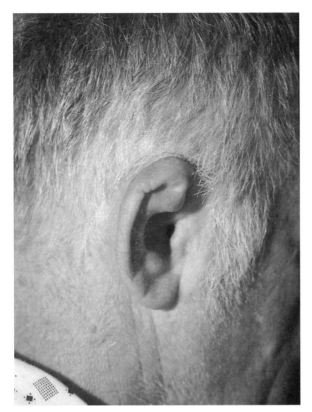

Fig 20.3 Fibrosis of the ear after a human bite. This retarded patient has been bitten several times, and is left with a deformed auricle.

Common causes of minor lacerations include earrings being torn from the ear lobe, and animal or human bites to the pinna (Fig 20.3). Ear lobe lacerations develop in one of two ways. Heavy earrings may, over time, cut through the ear lobe. More acutely, the earring may be torn out accidentally as an infant grabs for the shiny bauble. The ear lobe is devoid of cartilage and is well vascularized. Infection is therefore rare. Repair of a torn ear lobe usually takes place some time after the injury when the edges of the tear are healed. Reconstruction may vary from simple approximation to a Z-plasty or sliding flaps. The more complex repairs break up the line of tear and help to prevent re-injury should the patient wish to repierce the ear for earrings.

Bites may cause lacerations or punctures, and often involve the cartilaginous pinna. They are inflicted most often by small dogs, such as poodles or terriers, which are held in the lap. Human bites sustained during a brawl are the second most common source.

Bites are by definition infected wounds. The human mouth contains a variety of micro-organisms, most notably microaerophilic streptococci.

These wounds must therefore be irrigated, and topical antisepsis used. Tetanus toxoid must be given. A simple puncture wound may then be managed with topical antibiotic ointment. If more complicated, systemic prophylaxis should be considered.

Bites may also cause lacerations, but significant lacerations occur more commonly after a motor vehicle accident or industrial injury. A laceration or partial avulsion needs to be repaired. After copious irrigation, the wound should be surgically debrided to remove non-viable tissue. Exposed cartilage must be addressed. A small edge of exposed cartilage should be trimmed back, so that overlying skin and soft-tissue cover is present. The incision can then be closed. If a large area of cartilage has become exposed by means of a tear or shearing injury, it is worthwhile to embed the cartilage in a postauricular surgical pocket. An incision is made over the mastoid, and a subcutaneous space is created. The exposed cartilage is then buried in this pocket. In some cases, this restores vascularity in a sterile environment. After initial healing is complete, the surgeon can then excise the cartilage with its attached skin cover, and reconstruct the auricle. The postauricular defect can be closed using small sliding or rotational flaps. Even in the absence of overt infection, the initial repair or laceration should be covered by oral antibiotics.

The auricle has a generous blood supply with ample cross anastomoses. Surgeons know that the auricle remains viable even after a Heermann incision, which combines an endaural and postauricular incision, transects three-quarters of the ear's attachments, and pedicles the auricle inferiorly on the postauricular vessels.[1] Even auricles that have been totally avulsed and reattached as a free graft have on occasion survived without the need for microvascular anastomoses.[2] It is therefore recommended that most avulsions, no matter how extensive, be treated by immediate reattachment. If the auricle is severely mangled or overtly infected, this practice should not be followed, although the surgeon should consider salvaging as much cartilage as possible by meticulous debridement and postauricular implantation for later use

Thermal injury and injuries from cold

Cold and heat injuries of the auricle are in some ways similar. Both may exhibit different degrees of severity, resulting in reversible or irreversible tissue damage and cell death.

Burns are traditionally classified in three degrees of severity: erythema (first degree), blistering (second degree) and full-thickness destruction (third degree). The first two are accompanied by pain, whereas a full-thickness burn destroys the nerve endings and is therefore anaesthetic. The commonest burns to the auricle are due to sun exposure. The ultraviolet type-B rays emitted by the sun cause acute and chronic skin damage. Acute sunburn or solar dermatitis results in erythema and a sensation of heat or discomfort. Depending on the severity of exposure, there may be blistering of the skin, most commonly over the helix. These first and second degree burns are best treated by cool compresses and oral anti-inflammatory analgesics. Such milder burns resolve completely; however, repeated or chronic sun exposure will lead to a variety of disorders, including actinic keratoses and skin cancer.

Burns due to scalding liquids or fire are often full thickness. Untreated, they may lead to perichondritis. Prophylactic use of antipseudomonal antibiotics has been recommended. The antibiotic may be injected subperichondrially in six to eight different injection sites distributed over the anterior and posterior surfaces of the auricle.

Compresses saturated with 5 per cent silver nitrate solution are then applied. If bacterial perichondritis develops despite these measures, the infected areas should be surgically opened. Indwelling catheters are then placed, and the site irrigated with a dilute solution of antipseudomonal antibiotics.[3]

Electric burns are particularly destructive, with deep tissue damage and loss of cartilage. The burn should be kept free of infection, and definitive debridement delayed until eschar formation ensues and the demarcation between viable and dead tissue is manifest.

Thermal injury to the ear canal and tympanic membrane is most commonly due to accidental scalding with hot liquids. As the skin of the bony canal and tympanic membrane is thin, the 'heat sink' ability of these tissues is limited. Unlike the auricle, the ear canal tends to retain the hot liquid. For both these reasons, thermal injuries of the ear canal are often more serious than those seen on the surface of the ear.

A specific type of thermal injury in this area is hot slag penetration. Slag, a small hot metal particle generated during smelting, may puncture the eardrum. Mechanical rupture of the membrane is compounded by thermal injury and the slag particle often lodges against the promontory of the middle ear. Otitis media may be produced by the foreign body. Treatment of slag injuries may require removal of the particle and repair of the tympanic membrane.

The auricle is particularly susceptible to frostbite because of its exposed location.[4] The effect of cold is increased by exposure to the wind and by the presence of moisture on the exposed part. These circumstances may be readily present during winter sports activities. The anaesthesia that develops in areas exposed to severe cold allows significant damage to occur 'silently'.

Tissue damage from extreme cold is similar in appearance to heat injury, although the mechanism is different. Heat produces initial vasodilatation and eventual cell death due to heat denaturation of tissue proteins. Exposure to cold results in capillary ischaemia due to prolonged arteriolar vasoconstriction. Over time, this leads to anoxic cell damage. As the ear is rewarmed, profound vasodilatation ensues. The ear becomes erythematous and resembles a first degree burn. There is often an accompanying sensation of burning or itching of the auricle during rewarming.

More profound cold can cause disruption of cell walls as a result of ice crystal formation. Rubbing a frostbitten ear is ill advised, as this will only aggravate the mechanical damage to the tissues. The frostbitten ear may develop bullae, resembling a second degree burn (Fig 20.4). As already mentioned, the

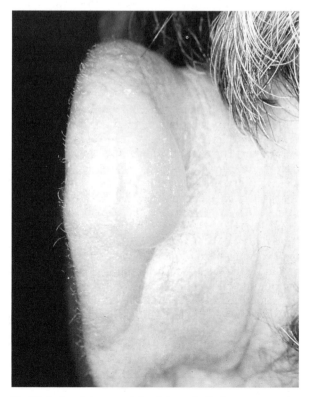

Fig 20.4 Frostbitten auricle. A large bulla is seen over the posterior aspect of the helix. The appearance is reminiscent of a second degree burn.

frost-damaged ear should be rewarmed gradually in a warm room. Rapid reheating, rubbing or mechanical trauma will worsen the damage.

Dystrophic calcification and heterotrophic ossification of the auricular cartilage may develop as a delayed sequel to severe frostbite. When this occurs, the pinna is bony hard to palpation, and an X-ray of the pinna reveals radiopaque areas in the auricular cartilage.[3]

Acid burn of the auricle

Industrial strength acids, when spilled on the side of the face, may cause severe injury to the auricle. This may occur accidentally or in the course of a criminal assault. The result is massive denaturation of protein, with an effective 'melting' of the auricle. Healing is usually accompanied by fibrosis, and there may be a resultant obliteration of the ear canal (Fig 20.5 and Plate section).

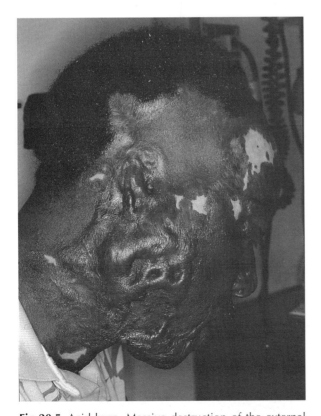

Fig 20.5 Acid burn. Massive destruction of the external ear and ear canal caused by criminal assault with sulphuric acid. Note keloid formation and vitiligo in this patient.

Radiation injury

Radiation injury of the ear canal may be seen after radiotherapy for malignancies of the skull base. These injuries range from radiation dermatitis to osteitis and sequestration of parts of the tympanic bone. Treatment is topical and not always curative. Curettage of the sequestered bone may lead to healing by secondary epithelialization; however, in some cases a patch of persistent eburnated bone remains.

Mechanical injuries of the ear canal

As discussed at the beginning of this chapter, the ear canal has several curves that normally deflect a 'direct hit' from the tympanic membrane. The price, however, is paid by the ear canal, and mechanical trauma will often cause contusion or laceration of the canal wall. These injuries are most often due to cotton swabs (despite the manufacturer's hypocritical injunction that they are only to be used externally). Injudicious irrigation of impacted wax may also lead to a laceration.

Lacerations normally occur along the floor of the canal. This is due to the shape of the canal and the thinness of the skin along the floor. The patient notes pain, followed by bleeding. Initial examination is usually hampered by blood clots, which often fill the entire canal. Treatment of such lacerations should be conservative. Careful partial debridement of the canal may be attempted, although complete removal of the clot usually results in further bleeding. Once the passage is partially opened, ear drops should be given. Over time, the laceration usually heals, and the scab separates and is carried laterally. Initial assessment should include consideration of possible damage to the middle and inner ear. Tinnitus, vertigo or obvious laceration or contusion of the tympanic membrane require an audiogram.

Seemingly minor lacerations of the ear canal can result in localized areas of persistent infection and granulation. This condition is due to a keratin implantation granuloma.[5] Surface keratin is accidentally implanted below the surface and provokes a foreign body reaction. These granulomas are easily treated by curettage. If viable epidermis is buried, as may occur after a tympanoplasty, the patient will, over time, develop keratin pearls. These pearls may be seen in the deep canal, or through the surface of the onlay-grafted tympanic membrane. Such keratin pearls are harmless, and treatment, if deemed necessary, requires uncapping the cyst into the ear canal with a curette.

Surgical trauma to the ear canal is inevitable during endaural or endomeatal incisions. Endaural incisions may become complicated if the auricular cartilage is exposed and then becomes devitalized through rough handling or thermal damage from the cautery. If the helical or tragal cartilage is accidentally exposed or transsected, it should be conservatively removed before closing the incision. Cautery should be used only sparingly within the ear canal, as the bone may become devitalized and lead to a prolonged postoperative course of recurrent infections and granulations.

Twigs and other foreign objects may also enter the ear canal. The cause may be accidental or, in the case of curious young children, experimental. When the object is organic in origin, such as a splinter or a bean, the entire object must be removed to prevent secondary inflammation due to a foreign body reaction. Injudicious attempts at removal of foreign bodies from the ears of squirming children probably cause more lacerations than the foreign bodies themselves.

Occasionally, insects will enter the ear canal seeking warmth. The frequency of this occurrence is not necessarily related to socioeconomic status: some years ago, I removed a cockroach from the ear of a prominent Wall Street stockbroker. The patient will complain of discomfort and scratching or buzzing in the ear canal. If on examination the insect is alive, it should be killed by instillation of warm olive oil. Once the insect is dead, it should be removed using a microscope. Care is taken to remove all parts of the insect, which typically fragments in the course of extraction.

Fractures of the external ear canal

Extensive injuries of the ear canal may occur in an accident. A strong blow to the jaw (particularly the chin) can drive the mandibular condyles into the ear canal resulting in a laceration or fracture of the anterior canal. The diagnosis is confirmed by observing the ear canal during passive movements of the mandible. If the laceration is large, or if tissue is partially avulsed, this should be repositioned and the canal gently packed with antibiotic-saturated gauze. Suturing is difficult and usually not necessary. As the fracture heals, the patient is often left with a protruding spicule of bone projecting from the anterior ear canal.

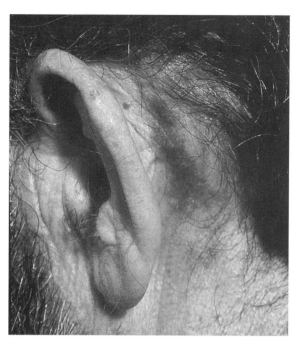

Fig 20.6 Battle's sign: bruising over the mastoid area, which developed 3 days after a transverse fracture of the temporal bone.

Longitudinal temporal bone fractures may extend into the bony ear canal. These fractures follow lines of relative structural weakness, and usually pass through the bony tympanic ring at the junction of the scutum and the tympanomastoid suture. Bleeding from the deep posterosuperior ear canal is seen, usually in conjunction with a tear of the tympanic membrane. These fractures normally heal spontaneously; however, a persistent diastasis or 'step' in the bony annulus will remain.[6] The real concern with these fractures relates to ossicular damage in the attic, and is discussed in Chapter 32. Battle's sign, an area of ecchymosis over the mastoid, may be the only visible evidence of a temporal bone fracture (Fig 20.6 and Plate section). This sign usually develops several days after the injury, and is seen with longitudinal and transverse fractures of the temporal bone.

References

1. Heermann H, Heermann J. *Endaural surgery*. Munich: Urban & Schwarzenberg, 1964.
2. Salyapongse A, Maun LP Suthunyarat P. Succssful replantation of a totally severed ear. *Plastic Reconstructive Surgery* 1979; **64**:706–10.

3. Hawke M, Jahn AF. *Diseases of the ear. Clinical and pathologic aspects*. London: Gower, 1987.

4. Sessions DG, Stallings JO, *et al*. Frostbite of the ear. *Laryngoscope* 1971; **81**:1223–32.

5. Hawke M, Jahn AF. Keratin implantation granuloma in the external ear canal. *Archives of Otology* 1974; **100**:317–8.

6. Schuknecht HF. *Pathology of the ear, 2nd edn*. Philadelphia: Lea & Febiger, 1993.

CHAPTER 21

Infection and inflammation of the external ear

ANTHONY F JAHN

Introduction

The external ear, comprising the auricle, ear canal and tympanic membrane, consists of a 'skeleton' of cartilage, bone and fibrous tissue covered by skin. Inflammation may involve any of these tissues, either regionally or as part of a generalized disorder of skin and connective tissue. These inflammatory disorders in turn may be characterized as infectious or non-infectious. Infections include bacterial, viral and fungal diseases, and only rarely other organisms. Non-infectious inflammations may be primary or reactive (secondary). As a comprehensive treatment of inflammatory conditions would require a synopsis of dermatology, this chapter deals only with those conditions most frequently encountered in clinical otolaryngology.

Protective mechanisms of the skin in infection and inflammation

The skin of the external parts of the ear is contiguous with the skin covering the body. It is therefore part of the interface between an often hostile physical and microbial environment and the precariously maintained 'milieu interieur' of the body. The skin covering the auricle and lining the ear canal, like skin elsewhere, has evolved numerous protective mechanisms that minimize the likelihood of infection. These are discussed below in order to emphasize how the breakdown of cutaneous defences may precipitate infection.

The epidermis is a multicellular layer. Its cells originate from rapidly dividing cells in the stratum basale, which lie at the interface of epidermis and dermis. As the basal cells proliferate and migrate towards the surface, their physical characteristics change. Most importantly, they become transformed from living and dividing cells to flat flakes of keratin. This process of maturation is normally coordinated with the rate of migration, so that by the time cells reach the surface they have lost their nuclei and have flattened into tightly joined squamous cells that form a nearly seamless cover. These squamous cells then die and their remnants form keratin. Keratin initially begins as small intracellular keratohyalin granules. It is a sulphated protein that, through secondary cross-linking of sulphydryl bonds, alters its stereoconfiguration and becomes a material that is 'foreign' and no longer recognized by the body; if keratin is implanted below the surface of skin, it evokes a foreign body reaction, complete with ovoid clefts and foreign body giant cells. Keratin is a tough and relatively impermeable shield that forms a physical protective barrier against the environment. The double layer of tightly joined squamous cells and its 'horny' keratin cover form an important defence against infection. The epidermis also features non-keratinizing cells, such as melanocytes, Merkel cells and Langerhans cells. These aid in defence against actinic damage (sunlight), noxious mechanical stimuli and antigenic elements, respectively, but cannot be covered in this brief overview.

Skin appendages also play a defensive role. Hairs may be involved in defence. Traditional teaching suggests that the outward facing hairs in the cartilaginous part of the ear canal hinder the entry of invaders such as insects. Numerous apocrine and eccrine glands lubricate the skin surface. They keep the surface supple and water-repellent. These secretions, mainly sebum and cerumen, form an additional physical barrier. Cerumen also contains lysozyme, which has antimicrobial properties.

As more keratin is produced, the sheets, initially adherent to the underlying squamous cells, become detached and are shed from the body surface. This constant desquamation presents a renewed protective surface cover. Furthermore, as keratin, especially wet keratin, offers a potentially favourable environment to microbial colonizers, the constant flaking away of dead cells and keratin helps to keep commensal microbial populations at a non-pathogenic level. As keratin is carried away laterally, the laterally directed hairs may aid in this separation.

The acidic pH of the skin surface is another microbial deterrent. The pH of the external ear canal is normally 6.5–6.8, significantly below the optimal pH (7 or higher) for the growth of pathogenic microbes.[1]

In addition to the epidermal defences discussed above, the dermis and subdermis also play important roles. The vascular supply to the skin is extensive, with ample collateral circulation. Cell-mediated and humoral immunity comes into play in these deeper skin layers and serves to contain and eliminate infection.

The inflammatory response of the skin involves all layers. Acute inflammation is usually triggered by inflammatory mediators such as histamine and results in increased vascular permeability and tissue oedema. This facilitates access for leucocytes and other mediators of immunity. Chronic inflammation is characterized by a more diffuse infiltrate of small round cells against a background of subepithelial oedema or fibrosis. The inflammatory cells may infiltrate the epidermis. Inflammation also accelerates cell turnover in the epithelium, often with a thickened epidermis, abnormal retention of nuclei (parakeratosis) and adherence of keratin. These general features of inflammation may be specifically modified, depending on the aetiology of the particular disorder.

Inflammatory disorders of the auricle

Infections of the external ear may involve the auricle, the external ear canal or the tympanic membrane. The infection may be localized to any of these areas or may extend to adjacent parts; it may be acute or chronic. The infectious agent may be bacterial, viral or fungal. Less commonly, skin lesions caused by mycobacteria, rickettsia or parasites have also been described. Mixed infections are common, particularly in indolent cases. In chronic infections non-infectious inflammation may also play a significant role, the actual micro-organism being a relatively minor factor.

CELLULITIS OF THE AURICLE

Cellulitis is a bacterial infection that may involve the auricle. It usually begins with an abrasion or laceration and progresses to a bacterial infection of the epidermis and dermis. The ear is red, swollen and tender to manipulation. Regional neck nodes may be palpable. Malaise or fever are uncommon. The condition is usually localized to the auricle.

Cellulitis is usually caused by Gram-positive cocci, rarely Pseudomonadaceae or other organisms.[2] A history of trauma is usually present. In the absence of trauma, the physician should consider a topical allergic reaction or less common, a local manifestation of a systemic disorder such as relapsing polychondritis. Initial treatment includes high-dose oral antibiotics active against Gram-positive organisms, topical soaks with 4–6 per cent aluminium acetate (dilute Burow's solution), and analgesics. If the infection fails to respond or worsens, intravenous antibiotics should be used.

ALLERGIC DERMATITIS OF THE AURICLE

Allergic dermatitis of the auricle is a reactive inflammation of the outer ear. The auricle is red, shiny and may demonstrate areas of 'peau d'orange' due to lymphoedema (Fig 21.1 and Plate section). Allergic or contact dermatitis is distinguished from bacterial cellulitis in several ways. There is usually no history of trauma. The inflammation is often localized to the area of allergen exposure; for example, a patient with nickel allergy may demonstrate erythema and oedema of the part of the lobule that is in contact with earrings. A patient allergic to neomycin who is using ear drops for otitis externa will demonstrate dermatitis in the dependent parts of the auricle, corresponding to the areas exposed to the ear drops as they trickle out of the ear canal. With sensitivity to cosmetics, the inflamed area may extend to adjacent parts of the face. The ear is swollen, often shiny and itchy. Unlike with infectious external otitis, there is no

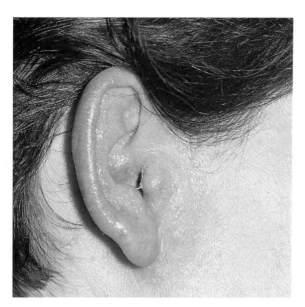

Fig 21.1 Contact dermatitis of the auricle caused by ear drops. The auricle is shiny, red and oedematous.

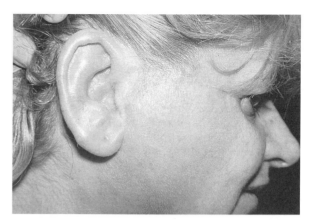

Fig 21.2 Erysipelas of the auricle and adjacent cheek. Note the red, raised area with a clearly demarcated advancing margin.

pain or real tenderness and the patient typically complains of itching.

Some forms of contact allergy may be inherited, although the mechanism is not clear.[3] Repeated exposure may result in sensitization and a more marked reaction. Unlike for inhalant allergies, desensitization for contact allergies is generally believed to be unsuccessful.[4]

Treatment begins with identifying and removing the allergen. When patients require ear drops these should be changed to 4% aluminium acetate or dilute table vinegar. Acute vesicular eruptions benefit from topical soaks of aluminium acetate, applied with saturated cotton-wool balls. If no secondary infection is present, topical steroid cream may be applied. Oral antihistamines offer additional relief.

ERYSIPELAS OF THE AURICLE

Erysipelas is a characteristic superficial cellulitis that may involve the auricle. It is usually caused by group-A streptococcus. The condition may begin with an abrasion or laceration that is inadvertently inoculated with the bacterium. Unlike localized cellulitis or an allergic reaction, erysipelas is marked by systemic toxicity, including fever and chills. Clinically the auricle is diffusely bright red, hot, shiny and tender. Brawny oedema or peau d'orange are signs of marked lymphatic vessel involvement. The infection may spread to the adjacent face, and its advancing margin is raised and clearly demarcated (Fig 21.2 and Plate section).

Erysipelas is contagious and should be treated accordingly. The patient requires high-dose systemic antibiotics such as erythromycin. There is usually good response to oral medications, but parenteral therapy should be considered if necessary. Topical therapy again includes soaks with aluminium acetate solution.

INFECTIOUS PERICHONDRITIS AND CHONDRITIS OF THE AURICLE

Bacterial infection involving the cartilage of the auricle leads to perichondritis and chondritis. Perichondritis may develop as an inadequately treated bacterial cellulitis extends to the deeper tissues.

Chondritis is usually caused by trauma, either accidental or surgical. Exposed cartilage, particularly if devitalized, may become inoculated during such trauma and give rise to infection. The infective organisms include *Pseudomonas, Staphylococcus aureus* and *Streptococcus*.[5] Chondritis may begin if the cartilage is inadvertently cut during an endaural incision, especially in the presence of a chronically infected middle ear or mastoid. Inadequately cleaned accidental lacerations or bites are another cause. Clinically the auricle appears swollen and inflamed. As the infection is deeper, there is no lymphoedema. Because of the inflammation of the highly sensitive perichondrium, touch and particularly deflection of the auricle are painful. This sign distinguishes perichondritis from more superficial infections, and also alerts the physician that a superficial infection is invading more deeply. The ear is acutely swollen, red and stiff. The incision or laceration is open, infected and often draining pus or infected tissue fluid (Fig 21.3 and Plate section).

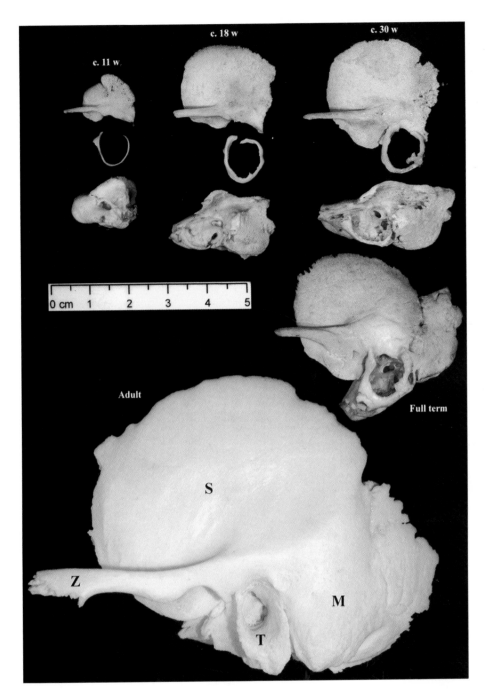

Fig. 1.4 Stages in the development of the temporal bone. The illustrations are of lateral views of the temporal bone and the first three are of ancient fetal remains. The very early stages have the separate elements of the developing bone clearly displayed as the flattened squamous portion, the tympanic ring and the petrous segment. At birth the three elements are fused although still very underdeveloped. The oval window for the stapes can be identified and it should be noted that the facial nerve canal is absent in the early bones. The fourth bone is from a term infant. The facial nerve is covered by a bony canal at birth but the stylomastoid foramen is very superficial. It is not until the growth of the mastoid process that the foramen becomes buried in the base of the skull. The full-grown adult temporal bone is shown to illustrate the remarkable growth that occurs postnatally. S, squamous portion; M, petromastoid; T, tympanic ring; Z, zygomatic arch;. The styloid process is missing in this specimen. (I am very grateful to Dr Louise Scheuer PhD, Senior Lecturer in Anatomy and Developmental Biology at the Royal Free Hospital School of Medicine, for permission to image these Roman bones digitally and to use the images. These and other images are available for study on the web at www.vml.ucl.ac.uk)

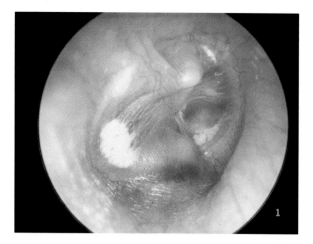

Fig 18.7 An endoscopic photograph of the right tympanic membrane. The patient was an achondroplastic dwarf and had as an incidental finding this high and exposed jugular bulb in the right middle ear.

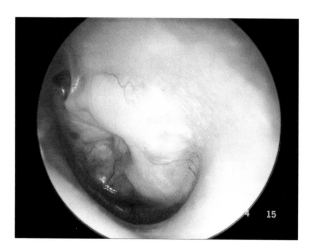

Fig. 18.8 An endoscopic photograph of the left tympanic membrane of a 4-year-old child who presented with a unilateral hearing loss detected at a routine school screening, when headphones rather than free-field testing were used. The intact membrane is bulging with a white mass present in the middle ear. The attic is intact and the mass was soft on palpation with a Jobson-Horne probe.

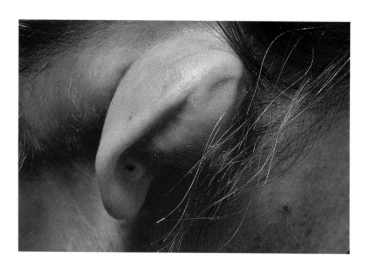

Fig. 20.1 Haematoma of the auricle. There is a subperichondral extravasation of blood along both surfaces of the auricle, suggestive of a fractured cartilage.

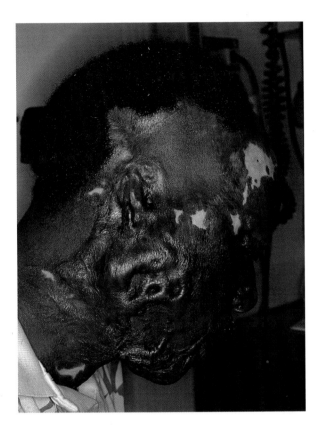

Fig. 20.5 Acid burn. Massive destruction of the external ear and ear canal caused by criminal assault with sulphuric acid. Note keloid formation and vitiligo in this patient.

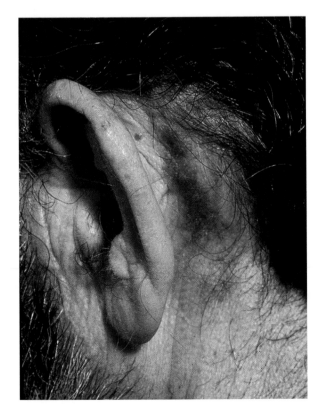

Fig. 20.6 Battle's sign: bruising over the mastoid area, which developed 3 days after a transverse fracture of the temporal bone.

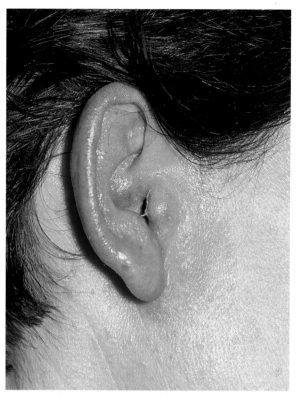

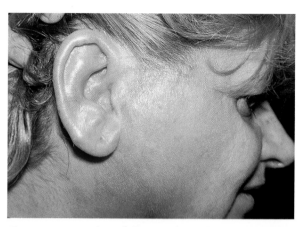

Fig. 21.2 Erysipelas of the auricle and adjacent cheek. Note the red, raised area with a clearly demarcated advancing margin.

Fig. 21.1 Contact dermatitis of the auricle caused by ear drops. The auricle is shiny, red and oedematous.

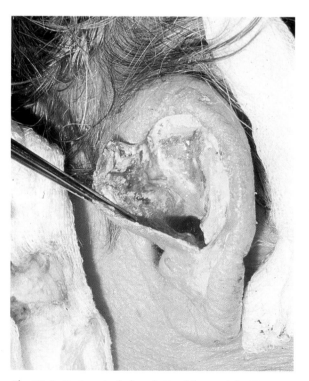

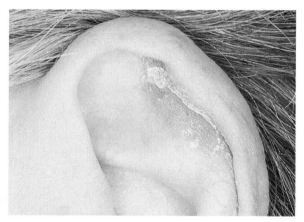

Fig. 21.4 Psoriasis involving the scapha of the auricle. Silvery flakes adhere to an inflamed base with evidence of punctate haemorrhage (Auspitzís sign).

Fig. 21.3 Postsurgical chondritis of the auricle. The cartilage has been exposed and is diffusely coated with pus.

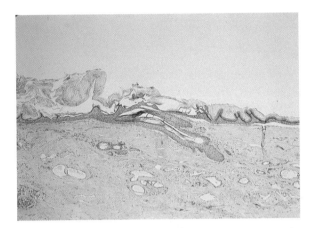

Fig. 21.5 Histological section of the ear canal along its long axis, demonstrating the separation of keratin sheets. As the keratin is pushed laterally, the separation is aided by the outward-pointing hairs.

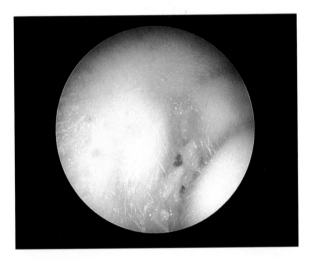

Fig. 21.6 Acute diffuse otitis externa. The meatus is narrowed as a result of oedema, and the lumen is filled by an infected sticky secretion.

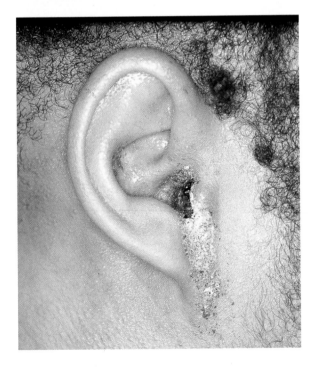

Fig. 21.7 Pseudomonas otitis externa in a diabetic. In this patient, the infection is characterized by a copious discharge of blue-green pus (i.e. pyocyaneus).

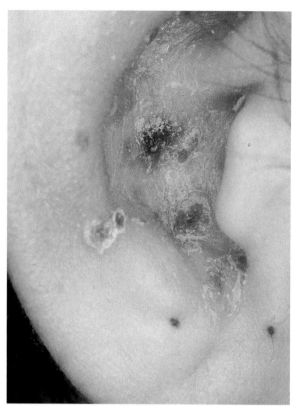

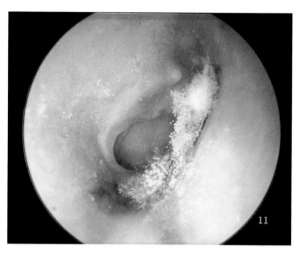

Fig. 21.9 Otomycosis due to to Aspergillus species. Dots, representing fungal spores, are scattered across the deep canal. The stalks and fruiting heads (conidiophores) of the mature fungus can be discerned.

Fig. 21.8 Herpes zoster of the concha. The vesicles are crusted and drying. This patient also had a vesicle on the tympanic membrane.

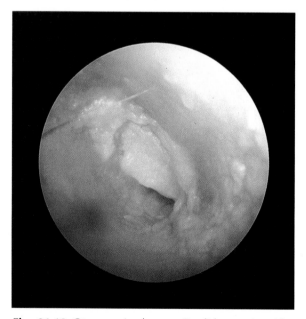

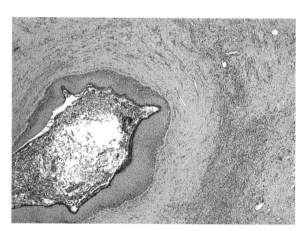

Fig. 21.11 Histological cross-section of the ear canal demonstrating postinflammatory stenosis. The epidermis is thickened and lies on a markedly scarred dermal layer. The deeper tissues are chronically inflamed.

Fig. 21.10 Otomycosis due to Candida species. The white curd-like material coats the ear canal.

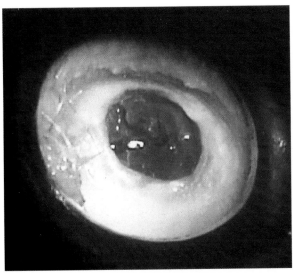

Fig. 21.12 Inflammatory obliteration of the ear canal (operative image). The deep canal is filled with fresh granulation tissue. Covering epithelium is growing in from the periphery. When the epithelialization is complete, the patient will have developed a false fundus.

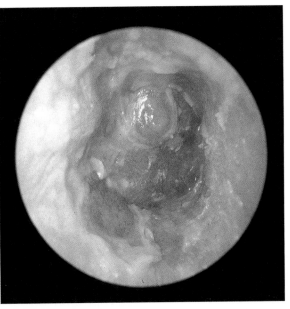

Fig. 21.14 Granular myringitis. The typanic membrane is thickened and red and demonstrates nubbins of granulation tissue. Secondary infection may be responsible for the erythema and exudate.

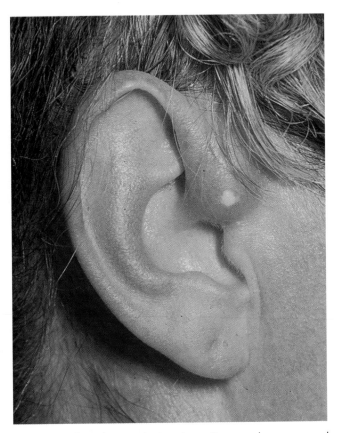

Fig 22.2 Infected preauricular sinus. Pressure has expressed creamy pus.

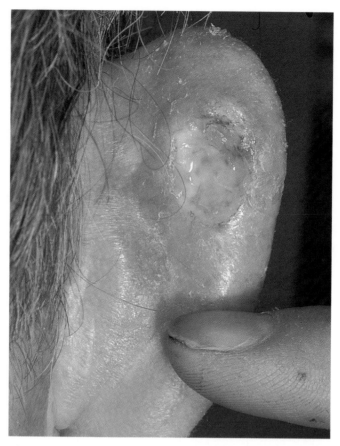

Fig. 22.4 Keratoacanthoma: a large raised painless lesion with a central crater.

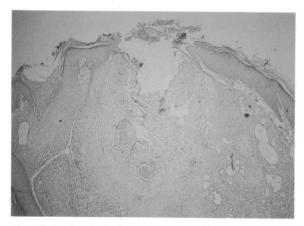

Fig. 22.5 Histological cross-section of keratoacanthoma demonstrates the calyx filled with sheets of parakeratotic cells and keratin debris.

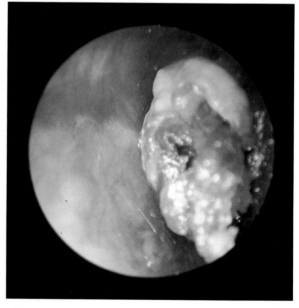

Fig. 22.7 Keratosis obturans: the deep canal is filled with a white plug of keratin.

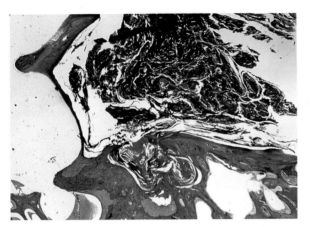

Fig. 22.8 Cholesteatoma of the external ear canal. Note the bony erosion of the floor of the ear canal, a feature that distinguishes this condition from keratosis obturans.

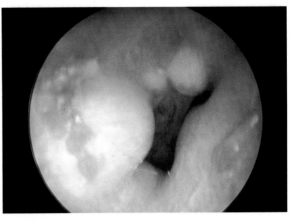

Fig. 22.9 Exostoses anteriorly and posteriorly, obliterate most of this ear canal, leaving only a narrow passage.

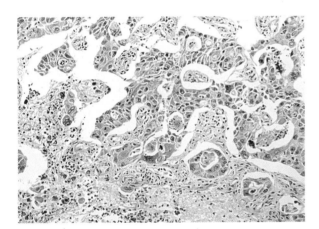

Fig. 22.11 Malignant ceruminoma of the ear canal. The cells demonstrate a clearly malignant morphology, and the cribriform arrangement is similar to adenoid cystic carcinoma.

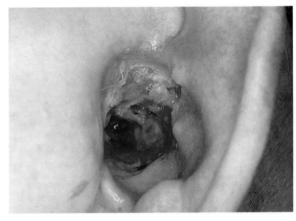

Fig. 22.12 Squamous cell carcinoma of the ear canal. Deep erosion of cartilage and bone are an ominous sign.

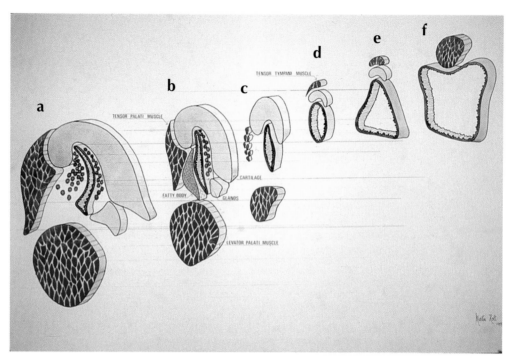

Fig. 24.1 a-f Six different regions of the Eustachian tube. The 'bellows' region is made of three parts, all of which are related to the palatal musculature. The post isthmus has the tensor tympani running along its roof in a separate canal. (a) pharyngeal (b) midportion - pre isthmus (c) Isthmus - which is the joining link with the non-collapsible part of the Eustachian tube (d) Post-isthmus (e) Mid-portion - post-isthmus (f) Mesotympanic.

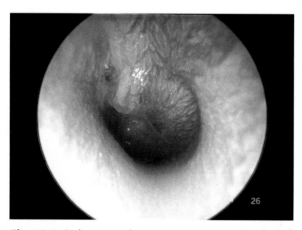

Fig. 25.3 Early stage of acute suppurative otitis media: Note the erythema of the tympanic membrane and presence of a middle ear exudate that is not under pressure (with permission of A. Wright, Institute of Laryngology and Otology, London).

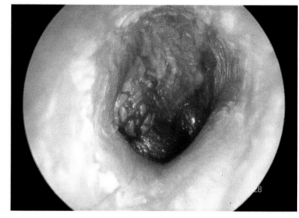

Fig. 25.4 Full-blown acute suppurative otitis media. Note the bulging of the tympanic membrane and the presence of purulent middle ear fluid (with permission of A. Wright, Institute of Laryngology and Otology, London).

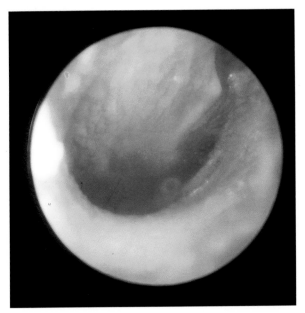

Fig. 26.3 Right tympanic membrane, viewed by otoscope, showing mild changes of chronic secretory otitis media with polypoid mucosa on the medial aspect.

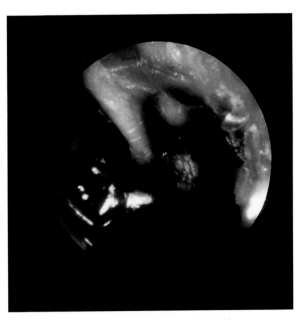

Fig. 26.4 Left tympanic membrane, viewed by otoscope, showing marked retraction of tympanic membrane and dark middle ear effusion.

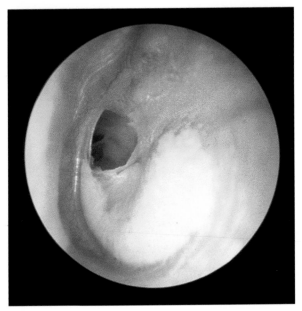

Fig. 27.1 Anterior perforation of the left tympanic membrane.

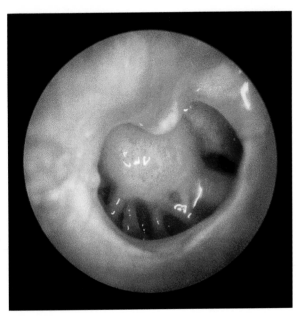

Fig. 27.2 Subtotal perforation of the right tympanic membrane.

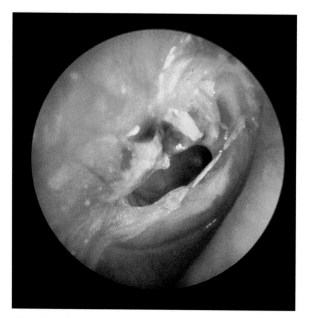

Fig. 27.3 Marginal perforation of the right tympanic membrane.

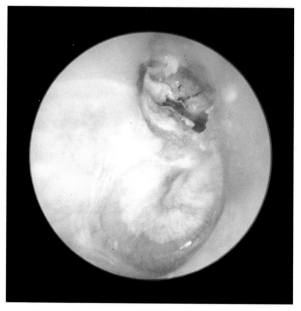

Fig. 27.4 Attic perforation of right tympanic membrane.

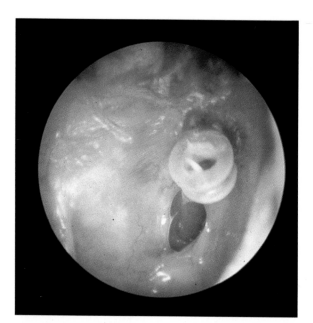

Fig. 27.7 An extruding ventilation tube with a residual perforation of the right tympanic membrane.

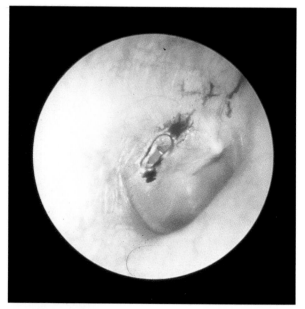

Fig. 27.8 Healing traumatic perforation of the right tympanic membrane.

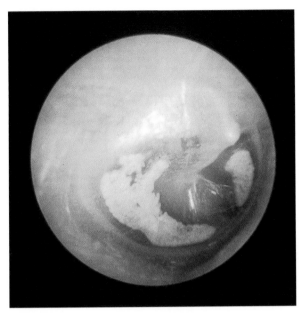

Fig. 27.13 Tympanosclerosis of the right tympanic membrane.

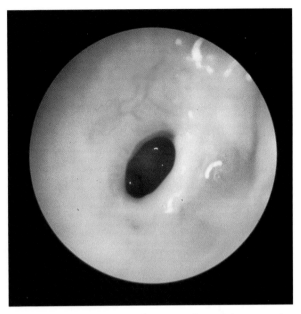

Fig. 27.14 Discharging right tympanic membrane perforation.

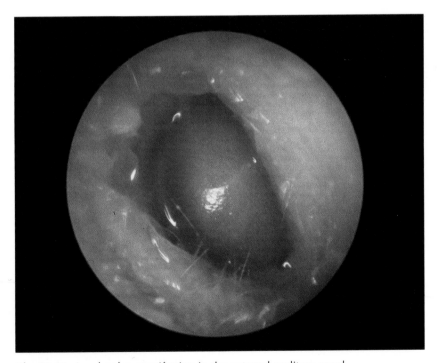

Fig. 27.15 Aural polyp manifesting in the external auditory canal.

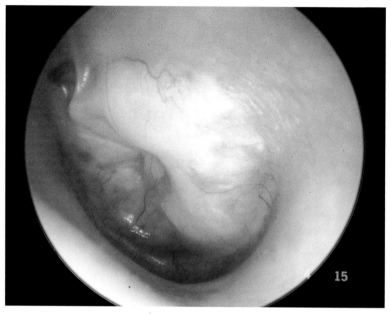

Fig. 28.3 Occult cholesteatoma of the left middle ear. (Reproduced with permission of A. Wright, Institute of Laryngology and Otology, London.)

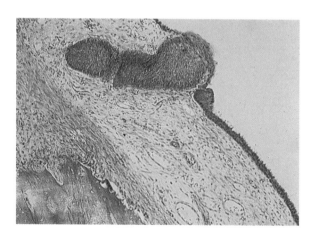

Fig. 28.4 Photomicrograph of the epidermoid formation in the developing middle ear. (Reproduced with permission of Professor L. Michaels.)

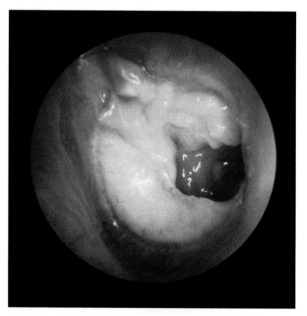

Fig. 28.10 Pars tensa cholesteatoma of the left ear.

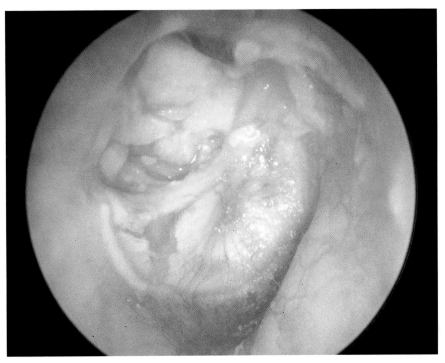

Fig. 28.11 Pars flaccida cholesteatoma of the right ear. (Reproduced with permission of A. Wright, Institute of Laryngology and Otology, London.)

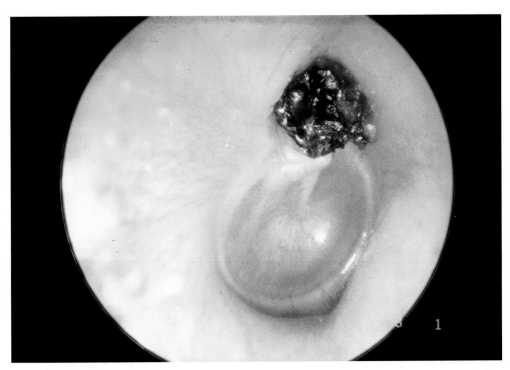

Fig. 28.13 Crust in the right attic overlying a cholesteatoma. (Reproduced with permission of A. Wright, Institute of Laryngology and Otology, London.)

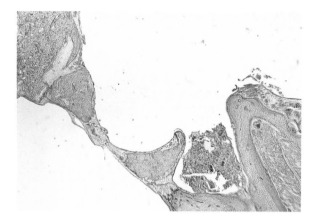

Fig. 33.1 Stapes ankylosis by an otosclerotic focus (from an ear subject to a previous stapedectomy). Note anterior focus, area of new membrane over fenestra, remains of posterior crus and, posteriorly, the stapedius muscle in the pyramid. (Reproduced with permission of Professor A. Wright.)

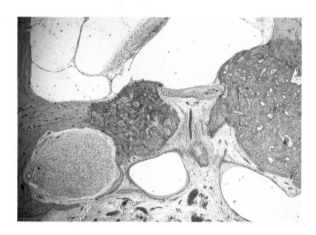

Fig. 33.2 Active otospongiotic lesion and associated sclerotic lesion. (Reproduced with permission of Professor A. Wright.)

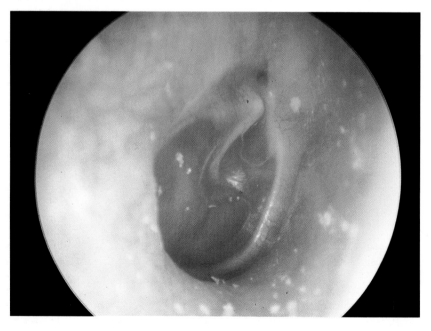

Fig. 34.2(b) Otoscopic photograph of the tumour shown in Fig. 34.2(a).

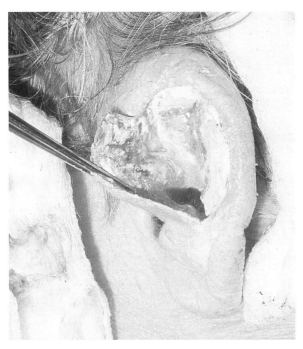

Fig 21.3 Postsurgical chondritis of the auricle. The cartilage has been exposed and is diffusely coated with pus.

Chondritis of the auricle is a potentially serious infection and must be treated aggressively. The purpose of treatment is to minimize loss of tissue and to contain the infection. The incision or laceration should be cultured. If pus is present, it should be evacuated, and devitalized skin and cartilage should be resected. Intravenous antibiotics should be started to cover Gram-positive and Gram-negative organisms. Topical antibiotic irrigation with indwelling catheters has been suggested as an ancillary measure. If the infection cannot be controlled, more aggressive measures, including hyperbaric oxygen and further excision, may be necessary.

RELAPSING POLYCHONDRITIS

Relapsing polychondritis is an autoimmune disease manifesting as recurring episodes of inflammation that involve cartilaginous tissue throughout the body. It is currently believed to be due an autoimmune response to type-II collagen.[6] According to McAdam *et al.*[7] 85–90 per cent of patients with relapsing polychondritis develop inflammation of the auricular cartilage. Nasal and laryngeal cartilages are less frequently involved.

The external ear becomes red, warm, swollen and tender. The lobule is characteristically spared and the condition may involve only one ear. Recurrent episodes may leave the auricular cartilage damaged, resulting in a floppy or cauliflower ear. Destruction of the septum may lead to a saddle deformity.

Treatment of relapsing polychondritis includes systemic corticosteroids for acute episodes. Dapsone and indomethacin have been suggested for chronic systemic manifestations.[8]

CHRONIC CONCHAL INFLAMMATION

Chronic conchal inflammation, involving the cavum conchae, usually has a combination of causes. Typically the patient wears a hearing aid on the affected ear. The conchal bowl is red, and demonstrates oedema and lymphoedema. The inflammation is clearly demarcated and limited to the cavum conchae.

Chronic inflammation of the conchae may be caused by allergy or infection, or may be self-induced (neurodermatitis, or dermatitis artefacta). Often two or more factors are involved. If the patient is allergic to the earmould, a topical reaction occurs. Even in the absence of hypersensitivity, constant occlusion of the area may result in moisture and a secondary infection develops. This may be bacterial, but is more often candida. The itching and irritation may in turn lead to scratching, resulting in abrasion, areas of punctate haemorrhage and further injury to the skin.

The multifactorial aetiology of this condition must be appreciated for proper treatment. The patient should be instructed to avoid wearing the hearing aid. Topical therapy is begun using an anti-fungal cortisone cream. The patient should be instructed to keep the nails short and not to scratch the area. Once the condition has resolved, a hypo-allergenic earmould should be made. The patient should be instructed to wear the aid as little as necessary, and to clean it with an alcohol wipe before reinsertion.

SEBORRHOEA

Seborrhoeic dermatitis is a disorder usually associated with oily skin. It manifests as scaling patches that are typically oily and slightly yellow. Seborrhoea of the ear occurs most frequently in the retroauricular area. The postauricular crease may be erythematous and weeping. When seborrhoea of the ear canal is suspected, the retroauricular area is also usually involved, which helps with the diagnosis. These patients usually have seborrhoea of the scalp also, manifesting as diffuse dandruff. Seborrhoea may also involve the face. This diffuse distribution distinguishes seborrhoea from psoriasis, which is usually localized to areas of predilection.

There is controversy over the aetiology of seborrhoea. Bacteria and yeast are felt to play a facilitative rather than causative role.[9] Neuropsychological factors and seasonal variations in temperature and humidity have also been implicated.

Seborrhoea cannot be cured, only controlled. Topical steroids in a gel or propylene glycol base are recommended in brief doses. Oily based preparations should be avoided.

ECZEMA

Eczema or eczematous dermatitis is an inflammatory disorder of the skin characterized by erythema and oedema, oozing and vesiculation, crusting and scaling. Constant itching leads to scratching, and eventually results in lichenification, thickening or pigmentary changes of the skin. Eczema may involve the auricle or the external ear canal, and may be a significant component of chronic otitis externa, especially when this condition is refractory to antibiotic drops. Patients with eczematoid dermatitis are more prone to develop skin sensitization, and eczema of the ear may therefore worsen, rather than improve, with topical medications.

PSORIASIS

Psoriasis is a generalized dermatological disorder that may affect the external ear. Its cause is not known, although it appears to be inherited.[10] The involvement of immune mechanisms in psoriasis and its frequent coexistence with autoimmune diseases such as arthritis are suggestive of an immunological cause.[11]

The pathological process consists of an increased turnover of skin, with the formation of silvery adherent flakes of keratin (Fig 21.4 and Plate section). The silvery flakes, adherent to an inflamed base, characterize the condition. If the flakes are removed, punctate haemorrhage (Auspitz's sign) is seen at the base.

When psoriasis affects the ear, there are usually psoriatic lesions in more characteristic areas such as the elbows or legs. At times, the ears appear to be the most obviously involved. Psoriasis of the external ear usually involves the concha and the external ear canal. Less commonly smaller lesions may be seen on the scapha. The diagnosis is made by history, the presence of lesions elsewhere, and the clinical appearance.

Volumes have been written on the treatment of psoriasis, which is generally effective in the short

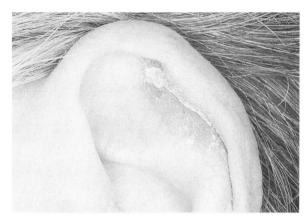

Fig 21.4 Psoriasis involving the scapha of the auricle. Silvery flakes adhere to an inflamed base with evidence of punctate haemorrhage (Auspitz's sign).

term but not curative. In the ear, most useful are creams containing steroids, salicylate or coal tar. Care should be taken not to occlude the ear canal with the resulting plug of ointment and keratin debris. More aggressive measures, including ultraviolet light and methotrexate,[12] are reserved for severe and disseminated cases.

Inflammatory disorders of the external ear canal

DEFENCE MECHANISMS OF THE EXTERNAL EAR CANAL

In addition to the normal skin defences described at the beginning of this chapter, the external ear canal has evolved several additional mechanisms to ensure proper function. The self-cleansing mechanism of the eardrum and ear canal is unique. Rapid cell turnover on the surface of the eardrum results in a constant centrifugal migration of skin. Skin moves laterally from the eardrum onto the deep canal wall, and then outwards. The skin desquamates, and keratin stacks are carried laterally like dishes on a conveyer belt and eventually shed into the lumen of the canal. As the skin moves past the hair follicles, the keratin is peeled away from the skin surface by the outward-pointing hairs. These hairs act as ramps, or wedges, separating keratin from skin (Fig 21.5 and Plate section). The keratin is trapped in the cerumen lining the lateral canal.[13] Although the primary purpose of this unique mechanism is to keep the lumen of the canal open for

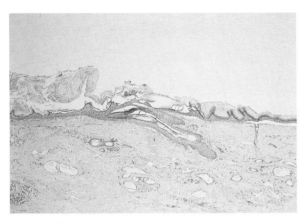

Fig 21.5 Histological section of the ear canal along its long axis, demonstrating the separation of keratin sheets. As the keratin is pushed laterally, the separation is aided by the outward-pointing hairs.

hearing, it clearly functions to reduce bacterial colonization and infection. The outward-pointing hairs and convolutions of the lateral canal are also said to hinder the entrance of foreign material and insects.

Cerumen, a modified sebaceous secretion, is formed by the ceruminous glands. These glands (which are modified sebaceous glands), sweat glands and hairs are present only in the lateral (cartilaginous) portion of the canal. The medial (bony) canal is lined by thin skin that is devoid of epidermal appendages. Cerumen serves primarily to trap and dispose of keratin debris that is shed by the ear canal. Its secondary functions include lubrication of the canal. Cerumen contains lysozyme and is considered bacteriostatic. Despite this, in some cases of

otomycosis it is common to see lush tufts of *Aspergillus* growing undisturbed on cerumen.

ACUTE LOCALIZED OTITIS EXTERNA (FURUNCLE)

A furuncle is a small abscess, which usually develops in a hair follicle. In the ear canal furuncles are therefore invariably in the lateral canal, and usually at the meatus. They appears as exquisitely tender small pimples. They may be diffusely red or highly localized and pointing, with a demarcated pustule. If the furuncle is ready to rupture, it should be gently opened with the tip of a sterile needle. The area can then be covered with an antibiotic ointment. Oral antibiotics are usually not necessary.

ACUTE DIFFUSE EXTERNAL OTITIS (SWIMMER'S EAR)

Acute external otitis is a diffuse bacterial infection of the ear canal. The causative organism is usually *Pseudomonas aeruginosa*. Often there is a history of prolonged water exposure or trauma to the ear canal (Q-tips, paper clips or hair pins).The patient presents with hearing loss, pressure, itching and pain in the area of the ear canal. A classic sign of acute external otitis is pain elicited by pulling the auricle upward and backward. An earlier finding is tenderness when the examiner pushes up on the cartilage of the ear canal, under the lobule.

Acute otitis externa usually starts in the lateral canal and even in severe cases may not extend into the bony portion. A characteristic finding, even in milder cases, is the absence of cerumen. More typically the ear canal is narrowed, the skin red and oedematous. Oedema may be marked, to the point of complete obliteration of the lumen. There is no discharge, but a sticky yellowish-clear exudate may be present (Fig 21.6 and Plate section). The infection is localized to the ear canal; it does not extend to the auricle, and cervical lymphadenopathy is rare.

The usual cause of swimmer's ear is *Pseudomonas aeruginosa*. Repeated water exposure has been shown to cause a shift in the flora of the external ear from predominantly Gram-positive to Gram-neative bacteria, mostly *Pseudomonas* and *Enterobacter*, in only 5 days.[14]

Treatment for acute otitis externa is primarily topical. The ear canal is gently debrided using a paediatric speculum and suction. A self-expanding wick, saturated with aluminium actetate solution or topical ear drops, is gently advanced into the ear canal with alligator forceps. This wick is kept in

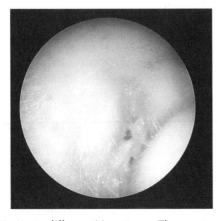

Fig 21.6 Acute diffuse otitis externa. The meatus is narrowed as a result of oedema, and the lumen is filled by an infected sticky secretion.

place for 3 days and kept constantly moist with frequent applications of ear drops, after which it is removed and the canal is again suctioned. If an adequate lumen has been re-established, drops are continued in the conventional fashion for 7 days. The ear is protected from water exposure for at least 2 weeks.

A variety of ear drops is available for treatment. Early work by Jones[1,15] demonstrated that simple vinegar is cidal for *Pseudomonas*. Indeed, native 'doctors' in the Caribbean still treat earache with a simple but effective mixture of vinegar and honey, which has the double virtue of being acidic and hyperosmotic. Drops most frequently used contain a combination of antibiotics and steroids. Otic and ophthalmic drops are both effective; however, the latter are less viscous, pH neutral and come in a wider variety of preparations. They may be especially useful if the canal is swollen shut, or if a patient complains of burning with the more acidic otic preparations. In most cases, any of the combination drops work well.

In cases of neomycin sensitivity or concern about steroids, dilute acetic acid or aluminium acetate drops are recommended.[16]

Adjunctive therapy includes systemic antibiotics for severe cases. The best currently available oral antipseudomonal antibiotic is ciprofloxacin. It is a matter of personal preference whether the physician prefers to use this antibiotic, or to reserve it for more serious or systemic infections. There is considerable pain associated with this condition, and analgesics, and at times narcotics, may be needed.

Some patients, classically swimmers, are prone to recurrent external otitis. They should consider using swim plugs and instilling alcohol or boric acid drops into the ear canals after swimming. Other patients develop recurrent external otitis, even in the absence of self-inflicted trauma or water exposure. The cause for this is not known, but it may relate to inadequate acidity of the skin surface. Lack of cerumen may also be a factor. These patients should be advised to instil acetic acid drops into the ear canals once a week.

NECROTIZING (MALIGNANT) OTITIS EXTERNA

Necrotizing otitis externa is an invasive pseudomonas infection of the external ear canal, which may lead to osteomyelitis of the temporal bone, multiple cranial nerve palsies and death. Initially described in 1968 by Chandler,[17] malignant otitis externa, which usually arises in diabetics has since been diagnosed in a variety of immune depressed states, including lymphoma and renal

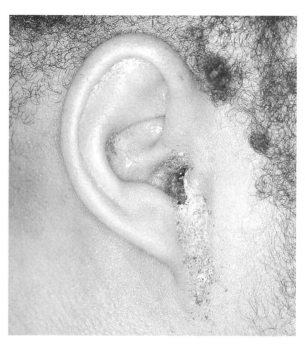

Fig 21.7 Pseudomonas otitis externa in a diabetic. In this patient, the infection is characterized by a copious discharge of blue-green pus (i.e. pyocyaneus).

transplant patients.[18] Surprisingly, it is not thus far a significant feature of HIV infections. Necrotizing otitis externa is most ominous in the elderly insulin-dependent diabetic, but it may occur in milder forms of hyperglycaemia as well. The initial presentation is a diffuse pseudomonas external otitis, much like swimmer's ear, often after a minor laceration (Fig 21.7 and Plate section). It does not, however, respond to conventional topical measures. The true nature of the condition emerges as the patient develops constant pain, which is most marked at night.[19] Examination may reveal granulation tissue on the floor of the ear canal, just lateral to the bony–cartilaginous junction. Instrumental sounding of the area often reveals a small pocket with exposed bone at its base. This finding represents focal osteitis of the lateral lip of the tympanic ring, and is often the first sign of deeper invasion.

Bacteria invade the deeper tissues of the floor of the ear canal at this bony–cartilaginous junction. Some authors believe that invasion also occurs through the fissures of Santorini, transverse slits in the cartilaginous canal floor that normally transmit small vessels. At this stage, the patient's discomfort grows and there may be a serous or blood-tinged discharge from the ear canal.

If the infection continues unchecked, it travels medially through the soft tissues under the bony canal floor and posteriorly to the stylomastoid foramen. Facial paralysis may now develop, accompanied by opacification of the mastoid. Abscess formation is not common.

In the final stages of the infection, osteomyelitis of the temporal bone develops, which may become intractable and may extend across the base of the skull.[20] Multiple lower cranial nerve palsies accompany this stage, which usually ends in death.

Diagnosis and investigation of malignant otitis externa

A high level of suspicion should attend the management of any diabetic or immunocomprised patient with pseudomonas external otitis, especially when pain is prominent. In the earliest stages no tests are specific, and treatment must be initiated solely on the grounds of clinical concern.

Investigations should include high resolution, fine cut CT scanning, looking at bone window settings for evidence of erosion; however, changes of osteomyelitis may not become evident until a week or more after the onset.

Radionuclide scanning (scintigraphy) can be useful. Technetium isotopes, as phosphate analogues (methyl diphosphonate – MDP), are taken up by proliferating fibroblasts and may show 'hot spots' within 1 or 2 days of the start of osteomyelitis. Gallium isotopes shows areas of actively dividing white blood cells, and gallium scanning can be used to monitor the resolution of infection, watching for the fading of residual 'hot spots'.

Treatment of malignant otitis externa

Topical preparations include acetic acid solutions, and gentamicin drops may be used. My personal preference is to avoid steroid-containing drops. Pain may become severe and require narcotic analgesia. If granulation tissue signals early osteitis of the bony canal, this may be curetted down to viable bone and topical medications applied. The patient must also be placed on a maximal dose of ciprofloxacin by mouth.[21] The third component of therapy is rigorous control of the diabetes. A vicious cycle develops: infection leads to hyperglycaemia, which in turn exacerbates the infection. Malignant otitis externa cannot be cured without strict diabetic control. Patients may need to be temporarily changed from oral hypoglycaemics to insulin, and the insulin may need to be continually adjusted by reaction.

If the infection fails to respond, or worsens, as signalled by severe pain, the patient must begin long-term intravenous antibiotic therapy with an aminoglycoside. Depending on clinical and radiological changes, a mastoidectomy may be necessary with facial nerve decompression, or even a partial temporal bone resection. Adjunctive hyperbaric oxygen has also been used in severe cases.[22]

The first sign of clinical response is a lessening of pain. If analgesics are less frequently requested or if the patient begins to sleep through the night, the infection has begun to yield to therapy. Intravenous antibiotics and insulin must be continued for at least 6 weeks to avoid relapse.[23] Once the patient has recovered, they should consider antipseudomonas prophylaxis, which consists of a weekly installation of acidic drops.

HERPES ZOSTER OF THE EXTERNAL EAR

Herpes zoster is a localized form of shingles that affects the external ear. The herpes zoster virus, related to the varicella virus, may lie dormant in the sensory ganglia of some patients with a past history of chicken pox infection. It becomes reactivated under conditions of decreased immune vigilance. The virus travels down the nerve roots, and expresses itself as a herpetic blister on the skin. Herpes zoster is confined to specific dermatomes, which may encompass the auricle, the external ear canal and even the lateral surface of the tympanic membrane.

The herpetic lesions typically appear as round reddish raised lesions that vesiculate, rupture, dry, crust and heal (Fig 21.8 and Plate section). On the ear the diagnosis may be missed as the blisters may be few and not in crops, as is seen on the trunk. Some patients with herpes zoster oticus also suffer involvement of the cochleovestibular and facial nerves. This clinical complex of hearing loss, vertigo and facial paralysis due to herpes zoster is called herpes zoster oticus or the Ramsay Hunt syndrome. A full description of this condition is presented in Chapter 17. Suffice it to say here that the connection of hearing loss, vertigo and facial paralysis to herpes zoster is often missed as, by the time the patient presents to the physician, the skin lesions have healed. Only persistent questioning of an observant patient will yield the correct diagnosis. Another confusing clinical picture may develop when herpetic vesicles develop a secondary bacterial infection and this is mistaken for malignant external otitis.

Because herpes zoster reactivation is a symptom of decreased immune competence, it may occur during times of stress or concurrent illness. It has classically been considered a warning sign of an occult malignancy,[24] and may be more frequent among HIV-infected patients.

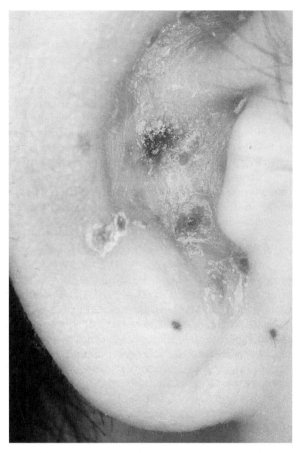

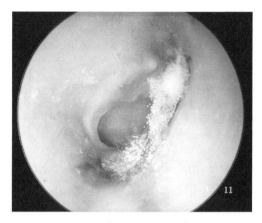

Fig 21.9 Otomycosis due to *Aspergillus* species. Dots, representing fungus, are scattered across the deep canal. The stalks and fruiting heads (conidiophores) of the mature fungus can be discerned.

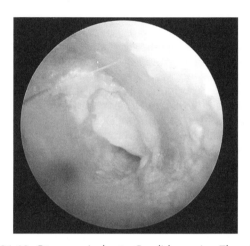

Fig 21.8 Herpes zoster of the concha. The vesicles are crusted and drying. This patient also had a vesicle on the tympanic membrane.

OTOMYCOSIS

Although fungi are known commensals in the ear canal, primary fungal infection of the ear canal is less frequent. The commonest fungi are *Aspergillus* species *(A. niger, A. flavus, A. fumigatus)*, and *Candida* species *(C. albicans, C. parapsilosis)*. These organisms are airborne in the spore form and may be indigenous to moist surfaces.

Fungi have been estimated to play a role in over 20 per cent of all cases of otitis externa.[25] Otomycosis develops most commonly in a chronically inflamed ear canal that has been treated with a variety of antibiotic or steroid drops. If the patient complains of itching and some moisture and the condition continues despite conventional treatment, otomycosis should be suspected.

Although aspergillosis and candidiasis of the ear canal are superficial infections, their clinical appearance differs considerably. Aspergillosis is characterized by a mild moist inflammation of the deep ear

Fig 21.10 Otomycosis due to *Candida* species. The white curd-like material coats the ear canal.

canal. The lumen is filled with large shed sheets of keratin that have a wet tissue-paper appearance. With the microscope, individual colonies of the flowering fungus may be discerned, complete with hyphae (stalks) and conidiophores (fruiting heads) (Fig 21.9 and Plate section). These may be yellow, grey or black, depending on the subspecies.

Candida usually causes greater oedema and maceration of the deep ear canal. The lumen may be filled with a curd-like material (Fig 21.10 and Plate section). *Candida* is a dimorphic fungus and may exist in either the budding yeast or the pseudo-hyphaenated form. At times, the distinction between these two fungi, and indeed the diagnosis of otomycosis itself, is not clear and must be made by elimination.

Treatment involves elimination of predisposing factors. Topical ear drops must be stopped. The optimal pH for fungi is lower than for bacteria, hence acidification of the ear canal may not be curative.

The patient's nails should be inspected. Onychomycosis is a potential source of repeated autoinoculation. If the nails are thickened, white and crumbling, they should be trimmed and sent for culture and systemic therapy should be considered. Some women with recurrent vaginal candidiasis also develop recurrent candidal otomycosis. The flare-ups in these cases are hormonally related and also require systemic therapy.

With the exception of onychomycosis and recurrent vaginal candidiasis, treatment for otomycosis is topical. The ear canal is microscopically debrided of all visible debris. Fungicidal drops may be prescribed, or the eardrum and deep canal may be covered with a fungicidal cream. This is layered on using a hypodermic syringe attached to a blunt cannula. A readily available and usually effective preparation for *Candida* is tolnaftate, available over the counter for the treatment of athlete's foot.[26] This may be instilled as a cream, insufflated as a powder or given as drops. Nizoral in topical and oral form may be useful for candidal otomycosis.[27] The newer imidazole derivatives, such as econazole or miconazole, are particularly effective as they are produced in water-based solutions. If several preparations have been tried in vain, the physician may paint the affected areas with 1% aqueous gentian violet before considering long-term systemic therapy.

Atypical otomycosis is occasionally seen in patients with AIDS. Although the organism is usually *Aspergillus*, the infection in these patients is invasive, clinically resembling mucormycosis.[28] The patient complains of severe pain. Examination reveals macerated bleeding tissue in the deep canal, which cannot be adequately removed in the surgery. These patients clearly require more aggressive treatment, including surgical debridement and parenteral amphotericin B.[29]

CHRONIC NON-SPECIFIC EXTERNAL OTITIS

Patients with chronic non-specific external otitis complain of chronic itching and will resort to any instrument 'smaller than an elbow' to obtain relief. Often there has been repeated treatment with conventional ear drops and ancillary measures, including steroids, antihistamines and analgesics. Physical examination reveals an ear canal that is devoid of cerumen and lined by skin that is thinned and often shiny. Scaling and erythema may be present. Small bloody crusts bear witness to the patient's incessant need to scratch.

The primary condition quite often is seborrhoeic dermatitis. Neurodermatitis (dermatitis factitia) may be an exacerbating component. Culture may be non-specific, even misleading. It may grow a commensal or a fungus that is a secondary colonizer and not the primary pathogen.

The most important initial treatment for these patients is to provide relief from the itch. Irrigation with boric acid or aluminium acetate solution is often helpful, along with systemic antihistamines or hydroxyzine. A sleeping pill prevents inadvertent nocturnal manipulation. Once secondary infection has been addressed with ear drops, the patient should be tried on a strong semisynthetic steroid ointment. This treatment must be continued daily for several weeks, regardless of any apparent early response. The itch is often exacerbated by chronic lymphoedema, and this condition will not disappear in a few days. Once the inflammation has resolved, the patient should consider weekly preventive treatment with acidic ear drops or a steroid cream.

Despite the most rigorous measures, however, some cases of chronic non-specific otitis externa recur or fail to resolve altogether.

POSTINFLAMMATORY STENOSIS OF THE EAR CANAL

Postinflammatory stenosis is a rare but troublesome result of chronic otitis externa. The condition may begin with hypertrophic changes. There may be marked lymphoedema of the meatus, called by some 'elephantiasis' of the ear.[30] The chronic

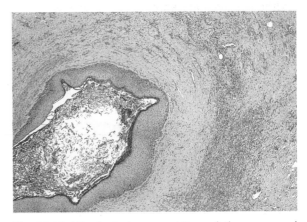

Fig 21.11 Histological cross-section of the ear canal demonstrating postinflammatory stenosis. The epidermis is thickened and lies on a markedly scarred dermal layer. The deeper tissues are chronically inflamed.

inflammation brings about subepithelial fibrosis with progressive narrowing of the ear canal (Fig 21.11 and Plate section). Medial meatal stenosis may nearly obliterate the bony canal, leaving only a pinpoint lumen.

Postinflammatory stenosis has several adverse consequences: it impedes topical or systemic therapy of the inflamed lining, facilitates *de novo* infection or obstruction of the lumen, and ultimately causes hearing loss. Otoscopy reveals a funnel-like narrowing of the ear canal. Histologically, dense scar invests the bony canal circumferentially, narrowing the lumen.

Early management of postinflammatory stenosis includes local injection of steroids and systemic steroids. Once the scar has matured, however, definitive treatment requires excision of the tissue and split-thickness skin grafting.

INFLAMMATORY OBLITERATION OF THE EAR CANAL

Inflammatory obliteration of the ear canal is a most troublesome disorder that often begins as granular myringitis. The lateral surface of the tympanic membrane becomes partially denuded and

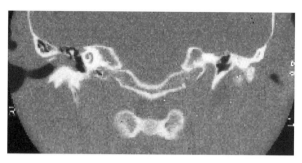

Fig 21.13 Coronal CT image demonstrating a 'false fundus'. The deep canal is completely obliterated. The inflammatory tissue has incorporated the tympanic membrane.

covered with granulations. These may remain isolated and confined to the membrane, but in some cases they become confluent and extend to the deep bony canal. The fundus of the canal becomes filled with granulations that recur and progress despite drops, outpatient debridement and silver nitrate cautery. Eventually the granulations fill most of the bony canal. Just lateral to the involved area, a gradual circumferential stenosis develops. A thin layer of skin, originating along the canal wall, forms a ring-like diaphragm that eventually covers the granulations (Fig 21.12 and Plate section). The patient with this condition in its healed state appears to have a shortened ear canal ending with a featureless blind pocket; this has been described as a 'false fundus' (Fig 21.13 and Plate section).[31] The depth of the scar plug varies and may be approximated by measuring the distance from the fundus to the tragus and comparing it with the normal side. Full evaluation requires a CT scan, specifically to assess depth and involvement of the tympanic membrane.

Although this condition has been repeatedly described, an aetiology and reliable treatment are still lacking. Culture of the granulations may yield bacteria or fungi, but antimicrobial treatment usually does not arrest the process. Aggressive steroid therapy should be tried, orally and with intralesional injections. Once the false fundus has developed, it is best to wait at least 1 year for the granulations to mature before attempting excision. Even with this conservative stance, the stenosis may recur after resection, regardless of whether the tissue was removed with cold knife or laser and whether the area was stented or skin grafted. Despite repeated resections, some of these patients are left with a dense obliterating plug of scar tissue, and some are best managed with a hearing aid.

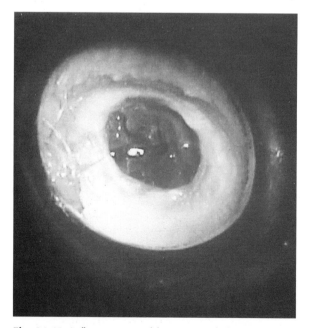

Fig 21.12 Inflammatory obliteration of the ear canal (operative image). The deep canal is filled with fresh granulation tissue. Covering epithelium is growing in from the periphery. When the epithelialization is complete, the patient will have developed a 'false fundus'.

Inflammatory disorders of the tympanic membrane

MYRINGITIS BULLOSA HAEMORRHAGICA

Bullous myringitis (myringitis bullosa haemorrhagica) is a painful infection of the tympanic membrane. The causative organism has not been defined; possible suspects have included viruses, mycoplasma and bacteria. Bullous myrinigitis has a seasonal predilection, occurring mostly in the autumn. The condition develops rapidly with severe pain and at times some aural fullness. Examination reveals blisters of varying sizes on the tympanic membrane and adjacent deep ear canal. The bullae may be filled with a serous or haemorrhagic fluid. The condition often involves both ears in sequence.

Treatment of bullous myringitis requires analgesia. The condition is benign and self-limiting. Ancillary measures include topical antibiotic or steroid drops. Rupturing the blisters to hasten pain relief has also been advocated, but is probably of no benefit once the bullae are fully formed.

GRANULAR MYRINGITIS

Granular myringitis is an inflammation of the tympanic membrane. It manifests as separate or con-

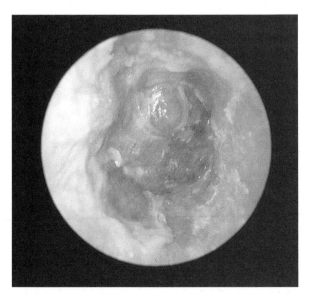

Fig 21.14 Granular myringitis. The tympanic membrane is thickened and red and demonstrates nubbins of granulation tissue. Secondary infection may be responsible for the erythema and exudate.

fluent granulations on the surface of the drum. The eardrum is thickened, inflamed, and moist (Fig 21.14 and Plate section). Loss of sensation on the surface of the tympanic membrane accompanies the inflammation. Although culture may implicate an organism, the actual cause is not known. Treatment includes topical drops and superficial curettage. Although most cases respond to treatment, some progress to an inflammatory obliteration of the deep ear canal (see above).

References

1. Jones EH. *Otitis externa - diagnosis and treatment.* Springfield, IL: Charles C. Thomas, 1965.
2. Granoff DM, Nankervis GA. Cellulitis due to *Hemophilus influenzae* type b antigenemia and antibody responses. *American Journal of Diseases of Childhood* 1976; **130**:1211–4.
3. Valsecchi R, Bontempelli M, Vicari O, Scudeller G, Cainelli T. HLA antigens and contact sensitivity. *Archives of Dermatology* 1982; **118**:533–4.
4. Kligman AM. Hyposensitization against *Rhus* dermatitis. *Archives of Dermatology* 1958; **78**:47–72.
5. Bassiouny A. Perichondritis of the auricle. *Laryngoscope* 1981; **91**:422–31.
6. Foidart JM, Abe S, Martin GR, *et al.* Antibodies to type II collagen in relapsing polychondritis. *New England Journal of Medicine* 1978; **299**:1203–7.
7. McAdam LP, O'Hanlan MA, Bluestone R. Relapsing polychondritis. Prospective study of 23 patients, and a review of the literature. *Medicine* 1976; **55**:193–215.
8. Barranco VP, Minor DB, Soloman H. Treatment of relapsing polychondritis with dapsone. *Archives of Dermatology* 1976; **112**:1286–8.
9. Green CA, Farr PM, Shuster S. Treatment of seborrhoeic dermatitis with ketoconazole. II. Response of seborrhoeic dermatitis of the face, scalp and trunk with topical ketoconazole. *British Journal of Dermatology* 1987; **116**:217–21.
10. Watson W, Cann HM, Farber EM, Nall ML. The genetics of psoriasis. *Archives of Dermatology* 1972; **105**:197–207.
11. Cooper KD, Baadsgaard O. Immunologic features of psoriasis. In: Jordan RE, ed. *Immunologic diseases of the skin*, Norwalk: Appleton and Lange, 1990.
12. Walsdorfer W, Christophers E, Schroder JM. Methotrexate inhibits polymorphonuclear leucocyte chemotaxis in psoriasis. *British Journal of Dermatology* 1983; **108**:451–6.
13. Johnson A, Hawke M. The nonauditory physiology of the external ear canal. In: Jahn AF, Santos-Sacchi J, eds. *Physiology of the ear*. New York: Raven Press, 1988.
14. Wright DN, Alexander, JM. Effect of water on the bacterial flora in Swimmer's ear. *Archives of Otolaryngology* 1974; **99**:15–8.
15. Jones EH, Norman TD. The pathogenesis of acute external otitis. *Trans AAOO* 1959; **63**:63–78.

16. Jahn AF, Hawke M. Otitis externa: a rationale for treatment. *Canadian Fam Phys* 1977; **23**:1388–95.

17. Chandler J, Ryan. Malignant external otitis. *Layngoscope* 1968; **78**:1257–94.

18. Britigan BE, Blythe WB. Malignant external otitis in a diabetic renal transplant patient: successful treatment without discontinuation of immunosuppressive therapy. *Transplantation* 1987; **43**:769–71.

19. Doroghazi RM, Nadol JB, Hyslop NE, *et al.* Invasive external otitis. Report of 21 cases and review of the literature. *American Journal of Medicine* 1976; **71**:603–14.

20. Chandler JR. Malignant external otitis and osteomyelitis of the base of the skull. *American Journal of Otology* 1989; **10**:108–10.

21. Lang R, Goshen S, Kitzes-Cohen R, Sade J. Successful treatment of malignant external otitis with oral ciprofloxacin: report of experience with 23 patients. *Journal of Infectious Diseases* 1990; **161**:537–40.

22. Shupak A, Greenberg E, Hardoff R, Gordon C, Melamed Y, Meyer WS. Hyperbaric oxygenation for necrotizing (malignant) otitis externa. *Archives of Otolaryngology – Head and Neck Surgery* 1989; **115**:1470–5.

23. Uri N, Kitzes R, Meyer W, Schuchman G. Necrotizing external otitis: the importance of prolonged drug therapy. *Journal of Laryngology and Otology* 1984; **98**:1083–5.

24. Schimpff S, Senpick A, Stoter B, Rumack B, Mellin H, Joseph JM. Varicella zoster infection in patients with cancer. *Annals of Internal Medicine* 1972; **76**:241–54.

25. Grigoriu D, Bambule J, Delacretaz J, Savary M. Les otomycoses. *Dermatologica* 1979; **159(suppl 1)**:175–9.

26. Liston SL, Siegel LG. Tinactin in the treatment of fungal otitis externa. *Laryngoscope* 1986; **96**:699.

27. Zelen B. Treatment of otolaryngological mycoses with Nizoral. *Ther Hung* 1985; **33**:156–9.

28. Bickley LS, Betts RF, Parkins CW. Atypical invasive external otitis from Aspergillus. *Archives of Otolaryngology – Head and Neck Surgery* 1988; **114**:1024.

29. Pursell KJ, Telzak EE, Armstrong D. *Aspergillus* species colonization and invasive disease in patients with AIDS. *Clinical Infectious Diseases* 1992; **14**:141–8.

30. Hawke M, Jahn AF. *Diseases of the ear: clinical and pathologic aspects*. Philadelphia: Lea & Febiger, 1987.

31. Schuknecht HF. *Pathology of the ear, 2nd edn*. Philadelphia: Lea & Febiger, 1993.

CHAPTER 22

Non-inflammatory lesions of the external ear

ANTHONY F JAHN

The auricle and external ear canal may give rise to a variety of lesions that are not primarily inflammatory in nature, although infection or inflammation may be a secondary feature. Some of these conditions are inherited or are developmental malformations; others are local manifestations of systemic disorders. Still others are true neoplasms, which may be benign or malignant.

Although the auricle and external ear canal are readily accessible to physical examination, lesions in this area are often overlooked. As an asymptomatic lesion in this area, such as a basal cell skin cancer, may nonetheless be significant, systematic examination of the auricle and periauricular skin should precede every otoscopic examination.

Lesions of the auricle

MICROTIA

Microtia refers to a congenital deformity of the auricle that can range in severity from almost no external ear (anotia) to a minor underdevelopment. The external canal develops from the first branchial cleft, and the auricle forms when six cartilage mounds (so-called hillocks of His) coalesce around the cleft. Failure of the hillocks to fuse properly leads to a diminution and malformation of the auricle. Microtia is often accompanied by stenosis or atresia of the external ear canal.[1] The malformed auricle itself may be low set along the side of the head, signifying failure of ascent to its proper position. Microtia may be unilateral, and related to

arrest of intrauterine development. When bilateral, it may be due to toxicity, such as seen with Accutane or thalidomide,[2] and associated with central nervous system malformations or limb defects, respectively (Fig 22.1).

Microtia may also be associated with regional field defects, such as hemifacial microsomia and middle ear malformations.[3]

Treatment of microtia depends on the severity. A minor malformation can be surgically corrected using local excision and flaps. If more tissue is missing, an implant of autogenous rib cartilage or a synthetic template may be required. In the presence of canal atresia, the ear canal and auricle are usually corrected in separate procedures.

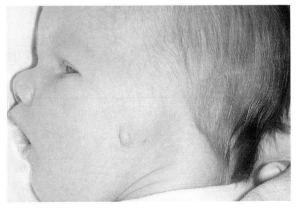

Fig 22.1 Severe microtia in an infant. The mother took Accutane for acne during the first trimester of pregnancy.

PRE-AURICULAR TAGS AND ACCESSORY AURICLES

These are small nodular masses, usually anterior to the tragus. They may consist of skin and fat only, in which case they are called pre-auricular tags. If they also contain a nubbin of cartilage, they are considered an ectopic remnant of auricular tissue, that is, an accessory auricle. They are often bilateral and may be hereditary. Excision is simple and may be carried out for cosmetic reasons. However, it is necessary to be aware of the facial nerve, which is very superficial in children and may be involved in the root of the accessory auricle. Removal is not an outpatient procedure.

PRE-AURICULAR PITS AND SINUSES

Pits are skin-lined depressions that are found on or just anterior to the anterior crus of the helix. They may be shallow or may extend down to the cartilage. Pre-auricular pits are inherited through an autosomal dominant gene with incomplete penetrance. They are usually bilateral. Pre-auricular pits are usually asymptomatic, although they may

contain a small amount of cheesy keratin debris. If infected, a pre-auricular pit may develop erythema and a purulent discharge (Fig 22.2 and Plate section). Treatment is by excision. Complete excision usually requires removal of a small oval of helical cartilage at the base of the tract.

A pre-auricular sinus is deeper, a distinction made with a lachrymal probe. It is lined with squamous or columnar epithelium and extends medially, usually ending blindly at the tympanic ring. Recurrent infection may necessitate excision. Again, complete excision of the epithelial tract is needed to prevent recurrence.

CUTANEOUS CYSTS

Cutaneous cysts are usually developmental and may arise from the epidermis (epidermal or epidermal inclusion cyst) or the root sheath of a hair follicle (trichilemmal or pilar cyst). Trichilemmal cysts account for 10–20 per cent of keratinizing cysts submitted to pathology.

Cutaneous cysts may arise anywhere around the ear, although they are seen most commonly in the postauricular skin. Milia are tiny seed-like keratin-containing cysts seen more commonly around the eye. Epidermal inclusion cysts may develop from implanted keratinizing epidermis and may be associated with an earring tract in the lobule. These cysts are normally slow to grow, soft to firm and non-tender. The cyst may become inflamed if it ruptures or becomes infected. A ruptured epidermal cyst spills keratin into the subcutaneous tissues and evokes a foreign body reaction with inflammation, tenderness and erythema. A cyst may become infected once it has ruptured or been opened. Infected cysts are red, tense, tender and may be discharging.

Cutaneous cysts may be excised. This is best done when they are quiescent. If inflamed or infected, initial treatment should be medical using oral and topical antibiotics and topical soaks.

WINKLER'S NODULE (CHONDRO-DERMATITIS NODULARIS CHRONICA HELICIS)

Winkler's nodule is a benign lesion that usually (but not invariably) occurs on the rim of the helix in older men. Sunlight is believed to cause a breakdown of elastin fibres, and trauma initiates chronic inflammation that extends down to the perichondrium. Secondary epithelial changes develop leading to transdermal elimination of degenerated connective tissue.[5] Clinically the lesion is a red,

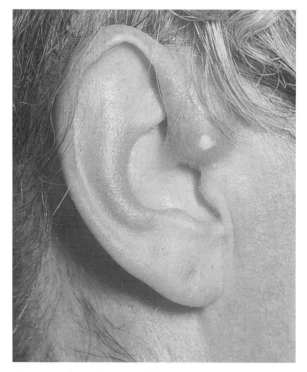

Fig 22.2 Infected pre-auricular pit. Pressure has expressed creamy pus.

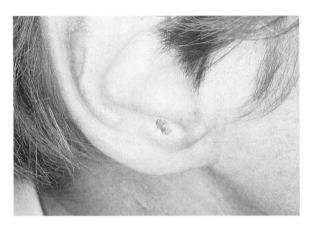

Fig 22.3 Winkler's nodule along the inner curvature of the helix. The raised inflamed lesion has a crater-like centre that mimics carcinoma.

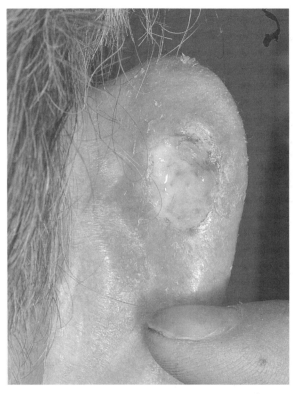

Fig 22.4 Keratoacanthoma: a large raised painless lesion with a central crater.

raised and tender nodule, usually with a central depression or crater (Fig 22.3). The fundus of the crater is cartilage or perichondrium, accounting for the exquisite tenderness of the lesion. Patients often complain that they cannot sleep if the ear touches the pillow. This tenderness helps to distinguish Winkler's nodule from lesions such as senile keratosis, keratoacanthoma, cutaneous horn and carcinoma, which are usually painless.

Definitive treatment of Winkler's nodule requires full-thickness excision, which includes a wedge of cartilage. The defect may be closed by local advancement flaps to minimize the cosmetic deformity.[6] Temporizing measures include topical steroids[7] and an adhesive bandage worn at night to minimize contact.

GOUTY TOPHI OF THE AURICLE

Gouty tophi of the ear may be seen in cases of hyperuricaemia. The uric acid crystallizes to form subcutaneous nodules, most commonly over the helix of the ear. The nodule appears yellowish or salmon pink and is hard and gritty to the touch. There is often erythema of the overlying skin and tenderness. Histological findings reveal needle-shaped crystals of monosodium urate accompanied by an inflammatory reaction in the surrounding tissues. Although the appearance of a tophus in the absence of gouty arthropathy is rare, gout should be part of the differential diagnosis of a tender sclerotic nodule. Management requires dietary control of serum uric acid levels and administration of allopurinol, colchicine and adjunctive anti-inflammatory medications.[8]

KERATOACANTHOMA

Keratoacanthoma or 'self-healing basal cell carcinoma' is a benign tumour believed to arise from the hair follicles.[9] It may form anywhere on the body and is believed to be related to actinic exposure.[10]

On the external ear, keratoacanthomas are most commonly seen anterior to the tragus. Keratoacanthoma is a rapidly growing painless tumour that is red, raised and circular. The tumour is further characterized by a central crater that often contains a keratin plug (Fig 22.4 and Plate section). Histologically this crater is seen as a calyx filled with parakeratotic cells and desquamated debris (Fig 22.5 and Plate section).

Even a classic keratoacanthoma may strongly resemble a squamous cell carcinoma. Keratoacanthoma may spontaneously involute and disappear. This involution sets it apart from malignancies, whereas its painless nature distinguishes it from Winkler's nodule.

Keratoacanthomas are usually excised for biopsy and treatment. If the diagnosis is not in doubt, the otologist may follow the tumour clinically and allow spontaneous resolution to take place.

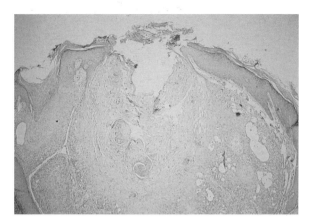

Fig 22.5 Histological cross-section of keratoacanthoma demonstrates the calyx filled with sheets of parakeratotic cells and keratin debris.

Topical 5% fluorouracil has also been recommended in the dermatological literature.[11]

HYPERTROPHIC SCARS AND KELOIDS

Hypertrophic scars and keloids represent an unchecked healing response to trauma. Whereas hypertrophic scars remain confined to the original site of injury, keloids often invade adjacent untraumatized tissue, thereby causing a greater cosmetic or functional deformity. The keloid differs also in its histology. In addition to focal areas of mature collagen seen in hypertrophic scars, keloids also demonstrate thick, acellular eosinophilic bundles of collagen with a nodular or concentric arrangement.

Keloids form more often in dark-skinned individuals and tend to occur most frequently in the upper part of the body.[12] The otologist most often encounters keloids of the lobule.[13] These usually result from ear piercing and may grow to enormous size (Fig 22.6).

A variety of treatments have been proposed for keloids. Small keloids are best left alone and the patient should be advised to avoid the use of earrings. Even clip-on earrings cause trauma.

Simple excision usually results in a more exuberant regrowth and should be discouraged. Topical injection of steroids has been recommended using triamcinolone acetate.[14] This may be of benefit in a fresh keloid but has less effect on mature scar tissue.

In my hands excision followed by topical steroids has been beneficial. The keloid is fully excised, undermining and preserving as much adjacent skin as possible. The area is closed with minimum trauma using fine non-absorbable sutures. Postoperatively the ear

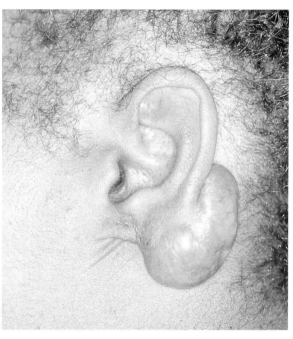

Fig 22.6 Keloid of the ear lobe due to repeated ear piercing.

is injected weekly with a mixture of triamcinolone and hyaluronidase. A Dermajet cutaneous injector is used to force a finely dispersed mixture directly into the superficial skin. The patient should be warned that the ear may show a deformity after excision and repeated injections and that no further piercing or surgery should be done. The use of γ interferon is promising as it appears to inhibit fibroblasts strongly. An injection of 5 million units in 1 ml, 1 week after excision of the keloid can prevent regrowth. An anti-inflammatory agent such as ibuprofen may be necessary to reduce systemic symptoms.

CARCINOMA OF THE AURICLE

Carcinoma of the auricle is seen most often in older men. These tumours reflect the end-stage of actinic-induced epidermal dysplasia. They are more common in light-haired fair-skinned individuals, particularly those who spend time outdoors. These patients often show varying degrees of actinic damage in other exposed areas of the head and neck and may develop carcinomas on the cheek, nose or lip.

Every susceptible individual should be carefully examined, as these tumours often arise in areas not readily visible to the patient. In the region of the external ear, such tumours are typically seen anterior to the tragus and over protruding portions of the auricle such as the helix and antihelix. Basal cell tumours are raised, pearly shiny nodules. Neovascularization is common. The surface of the early tumour is usually intact, and ulceration is a later and more ominous finding. By contrast, squamous cell cancers often show breakdown of the surface.

Histologically basal cell cancer is usually a localized tumour, with a gradual, pushing invasive deep margin. The tumour is normally easily resected, with an identifiable margin. A less easily excised variant is the sclerosing or morpheaform basal cell carcinoma. Clinically this cancer is cicatrizing, forming a whitish flat patch that is better appreciated by palpation than inspection.[15] Histologically this lesion is distinguished by less distinct infiltrating margins with fibrous tissue in surrounding nests of tumour cells. For these tumours, a clear margin requires a wider field of resection and recurrence is more frequent. Control of excision margins should be by frozen section appraisal, and the surgeon must be prepared to be left with a larger defect than originally anticipated.[16]

Although local excision is the treatment of choice, some tumours also respond to topical 5-fluorouracil cream, and this may be considered in cases in which small multiple or recurrent tumours or widespread actinic dysplasia makes resection problematic.

A less frequent but more threatening form of basal cell carcinoma arises in the postauricular skin over the mastoid process. These tumours, by virtue of their location, are frequently overlooked in the early stages. By the time the tumour is diagnosed, it has often invaded the mastoid periosteum. The invasive nature of these cancers, along with their avidity for underlying bone, is reminiscent of basal cell cancers of the inner canthus. In the older literature these postauricular tumours were called 'rodent ulcers', referring to their erosive and invasive behaviour. Treatment carried a high failure rate and gave rise to the descriptive name, '*noli me tangere*' (do not touch me), a clear warning to over enthusiastic surgeons.

Postauricular basal cell tumours require radiological evaluation of the underlying bone and the regional lymph nodes. Treatment involves wide-field resection with or without radiotherapy. Advanced cases are often not amenable to resection because of invasion of the marrow and the skull base and may be treated by full-course radiotherapy.

Squamous cell carcinoma shares a common aetiology with basal cell carcinoma (BCC). Although other factors, such as arsenic, radiation and previous scarring have been cited as causative, the location, age and sex predilection of squamous cell carcinoma (SCC) suggest that, around the ear, this tumour is related to sun damage. This tumour usually arises from solar keratosis and progresses through stages of dysplasia, in-situ carcinoma and invasive carcinoma. Although both squamous and basal cell tumours occur in sun-exposed skin, the relationship between ultraviolet radiation and squamous cell cancer is more direct.[17]

On the ear SCC usually arises on protuberant areas such as the helix. The appearance is of an indurated nodule, perhaps with an adherent keratotic scale and evidence of erosion or ulceration. The clinical appearance of SCC is often not pathognomonic and may be confused with BCC or solar keratosis. Early lesions should be fully excised, with direct or local flap closure. More advanced lesions need to be worked up for deep invasion and regional nodal metastases before definitive treatment.

OTHER MALIGNANCIES

The skin of the ear and peri-auricular region may give rise to any of the malignancies found elsewhere on the body. Melanoma, melanotic and amelanotic, may arise either primarily, from a pre-existing pigmented lesion, or by metastasis. Kaposi's sarcoma of the auricle, described as a rarity in 1960[18] is seen increasingly often in AIDS patients.

Lesions of the external ear canal

KERATOSIS OBTURANS AND CHOLESTEATOMA OF THE EXTERNAL EAR CANAL

Keratosis obturans is a disorder of keratin formation and disposal that involves the deep external ear canal. The patient presents with obstruction of the canal. On examination, the deep canal is filled with a large, adherent keratin plug, which can often be removed intact (Figs 22.7 and 22.8 and Plate section). The underlying skin looks normal. Pressure from the accumulated keratin may over time result in a remodelling of the bony canal.

The cause of keratosis obturans is not known. It is a clinical impression that the condition is often found in older male smokers with chronic obstructive lung disease.[19] No definitive treatment exists and management requires periodic debridement of the ear canal.

By contrast, cholesteatoma of the external ear canal probably starts with an injury of the skin overlying the bony canal. Focal osteitis develops with granulation tissue and a secondary hyperkeratotic

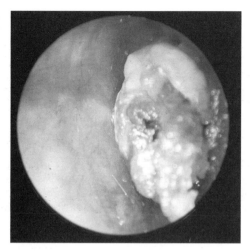

Fig 22.7 Keratosis obturans: the deep canal is filled with a white plug of keratin.

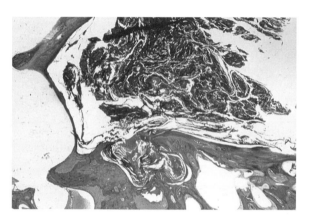

Fig 22.8 Cholesteatoma of the external ear canal. Note the bony erosion of the floor of the ear canal, a feature that distinguishes this condition from keratosis obturans.

skin reaction of the adjacent canal. Bone remodelling and destruction are common. Cholesteatoma of the ear canal manifests with obstruction, pain and otorrhoea. Debridement of the keratin discloses exposed bone.

Treatment of external ear canal cholesteatoma requires debridement of the accumulated keratin and the inflamed or devitalized bone. Topical antibiotics may be beneficial. Curettage of the osteitic bone may result in healing with an intact skin cover.

POSTMASTOIDECTOMY STENOSIS OF THE EAR CANAL

Older patients who had undergone cortical mastoidectomy in childhood may over the years develop stenosis of the ear canal. This narrowing typically involves the cartilaginous canal and at times leads to complete occlusion. Postmastoidectomy stenosis probably has several causes. The postauricular incision allows the auricle to move forwards, and the conchal cartilage slides across the meatus to cause a narrowing at the meatal entrance. Deposition of scar tissue between the skin of the ear canal and the underlying bone further narrows the lumen.

These patients often complain of hearing loss, which is relieved by retracting the auricle. Some patients are seen because they cannot be fitted with a hearing aid because of the collapsed canal.

Surgical repair of postmastoidectomy stenosis may be performed in several ways. The postauricular approach involves resection of scar tissue and cartilage followed by insertion of retention sutures and packing of the canal. Permeatal surgery requires the local excision of cartilage and scar tissue. My preferred technique for localized narrowing due to conchal displacement involves an incision over the edge between concha and meatus. The incision becomes the transverse part of a Z-plasty. After excision of cartilage and scar tissue, the Z-plasty is completed and the ear canal packed.

EXOSTOSIS AND OSTEOMA OF THE EAR CANAL

Exostoses and osteomas are benign bony growths of the deep ear canal. Although grouped together here, these lesions are distinct aetiologically, clinically and histologically.

Exostoses are in fact bony calluses or hyperostoses that arise from the tympanic ring. They may be flat or protuberant, but are usually multiple and sessile (Fig 22.9 and Plate section). They typically involve both ears, although often to a different degree. Exostoses may occur anywhere on the tympanic bone, but are usually most prominent on its two arms, in the area of the tympanomastoid and tympanosquamous suture. Exostoses are found typically in the deep bony canal, often just adjacent to the bony tympanic annulus. They never form on the scutum, the portion of the squamous bone that bridges the notch of Rivinus.

Exostoses grow slowly. They begin as a thickening of the bony wall with a deformity of its contour. The long-term effect of exostoses is a gradual narrowing of the ear canal, which may progress to complete obliteration.

Although exostoses of the ear were already known to Virchow over a century ago, their aetiology was not clear until 1942 when Fowler and

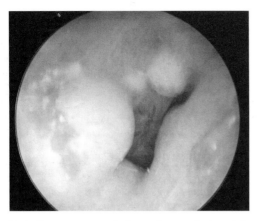

Fig 22.9 Exostoses anteriorly and posteriorly, obliterate most of this ear canal, leaving only a narrow passage.

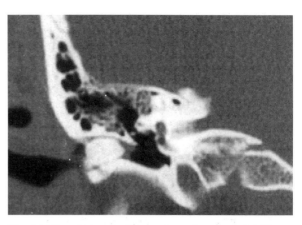

Fig 22.10 Coronal CT section demonstrating large osteoma of the ear canal. The soft tissue deep to the osteoma was an accumulation of keratin, which was pressing on the tympanic membrane.

Osmun[20] demonstrated their relationship to cold water exposure. It is theorized that cold water causes vasoconstriction in the periosteal vessels. This is followed by reflex vasodilatation and deposition of new bone. The histology of exostoses is in keeping with this theory. Sections demonstrate onion-like layers of compact lamellar bone generally devoid of blood vessels.

By contrast, osteomas are true neoplasms. They are solitary, often unilateral and seem to arise spontaneously. They may be pedunculated with only a tenuous attachment to the underlying bony canal, although in other cases they are broadly based. They often arise at the tympanosquamous suture and are usually attached more laterally than exostoses. Histologically they consist of cancellous bone with fibrovascular channels.[21] On thin section CT scan the osteoma may appear more heterogeneous than the invariably solid and dense exostosis (Fig 22.10).

The treatment of these bony lesions depends on the symptoms they cause. Small or medium size lesions are usually trouble-free and may be observed. If the growths become obstructive, they should be removed. Patients with obstructive exostoses or osteomas complain of recurrent hearing loss due to impaction of keratin or wax. Repeated trauma during ear cleaning may cause discomfort, obstruction by blood clot and even periosteitis with chronic pain. Some patients with unrelated nerve deafness will require removal of exostoses to allow proper fitting of a hearing aid.

As osteomas are usually pedunculated and solitary, they are easily removed using a drill or curette. Exostoses, by contrast, are multiple, more diffusely attached and closer to the tympanic membrane. A

postauricular or endaural incision frees both hands of the surgeon and is recommended. The bony canal should be opened using cutting and diamond burrs. Healing is facilitated by preserving as much canal skin as possible. If an exostosis is at the tympanic annulus, the middle ear may be inadvertently opened and the dehiscence must be repaired. A preoperative CT scan is helpful in noting the relationship of the exostoses to the tympanic annulus.

SOFT TISSUE TUMOURS OF THE EAR CANAL

There are a number of soft-tissue tumours that may arise in the ear canal. Polyps in the ear canal are usually based in the middle ear, and protrude through a perforation. These polyps are often associated with chronic otitis media or cholesteatoma. Although mucosal in origin, a chronic polyp may become covered with squamous epithelium and mimic a true external ear canal 'tumour'.

Rarely polyps arise in the external ear canal. A pyogenic granuloma of the ear canal typically arises after minor trauma. As the granuloma heals, a fibrotic tag may remain. Keratin implantation granulomas also arise from trauma. Subcutaneous implantation of keratin provokes a foreign body reaction with a inflammation and a granulation tissue polyp. These lesions may be simply removed.

Tumours of the external ear canal are generally rare. They usually arise from the skin or epidermal appendages. Ceruminomas are the commonest tumours found in this location.[22] The term 'ceruminoma' describes a tumour that arises from one of the 1000–2000 ceruminous glands present in the

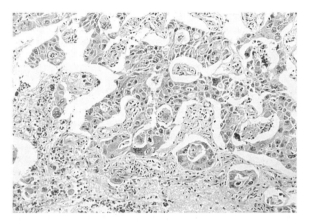

Fig 22.11 Malignant ceruminoma of the ear canal. The cells demonstrate a clearly malignant morphology, and the cribriform arrangement is similar to adenoid cystic carcinoma.

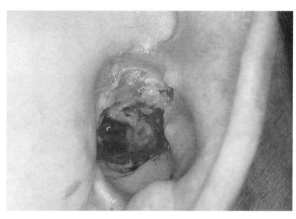

Fig 22.12 Squamous cell carcinoma of the ear canal. Deep erosion of cartilage and bone are an ominous sign.

external canal. The term alludes to the origin of the lesion and includes at least four different lesions, which vary from benign to malignant: ceruminal adenoma, ceruminal pleomorphic adenoma (mixed type tumour), ceruminal adenocarcinoma and adenoid cystic carcinoma. Primary adenocarcinoma of the ear canal is rare and a metastatic survey for other primary sites should be considered. In addition, it has been proposed that some cases of adenoid cystic carcinoma may in fact arise from salivary tissue in the adjacent parotid tail. Each type has its own histological pattern and clinical pattern of behaviour, including a proclivity to invade or metastasize (Fig 22.11 and Plate section).

Benign ceruminomas are often picked up incidentally in the course of a general examination. The commonest symptom is a sensation of blockage and hearing loss if obstruction of the lumen has occurred. Pain is an ominous symptom, more often seen with the malignant forms. The clinical appearance of the tumour varies from a subcutaneous nodule, polyp or area of granulation tissue to an ulcerated, painful and obviously malignant mass. Appearance is not always predictive, however, and even an innocent-appearing mass may be malignant.

Once the diagnosis of ceruminoma is entertained, based on either clinical suspicion or biopsy, the extent must be defined using mastoid films, tomograms or CT scans of the ear canal. Complete excision may be limited to the ear canal or may require a partial parotidectomy and upper neck dissection.

Squamous carcinomas may present as a *de novo* lesion. More often, however, they manifest as a change in symptoms in a chronically infected ear (Fig 22.12 and Plate section). Lewis,[23] in a study of carcinomas of the ear, showed that 50 per cent of all cases of ear canal carcinoma had a history of chronic suppurative external otitis or chronic otitis media of 10 years' duration or longer.

Pain, bleeding or facial paralysis are obvious alerting signs. The development of these signs or the discovery of a new or changed lesion in the ear canal mandates biopsy. If the biopsy is positive, the cancer is staged and treated.

The treatment of deep external ear canal carcinoma is lateral temporal bone resection, optionally followed by radiation therapy.[24] Carcinomas of the medial (bony) ear canal often involve the tympanic membrane and middle ear and therefore carry a worse prognosis. The outlook for 5-year survival is less than 25 per cent.[25]

References

1. Jahrsdoerfer RA. Congenital atresia of the ear. *Laryngoscope* 1978; **88(suppl 13)**:1–48.
2. Jahn AF, Ganti KM. Major auricular malformations due to Accutane (Isotretinoin). *Laryngoscope* 1987; **97**:832–5.
3. Caldarelli DD, Hutchinson JG, Pruzansky S, Valvassori GE. A comparison of microtia and temporal bone anomalies in hemifacial microsomia and mandibulofacial dysostosis. *Cleft Palate Journal* 1980; **17**:103–10.
4. Kaye WH. Chondrodermatitis nodularis chronica helicis. *Archives of Otolaryngology* 1966; **84**:403–5.
5. Goette DK. Chondrodermatitis nodularis chronica helicis: a perforating necrobiotic granuloma. *Journal of the American Academy of Dermatology* 1980; **2**:148–54.
6. Ceilley RI, Lillis PJ. Surgical treatment of chondrodermatitis nodularis chronica helicis. *Journal of Dermatology and Surgical Oncology* 1979; **5**:384–6.

7. Wade TR. Chondrodermatitis nodularis chronica helicis. A review with emphasis on steroid therapy. *Cutis* 1979; **24**:406–9.

8. Wyngaarden JB, Kelley WN. *Gout and hyperuricemia*. New York: Grune and Stratton, 1976.

9. Ghadially FN. The role of the hair follicle in origin and evolution of some cutaneous neoplasms in man and experimental animals. *Cancer* 1961; **14**:801.

10. Belisario JV. *Cancer of the skin*. London: Butterworth, 1959.

11. Goette DK. Treatment of keratoacanthoma with topical fluorouracil. *Archives of Dermatology* 1983; **119**:951–3.

12. Alhady SM, Sivanantharajah K. Keloids in various races. *Plastic Reconstructive Surgery* 1969; **44**:564–6.

13. Cheng LH. Keloid of the ear lobe. *Laryngoscope* 1972; **82**:673–81.

14. Griffith BH, Monroe CW, Mckinney P. A follow-up study on the treatment of keloids with riamicinolone acetonide. *Plastic Reconstructive Surgery* 1970; **46**:145–50.

15. Carter DM, Lin AN. Basal cell carcinoma. In: Fitzpatrick TB, Eisen AZ, Wolff K, *et al.*, eds. *Dermatology in general medicine, 4th ed*. New York: McGraw-Hill, 1993.

16. Swanson NA, Grekin RC, Baker SR. Mohs surgery: technique, indications, applications, and the future. *Archives of Dermatology* 1983; **119**:683–92.

17. Urbach F, Davies RF, Forbes PD. Ultraviolet radiation and skin cancer in man. In: Montagna W, Dobson RL, eds. *Advances in biology of skin, vol VII*. New York: Pergamon Press, 1966.

18. Naunton RF, Stoller FM. Kaposi's sarcoma of the auricle. *Laryngoscope* 1960; **70**:1535–40.

19. Hawke M, Jahn AF. *Diseases of the ear: clinical and pathologic aspects*. London: Gower, 1987.

20. Fowler EP Jr, Osmun PM. New bone growth due to cold water in the ears. *Archives of Otolaryngology* 1942; **36**:455–66.

21. Graham MD. Osteomas and exostoses of the external auditory canal: a clinical, histopathological and scanning electron microscopic study. *Annals of Otology, Rhinology and Laryngology* 1979; **88**:566.

22. Batsakis JG, Hardy GC, Hishiyama RH. Ceruminous gland tumours. *Archives of Otolaryngology* 1967; **86**:66–72.

23. Lewis JS. Squamous carcinoma of the ear. *Archives of Otolaryngolology* 1973; **97**:41–2.

24. Tabb HC, Komet H, McLaurin JW. Cancer of the external auditory canal: Treatment with radical mastoidectomy and irradiation. *Laryngoscope* 1964; **74**:634–43.

25. Johns ME, Headington JT. Squamous cell carcinoma of the external auditory canal: a clinical study of 20 cases. *Archives of Otolaryngology* 1974; **100**:45–9.

PART V

Acquired middle ear disease

CHAPTER 23

Introduction to middle ear and mastoid disease

TONY WRIGHT AND HAROLD LUDMAN

This section of the book deals with acute and chronic diseases of the middle ear cleft, which comprises the Eustachian tube, the middle ear air space, the mastoid antrum and mastoid air cells. The range and complexity of the problems that can arise provide a subject full of fascination with sometimes only subtle clues leading to the discovery of extensive disease. Operations on the diseased middle ear and mastoid, when correctly indicated, must be meticulous and precise and are often very demanding. When successful, the outcomes of a dry, pain-free ear, an improvement in hearing, freedom from vertigo and possibly the reversal of a facial palsy or removal of other threats are extremely satisfying for patient and surgeon alike. There are still many problems to be overcome. These include disease in the sinus tympani and extensive, bilateral mucosal disease involving the Eustachian tube and mastoid, especially when the middle ear cleft is open to the exterior.

To discuss these problems a simple but robust system of nomenclature for the classes of disease is necessary. All too often different writers use names picked almost at random from the bewildering catalogue of possible synonyms, some of which are based on clinical, others on histopathological and yet others on prognostic features. Black[1] for example (1984) provided a list of 25 different names for what was presumably meant to be chronic secretory otitis media (Table 23.1).

With many of these terms being only loosely defined or not defined at all it is impossible to know how treatment of say condition A relates to that of condition B. Thus, one of the more powerful tools

Table 23.1 Glue ear terminology – some examples between 1869 and 1982

Year of first published usage	Name
1869	Otitis media catarrhal
	Phlegmonous inflammation of the middle ear
1873	Subacute catarrh of middle ear
	Chronic internal catarrh
1874	Mucous aural catarrh
	Catarrhal otitis media
1912	Exudative catarrh
	Serous catarrh of middle ear
	Seromucous catarrah
1921	Adhesive catarrh
1924	Chronic middle ear exudate catarrh
1927	Secretory otitis media
1938	Chronic non-suppurative otitis media
1943	Serous otitis media
	Hydrotympanum
1949	Otitis media with effusion
	Secretory exudative otitis media
1951	The hypersecretory ear
1952	Tympanic hydrops
1960	Glue ear
1962	Otitis media ex vacuo
1963	Exudative otitis media
1967	Indolent otitis media
1978	Seromucinous otitis media
1982	Mucoid otitis media

Reproduced from Black[1] with permission.

of statistics – meta analysis – cannot be used to make sense of the published data. We feel that using terms such as 'acute otitis media' in publications without precise definition serves only to make the problem worse even though we accept that accurate classification can be difficult in the early stages of many diseases. This problem was highlighted in the report of the Fifth Research Conference on Recent Advances in Otitis Media (1994), which suggested that there was a 'need for consistency in definition of disease. All studies should indicate specific criteria used for various components of the spectrum of OM', and yet did not itself define what was meant by acute otitis media or by otitis media with effusion.

Throughout this book we have adopted a nomenclature that runs as consistently as possible throughout all the chapters, despite different usages initially presented by the contributing authors. Some of our contributors may dislike or even resent our choices, but our readers will be exposed to consistency. We have avoided abbreviations, as they are often confusing.

Otitis media as a term means inflammation of the middle ear cleft, and it is only broadly descriptive. It does not, nor can it, specify a cause or a duration, and its use without further clarification is almost always unhelpful and ought to be avoided. Our scheme distinguishes between suppurative and secretory otitis media and divides each into acute and chronic forms.

Suppurative otitis media

The term suppurative otitis media means a purulent inflammation of the middle ear cleft. It implies the presence of pus, and in its original use indicated that the ear was making or discharging pus. The cause is often purely infective but other agents such as allergy, cholesteatoma, chemical irritants, malignancies, auto-immune diseases and others may underlie the discharge.

ACUTE SUPPURATIVE OTITIS MEDIA

This is an acute disease. By our definition it lasts less than 3 months from start to resolution and is typified by a short-lived infection that may first be viral then bacterial in origin, with pain, often with fever, and usually with some hearing loss. It may be accompanied by discharge from the ear. Rarely, an underlying condition such as a cholesteatoma may manifest as an acute suppurative otitis media and, once the infection has been

treated and settled, go undiagnosed until repeated infections occur and draw attention to the basic disease.

Synonyms (which we feel are better avoided) are

- acute otitis media
- AOM
- ASOM

CHRONIC SUPPURATIVE OTITIS MEDIA

The term chronic suppurative otitis media was established before antibiotics had been discovered and developed. It was likely that most chronically diseased ears did discharge, whereas only a few were 'silent' until a serious complication arose. The defining term – 'suppurative' – is therefore not fully appropriate to cover the range of conditions that the complete term now encompasses.

There is possibly scope for a term 'chronic non-suppurative, non-secretory otitis media' to include conditions such as non-infected cholesteatoma or masked mastoiditis but this is too cumbersome for everyday use.

A traditional way of subdividing chronic suppurative otitis media has been into 'safe' and 'unsafe' ear disease.

So-called 'safe' disease was characterized by a central perforation of the pars tensa and was also called tubo-tympanic disease to indicate disease of the Eustachian tube and tympanic cavity. The inflammatory process affected the mucosa of the middle ear cleft.

'Unsafe' disease was typified by a marginal perforation of the posterosuperior pars tensa or of the pars flaccida and was also called attico-antral disease. Cholesteatoma was almost always present and involved the attic (epitympanum) and mastoid antrum. Bone erosion, with potentially dangerous results, was an inherent pathological feature. Another synonym has been 'erosive middle ear disease'.

It is clear from the work of Browning[2] that previously described 'safe ears' do have a significant incidence of serious intracranial complication, so that this is not a reliably indicative description.

For simplicity and consistency we have subdivided chronic suppurative otitis media into

- mucosal disease
- cholesteatoma (and others)

Chronic suppurative otitis media – mucosal disease

Mucosal disease is typified by a bacterial infection of the middle ear cleft with the presence of pus, which discharges through a perforation in the pars tensa. The discharge is persistent for 3 months or more, although it may settle with appropriate treatment only to recur when the treatment has been withdrawn, so that the middle ear mucosa may never return to normal.

If the tympanic membrane is intact a similar disorder may be termed 'masked'. Over time, if fluid in the middle ear cleft becomes sterile, there may be a gradation to chronic secretory otitis media.

The following synonyms have been used:

- safe ear disease
- tubo-tympanic disease
- central perforations
- CSOM

Chronic suppurative otitis media – cholesteatoma (and others)

Acquired cholesteatoma arises from the skin of the tympanic membrane. Disease arising from the pars flaccida skin typically involves the epitympanum and mastoid antrum and can be very erosive, causing serious local complications. Retraction of the pars tensa can also give rise to accumulations of shed keratin, usually within the middle ear itself. This form of cholesteatoma is less erosive, although it may be more difficult to eradicate, and has been called cholesteatosis by many of the French otologists.

The following synonyms have been used:

- unsafe ear disease
- attico-antral disease
- marginal perforations
- CSOM
- erosive (or destructive) middle ear disease

Secretory otitis media

Secretory otitis media has been defined by Jacob Sadé as 'the presence of an effusion in the middle ear space without symptoms [and signs] of infection.' In other words, there is an effusion which may be free of pathogenic bacteria in the middle ear. There are many causes ranging from acute viral upper respiratory tract infections through allergy to barotrauma, which is the trauma related to major changes in external pressure.

ACUTE SECRETORY OTITIS MEDIA

Acute secretory otitis media is a very common condition that usually follows upper respiratory tract infections and is defined as the presence of an effusion (which may be sterile) in the middle ear, which resolves within 3 months. It frequently arises from some combination of altered production of mucus in the middle ear, both in quantity and quality; mucosal congestion and changes in the ciliary clearance mechanisms.

Once the initiating factors have cleared, self-resolution occurs and the middle ear returns to normal. Children seem particularly prone to recurrent bouts of acute secretory otitis media, which are often painful, and some of these attacks progress to an acute suppurative otitis media. Some children may subsequently develop chronic secretory otitis media.

The following synonyms have been used:

- acute otitis media
- AOM
- ASOM

CHRONIC SECRETORY OTITIS MEDIA

If a sterile effusion has been present for 3 months without clearing, then the effusion is no longer acute and should be called chronic. Acute suppurative episodes may superimpose themselves on a background of the chronic secretory state, but once an acute infective episode has cleared the effusion persists.

The following synonyms have been used:

- glue ear
- OME (otitis media with effusion)
- MEE (middle ear effusion)
- presumably all the other terms set out in Table 23.1.

Throughout this book we consistently apply this simple terminology, which we believe avoids confusion. If you, the reader, choose to use other terms in your writings and presentations, then we would urge you to define them so that your meaning is clear.

References

1. Black NA. Is glue ear a modern phenomenon? A historical review of the medical literature. *Clinical Otolaryngology* 1984; **9**:155–63.
2. Nunez DA, Browning GG. Risks of developing an otogenic intracranial abscess. *Journal of Laryngology and Otology* 1990; **104**:468–72.

CHAPTER 24

The Eustachian tube

JACOB SADÉ AND AMOS AR

Introduction

All land-living vertebrates – reptiles, birds and mammals – have developed some form of middle ear transformer mechanism to convert airborne sound waves into pressure changes suitable for transmission within the fluids of the inner ear. Despite divergent evolution of the various orders, the middle ear mechanism has achieved a remarkable homology with a tympanic membrane coupled by one or more ossicles to a mobile platform in contact with the perilymph. The middle ear is gas filled and so there is minimal frictional resistance to the movement of the ossicles, and the middle ear gas pressure is approximately equal to external pressure, which allows optimal transfer by the tympanic membrane.

The middle ear is, in effect, a gas pocket. Biological gas pockets are found in birds as respiratory air sacs and in fish as buoyancy bladders and elsewhere as in the paranasal sinuses and the pleural cavities.

Some biological gas pockets are equipped with elaborate mechanisms to maintain their total pressure or even to increase it. Fish possess an organelle called the rete mirabile, which can actively pump gas from the circulation into the buoyancy bladder to equilibrate its pressure with that of the surrounding water.

All biological gas pockets face two special problems: the need to overcome shrinkage or reduced pressure because of a net loss of gases into the surrounding circulation, and the need to keep the inside of the sac clean. In the middle ear these two problems have been overcome by 'gas inhalation' or ventilation through the Eustachian tube and by a mucociliary transport mechanism to clear mucus and debris from the middle ear towards the nasopharynx.

General principles regulating the gas economy of a biological gas pocket

The number of molecules in a specific gas (Gi) in a volume containing a mixture of gases, is expressed by its partial pressure (pGi). All the different partial pressures of the various gases (Gi, Gii...Gx) present in this mixture together exert the total gas pressure (pB) of that mixture. Under usual conditions the five major gases, which constitute air, that is, nitrogen (N_2), argon (Ar), oxygen (O_2), carbon dioxide (CO_2) and water vapour (H_2O), also constitute the gases dissolved in the blood and in any biological gas pocket. However, the proportion of each of these gases and the total pressure they exert may be different in air, arteries, veins and biological gas pockets.

The pB of air at sea level and at 20°C is approximately 10 000 mmH$_2$O, which is equal to 760 mmHg, and 1 mmHg (1 Torr) is approximately equal to 13.6 mmH$_2$O.

At 37°C and at sea level the composition of air when saturated with water vapour is

- pO$_2$ 150 mmHg
- pCO$_2$ approximately zero
- pN$_2$ (plus pAr)   563 mmHg
- pH$_2$O   47 mmHg
  Making a total of   760 mmHg.

The amount of water vapour, which varies from one situation to another, may 'dilute' or 'concentrate' the other gases depending on the degree of saturation and temperature. Thus, in biological systems water vapour may constitute up to 50 mmHg of the total pressure.

Both the partial and the total pressures of the gases in the lung alveoli are nearly in equilibrium with those in the arterial blood leaving the alveolar capillaries. As this arterial blood passes through the tissues at capillary level, large changes occur. Usually more oxygen, by volume, is absorbed than carbon dioxide is produced. (At the cellular level this is expressed as the respiratory quotient, which is the CO_2 to O_2 exchanged volume ratio).

The pCO_2 in blood increases less than the pO_2 decreases, because carbon dioxide is much more soluble in blood than oxygen. This asymmetry between the solubilities and the shapes of the oxygen and carbon dioxide saturation curves results in a marked decrease in the blood pO_2 and only a moderate increase in pCO_2, leaving a gas pressure deficit of about 50 mmHg in venous blood relative to air. The pN_2 and pH_2O barely change. Table 24.1 quantifies the changes.

Thus in venous blood there exists a lower total gas pressure than in air or arterial blood. Gas molecules tend to pass from a high to a low partial pressure environment until equilibrium is reached. This is true for each individual gas in a mixture, independent of the partial pressure of the other gases. The passage of a gas from a high to a low partial pressure region occurs across liquid, tissue, and blood vessel walls by diffusion. The rate of transfer varies for different gases.

In the middle ear lumen the gases 'strive' to reach equilibrium with their corresponding gas pressures in the surrounding capillaries. The middle ear oxygen, carbon dioxide and water vapour are in equilibrium with the blood leaving the middle ear, as they move relatively quickly across the various barriers. Assuming that the venous blood draining the middle ear has a gas composition similar to that of mixed venous blood, then a steady state situation would finally evolve in which the total middle ear gas pressure would be lower than that of the atmosphere by about 56 mmHg ($760 - 704 = 56$). This would result in a large pressure gradient across the tympanic membrane, which would compromise its impedance matching properties. For the middle ear to reach a total pressure equal to atmospheric, some compensation is needed and this is provided by the periodic supply of gas from the nasopharynx through the Eustachian tube. The partial pressure deficit is made up mainly by nitrogen, which is relatively slow to diffuse across capillary walls, so that the middle ear pN_2 is higher than in the blood and serves to maintain an overall total pressure of about 760 mmHg in the normal middle ear.

Table 24.1 Partial and total pressures in air, blood and middle ear lumen at sea level

	Saturated air at 37°C	Alveolar	Arterial	Mixed venous blood	Middle ear*
pO_2	150	102	93	38	40
pCO_2	0	39	39	44	50
pH_2O	47	47	47	47	47
pN_2**	563	572	575	575	623
pB	760	760	754	704	760

Pressures given in mmHg. *, average multiple measurements; **, N_2 represents nitrogen and other inner gases.
Reproduced from Dejours[1] with permission.

The gas that enters the middle ear from the nasopharynx is not atmospheric air, but has the composition of expired air, as swallowing normally occurs after an individual has breathed out when the nasopharynx is full of oxygen-depleted and carbon dioxide rich gas ($pO_2 = 99$; $pCO_2 = 36$; $pN_2 = 578$; $pH_2O = 47$ mmHg).

With a relatively high pN_2 in the middle ear nitrogen is driven into the blood, albeit slowly, so that the middle ear pressure drops a little until a new aliquot of gas is admitted via the Eustachian tube, thereby maintaining an overall pressure equivalent to atmospheric.

Should the middle ear, for whatever reason, have a ventilation rate lower than the rate of gas loss, then the total middle ear pressure will decrease. Negative middle ear pressure and the factors that cause it are the basis of much middle ear pathology.

Gas transfer from the nasopharynx into the middle ear

Not enough is known about the qualitative and quantitive physiological variables that govern gas transfer from the nasopharynx through the Eustachian tube into the middle ear. These are important if we wish to identify and compare ventilation in healthy and diseased ears. The equivalent of ventilation in the lung (tidal volume × respiratory rate) for the middle ear is the ventilation volume multiplied by the number of gas admissions per unit of time. The human Eustachian tube is 3–4 cm long and can be thought of as two cone-like structures fused together by a narrow ring, the isthmus (Fig 24.1 and Plate section).

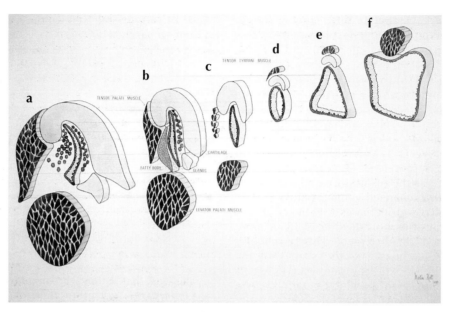

Fig 24.1 Six different regions of the Eustachian tube. The 'bellows' region is made of three parts, all of which are related to the palatal musculature. The post-isthmus has the tensor tympani running along its roof in a separate canal.

(a) Pharyngeal
(b) Midportion – pre-isthmus
(c) Isthmus – which is the joining link with
the non-collapsible part of the Eustachian tube

(d) Post-isthmus
(e) Midportion – post-isthmus
(f) Mesotympanic

The medial cone-like structure that joins the nasopharynx is collapsible and, indeed, is collapsed most of the time. This section can be thought of as the 'Eustachian tube bellows'. The lateral cone that joins the middle ear is bony and rigid and is an extension of the middle ear itself. The 'bellows' and the lateral cone meet at the isthmus, which is a 1–2 mm long segment of about 0.6–1.2 mm diameter. The bellows are actively opened by the tensor palati muscle during swallowing, yawning or movements of the jaw. The bellows open for nearly 0.2 seconds once every 1–2 minutes, that is for a total of about 3–4 minutes per 24 hours – a rather short time. In general, gas flows from one place to another in accordance with the total pressure difference existing between the two places. This is in contrast to the diffusion of individual gases within a mixture, which move according to partial pressure differences between one place and another. When passing through the Eustachian tube, gas flow is hampered by the isthmus. The Eustachian tube is therefore not so much a tube as a bellows at the end of which is the narrow isthmus. Once gas passes the isthmus it is in the middle ear. The structure of the Eustachian tube is such that, normally, the mucociliary clearance and ventilation functions do not interfere with one another. Mucus streams along the floor of the tube and, indeed, only the floor is paved with ciliated cells. Air flows above it, provided the Eustachian tube is not blocked with mucus. The amount of gas that will pass through the isthmus is a function of the pressure difference between the nasopharynx and the middle ear, the time the isthmus is opened and the length and diameter of the isthmus. Elner[2] estimated that under physiological and steady state conditions, about 1–2 ml gas enter the middle ear every 24 hours. This amount equals the net amount of gas lost per day by diffusion from the middle ear cleft through the mucosa into the blood.

Although pressure fluctuations in the nasopharynx exist when we breathe, only insignificant pressure fluctuations occur when we swallow, which is the period when the Eustachian tube opens. Thus, at a physiological steady state the main, if not the only, pressure difference between the Eustachian tube and the nasopharynx results from regular gas loss from the middle ear into the circulation. Thus, if we lose 1–2 ml gas per day into the circulation and swallow about 1000 times per day, about 1–2 µl should be expected to be lost by diffusion every 1–2 minutes and to be regained by swallowing.

The negative pressure difference created between the middle ear and the nasopharynx by the loss of 1–2 μl per 1–2 minutes depends on the size of the middle ear cavity, which in turn depends on the volume of the mastoid cavity. In a normal cellular mastoid, which has been estimated to have an average volume of about 12 ml, the negative pressure difference developed when 1–2 μl gas are lost is about 1–2 mmH$_2$O. This pressure difference is so small that it is questionable whether gas can pass passively through the 1 mm diameter opening of the 1–2 mm long isthmus during 0.2 seconds. The volume of the narrow hole that constitutes the isthmus is also about 1–3 μl. Consideration should therefore be given to the possibility that air normally passes through the Eustachian tube not passively down a pressure gradient, but by some active mechanism.

When the tensor palati contracts during swallowing or yawning it opens the collapsed bellows. In turn, the opening of the bellows creates a new volume with a lower pressure than that found in the nasopharynx or in the middle ear. Air will now stream into this newly created volume, most probably from the nasopharynx as the resistance to flow is less than at the isthmus. The second phase is the passage of air from the bellows through the isthmus. This may happen by return of the bellows to its collapsed and natural position, possibly aided by the contraction of the levator palati muscle. This muscle is larger than the tensor and lies along the floor of the Eustachian tube. It contracts for twice as long as the tensor does, that is, 0.45 seconds and its precise role has not yet been completely established.

The above explanation of an active process pumping gas into the middle ear becomes relevant when we remember that a considerable number of atelectatic ears appear at times with a bulging, hyperinflated tympanic membrane (Fig 24.2). Bulging indicates a total middle ear pressure higher than atmospheric. This can be explained either by a high concentration of CO$_2$ in the middle ear circulation or by gas being actively introduced into the middle ear through the Eustachian tube with a positive pressure.

Gas diffusion between the middle ear and the circulation

The middle ear lumen is separated from the blood by the middle ear epithelium, the lining of the blood vessels and some connective tissue between them. Gas diffuses passively from the blood vessels into the middle ear and vice versa, according to the difference of partial pressures of the individual gases in question. The gaseous steady state may change by

- an increase or decrease of the thickness of the middle ear lining, which correspondingly decreases or increases gas exchange at a given partial pressure difference
- an alteration in the blood flow (perfusion)
- a change in the permeability of the blood vessels

In general, increased perfusion rates may change the rate of gas supply or elimination from the system and thus may influence gas levels by 'washing out' nitrogen or promoting carbon dioxide diffusion into the middle ear. Decreased perfusion will halt gas diffusion whereas increased perfusion will accelerate it. Other factors that may influence the steady state are partial gas pressure changes in the blood such as those associated with sleeping, exercise or variations in altitude.

The mechanisms that regulate and keep the middle ear pressure in a near equilibrium are so far unknown. The question as to how such an equilibrium is disturbed in the 'chronic ear syndrome' is

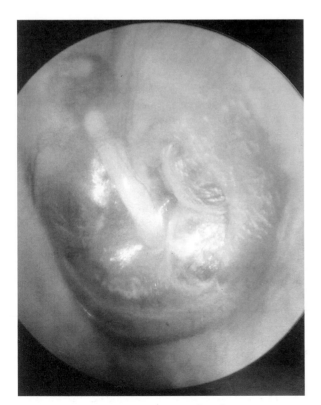

Fig 24.2 Anti-atelectasis. A hyperinflated tympanic membrane indicates a situation in which the pressure in the middle ear is higher than that of the atmosphere.

equally difficult to answer and awaits further research. Some of the information regarding this critical question is discussed in the rest of this chapter.

Changes in the physiological steady state – gas loss in the middle ear

Patients with chronic secretory otitis media, chronic suppurative otitis media, atelectatic tympanic membranes, retraction pockets and retraction pocket cholesteatomas may all be viewed as belonging to one family: the 'chronic ear syndrome'. All such patients will have had a lower than atmospheric pressure in their middle ears at some time. This negative pressure is considered important in the pathogenesis of the 'chronic ear syndrome'. Patients with acute suppurative otitis media and acute secretory otitis media may also have had a gas

deficiency in their middle ears. These two conditions, however, are a group apart as they are primarily inflammatory or infectious conditions. The classic example of the chronic ear syndrome is the ateletactic drum, which is typically retracted towards the promontory (Fig 24.3) and which can serve as a model for the study and understanding of the pathogenesis.

When a small hole is made through a retracted tympanic membrane, the latter usually returns to its physiological level, sometimes within minutes. This indicates that the tympanic membrane was retracted because of a low middle ear pressure. Once there is a passage for gas flow through the tympanic membrane, the pressure in the middle ear becomes atmospheric. An important question is: 'What mechanism is responsible for there being fewer gas molecules in the middle ear and what are the pathological conditions that lead to the atelectatic state?' It is interesting to note that atelectatic ears, besides classically manifesting as indrawn tympanic membranes, have several puzzling characteristics.

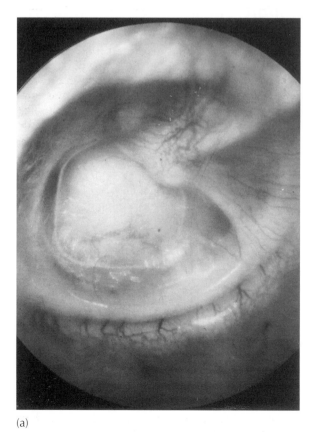

(a)

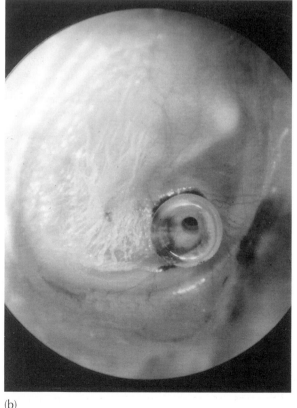

(b)

Fig 24.3 (a) Atelectasis grade III: the tympanic membrane is retracted and touching the promontory. (b) The same ear 1 hour after the insertion of a ventilation tube.

- An atelectatic ear usually persists in the same position for weeks, months or years as it has acquired a stable state.
- This new steady state is most often somewhere between the physiological state and total retraction. Only in a minority of ears is all gas lost from the middle ear.
- Atelectatic ears may recover and return to their normal position spontaneously.
- Atelectatic ears may change in the other direction and reach a new steady state, with a gradual step-wise progression towards a retraction pocket or retraction pocket cholesteatoma.
- A tympanic membrane that has at one time been indrawn and atelectatic may subsequently appear ballooned out, that is, anti-atelectatic. This denotes a higher middle ear pressure than that in the atmosphere.

There are several theories that have been suggested in an attempt to explain gas deficiency in the middle ear: ventilation deficiency – Eustachian tube dysfunction; sniffing and increased airflow through the nasopharynx; and diffusion defects.

VENTILATION DEFICIENCY

The most popular explanation for a lower middle ear gas pressure is that there is a relatively low supply of gas through the Eustachian tube. Inborn or acquired obstruction, or narrowing of the lumen of the Eustachian tube, or obstruction of the opening of the Eustachian tube by adenoids has often been suggested. This is one example where theory, repeatedly stated, finally becomes accepted as fact without the supposed evidence ever being carefully examined. Over 30 experiments involving obstruction of the Eustachian tube have been reported. Most resulted in some sort of acute otitis media. Although these experiments were often considered an adequate explanation for Eustachian tube obstruction being the cause of ventilation deficiency, the pathological results never even remotely resembled any of the forms of otitis media that are encountered clinically. Furthermore, practically all patients with atelectasis can have air passed through their Eustachian tubes by direct cannulation. As for the obstructing adenoids, these are hardly ever found in patients with the 'chronic ear syndrome'. Most patients are adults at an age when the adenoids have already atrophied. Furthermore, serial sections of temporal bones cut along the line of the Eustachian tube in specimens from patients with various types of secretory or suppurative otitis media showed no obstruction or narrowing of the lumen of the Eustachian tube (Fig 24.4).

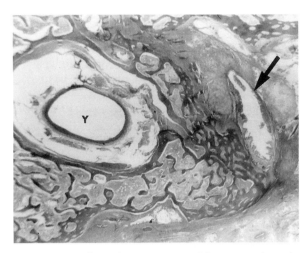

Fig 24.4 Histological cross-section of the petrous bone in the region of the isthmus of the Eustachian tube from a patient with atelectasis. Note that the lumen of the isthmus, which is marked by the arrow, is not obstructed. The carotid canal is marked with a Y.

As in the case of chronic secretory otitis media, so also in other chronic ear disorders, meticulous fibreoptic inspection of the Eustachian tube has failed to show any obstruction or narrowing of the lumen.

After the Eustachian tube obstruction theory was given up by some, but not all, a hypothesis suggesting a functional disorder was proposed. The Eustachian tube muscles were considered to be inadequate thus causing a condition in which the presence of a negative middle ear pressure along with the positive atmospheric pressure blocked the opening of the tube and the ventilation of the middle ear. Great effort went into various tests to try to support this theory. Patients were examined in pressurized chambers in high positive or negative pressures and were then asked to equilibrate these artificially induced pressures. The pressures used in these tests were of the order of several hundred mmH_2O. Measures of the ease with which the individuals were able to equilibrate their pressures were used to decide whether they had sufficient or insufficient 'tubal function'. Of course under normal physiological conditions no such major pressure differences between the middle ear and the atmosphere occur. The pressure difference between the middle ear and the nasopharynx is, at most, a few mmH_2O and the negative middle ear pressure in atelectatic conditions is also small. Furthermore, people with 'chronic ear syndrome' do not suffer more than the average person does from barotrauma and those who usually suffer from barotrauma usually do not have any chronic ear disease. The so-called Eustachian tube function tests do not seem to simulate realistic conditions, nor do they explain the differences between a middle ear with or without an atelectatic tympanic membrane.

One of the main incentives for a search for a test of Eustachian tube function has been to predict the outcome of middle ear surgery, especially grafting tympanic membranes. It was assumed that failure of tympanoplasty was due to insufficient aeration of the ears and it was hoped that a reliable test would identify the 'bad cases' preoperatively. A comparison of the postoperative behaviour of such ears showed no difference between those that failed the test and those that did not.[3]

Deficient ventilation with a steady loss of gas through diffusion should, sooner or later, result in zero gas in the middle ear cleft because of retraction of the tympanic membrane in response to the pressure difference across it. What is found is somewhat different. Most atelectatic ears present in a new steady state condition as if the ear 'requires' a lower pressure of only a few mmH$_2$O to stay for weeks, months or years without further progression. This is possibly because the reduced pressure also reduces the pN$_2$ in the middle ear and this, in turn, reduces the rate of nitrogen diffusion to the blood to a degree that now matches the ventilation. It is also possible that the residual elasticity of the tympanic membrane is sufficient to counteract the pressure gradient. Furthermore, it is very difficult to accept that the 'deficient ventilation' theory is the whole explanation of the atelectatic syndrome when one observes the clinical characteristics described earlier.

THE SNIFF THEORY

The observation that the Eustachian tube is not obstructed in patients with chronic ear syndrome has led to an opposite explanation for a deficit in the middle ear gases. It has been postulated that the Eustachian tube in diseased ears is more 'open' than in the physiological state. Magnuson[4] thought that the atelectatic condition was a result of middle ear gases being 'sucked out' along the Eustachian tube by the patients themselves, who were believed to sniff compulsively. As airflow through a channel increases, the pressure at right angles to that flow decreases. This, when expressed mathematically, is Bernouilli's theorem and the practical expression is the Venturi effect, which is used during anaesthesia for laryngoscopy and bronchoscopy in the form of jet ventilation. Sniffing may indeed lower the nasopharyngeal pressure and, in the presence of an

excessively open (patulous) Eustachian tube, this may induce the sucking out of gas from the middle ear. Although there is no doubt that some chronic ear patients have patulous tubes, and that some are compulsive sniffers, most are not, and it is not known what percentage of the healthy population are sniffers. (*Editors commentary*: this theory would explain the role of enlarged adenoids in the causation of secretory otitis media. As the volume of the nasopharynx decreases with increasing adenoid size, airflow speeds up during inspiration, thus the Eustachian tubes, which lie obliquely to the direction of airflow, are exposed to a greater negative pressure in children with enlarged adenoids than in those with small ones.)

In an attempt to establish whether sniffing is associated with a deficit in the middle ear gases, an experiment was performed in which various gases were blown through the Eustachian tube with a Politzer bag into atelectatic ears.[5] It is well known that politzerization abolishes atelectasis for only a limited period as the tympanic membrane retracts again quite quickly. This is because these ears quickly eliminate the excess gas.

It was theorized that if these atelectatic middle ears arise from sniffing, then the excess gas in the middle ear would be sniffed out and the atelectasis would return to its original position at time intervals that would be the same for each of the different gases used. However, the experiment showed that the atelectatic middle ears that were hyperinflated with different gases returned to their previous state after a period of time that was proportional to the diffusion coefficient of each specific gas. Thus, an ear ballooned with carbon dioxide by politzerization returned to its atelectatic condition after an average of 6 minutes, whereas those ballooned with nitrogen took 2 hours. This ratio of 1 : 20 is close to the ratio of the permeabilities of the two gases in water and thus in tissue. This experiment throws doubt on the sniffing theory as a key pathogenic explanation for the atelectatic tympanic membrane and indicates the important role that the diffusion process may play in the regulation of middle ear pressure.

EXCESS DIFFUSION

A third possibility that might explain the origin of the middle ear gas deficiency is an increased loss of gas through excessive diffusion into the surrounding tissues and blood despite steady state ventilation through the Eustachian tube. As we have already seen, oxygen, carbon dioxide and water have about the same partial pressure in the middle ear as in the surrounding tissues of venous blood, and have little drive, therefore, to diffuse from one of these compartments to the other. An exception is at night, when the carbon dioxide increases in blood and the oxygen decreases. However, nitrogen always has a higher pressure in the middle ear and, therefore, steadily diffuses into the tissues and circulation only to be replenished by ventilation through the Eustachian tube. Under inflammatory conditions, when the vascularity of mucosa increases many times, perfusion increases and nitrogen clearance into the blood may exceed the normal rate. This may result in an increased loss of nitrogen without a concomitant increase in the supply of nitrogen through the Eustachian tube. Consequently, a negative middle ear pressure can result. To increase the nitrogen supply through an increased swallowing rate is virtually impossible. Although the amount of gas entering the middle ear each time the Eustachian tube is opened may increase because of the increased pressure difference between the middle ear and the nasopharynx, in reality the pressure differences in chronic ears remain small because it is the volume and not the pressure that is reduced as the tympanic membrane becomes atelectatic. This effect means that the pressure gradient may be of little help in increasing ventilation.

The following experiment was performed to elucidate the possible role of increased nitrogen loss through increased perfusion in humans whose eardrums were perforated. The external canal of the relevant ear was sealed thereby converting the middle and external ear into one gas pocket. A mass spectrometer probe was inserted through the seal into the external ear canal (Fig 24.5). The experiment lasted 1–2 hours.

Initially gas measurement showed pCO_2, pO_2 and pN_2 to be quite similar to those of air. After a while pCO_2 increased and pO_2 decreased until both

reached normal middle ear values. The rate at which pCO_2 reached normal values was found to be seven times faster in ears with inflamed mucosa than in dry ears. The fast equilibration of carbon dioxide in ears with inflamed mucosa is attributed to an increase in mucosal perfusion and therefore to a higher gas diffusion rate. The same effect of increased perfusion might also apply to nitrogen moving in the opposite direction. The consequence may be a net deficit of middle ear pressure that cannot be replaced by ventilation along the Eustachian tube. Further support for a diffusional process playing some role in excessive gas loss from the middle ear was found when radioactive xenon was inflated through the Eustachian tube into the middle ear and was seen to diffuse out faster from inflamed ears than from dry ears.

The process of excessive gas diffusion may have a cumulative effect on nitrogen loss and this may well play a role in the riddle we are trying to solve. It does not provide the complete solution by itself and we are still missing at least one factor.

In any steady state, ventilation is balanced by a loss of gas and therefore what we should be focusing on is what happens as a result of a transition from the period during which an atmospheric pressure dominates the middle ear to that when a negative pressure applies.

The mastoid as a physiological buffer for the middle ear

The effect of a gas balance deficit in respect of the total pressure of an air pocket such as the middle ear depends on the amount lost in relation to the initial size of the gas pocket. Although the human middle ear proper gas volume is about 0.5 ml, the volume of the entire middle ear cleft differs greatly among individuals as it includes mastoid cavities of variable volume. The mastoid pneumatic system varies from about 1 ml to 30 ml. Therefore, a given gas deficit (or excess) will manifest itself differently in well pneumatized and in poorly pneumatized mastoids. A 20 µl volume change will result in a 100 mmH$_2$O pressure change in a 2 ml middle ear cleft, but will exert only a 10 mmH$_2$O pressure change in a 20 ml middle ear cleft. This pressure difference may be pathological in the small volume middle ear but non-significant in the other. It is not surprising, therefore, that most ears afflicted with the 'chronic ear syndrome' have a hypopneumatized, acellular or sclerotic mastoid. Ears with well pneumatized mastoids rarely exhibit any of the 'chronic otitis media' conditions and probably

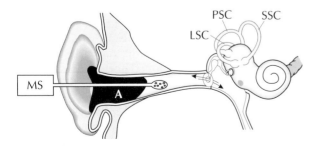

Fig 24.5 Schematic drawing of an ear in which the ear canal is plugged at A. Through the plug a probe is connected to a mass spectrometer (MS) and protrudes into the deep ear canal. The external ear canal and the middle ear now form, in effect, a single gas pocket.

rarely develop a negative middle ear pressure. The explanation for the protective effect of an adequately pneumatized mastoid is quite simple: its volume serves as a pressure buffer.

Hellstrom and Stenfors[6] showed that when pressure was exerted in the bulla of rats the pars flaccida retracted or ballooned to a degree that was proportional to the pressure exerted in the bulla. The correlation between the size of the mastoid pneumatization and middle ear pressure was also nicely demonstrated when our detailed observations showed that well pneumatized mastoids are associated with a pars flaccida that is not usually retracted, whereas a retracted pars flaccida was usually associated with a sclerotic mastoid.[7] This suggested the association of a non-pneumatized mastoid system with a negative middle ear pressure.

The effect of mastoid pneumatization on middle ear total pressure changes has also been demonstrated during anaesthesia with nitrous oxide.[8] This gas diffuses quickly into the middle ear, and it is found that the pressure in human middle ears increases more rapidly and attains higher values in those with small mastoids than in those with large ones. The observation shows that extensive pneumatization could buffer pressure changes, whereas small mastoid air volumes could not.

Mastoid cavities develop only after birth and grow almost to reach their adult size by the age of 5 years. Their final size is achieved when the skeleton matures, that is, between 15 and 20 years of age. Infants who lack adequate mastoid pneumatization do seem to suffer from acute suppurative otitis media and chronic secretory otitis media much more frequently than adults, although as the mastoid volume increases they 'grow out' of this problem. The reason some children suffer for a longer time than others probably depends on a slow rate of the development of the air-cell system. Ears with recurrent acute suppurative otitis media and chronic secretory otitis media can be shown radiologically to have delayed mastoid pneumatization. Histologically the primitive mesenchyme, which in development fills the middle ear and mastoid, seems to linger for longer in the mastoids of those ears with recurrent acute suppurative and secretory otitis media. In some patients mastoid pneumatization develops late and is incomplete. These individuals constitute the group most at risk of the entire chronic ear syndrome (Fig 24.6).[7]

The reasons why the mastoid matures more slowly in some individuals than others and why these individuals end up with a small volume mastoid cavity have been widely discussed. Some like Wittmaack[9] and Tos *et al.*[10] maintain that infections in childhood inhibit the growth of the mastoid cell system. This notion was based on the clinical

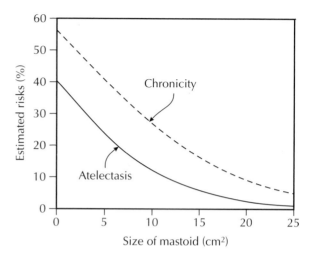

Fig 24.6 The estimated risk of developing atelectasis of the tympanic membrane is related to mastoid size and compared with the risk of chronic secretory otitis media requiring at least two ventilation tubes. Overall the frequency of chronic middle ear disease is related to mastoid area and therefore to mastoid volume.

impression that many adults with chronic ears and a sclerotic mastoid recall episodes of acute suppurative otitis media in childhood.

Diamant[11] leads another school of thought that sees the Gaussian distribution of degrees of mastoid pneumatization as a normal distribution of organ size variation. He does not associate the sclerotic mastoid with previous infection. The statistical linkage of the size of the mastoid cavity in twins, especially identical twins, also lends credibility to the concept that genotype is perhaps the dominant factor in shaping the final size of the mastoid air-cell system. The genetic linkage of an especially large pneumatic system with cystic fibrosis, otosclerosis and some congenital anomalies also supports a genetic influence on the final size of mastoid pneumatization. This contention is also based on the fact that many of those who suffered from recurrent acute secretory or suppurative otitis media in childhood developed normal pneumatization even though they suffered from mastoiditis and even when this condition was severe enough to require a cortical mastoidectomy. On the other hand, there are many adults with sclerotic mastoids who never suffered from an acute otitis media in childhood. If we take into account that about 90 per cent of all children have some form of acute otitis media in infancy, we can see how problematic it is to relate childhood otitis media to sclerotic mastoids in adults.

In summary, we may view the middle ear as a poorly ventilated biological gas pocket exhibiting pressure fluctuations and with a tendency to slip into a gas deficit condition that may or may not induce a negative middle ear pressure. For this purpose about 90 per cent of the population are 'equipped' with a built-in compensating pressure buffer – the pneumatic system of the mastoid. The other 10 per cent, who have an inadequate pneumatic system, constitute the group at risk of developing negative middle ear gas pressure, although the precise mechanisms by which this occurs are not known.

The reaction of the middle ear to negative pressures

When a negative pressure develops in the middle ear, the atmospheric pressure on the outside compresses the tympanic membranes at its weakest points, which

therefore retract. The pars flaccida retracts first because of its elasticity. Its sensitivity to pressure is high and it will retract in response to even minor changes. The amount of negative pressure that is damped by retraction of the pars flaccida depends on the buffering action of the mastoid cavity. Hellstrom and Stenfors[6] found that in rats the retracted or ballooned pars flaccida may change the middle ear volume by up to 0.5 per cent in the face of a 50 mmH$_2$O pressure gradient. When the pars flaccida had retracted to its maximum, a further decrease in middle ear pressure caused the relatively non-flexible pars tensa to retract. If the pressure continues to decrease after the final retraction of the pars flaccida and pars tensa, the Eustachian tube may open when gas from the nasopharynx enters the middle ear and abolishes the negative pressure. This is what happens during aircraft descent, but if equilibration does not occur and the negative pressure continues to increase then, when it reaches 50–90 mmH$_2$O, a transudate from the blood vessels lying in the middle ear fills the cavity. This transudate by itself diminishes the middle

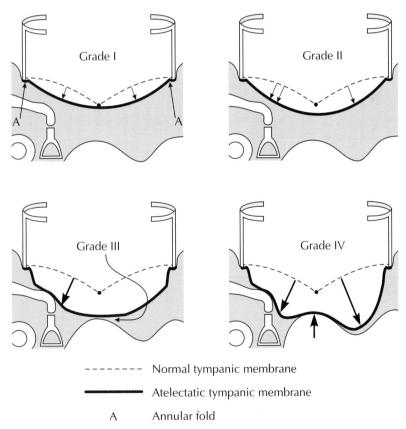

------- Normal tympanic membrane

—— Atelectatic tympanic membrane

A   Annular fold

Fig 24.7 The various atelectatic grades of the pars tensa. Grade I: a slight retraction of the tympanic membrane over the annulus. Grade II: the tympanic membrane touches the long process of the incus. Grade III: the tympanic membrane touches the promontory. Grade IV: the tympanic membrane is adherent to the promontory.

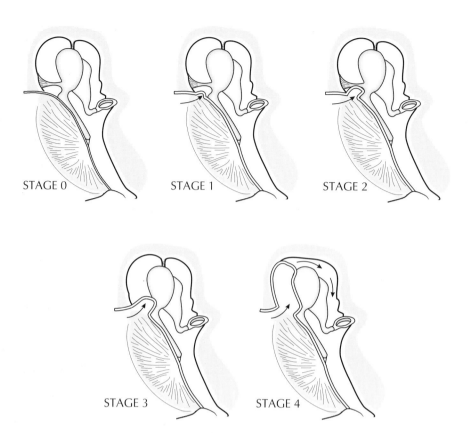

Fig 24.8 The various atelectatic grades of the pars flaccida. Stage 0: normal. Stage 1: a slight dimple. Stage 2: Shrapnell's membrane (i.e. the pars flaccida) is retracted maximally and is draped over the neck of the malleus. Stage 3: as stage 2, but with erosion of the outer attic wall (the scutum). Stage 4: the retraction is now deep and accumulated keratin cannot be reached by suction clearance. This last stage is a full-blown attic retraction pocket.

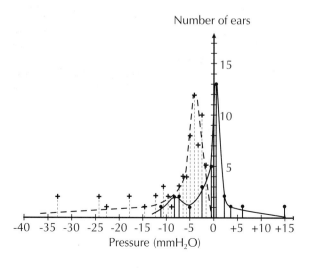

Fig 24.9 Middle ear pressures, that is, the difference from atmospheric pressure, in secretory otitis media as measured by Sadé *et al.*[13] (indicated by the dark line) and by Buckingham and Ferrer[12] (indicated by the broken line). Although not shown here, similar measurements in atelectatic ears gave similar results, that is, the middle ear pressures were not negative and hovered around atmospheric, although there was a short tail of the distribution into the slightly negative pressure regions.

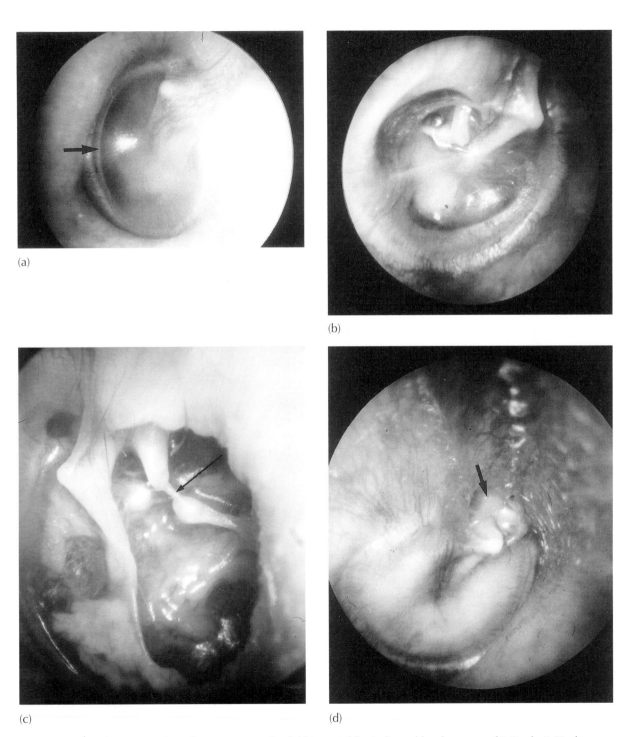

Fig 24.10 (a) Atelectasis grade I: there is an annular fold just visible, indicated by the arrow. (b) Grade II–III: the tympanic membrane is retracted onto the long process of the incus and almost touches the promontory. (c) Grade IV atelectasis of the posterior portion of the tympanic membrane. Note how the long process of the incus has been replaced by a narrow fibrous band. (d) Retraction of the pars flaccida over the neck of the malleus as indicated by the arrow; this is stage 2.

ear volume and prevents a further decrease in its pressure. These changes constitute barotrauma.

In humans the volume displaced by total retraction of the pars flaccida is about 0.05 ml. Total retraction will therefore damp pressure differences of about 50 mmH$_2$O in a small middle ear cleft whose entire volume is 1 ml. In a normal middle ear cleft of about 10 ml only 5 mmH$_2$O will be compensated by a total retraction of the pars flaccida. It seems likely that regular physiological pressure fluctuations are of the order of 5 mmH$_2$O, and that such small pressure changes are readily equalized by retraction of the pars flaccida. If negative pressure persists, then the more rigid tympanic membrane starts to retract. This compensating mechanism may not neutralize the entire negative pressure, but usually keeps it a few mmH$_2$O below atmospheric, as has been measured by Buckingham and Ferrer[12] and Sadé *et al.*[13] If further gas depletion continues there are several possible consequences. Damage to the collagenous skeleton of the pars tensa will convert it to an elastic membrane with properties similar to the pars flaccida. The new structure of the pars tensa will allow for further retraction and deep atelectatic pockets. It is the ear with the sclerotic mastoid that normally succumbs to consistent negative pressures.

The classification of atelectasis and retraction for the pars tensa and pars flaccida is given in Figures 24.7 and 24.8, respectively.

The volume of the middle ear may be reduced by swelling of the mucosa or engorgement of the blood vessels. Middle ear gas volume is also reduced by 'flooding' the middle ear space by an effusion. This is usually seen in acute and chronic secretory otitis media, but also in 20 per cent of atelectatic middle ears. Under these conditions the middle ear cavity can be partly or even entirely filled with an effusion, leaving little or no gas pocket free to develop a negative pressure. Indeed, at times so much exudate is formed that the pressure becomes positive – as seen when the exudate spills out through the edge of a myringotomy.

Thus, although atelectatic ears and those with a secretory otitis media may develop significant negative pressure during their formation, reduction of the middle ear volume in one way or another leaves a pressure that is only a few mmH$_2$O below (or above) that of the atmosphere (Fig 24.9).

The middle ear exudate in acute and chronic secretory otitis media can be viewed as a mechanism protecting the tympanic membrane from prolonged negative pressure. The price of this protection is a relatively small conductive hearing loss.

A prolonged and uncompensated negative pressure can damage middle ear structures. Changes in the collagenous layer of the tympanic membrane have been mentioned already, but the ossicular chain, especially the long process of the incus, can also disintegrate (Fig 24.10).

The mucociliary clearance system

The middle ear and the Eustachian tube are lined by a mucociliary system, as found elsewhere in the respiratory tract (Fig 24.11). A thin mucoglycoprotein layer is excreted by the mucosal cells and lies on top of the cilia that beat continuously and convey it and any debris from the middle ear through the Eustachian tube and into the nasopharynx. In spite of the system, micro-organisms may still reach the middle ear from the nasopharynx through the Eustachian tube in a way that still

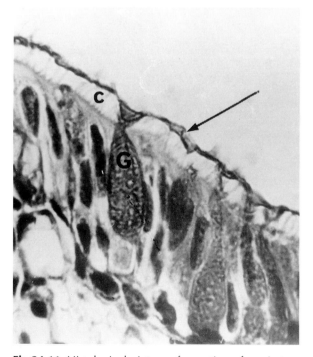

Fig 24.11 Histological picture of a section of respiratory mucosa as usually present in the anteroinferior part of the middle ear. Note the cilia (C) that project from the upper edge of the epithelium. A mucus-synthesizing cell, i.e. a goblet cell (G), is producing mucus, which spreads like a blanket (arrow) over the ciliary carpet.

awaits study. The reaction that ensues leads to the formation of an inflammatory exudate and usually causes the goblet cells to synthesize more mucus than usual.

Long-standing inflammation results in a proliferation of goblet cells and the formation of mucus glands and mucus cysts. Some of these are found in otherwise healthy ears, as most ears have been inflamed at one time or another. The metaplastic changes that bring about an increase in mucus secretion may result in the entire middle ear being filled with mucus. Why large amounts of mucus are not cleared swiftly from the middle ear by ciliary action has been an intriguing question for some while, especially as ciliated cells are rather sturdy. It was initially thought that the failure to clear the mucus was secondary to an obstruction of the Eustachian tube opening by enlarged adenoids. This seemed logical as large adenoids are frequently found in children with chronic secretory otitis media and their removal seemed to help the resolution of the condition. An alternative explanation was that the Eustachian tube lumen itself was either narrow or affected by an inflammatory oedema.

The obstructive role of the adenoids has been questioned as many patients continue to have a chronic secretory otitis media despite adenoidectomy. Furthermore, many children with large adenoids have no problems. In other children the space-occupying lesions in the nasopharynx, such as choanal polyps or juvenile angiofibromata, rarely exhibit chronic secretory otitis media. More recently histological and direct fibreoptic examinations of the Eustachian tube lumen have shown that the tube is neither narrower nor obstructed in children with chronic secretory otitis media. The only finding was that the lumen was filled with mucus.[5]

The mechanism of the process of the failure to clear mucus was demonstrated experimentally by Hilding[14] who filled the isolated hen's trachea with mucus. One end of the trachea was left free, whereas the other was plugged and a manometer inserted through the plug (Fig 24.12). Mucus was observed to start streaming along the trachea only to slow down within a short time, and finally to stop despite continued ciliary action. At this stage the manometer showed that a negative pressure difference of up to $50\,mmH_2O$ existed in the trachea between the mucus and the manometer. It was this pressure that balanced the force of ciliary action and stopped the mucus from being propelled. Hilding then made a small hole in the pipe leading from the manometer to the trachea, which promptly relieved the negative pressure and allowed the mucus to flow again.

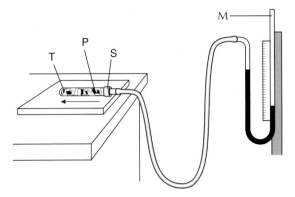

Fig 24.12 Hilding's experiment. T, Trachea; P, Mucus in trachea; S, Stop cork; M, Manometer.

Hilding's experiment (which was done in the basement of his home) may be regarded as analogous to what happens in secretory otitis media. Once the Eustachian tube is plugged with mucus, a negative pressure develops in the middle ear and the mucus becomes stagnant despite ciliary action. The negative pressure in the middle ear may increase further by loss of gas from the middle ear cavity, which is not replenished by gas from the Eustachian tube blocked by mucus. The problem then is not a primary obstruction of the Eustachian tube causing the middle ear effusion nor a 'hydrops ex vacuo' mechanism, but a secondary obstruction of the Eustachian tube by a mucus plug that is formed primarily by a middle ear inflammatory process and held in place by the negative pressure. The stagnation of the mucus in the Eustachian tube cannot be overcome unless the negative middle ear pressure is relieved. When a small hole is made in the eardrum by the introduction of a ventilation tube, then the pressure in the middle ear equalizes with that of the atmosphere and the mucus can now be propelled by ciliary action into the nasopharynx (Fig 24.13). Note that in the above situation there are two sources of the pressure difference across the tympanic membrane: the ciliary action on the mucus plug and the gas loss from its lumen.

Defects of the cilia are hardly ever responsible for deficient mucus clearance, the exception being the rare Kartagene syndrome in which the cilia are defective from birth. The production of an effusion in the middle ear can be traced in some 70 per cent of patients to an upper respiratory tract infection. The rest may possibly be a reaction of the middle ear mucosal cells to a negative pressure of unknown origin. This second form of response seems particularly marked in children.

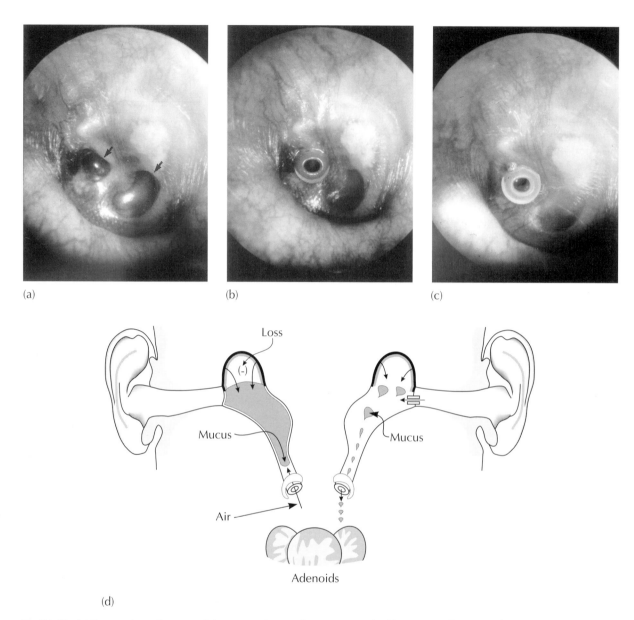

(a)   (b)   (c)

(d)

Fig 24.13 (a) Two atelectatic areas of the tympanic membrane are marked by arrows. (b) A ventilation tube was inserted under local anaesthetic and no attempt was made to aspirate the mucus. (c) The next day the tympanic membrane has returned to its neutral position and all the mucus has drained down the Eustachian tube. (d) Diagram showing the right middle ear filled with mucus, which is blocking the Eustachian tube. The action of the cilia induces a negative middle ear pressure as the mucus is moved en bloc along the tube. The left middle ear has a ventilation tube inserted and as the negative pressure is relieved the ciliary action is able to move the mucus into the nasopharynx.

Conclusion

The normal middle ear has an inherent tendency to lose gas by diffusion into the surrounding tissues and circulation. This loss is compensated by the Eustachian tube, which admits just enough gas to maintain the middle ear gas pressure at close to atmospheric. When this system fails to function properly, a negative gas pressure develops in the middle ear. The reasons for failure of the system and its slipping into a state of undecompensated negative middle ear pressure are not entirely clear. There seems to be as yet no evidence for the conventional explanation of Eustachian tube dysfunction as the sole cause of the problem. Some evidence does exist that the middle ear gas deficit may involve excessive net gas loss through increased gas diffusion into the surrounding middle ear circulation. The total pressure in the middle ear may fluctuate dynamically between atmospheric, negative and positive values, suggesting the involvement of undiscovered factors in the pathogenesis. When middle ear gas balance is disturbed, the negative pressure that results is usually successfully buffered by the pneumatized mastoid system. In individuals with a sclerotic mastoid this buffering effect may be ineffective and a long-term negative middle ear pressure may ensue. When a negative pressure is established, the middle ear responds by a reduction of gas volume to equalize the pressure. This response may take the form of tympanic membrane retraction, swelling of the mucosa or 'flooding' the middle ear space with an effusion.

A middle ear effusion, however, is most commonly the result of an upper respiratory tract infection, which provokes the production of an inflammatory exudate.

Our present knowledge is such that in most patients we can deal surgically with the results of negative middle ear pressure by inserting a ventilation tube, but cannot prevent or change the reasons for such a condition developing.

Discussion of the Eustachian tube would be incomplete without mention of three further topics that, although not related directly to the 'chronic ear syndrome', nevertheless have features about them that are of relevance.

The patulous Eustachian tube

Whereas the Eustachian tube bellows are usually collapsed and only open on swallowing or yawning, some people have a Eustachian tube whose bellows seem permanently open. This condition is termed a patulous Eustachian tube. A patulous tube can be diagnosed by sonotubometry, a method by which sound is made at the nostril and detected in the ear canal. When the Eustachian tube is open the sound is louder than when it is closed. This method, which has been used to study the duration and frequency of the opening of the Eustachian tube, may also demonstrate that the tube is permanently open. A patulous Eustachian tube can also be diagnosed by using the operating microscope to observe the tympanic membrane during respiration. Movement is more easily seen when the tympanic membrane has undergone an atrophic change and when it is thinner and some-

times wrinkled compared with the normal tympanic membrane. When patients with patulous Eustachian tubes are asked to swallow with their noses pinched, that is, to perform a Toynbee manoeuvre, which induces relatively high positive pressures in the nasopharynx, the drum is seen to bulge. Conversely, on sniffing, when a negative pressure is usually formed in the nasopharynx, the bulging tympanic membrane sinks back to its previous position. The percentage of people with a permanently open Eustachian tube is not known, but has been estimated to be about 0.5 per cent of the entire population. The patulous Eustachian tube is usually accompanied by a normal tympanic membrane, although it is sometimes associated with some form of atelectasis. A patulous tube is a condition that is usually asymptomatic, although a minority feel their voice creeping through the Eustachian tube to be heard in the ear. This is autophony. It may occasionally be accompanied by various bizarre symptoms that are described by the patients as blocked ears, but which do not show any corresponding audiological abnormalities and usually show no tympanometric changes. Those with autophony may be deeply distressed by the symptoms or the feeling of some unusual middle ear pressure or blockage. Unfortunately, no satisfactory treatment has been described for those who do suffer from such symptoms; insertion of a ventilation tube rarely helps and much more frequently makes the patient feel even worse.

One of the most interesting aspects of the patulous Eustachian tube is related to the occasional patient who has a patulous Eustachian tube and an atelectatic tympanic membrane or even a cholesteatoma. There is no simple explanation of the mechanism that will produce both a negative pressure, causing retraction, and a patulous tube, which is supposed to be accompanied by hyperventilation of the middle ear. It is just possible that a Bernouilli effect, as described earlier, is depriving the middle ear of some gas on each inspiration and expiration. Magnuson[4] sees this possibility as being a major pathogenic factor in atelectatic drums and cholesteatoma. However, although some patients with atelectasis are compulsive sniffers, most are not and the experiments described earlier throw doubt on the validity of this interesting theory.

Nasopharyngeal carcinoma and the Eustachian tube

Patients suffering from nasopharyngeal carcinoma often exhibit a middle ear effusion as a first symptom. The mechanism of the effusion has usually been ascribed to poor ventilation through the Eustachian tube. At first it was assumed that the carcinoma obstructed the Eustachian tube opening, thereby preventing gas inhalation. The middle ear in the face of a continuous loss of gas by diffusion would develop a negative pressure and this would result in a 'hydrops ex vacuo' effusion, that is, a transudate from the vessels lining the middle ear. However, it became apparent that the middle ear effusion often occurred when the carcinoma was very small and could not obstruct the Eustachian tube opening. Histological studies showed that the lumen of the Eustachian tube was usually unaffected. Further histological examination revealed that these patients had carcinomatous infiltration confined to the Eustachian tube muscles deep in the skull base. Indeed, after maxillectomy or other operations in which these muscles may be damaged a middle ear effusion can appear without any nasopharyngeal pathology.[15] In these cases a ventilation tube will usually clear the fluid to the relief of the patient. A similar situation, at least from a functional point of view, was produced in monkeys by Casselbrant *et al.*[16] who injected botulinum poison into the Eustachian tube muscles of monkeys. These findings seemed to strengthen the argument that some functional but undefined disorder of the Eustachian tube muscles may be connected to the chronic ear syndrome. However, when histological sections of the Eustachian tube muscles were measured in healthy ears and compared with specimens coming from patients with chronic secretory otitis media, no difference was found.[17]

Whether the higher frequency of various forms of otitis media in patients with cleft palates is due to some innate damage to their palatal muscles, which are indeed different at the palatal level from normal, is a moot point. Although cleft palate patients are often afflicted by middle ear disease, they also belong to the population group whose mastoids mature later than normal and often stay poorly pneumatized for life.

In conclusion, we can see that a disturbance of the function of the Eustachian tube muscles possibly plays a role in the development of a middle ear effusion in nasopharyngeal carcinoma. Although the middle ear effusion associated with this is often presented as a model that can explain the mechanism for the formation of an effusion in secretory otitis media, it should be noted that the pathogenic factors are basically different. Furthermore, atelectasis hardly ever accompanies the fluid formation in cases of nasopharyngeal carcinoma.

Barotrauma

People who reach altitudes where the total gas pressure is much lower than that at sea level must reduce their middle ear pressures in order to equilibrate with the external pressure. The difference between the two sides of the Eustachian tube at high altitudes is large and even in pressurized aircraft may reach hundreds of mmH$_2$O. Under these circumstances equilibrium is usually achieved easily by gas escaping from the middle ear through the Eustachian tube to the nasopharynx because of the relatively large differences of pressure between the two.

On descent to sea level a reverse situation occurs and pressure equalization takes place by ventilation when the Eustachian tube opens periodically and gas streams from the nasopharynx into the middle ear. However, equilibration of a low middle ear pressure with an increasing atmospheric pressure (on descent) is more difficult than ventilation on an ascent because of the elastic lips of the Eustachian tube on the nasopharyngeal side of the isthmus, which may be squeezed together and closed by the relatively high nasopharyngeal pressure.

Scuba divers encounter a situation similar to descent from high altitude as they dive towards a higher pressure environment. On descent they must ventilate the middle ear by forcing air into it. This manoeuvre does not happen spontaneously or easily, and scuba divers are trained to deal with this situation. On ascending from deep water the higher than ambient middle ear pressure escapes almost spontaneously and easily via the Eustachian tube. However, occasionally during emergency ascents the middle ear pressure is not released fast enough and this results in explosive rupture of the tympanic membrane.

Most people equilibrate the differences of pressure with ease whether on descent or ascent, although some require autoinflation. When this procedure fails on aircraft descent or while diving, a negative middle ear pressure may develop and is occasionally great enough to bring about the transudation of serum or sometimes blood, from the circulation into the middle ear. The symptoms are fullness and earache. Otoscopy shows an effusion that may be haemorrhagic. A retraction of the pars flaccida and pars tensa, which denotes negative pressure, is sometimes also present. This condition is called barotrauma.

Why some people are able and others are unable to equilibrate these higher pressures is unknown. When experiments are performed on large normal cohorts as to the level of pressure they can equilibrate, the differences are large, with some individuals being able to inflate or deflate their ears with ease whereas others, who otherwise have perfectly healthy ears, cannot do so either passively or actively. No anatomical or physiological difference between the ears has been found so far to explain the susceptibility of some individuals to barotrauma.

Barotrauma has been viewed as being basically similar to the chronic ear syndrome. However, the effusion in barotrauma is a haemorrhagic transudate, whereas in the chronic ear syndrome it is practically never haemorrhagic and has the characteristics of an inflammatory exudate. Barotrauma is a situation in which a negative pressure is provoked within minutes or hours, whereas in chronic ears this develops relatively slowly.

In barotrauma the actual negative pressure in the middle ear can be expected to exceed 60–90 mmH$_2$O because it is at this level that a middle ear transudate appears. In chronic ears, the pressure difference when measured directly is found to be only a few mmH$_2$O below atmospheric.

Delayed barotrauma

Divers who use oxygen in their tanks may exhibit a delayed barotrauma. When a diver descends, their middle ear is filled mainly with oxygen. When they ascend, the oxygen will diffuse into the circulation so that the pO$_2$ falls before its place in the middle ear has been taken by 'inhaled' nitrogen. After some hours, especially after sleep, this may provoke a significant middle ear gas deficit and consequently a negative pressure severe enough to bring about the symptoms and signs of barotrauma.

References

1. Dejours P. *Principles of comparative respiratory physiology, 2nd ed.* Amsterdam: Elsevier, 1981.
2. Elner A. Normal gas change in human middle ear. *Annals of Otology, Rhinology and Laryngology* 1976; **85**:161–4.
3. Palva A, Karja J. Eustachian tube patency in chronic ears. *Acta Otolaryngologica* 1969; **(Suppl 263)**:25–8.
4. Magnuson B. Tubal closing failure in retraction type cholesteatoma and adhesive middle ear lesions. *Acta Otolaryngologica* 1978; **86**:408–17.
5. Sadé J, Luntz M. Gaseous pathways in atelectatic ears. *Annals of Otology, Rhinology and Laryngology* 1989; **99**:355–8.
6. Hellstrom S, Stenfors LE. The pressure equilibration function of the pars flaccida in the middle ear mechanism. *Acta Physiologica Scandinavica* 1983; **118**:337–41.
7. Sadé J, Fuchs C. Secretory otitis media in adults. Mastoid pneumatization as a prognostic factor. *Annals of Otology, Rhinology and Laryngology* 1997; **106**:37–40.
8. Sadé J, Fuchs C, Luntz M. The pars flaccida middle ear pressure and mastoid pneumatization index. *Acta Otolaryngologica* 1996; **116**:284–7.
9. Wittmaack K. Uber die Entstehung der Schleimhautkonstitution des mittelhors. *Acta Otolaryngologica* 1937; **25**:414–29.
10. Tos M, Stangerup SE, Hvid G. Mastoid pneumatization. *Archives of Otolaryngology* 1984; **110**:502–7.
11. Diamant M. *Chronic otitis.* New York: Karger, 1952.
12. Buckingham RA, Ferrer JL. Middle ear pressures in Eustachian tube malfunction, manometric studies. *Laryngoscope* 1973; **83**:1585–93.
13. Sadé J, Halevy A, Hadas E. Clearance of middle ear effusions and middle ear pressure. *Annals of Otology, Rhinology and Laryngology* 1976; **85(suppl 25)**:58–62.
14. Hilding AC. Role of ciliary action in production of pulmonary atelectasis vacuum in paranasal sinuses and in otitus media. *Transactions of the Academy of Ophthalmology and Otology* 1944; **July/Aug**:7–12.
15. Myers EN, Beery QC, Bluestone CD, Rood SR, Sigler BA. Effect of certain head and neck tumors and their management on the ventilatory function of the Eustachian tube. *Annals of Otology, Rhinology and Laryngology* 1984; **114**:3–16.
16. Casselbrant ML, Cantekin EI, Dirkmaat DC, Doyle WY, Bluestone CD. Experimental paralysis of tensor veli platini muscle. *Acta Otolaryngologica* 1988; **106**:178–85.
17. Sadé J, Shatz A, Luntz M, Fuchs C. Eustachian tube muscles in otitis media. *Acta Otolaryngologica* 1988; **105**:543–8.

Suggested reading

Eden AR, Gannon PJ. Neural control of middle ear aeration. *Archives of Otolaryngology – Head and Neck Surgery* 1987; **113**:133–7.

Flisberg K, Ingelstedt S, Ortegren U. On middle ear pressure. *Acta Otolaryngologica* 1963; **182**:43–56.

Hergils L, Magnuson B. Analysis of middle ear gas composition by mass spectrometer. In: Sadé J ed. *The Eustachian tube, basic aspects.* Amsterdam: Kugler and Ghenidi, 1991:295–8.

Ikarashi H, Nakamo Y. The effect of chronic middle ear inflammation on the pneumatization of the tympanic bulla in pigs. *Acta Otolaryngologica* 1987; **104**:13–7.

Maw RA. *Glue ear in childhood.* MacKeith Press and Cambridge University Press, 1995.

Richards SH, O'Neill G, Wilson F. Middle ear pressure variations during general anaesthesia. *Journal of Laryngology and Otolaryngology* 1982; **96**:883–92.

Ruah CB, Schachern PA, Zelterman D, Paparella MM, Yoon TH. Age related morphological changes in human tympanic membrane. *Archives of Otolaryngology – Head and Neck Surgery* 1991; **117**:627–34.

Sadé J. *Secretory otitis media and its sequelae.* New York: Churchill Livingstone, 1979.

Sadé J. Atelectatic tympanic membrane. *Annals of Otolology, Rhinology and Laryngology* 1993; **102**:712–6.

Sadé J. The nasopharynx Eustachian tube and otitis media. *Journal of Laryngology and Otolaryngology* 1994; **108**:95–100.

Sadé J. Pathology and pathogenesis of serous otitis media. *Archives of Otolaryngology* 1996; **84**:297–305.

Sadé J. Ciliary activity and middle ear clearance. *Archives of Otolaryngology* 1967; **86**:128–35.

Sadé J, Luntz M. The Eustachian tube lumen: a comparison between normal and inflamed specimens. *Annals of Otology, Rhinology and Laryngology* 1989; **98**:630–4.

Sadé J, Meyer FA, King M, Silberberg A. Clearance of middle ear effusions by mucociliary system. *Acta Otolaryngologica* 1975; **79**:277–82.

CHAPTER 25

Acute suppurative otitis media

PAUL B VAN CAUWENBERGE, STEFAN EG DE MOOR AND INGEBORG DHOOGE

Introduction

Acute suppurative otitis media is a very frequent diagnosis in infants and children attending a physician because of illness. Of the 120 million prescriptions written for oral antibiotics each year in the USA, more than 25 per cent are for the treatment of otitis media. More than 40 per cent of all children have three or more episodes of acute suppurative otitis media during the first 3 years of life.[1] Until the advent of antimicrobial therapy, acute suppurative otitis media and its sequelae were a major concern of physicians active in the field of otology. Nowadays, the disease is well controlled in the majority of patients and although life-threatening intracranial complications are uncommon, complications within the middle ear are still prevalent. Some patients do not respond well to medical therapy and require surgery in the prevention or management of these complications.

Definition and classification

Otitis media is an inflammation of the middle ear, without reference to aetiology or pathogenesis.
    There are many forms of otitis media concerning the aetiology, pathophysiology, clinical manifestations and duration. We use the following classification.[2,3]

MYRINGITIS

Myringitis is an inflammation of the tympanic membrane that occurs alone or in association with external otitis or suppurative otitis media.

OTITIS MEDIA WITHOUT EFFUSION

In this form of otitis media inflammation of the middle ear mucous membrane and tympanic membrane is present without effusion in the tympanum. This type of otitis is usually present in the early stages of acute suppurative otitis media or in the stage of resolution. Otoscopic examination of this disorder shows an inflammation of the tympanic membrane, with erythema or opacification, or both, but with normal mobility of the eardrum.

ACUTE SUPPURATIVE OTITIS MEDIA

Acute suppurative otitis media is an infectious disorder of the middle ear and tympanic membrane with signs and symptoms of inflammation of the tympanum. Acute suppurative otitis media is characterized by the presence of a middle ear effusion in combination with local or systemic signs, or both, such as otalgia, otorrhoea (in case of perforation of the eardrum), fever and irritability.

RECURRENT ACUTE SUPPURATIVE OTITIS MEDIA

Recurrent acute suppurative otitis media is defined as three or more acute infections of the middle ear in a 6-month period or four or more episodes in a 12-month period. In order to make this diagnosis the infection should clear between episodes.

CHRONIC SUPPURATIVE OTITIS MEDIA

Chronic suppurative otitis media (see Chapters 27 and 28) is an infection of the middle ear that lasts for more than 3 months and is accompanied by a perforation of the tympanic membrane.

SECRETORY OTITIS MEDIA

Secretory otitis media (see Chapter 26) is a middle ear disorder in which an effusion fills the middle ear cleft. By this definition the effusion can be serous or mucoid, and only rarely purulent. The effusion is usually not sterile. The duration may be acute (less than 3 weeks), subacute (3 weeks to 3 months) or chronic (more than 3 months).

Epidemiology

INCIDENCE

Acute suppurative otitis media is one of the most common infectious diseases in childhood. In a survey of the frequency of infectious diseases during the first year of life only the common cold was more frequent.[4] The US Food and Drug Administration reports that approximately one-half of the courses of antibiotics prescribed for children less than 10 years of age were administered for acute suppurative otitis media in 1986.

A study by Stangerup and Tos[5] in 1986 of Danish children followed from birth to the age 9 years showed an incidence of acute suppurative otitis media of 22 per cent during the first year of life, 15 per cent in the second year, 10 per cent for the third and fourth year and only 2 per cent by the eighth year.

PREDISPOSING FACTORS

Many intrinsic and extrinsic factors have an influence on the incidence of acute suppurative otitis media.

Age

Acute suppurative otitis media is a very frequent infection in children under the age of 7 years. In newborns it is a disease that can be found as an isolated infection or associated with sepsis, meningitis and pneumonia, but it is uncommon. By the age of 6 months about 25 per cent of all children have had one or more episodes of acute suppurative otitis media. At the first birthday this figure has risen to 62 per cent, by 3 years to 81 per cent and at the age of 5 years to 91 per cent (Fig 25.1).[1] After the age of 7 years the incidence declines.

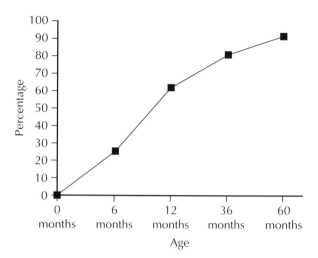

Fig 25.1 Percentage of all children who were observed with one or more episodes of acute suppurative otitis media at different ages.[1]

Several reasons account for the high incidence of acute suppurative otitis media in young children:

- the incidence of upper respiratory infections is high in young children
- the short and straight, immature Eustachian tube (in children younger than 1 year) allows more ready access of bacteria into the middle ear
- the abundant and/or chronically infected lymphoid tissue in the nasopharynx of children produces 'obstruction' of the Eustachian tube and ascending infections
- the immature immune system.

An early first acute suppurative otitis media episode may be the primary event that predisposes a child to recurrent and chronic suppurative otitis media by setting up an inflammatory process in the middle ear and Eustachian tube. Alternatively, an early attack may reflect an innate predisposition for middle ear disease, in which the early affliction is a marker for the underlying predisposing factors.

Gender

In most studies on the incidence of acute suppurative otitis media there is little difference between males and females. Teele *et al.*[1] however, reported a higher incidence in males.

Race

Few interracial studies have been done but there are some striking differences to be noted. American

Indians and Canadian Inuits have a strikingly high incidence of acute suppurative otitis media. In African and Australian aboriginal children the severity of middle ear infections has been noted. American black children seem to have fewer episodes of middle ear infections than American Caucasians. Most of these observations can probably be explained by differences in anatomy and function of the Eustachian tube.

Seasonal variations

There is a definite increase in the incidence of acute suppurative otitis media in the colder months. The peak incidence follows that of the upper respiratory tract infections.

Breastfeeding

Many studies have shown that breastfeeding has an influence on the occurrence of acute suppurative otitis media; the incidence of acute suppurative otitis media is lower in breastfed children. The effect is not as significant as it is on respiratory and gastrointestinal infections. Many hypotheses have been suggested to provide reasons for this effect: the presence of immunological and non-immunological antiviral and antibacterial factors in breast milk; allergy to cows milk or formula milk with resulting changes in the upper respiratory tract mucous membrane; difference in development of facial musculature between breastfed and bottle-fed children; difference in position between breast-feeding and bottle-feeding.

Daycare centres

Daycare is a major factor in the incidence of acute suppurative otitis media, presumably because of the increased exposure to infections. Upper airway hygiene in these children is poor and coughing, sneezing and nasal dripping contaminates the environment with bacteria and viruses.

Underlying disease

Anatomical changes (cleft palate, cleft uvula), immunological deficiencies (immunoglobulin deficiencies, AIDS, leukaemia, immunosuppressive drugs) and functional changes (barotrauma, patulous tube) have an important influence on the incidence of middle ear infections. Over 50 per cent of children with cleft palate have recurrent episodes of acute suppurative otitis media, often with subsequent complications.

The presence of adenoid hypertrophy with or without infection may be an important factor in the occurrence of recurrent attacks because of the close relationship between this lymphoid tissue with the Eustachian tube. Adenoid hypertrophy may block the tube and colonization of the adenoids with upper airway pathogens may be the main source of infection of the middle ear.[6]

Pathophysiology

Acute suppurative otitis media is essentially a self-limiting disease with a tendency towards spontaneous healing, even without therapy. Complications are, however, possible and in some patients the disease progresses towards chronicity. There are five stages and spontaneous healing can occur after any of them.[7]

STAGE OF HYPERAEMIA

The first stage of infection of the middle ear is characterized by hyperaemia of the mucous membrane of the tympanic cavity, the mastoid air cells and the Eustachian tube. The Eustachian tube becomes occluded in the narrowest portion (the isthmus), which leads to changes in the middle ear pressure. There are also changes in the mucociliary transport and changes in a surfactant-like substance in the Eustachian tube.

The changes in the tube may precede the middle ear hyperaemia. This is the case when the middle ear infection is preceded by an event that results in congestion of the respiratory mucosa throughout the (upper) respiratory tract, including the nasopharynx and auditory tube.

The pathogens (bacterial or viral) enter the middle ear via the Eustachian tube or, much less frequently, haematogenously.

STAGE OF EXUDATION

Serum, fibrin, red blood cells and polymorphonuclear leucocytes originating from the dilated capillaries of middle ear, antral and mastoid mucous membranes fill the cavity with an exudate. A part of the cuboidal epithelial cells of the middle ear change into mucus-producing goblet cells. In this stage the tympanic membrane thickens and sometimes bulges under the pressure of the exudate, which becomes mucopurulent.

STAGE OF SUPPURATION

Under the influence of toxic factors produced by bacteria and inflammatory cells, in combination with the pressure in the tympanic cavity, the tympanic membrane may perforate and drainage of the middle ear exudate appears. The perforation is small and is situated in the pars tensa of the drum.

STAGE OF COALESCENCE

Fewer than 5 per cent of all patients with acute suppurative otitis media will have persistent otorrhoea through a tympanic perforation for more than 2 weeks. In this small group progressive thickening of the middle ear mucous membranes begins to obstruct the drainage of mucopus in the epitympanum and in the smaller air cells around the antrum. The small air cells filled with pus under pressure begin to show decalcification and osteoclastic activity, leading to coalescence of these cells into larger, irregular cavities filled with pus, hypertrophic mucosa and granulation tissue.

STAGE OF COMPLICATION

When the osteoclastic erosion progresses to the bony limits of the tympanic or mastoid cavity, the bacterial infection may extend beyond the confines of the middle ear and mastoid. This may lead to the well known and sometimes life-threatening complications of acute suppurative otitis media, including periosteal mastoid abscess, extradural abscess, thrombophlebitis of the sigmoid sinus, brain abscess, petrositis, facial nerve palsy and suppurative labyrinthitis (see Chapter 29).

Microbiology

VIRUSES

Respiratory viral infections play an important role in the pathogenesis of acute suppurative otitis media. Most episodes of acute suppurative otitis media are preceded by a respiratory tract infection of viral origin. Respiratory viruses are present in 40 per cent of nasopharyngeal secretions at the time of diagnosis of acute suppurative otitis media.[8] Rhinovirus (24 per cent) and respiratory syncytial virus (13 per cent) are the most common. The prevalence of respiratory viruses may be even higher, considering the frequency of associated respiratory symptoms, but these are probably missed by the currently available virus detection tests. Respiratory syncytial virus and adenovirus are particularly involved in persistent purulent otitis.

BACTERIA

The bacterial causes of otitis media have been studied by culturing middle ear aspirates from acute suppurative otitis media. In 65–70 per cent a positive culture for bacteria is found, whereas 30–35 per cent of the aspirates show no growth. There is a remarkable consistency in the studies, which demonstrate the importance of the classic respiratory pathogen: *Streptococcus pneumoniae, Haemophilus influenzae* and *Moraxella catarrhalis*. Respective percentages of the main bacteria are represented in Figure 25.2.

Some anaerobic bacteria can be found in middle ear aspirate: *Bacteroides* species, peptococci and peptostreptococci; they are, however, uncommon and do not seem to play an important role. In young infants Gram-negative bacteria other than *H. influenzae* and *M. catarrhalis* are responsible for about 20 per cent of cases of acute suppurative otitis media, but they are rarely found in older children (in contrast to chronic suppurative otitis media in which Gram-negative species are common).

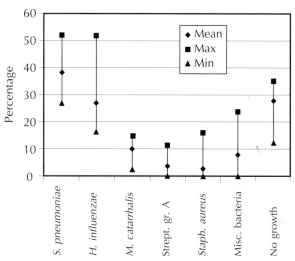

Bacterial pathogens isolated from middle ear aspirates in children with acute suppurative otitis media

Fig 25.2 Microbiology of middle ear aspirates in children with acute suppurative otitis media. Respective mean percentages and range of different bacteria are presented as they were described by Bluestone *et al.*[3]

A therapeutic problem is the important increase of antimicrobial resistance during the past 10 years. In the UK, *S. pneumoniae* shows a resistance for the following drugs: penicillin 3–8 per cent, erythromycin 7 per cent and tetracycline 8 per cent.[9,10] The resistance of *H. influenzae*, 90 per cent of which are non-typeable, for β-lactam antibiotics is steadily increasing; in the USA up to 44 per cent of cultured *H. influenzae* produce β-lactamase. In Europe more than 80 per cent of *M. catarrhalis* strains produce β-lactamase.[11]

In some patients cultures of both middle ears in bilateral acute suppurative otitis media show disparate or mixed results. This demonstrates that microbiological investigation of the middle ear should always include both ears.

In all studies on the microbiology of acute suppurative otitis media a significant portion of middle ear aspirates remains sterile. Different factors can be the cause of this finding: the causative agent is non-bacterial (viruses, chlamydia or mycoplasma); the pathogen does not grow in the classic conditions (anaerobic bacteria, mycobacterium); prior administration of antibiotics; growth suppression by immunological response of the host; a non-infectious form of disease caused by an immune response to a non-infectious agent.

Clinical manifestation

The earliest clinical manifestations of acute suppurative otitis media are related to the stage of tubal occlusion with subsequent changes in the middle ear pressure and hyperaemia of the mucous membrane. There is a sense of fullness in the ear together with some conductive hearing loss. Earache may be present but is not severe. Otoscopy shows a hyperaemic tympanic membrane that is not thickened and an aerated middle ear if there is no pre-existing secretory otitis media (Fig 25.3 and Plate section).

In the exudative stage the middle ear becomes filled with an exudate under pressure. The otalgia is marked and fever is usually high in children because of resorption of toxic products of inflammation by the middle ear mucosa. In smaller children systemic symptoms of infection can be present: anorexia, vomiting and diarrhoea. The tympanic membrane becomes thickened and bulges (Fig 25.4 and Plate section). There is a noticeable conductive hearing loss.

If the infection progresses, the tympanic membrane may perforate spontaneously with abundant otorrhoea (usually haemorrhagic at first, followed by a mucopurulent discharge). The reduction of the pressure by the perforation results in a reduction of the pain. Fever also starts to recede. Otoscopy shows a small perforation in the pars tensa, just large enough to let the middle ear drain. Most frequently this is the turning point in the infectious episode and from here there is progressive normalization of the middle ear mucosa and healing of the tympanic membrane.

In about 5 per cent of the cases the middle ear does not heal and evolves towards a stage of coalescence as described above. This stage is marked by fluctuating discharge and otalgia (not so intense as in the stage of exudation), low-grade fever,

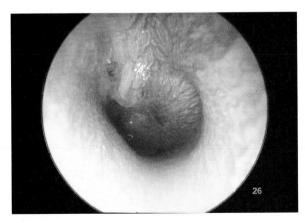

Fig 25.3 Early stage of acute suppurative otitis media. Note the erythema of the tympanic membrane and presence of a middle ear exudate that is not under pressure (with permission of A. Wright, Institute of Laryngology and Otology, London).

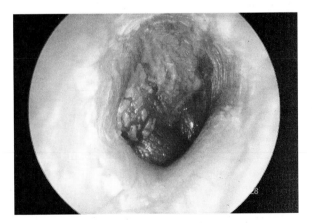

Fig 25.4 Full-blown acute suppurative otitis media. Note the bulging of the tympanic membrane and the presence of purulent middle ear fluid (with permission of A. Wright, Institute of Laryngology and Otology, London).

leucocytosis and conductive hearing loss. Complications can follow this stage, but may also arise in the stage of exudation when the antrum becomes blocked and pus under pressure is present in the mastoid cavity. The complications of acute suppurative otitis media are discussed in Chapter 29.

Diagnosis

The diagnosis of acute suppurative otitis media depends mainly on clinical symptoms and (pneumatic) otoscopic findings. A high index of suspicion is equally important in small children because specific otological symptoms can be absent. The classic clinical picture is that of a child with a respiratory tract infection for several days who develops otalgia, which may manifest as ear tugging in the younger child, hearing loss and fever. Otalgia may be absent; in a study by Casselbrant[12] 20 per cent of children with acute suppurative otitis media were without earache. Other systemic signs and symptoms, such as diarrhoea, anorexia, vomiting and irritability, may also be present. Alternatively all these clinical manifestations may be absent and an abnormal otoscopic appearance may be the only indication.

Examination with the otoscope reveals a hyperaemic, opaque, bulging tympanic membrane. Pneumatic otoscopy shows a reduced mobility. Erythema may be absent, especially when the bulging is marked. Mucopurulent otorrhoea is also a reliable sign. In children the diagnosis can be difficult because of a small ear canal and the presence of cerumen. Cleaning of the ear canal and manipulation of the ear speculum can also result in hyperaemia over the malleus handle. An audiogram usually shows a conductive hearing loss of 20–30 dB.

Culturing the discharge after spontaneous perforation is reliable in the first few hours only, because external ear canal flora contaminates the otorrhoea. The correlation between the bacterial cultures of the middle ear fluid and those of the nasopharynx and oropharynx is poor.

When determination of the causative agent is desired and the tympanic membrane is intact, aspiration of middle ear fluid may be performed. Indications for this are seriously ill or toxic children, poor response to antimicrobial therapy, presence of suppurative complications and acute suppurative otitis media in the newborn. In order not to culture commensal bacteria of the ear canal, the canal may be thoroughly rinsed and instilled with alcohol (70 per cent) for 1 minute. After aspiration of the alcohol a tympanocentesis is performed and the middle ear fluid is aspirated and kept in a sterile container (e.g. a syringe).

Treatment

There is a lot of controversy about the treatment of acute suppurative otitis media. Since the study of van Buchem *et al*.[13] in which it was shown that antibiotic treatment did not have any additional effect on the outcome of acute suppurative otitis media and that irregular courses were rare in children older than 2 years of age, some general practitioners, and even paediatricians and otolaryngologists, do not prescribe antibiotics routinely. This is especially the case in The Netherlands. In most other parts of the world, antibiotic treatment still is the classic treatment. It should be stressed, however, that for children younger than 2 years of age and for children in whom patient compliance or continuing medical supervision is not good enough, antibiotic treatment should be prescribed.

ANTIMICROBIAL TREATMENT

Most episodes of acute suppurative otitis media are caused by *S. pneumoniae*, *H. influenzae* and *M. catarrhalis*. These organisms were known to be sensitive to amoxycillin and ampicillin, but as *H. influenzae* and *M. catarrhalis* show an ever increasing β-lactamase activity, resistance is to be expected in more than 20 per cent of the patients; however, this differs between countries and even between regions. Therefore the first-line antimicrobial drug has become a β-lactamase-resistant one in many regions. Drugs of choice are amoxycillin (with or without clavulanate) and cefuroxime axetil. Other satisfactory regimens include trimethoprim–sulphamethoxazole and to a lesser degree the neo-macrolides (azithromycin, roxithromycin, clarithromycin). For a child who is allergic to penicillin these last two groups offer a valuable alternative.

Antimicrobial treatment has to be administered for at least 7 days. With the appropriate antibiotic therapy, most children improve significantly within 48–72 hours. If there is no improvement after that time, or when there is deterioration, a tympanocentesis with culture of the aspirate is advised. The causative organisms may be resistant to the administered antibiotic or a complication may have developed.

After resolution of the acute signs and symptoms, a residual middle ear effusion may be seen for 6 weeks or longer. Within 2–3 months the tympanic membrane should be entirely normal. A number of patients will show a persistent middle ear effusion, which will need appropriate therapy.

ADDITIONAL THERAPY

Adjunctive therapy for acute suppurative otitis media includes analgesics and antipyretics. Oral or topical decongestants, such as pseudoephedrine, may relieve nasal congestion. They have, however, no proven efficacy in the treatment of acute suppurative otitis media. There is a common belief that these drugs reduce congestion of the mucosa of the Eustachian tube. This may be true for less severe conditions, but in acute suppurative otitis media the effect is less significant. Moreover, side effects of these preparations are not uncommon.

MYRINGOTOMY

Myringotomy, the incision of the tympanic membrane, is the oldest surgical therapy for acute suppurative otitis media. Until the advent of antimicrobial therapy, myringotomy was the most widely used treatment. Nowadays it is reserved for some special cases. The main indications for myringotomy (Table 25.1) are severe otalgia or high fever, or both, as the incision of the tympanic membrane and subsequent drainage of the middle ear gives immediate relief of both symptoms.

Table 25.1 Indications for myringotomy

Severe otalgia or high fever
Toxic child
Presence of a suppurative complication
Poor response to antibiotic therapy
Acute suppurative otitis media occurring during antibiotic treatment
Newborns
Primary or secondary immunodeficiency

Ruuskanen *et al.*[14] nevertheless found no significant difference in symptomatic improvement or fluid resolution between a group treated with myringotomy and antibiotics and a group treated with antibiotics only. When myringotomy is performed a culture of the effusion can be taken, although this is not mandatory. Myringotomy is also indicated in 'toxic' children, in acute suppurative otitis media that has a poor response to antibiotics or occurs during antibiotherapy and in newborns or children with primary or secondary immunodeficiency, in whom an unusual organism may be present.

Technique of myringotomy

Myringotomy is the technique in which an incision is made in the tympanic membrane by a myringotomy knife in order to provide adequate drainage of the middle ear. The incision should be wide enough, circumferential and encompassing the anteroinferior quadrant of the tympanic membrane. The myringotomy can also be placed in the posteroinferior quadrant, but never in the posterosuperior quadrant as the incudostapedial joint could be damaged. Local anaesthesia (iontophoresis) does not provide adequate anaesthesia in acute suppurative otitis media, unlike in secretory otitis media.

Complications

The complications of a properly performed myringotomy are rare. Prolonged otorrhoea, in itself not a complication, can cause irritation of the external auditory canal and even otitis externa. Cleaning of the ear canal and ear drops containing an antibiotic and a mineralocorticoid will usually eliminate this problem. Serious complications are dislocation of the incudostapedial joint, severing the facial nerve or puncturing an exposed jugular bulb. These complications are extremely rare if the myringotomy is correctly performed.

More common but still infrequent sequelae are a persistent perforation, atrophic scar or myringosclerosis at the site of the incision. These do not outweigh the benefits of a myringotomy when indicated.

TREATMENT OF RECURRENT ACUTE SUPPURATIVE OTITIS MEDIA

An initial approach to the treatment of recurrent acute suppurative otitis media is the evaluation of the risk factors. Important underlying problems in older children are chronic sinus infections, nasopharyngeal obstruction (most frequently by enlarged and chronically infected adenoids) or cleft palate. Treating these (e.g. by adenoidectomy) may decrease the ear infections. In the absence of underlying problems one can also treat every individual episode and wait to see whether there is any spontaneous improvement over time.

Even in the absence of middle ear effusion, transtympanic ventilation tubes may be used in the prevention of recurrent acute suppurative otitis media. This therapy is effective, although the reasons are unclear, but has some side effects that should not be overlooked.

Antibiotic prophylaxis may be used. The same antibiotics are given as in the treatment of an acute attack but at half the daily therapeutic dose (single daily dose). The drugs are given for up to 6 months, especially in the winter. Side effects are low and there seems to be no increase in drug resistance of upper respiratory tract organisms.[9]

Systemic immunization may become an alternative choice for preventing recurrent acute suppurative otitis media. Pneumococcal vaccination (mainly polysaccharide conjugate vaccines) and *H. influenzae* vaccines have proved efficacious.[15]

References

1. Teele DW, Klein JO, Rosner B. Epidemiology of otitis media during the first seven years of life in children in greater Boston: a prospective, cohort study. *Journal of Infectious Diseases* 1989; **160**:83–94.
2. Goycoolea MV, Hueb MM, Ruah C. Definitions and terminology. *Otolaryngology Clinics of North America* 1991; **24**:757–61.
3. Bluestone CD, Stool SE, Scheetz MD. *Pediatric otolaryngology, vol 1*. Philadelphia: WB Saunders, 1990: 372–3.
4. Hoekelman R. Infectious illness during the first year of life. *Pediatrics* 1977; **59**:119–21.
5. Stangerup SE, Tos M. Epidemiology of acute suppurative otitis media. *American Journal of Otolaryngology* 1986; **7**:47–54.
6. Van Cauwenberge PB, Bellussi L, Maw AR, Paradise JL, Solow B. The adenoid as a key in upper airway infections. *International Journal of Pediatric Otorhinolaryngology* 1995; **32**:S71–S80.
7. Paparella MM, Shumrick DA, Gluckman JL, Meyerhoff WL. *Otolaryngology, vol 2, 3rd ed*. Philadelphia: WB Saunders, 1991:1306–9.
8. Arola M, Ruuskanen O, Ziegler T, *et al*. Clinical role of respiratory virus infection in acute otitis media. *Pediatrics* 1990; **86**:848–55.
9. Prellner K, Kahlmeter G, Marchisio P, Van Cauwenberge PB. Microbiology of acute otitis media and therapeutic consequences. *International Journal of Pediatric Otolaryngology* 1995; **32(suppl)**:S145–56.
10. Pichichero ME, Pichichero CL. Persistent acute otitis media: I. Causative pathogens. *Pediatric Infectious Diseases Journal* 1995; **14**:178–83.
11. Powell M, McVey D, Kassim M.H, *et al*. Antimicrobial susceptibility of *Streptococcus pneumoniae, Hemophilus influenzae* and *Moraxella (Branhamella) catarrhalis* isolated in the UK from sputa. *Journal of Antimicrobiology and Chemotherapy* 1991; **28**:249–59.
12. Casselbrant ML, Kaleida PH, Rockette HE, *et al*. Efficacy of antimicrobial profylaxis and of tympanostomy tube insertion for prevention of recurrent acute otitis media: results of a randomized clinical trial. *Pediatric Infectious Diseases Journal* 1992; **11**:278–86.
13. van Buchem FL, Dunk JHM, van't Hof MA. Therapy of acute otitis media: myringotomy, antibiotics or neither? A double-blind study in children. *Lancet* 1981; **ii**:883–7.
14. Ruuskanen O, Arola M, Ziegler T. Tympanocentesis in the treatment of acute otitis media. In: Lim DJ, *et al*. eds. *Abstracts of the Fifth International Symposium on Recent Advances in Otitis Media*. Fort Lauderdale, FL: 1991:162.
15. Ogra PL, Barenkamp SJ, Mogi G, *et al*. Microbiology, immunology, biochemistry, and vaccination. *Annals of Otology, Rhinology and Laryngology* 1994; **103(suppl 164)**:27–45.

CHAPTER 26

Secretory otitis media

A RICHARD MAW

Introduction

There are considerable interrelationships between acute suppurative otitis media, recurrent acute suppurative otitis media and chronic secretory otitis media. These include epidemiological and risk factors, causation and pathophysiological changes, and also diagnostic methodology and screening. Ultimately, however, the treatment methods differ significantly and there are different structural sequelae in the middle ear. At present it is difficult to define clearly the longer term effects on speech, language, cognition and behaviour in relation to each condition.

Chronic secretory otitis media is synonymously referred to as catarrhal, exudative, seromucinous or non-suppurative otitis media. The term secretory is appropriate in that it reflects a particular aspect of the pathological changes. Likewise the term otitis media with effusion allows differentiation of the type of effusion and facilitates distinction between acute and chronic forms. Chronic secretory otitis media may be defined as the prolonged presence within the middle ear cleft of an effusion that may be serous or mucoid but is not purulent.

Epidemiology

Reported studies show data for incidence and prevalence, including point and period prevalence. The rates for these vary in relation not only to the method of detection of the effusion but also to the ages of the children and whether it is the child or an individual ear that is assessed. Rates reflect whether high or low risk groups are investigated and finally there may be differing thresholds for diagnosis. International data are now available from several European countries, including Belgium, Holland, Denmark, Spain and the UK. There are also data from Japan, the USA, New Zealand and Saudi Arabia. Generally speaking, incidence of the disease fits a logarithmic regression curve with an annual incidence of 40 per cent in 2-year-olds and 2 per cent in 11-year-olds. Studies using serial tympanometry on nine consecutive occasions until 4 years of age showed an overall prevalence of 33 per cent of unilateral or bilateral disease in children and a rate of 25 per cent for ears. Most episodes were short-lived, 50 per cent resolved within 3 months and only 5 per cent persisted for more than 1 year. The combined results of selected published studies showed a bimodal prevalence curve with peaks of 20 per cent at age 2 years and 15 per cent at age 5 years (Fig 26.1).[1]

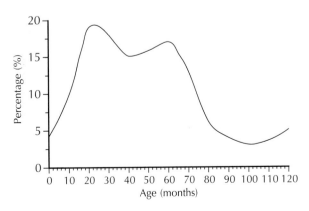

Fig 26.1 Bimodal prevalence of chronic secretory otitis media.

Table 26.1 Prevalence of middle ear effusions in different age bands

Age range (years)	Prevalence (%)	
	Ears	Children
2–6	4–25	5–38
7–8	–	3.6–9
9–11	–	1.1–4

Relapses and remissions occur and the median duration is less than 3 months. Ninety per cent of postinfective middle ear effusions are said to resolve within 3 months.

The international data for prevalence are summarized in Table 26.1.[2]

Risk factors

High and low risk cases are recognized; the former constitute an otitis-prone group. Risk factors may be defined as intrinsic or genetic, relating to the host, or extrinsic either environmental or aetiological. However, most risk factors represent associations and not causality. The factors are interrelated and there is comorbidity, for example the increase in frequency of daycare at a young age is reducing the ability to breastfeed. The factors may be divided into those that are now accepted as definite and proven and from those that are still unproven though possible.

Out of the proven risk factors, age and gender are without doubt. Relatively few children acquire clinical signs of chronic secretory otitis media after the age of 5 or 6 years and boys are more often affected than girls. There are seasonal risks. It is accepted that syndromic conditions such as Hurler, Hunter and Down syndromes are predisposed and that there may be infective and skull-based cofactors with Down syndrome. Children with palatal abnormalities invariably have chronic secretory otitis media. The racial differences may also represent anatomical factors but the reduced rates in North American black races may be the result of a lower rate of acceptance of medical care. Children with structural cilial abnormalities, such as the Kartagener syndrome, are predisposed. A family history of otitis media, particularly in siblings, and an early first episode of acute suppurative otitis media can identify increased susceptibility. The latter may indicate early colonization of the nasopharynx by

bacteria. The type of daycare and the age at which it is commenced probably relates to frequency of exposure to upper respiratory infections, and there may be some correlation with recurrent otitis and infections of the tonsils and sinuses.

Unproven but possible factors include low birth weight and parental smoking, both being interrelated. Bottle-feeding and daycare are also interrelated, and it seems that breast milk may have a protective effect. Maternal alcohol intake and HIV infection together with maternal blood group require further confirmation. The effect of sleeping position requires clarification as a change from prone to supine in infants has affected the incidence of subsequent ear-related symptoms. Atopy is certainly associated with chronic secretory otitis media, but as yet a causal role has not been confirmed.

Causation

A wide variety of risk factors indicates that there is no single cause for chronic secretory otitis media in children. However, in approximately one-half of the cases there appears to be an initial upper respiratory tract infection of viral origin, which is more likely in an otitis prone individual. Secondary bacterial colonization of the middle ear cleft occurs possibly in relation to nasopharyngeal infection. In some cases there may be primary bacterial colonization of both sites. The previously held ex-vacuo theory, which implicated tubal obstruction and dysfunction as a principal primary cause for chronic secretory otitis media is questionable, but a tubal component is likely to be involved (see Chapter 24). This is supported by the universality of chronic secretory otitis media in children with a cleft palate and the demonstration of effusions after experimental division of the tensor palati muscle. There is increasing evidence of involvement of a nasopharyngeal component in that reduced nasopharyngeal dimensions have been demonstrated in children with chronic secretory otitis media compared with controls (Fig 26.2).[3] A similar reduction in dimensions has recently been shown in children with recurrent acute suppurative otitis media. The adenoid tissue and other lymphoid tissue in the upper airway may act as a source of infection but factors in the nasopharynx, including pressure change and partial pressures of carbon dioxide, may be linked with tubal dysfunction. There is obviously comorbidity of the nasopharyngeal factors with other associated risk factors. Finally, there may be a cellular or humoral immune deficiency as a selective rather than a global deficit, for example, to

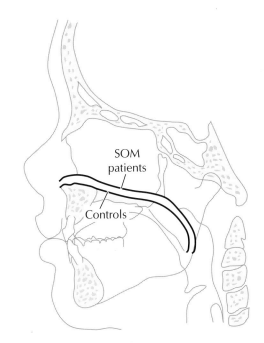

Fig 26.2 Overall difference in soft palate position and the nasopharyngeal airway in children with chronic secretory otitis media (SOM) compared with controls.

non-typeable *Haemophilus influenzae* infection in an otitis prone child.

Pathophysiological changes

The inflammatory and immunological mechanisms in chronic secretory otitis media are still ill understood. However, changes occur at a humoral and cellular level that result in obvious mucosal change where there is inflammation. Recent studies have defined the middle ear gas composition, which may be altered during the inflammatory reaction. There is continuing uncertainty in relation to the genetic or environmental cause for the changes in mastoid pneumatization associated with otitis media.

CELLULAR AND HUMORAL CHANGES

Inflammatory mediators and inflammatory cells are found in middle ear effusions together with adhesion molecules. Acute otitis media induced by viral infection initiates release of cytokines. Children with recurrent acute otitis media are poor producers of nasopharyngeal cytokines. Mast cell degranulation may be triggered by the viral infection occurring in acute otitis media. In addition to viral

induction of cytokines, adherence ligands have recently been shown. Mediators of the inflammatory cascade in the middle ear, such as interleukins, require further evaluation. T-cell lymphocyte activation occurs in the middle ear and in the blood of patients with chronic secretory otitis media and there may be specific binding factors in the middle ear that bind B lymphocytes. Immunological changes involve immunoglobulin G and immunoglobulin G subclasses. Thus an immune response occurs in the middle ear and nasopharynx to viral and bacterial invasion and there is lymphocyte migration to the middle ear, where adhesion occurs.

INFLAMMATORY CHANGES

Fifty to sixty per cent of the viral infections are caused by a respiratory syncytial virus and there is a seasonal component to this infection. Adenoviruses and influenza virus also occur. Bacterial infection is typically by *Streptococcus pneumoniae*, *H. influenzae*, *Moraxella catarrhalis* and *S. pyogenes*. Formation of an effusion requires living unattenuated bacteria but the effusion may be maintained by attenuated or unattenuated bacteria. Recently techniques based on the polymerase chain reaction have been used to demonstrate organisms within the sites of infection in the middle ear and the nasopharynx.

MUCOSAL CHANGES

Acute and later chronic inflammatory changes occur at a mucosal level and there is goblet cell proliferation with mucus production. There may be alteration of mucosal clearance mechanisms. The role of surfactant is still undefined. Functional effects on cilia are said to occur, but these may reflect a response to inflammatory change and could be due to environmental factors such as parental smoking.

ALLERGY

It does not appear that an immunoglobulin E mediated allergic response is the primary causal factor in the development of chronic secretory otitis media but it may occur as an association. Further studies are required, which should include full atopic histories, intradermal immediate hypersensitivity skin testing together with total immunoglobulin E estimation and specific RAST testing. Eosinophilic cationic protein, which is a histochemical marker for allergy, may further define the role of allergy in chronic secretory otitis media.

MIDDLE EAR CLEFT CHANGES ASSOCIATED WITH INFECTION

The association of reduced mastoid pneumatization with a preceding history of ear infection is without doubt. There is still uncertainty over whether this is due to a genetic predisposition or whether it is an environmental effect of the middle ear changes (see Chapter 24). Recent studies have suggested that pneumatization may occur into predetermined spaces that exist, for example, in relation to the development of the mastoid antrum. Bone absorption is said to occur during development in contrast to a process of active epithelial invasion. There is a correlation between middle ear volume and the degree of mastoid pneumatization. However, the normal increase in size of the middle ear with age does occur in patients who suffer from acute suppurative otitis media. Reduced pneumatization may be a risk factor for development of chronic secretory otitis media in adults and may account in part for the increased incidence of chronic secretory otitis media in Down syndrome.

MIDDLE EAR GAS COMPOSITION

Microanalysis techniques for estimation of middle ear gas composition are now available and mathematical models have been constructed to demonstrate gas changes within the middle ear cleft. Spectrometry studies show middle ear gas partial pressures of nitrogen at 82.4 per cent oxygen at 7.6 per cent and carbon dioxide at 10 per cent. These are different from levels in atmospheric air but closely resemble levels in mixed venous blood. Oxygen and nitrogen transfer from the ear to the blood; carbon dioxide transfers from the blood and the tissues to the ear. Current models do not reflect the pathological state in which increase in diffusion may occur as a result of the increased vascularization that accompanies middle ear mucosal inflammation. Sadé and Luntz[4] suggest that the middle ear gas deficiency in association with chronic secretory otitis media may be secondary not to Eustachian tube dysfunction but to excessive loss of middle ear gases by diffusion into the blood.

Middle ear gas composition and pressure may affect Eustachian tube ventilatory function by a feedback modulation mechanism. There may be a similar effect in the nasopharynx and it is likely that the partial pressure of carbon dioxide is particularly important. There is known to be an effect of sleep on middle ear gas partial pressure and it is accepted that the capacitance or volume of the middle ear mucosa can also be important in relation to overall gas composition. However, as yet we have no reliable test of Eustachian tube function in normal individuals and little indication of its function during disease.

Diagnosis and screening

Diagnosis and screening involve assessment of hearing ability, middle ear mechanical function and aspects of cochlear and possibly vestibular labyrinthine function.

DIAGNOSIS

Attention is drawn to the possibility of fluid within the middle ear by the hearing loss that it may cause or by its effects on speech, language, cognition and behaviour. The symptoms differ with age. Secondary acute infection of the middle ear fluid may lead to otalgia and sometimes otorrhoea. Frequently these episodes coincide with a cold, upper respiratory ttract infection or period of allergic rhinitis, or they may occur as a sequel to swimming. The presence of middle ear fluid may be covert and under these circumstances detection may occur during screening. Otoscopy is required visually to confirm the presence of an effusion. Pneumatic otoscopy should be performed, preferably using an instrument with a halogen light source. Examination under the microscope with magnification may further improve diagnostic accuracy. Tympanic membrane examination should have a high degree of specificity and sensitivity. Rates of approximately 75 per cent and 90 per cent, respectively, are quoted if a pneumatic otoscope is used. In clinical studies there should be interobserver vaildation of these variables (Figs 26.3 and 26.4 and Plate section).

Tympanometry provides an objective assessment of middle ear status. The equipment should elicit a pressure range of –600 to +200 decaPascal (daPa). Jerger's nomenclature has been modified by Fiellau-Nikolajsen[5] and can be used to produce four subgroups of tympanogram (Table 26.2).

A positive predictive value of 84 per cent may be achieved with a simple peak versus no-peak classification. Such qualitative measures are sufficient for clinical needs but quantitative measurements of static compliance and measurements of tympanometric peak, width, height and equivalent volume may allow severity to be assessed by measuring these

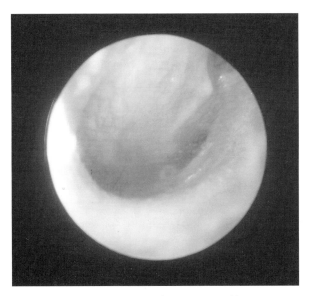

Fig 26.3 Right tympanic membrane, viewed by otoscope, showing mild changes of chronic secretory otitis media with polypoid mucosa on the medial aspect.

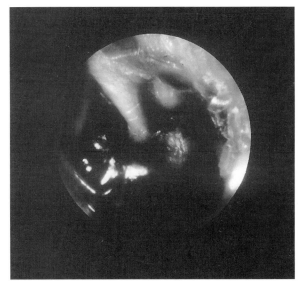

Fig 26.4 Left tympanic membrane, viewed by otoscope, showing marked retraction of tympanic membrane and dark middle ear effusion.

Table 26.2 Types of tympanograms

Type A	Middle ear pressure +200 to –99 daPa
Type C1	–100 to –199 daPa
Type C2	–200 to –400 daPa
Type B	Flat trace without well defined compliance peak

continuous variables. Tympanometry is unreliable in children under 6 months old. The reliability improves with age. There is a relationship between the type of tympanometric trace and audiometric hearing threshold. Type B traces are highly sensitive in detecting effusions with a greater than 25 dB hearing loss but are only 75 per cent specific. Only 2 per cent of children with a bilateral hearing loss greater than 25 dB do not have flat type B tympanograms.

Multifrequency tympanometry may further increase diagnostic ability. The inclusion of acoustic reflex measurements does not increase the ability of tympanometry to predict clinically significant hearing thresholds.

Newer microtympanometers and automatic impedance tympanoscopes may be suitable for use in general practice but may lead to over-referral of patients suspected of having chronic secretory otitis media. The development of acoustic reflectometry has not as yet further improved diagnostic ability.

Myringotomy and aspiration of the middle ear fluid is still the gold standard for diagnosis of chronic secretory otitis media. The so-called 'dry

tap' rates reported in clinical trials and acknowledged by otolaryngologists have several obvious causes. These include the length of time the patient has remained on the surgical waiting list; the presence or absence of preoperative tympanometry at pre-admission clinics; and the degree of negative pressure developed by tympanometers. Nitrous oxide anaesthesia may displace middle ear fluid and prevent aspiration at operation.

HEARING ASSESSMENT

Clinical voice tests fail to detect 20 per cent of children with hearing impairment of 20 dB or less and tuning fork tests are unreliable in young children. The results of behavioural observational tests and distraction testing rely on the experience of the testers. In younger children free-field audiometry may be used.

The introduction of the automated McCormick toy discrimination test allows more accurate assessment of hearing thresholds of children under 4 years of age. In older children pure tone audiometry should be performed across the speech frequency range, if necessary with estimation of bone and air conduction thresholds. Audiometry is not of diagnostic value but allows assessment of the severity of the condition and may be used to monitor progress. 'Dry' ears have been shown to have a mean hearing threshold of 17 dB; mild chronic secretory otitis media, 23 dB; moderate chronic secretory otitis media, 29 dB; and so-called impacted middle ears 34 dB.[5] The latter would appear to be a description of persistent chronic secretory otitis media as reported in other studies of clinical trials of treatment. More recently, high frequency audiometry from 10 to 14 kHz has demonstrated a high frequency loss as a consequence of chronic secretory otitis media. Special tests have also demonstrated a hearing loss in noise. Subtle interaural differences in children with chronic secretory otitis media occur with a failure to detect and recognize signals in noisy backgrounds.

SCREENING

Screening for hearing loss was initially developed with programmes for the early detection of sensorineural hearing loss. It was hoped that this would be detected particularly in at-risk children during the first year of life. In the UK, screening for hearing loss takes place at about 7 months and at school age. An intermediate screen at 3.5 years of age has been the practice of about 50 per cent of Health Authorities. A preschool or school screen is carried out before or at school entry, that is, in 4- to 5-year-olds. Although the 7-month screen is aimed at detection of sensorineural hearing loss, it will detect children with significant conductive loss and accounts for referral for otological opinions of children in their first year. The two subsequent screens mostly detect conductive hearing loss almost invariably due to chronic secretory otitis media. There is a higher failure rate

during the winter months. The most appropriate timing for re-testing is not clear, but depending on season should not be within 6–12 weeks and probably should be left for longer. Haggard and Hughes[6] have extensively reviewed and discussed the cost effectiveness of screening programmes.

There is a need to validate the diagnostic measures used for screening and then to assess the effect of these validated methods of detection.

Treatment

Any treatment regimen needs to take note not only of the severity of disease but also of the persistence of constant or intermittent disease, and whether the condition is symptomatic. Such symptoms may concern hearing loss or its secondary effects on speech, language, cognition and behaviour, or they may be a consequence of secondary infection within the middle ear. The possible effects of middle ear structural damage should be considered.

Treatment protocols should take into account epidemiological and other studies that have defined the natural history of the untreated condition. These are relatively few, but spontaneous resolution of severe persistent chronic secretory otitis media has been shown to occur in 20 per cent of patients at 1 year, 30 per cent of patients at 2 years, 50 per cent of at 3 years, 60 per cent at 4 years, 70 per cent at 5 years, 85 per cent at 7 years and 95 per cent at 10 years (Fig 26.5).[7] Clinicians treating children with chronic

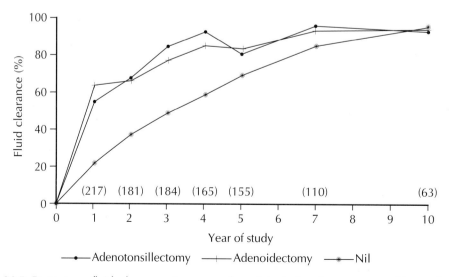

Fig 26.5 Percentage fluid clearance in cases of persistent chronic secretory otitis media after treatment by adenotonsillectomy, adenoidectomy and in the control ears that have received no treatment (nil).

Table 26.3 Percentage rates of intervention per capita population

	Holland	England & Wales	New Zealand
Myringotomy +/– ventilation tubes	0.29	0.1	0.31
Adenoidectomy Tonsillectomy Adenotonsillectomy	0.44	0.19	0.21

secretory otitis media should be aware of the results of trials of medical and surgical treatment and should also be aware of the criteria used for inclusion in such trials.

There is limited knowledge of the rates of intervention between surgeons, hospitals, districts, regions and across international borders. Few data are available at an international level, for there is often a failure to report daycase and inpatient surgical operations and those taking place within commercial and private systems. The rates of intervention in Holland, England and Wales and New Zealand during 1992 and 1993 have been calculated based on a per capita population estimate. These countries have among the best data collection systems for these conditions (Table 26.3).[2]

Treatment should aim to relieve the symptoms caused by the middle ear condition, it should resolve the underlying pathophysiological changes and it should prevent recurrence and development of sequelae. There may also be a need to treat coexistent conditions such as infection in the nose and sinuses and allergy.

MEDICAL TREATMENT

Decongestants and mucolytics

Neither topical nor systemic decongestants and antihistamines have any place in the treatment of persistent chronic secretory otitis media. Mucolytic preparations are still under investigation but as yet no trials have confirmed a significant long-term beneficial effect.

Antibiotics

Treatment with antibiotics may be therapeutic and prophylactic. The choice of antibiotics is wide. Simple penicillins V and G have been used for acute suppurative otitis media and chronic secretory otitis media, but on a worldwide basis one of the aminopenicillins, in particular amoxycillin rather than ampicillin, has been the treatment of choice. Augmented penicillins with anti-β-lactamase enzymatic activity, such as amoxycillin and clavulanate, have also been used. First, second and third generation cephalosporins and macrolides such as erythromycin have been used and tested in clinical trials. Quinolones such as ciprofloxacin are not recommended for children with chronic secretory otitis media. Erythromycin reduces cytokine action in addition to its antibiotic activity; thus its use in low doses on a long-term basis has been suggested. Finally it should be noted that viruses within the middle ear effusion may interfere with antibiotic treatment.

Antibiotic treatment is only effective in one out of four or five patients with chronic secretory otitis media and only in the short term. Meta-analysis has been used to show the effects of antibiotics for acute suppurative otitis media and prophylactically for recurrent acute suppurative otitis media. Similarly meta-analysis shows a limited short-term benefit for treatment of chronic secretory otitis media (Table 26.4).

There are increasing problems with penicillin-resistant strains of *S. pneumoniae*, which have now been reported in 28–61 per cent of patients. Multi-drug-resistant organisms are also reported and there is a continuing increase in the number of organisms that produce β-lactamase.

Antibiotics are associated with significant complications. Twenty-five per cent of patients develop a systemic effect, in particular gastrointestinal problems such as diarrhoea. A similar percentage may be prone to allergic reactions. These certainly reduce the effective range of medical treatment and may have fatal effects. Severe haematological complications with neutropenia and thrombocytopenic purpura also occur, particularly with sulphonamides.

Steroids

There have been only relatively few studies with small numbers of patients showing the effects of steroids, either alone or in combination with antibiotics for chronic secretory otitis media.

Table 26.4 Meta-analysis data for mean and range of short-term cure rates

	Mean (%)	Range (%)
Acute suppurative otitis media	14	8–19
Recurrent acute suppurative otitis media	11	3–19
Chronic secretory otitis media	14	3–30

Meta-analysis of these studies shows that for steroid treatment alone there is a short-term cure rate of 18–21 per cent (–2–43 per cent confidence interval). For steroids combined with antibiotics the range is 25–31 per cent (–9–71 per cent confidence interval). Thus the effect is not statistically significant. However, because only small numbers have been studied, the magnitude of any possible benefit may not have been detected.

Steroid treatment has the potential complication of adrenal suppression and the development of varicella. There may also be precipitation of episodes of acute suppurative otitis media.

Non-steroidal anti-inflammatory drugs

Aluminium ibuprofen for 2 weeks is less effective than trimethoprim with sulphamethoxazole or prednisolone when assessed after 4 or 12 weeks. There is as yet no report of any long-term benefit from non-steroidal anti-inflammatory drugs.

Autoinflation

A short-term benefit for up to 3 months with a two- to fivefold improvement in otoscopic and tympanometric outcome has been reported using an otovent device. The improvement is age-related and dependent on compliance (Fig 26.6).

Other treatments

There has been no evaluation with properly controlled studies of the use of hearing aids. No benefit has resulted from studies involving surfactant. As yet, vaccination has not become a commercial possibility. However, there is the possibility of trials using a non-typeable *H. influenzae* vaccine within the near future. Vaccination will be required in very young infants. There is a problem with multiple pneumococcal serotypes that makes this vaccine production difficult. Notwithstanding the problems, the massive effect on other infections such as acute epiglottitis that has been demonstrated after *H. influenzae* vaccination provides hope for the future.

SURGICAL TREATMENT

Myringotomy and ventilation tubes

Myringotomy alone with aspiration of the middle ear effusion has only a short-lived beneficial effect and is not recommended for persistent effusions. The introduction of ventilation tubes in 1954 by Armstrong[8] has transformed the surgical treatment of chronic secretory otitis media. Tubes may

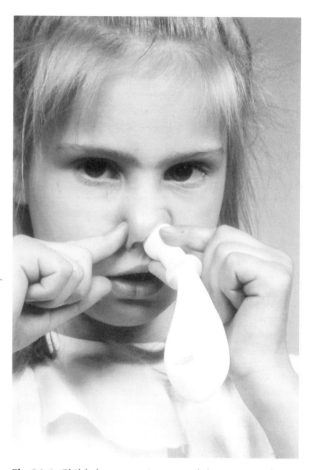

Fig 26.6 Child demonstrating use of the otovent device in the left nasal passage.

be either of a short-term type, which remain *in situ* for 9–12 months, or of the long-term type, which are retained for years. There are increasing reports of an unacceptably high rate of persistent tympanic membrane perforation after use of long-stay tubes, perhaps because these have been used in patients with tympanic membrane atelectasis in whom a perforation might be anticipated. Long-stay tubes are not recommended for uncomplicated cases of chronic secretory otitis media. There is uncertainty about the need to remove ventilation tubes and generally they should be left to extrude spontaneously. Under these circumstances the persistent perforation rate with short-stay tubes is in the order of 1–3 per cent. Children with tubes should be permitted to swim perhaps with restriction of diving or jumping into the water, which is prudent but often not adhered to. Children who swim with tubes appear to develop ear infections at a similar rate to those who swim and who do not have tubes.

There seems to be a need for re-treatment with tubes in approximately 30 per cent of patients. There may be an adjuvant effect of adenoidectomy on the need for re-treatment with tubes.[9] Ventilation tubes produce an immediate and short-term hearing gain with improvement of speech reception thresholds of 20 dB or less. Longer term studies, however, show less satisfactory hearing thresholds of 12 dB or less 12 months postoperatively. Tube insertion may be complicated by early postoperative otorrhoea and this seems more frequent if bacterial pathogens are present in the external auditory meatus or in the middle ear effusion. Late sequelae also occur as a result of the effusion and the ventilation tube insertion.

The indications for tube insertion depend on the duration, severity and laterality of disease. Generally, unilateral effusions require intervention less than if the fluid is bilateral. Acceptable indications would be persistence of bilateral chronic secretory otitis media confirmed by a validated otoscopist and supported by tympanometry, which should show a B or C2 curve rather than an A or C1 curve. There should be confirmation of hearing impairment by appropriate testing with behavioural tests or audiometry. Re-examination approximately 3 months after the initial diagnosis should be mandatory. Clinically there should also be confirmation of hearing loss or its effects and the child's age and seasonal variation should be taken into account.

Although a 'dry tap' rate of up to 30 per cent has been reported in some studies, with stricter criteria a rate of less than 10 per cent has been shown. This is probably acceptable, particularly if it includes patients listed for surgical treatment of recurrent acute suppurative otitis media in whom a dry ear might be anticipated at the time of operation. Tube insertion does not prevent development of attic retraction, outer attic wall erosion or atelectasis,[10] for which the cause remains unclear.

Adenoidectomy

The four most recent trials that have attempted to evaluate adenoidectomy using acceptable controls in a prospective manner have shown a beneficial effect.[7,11–13] Adenoidectomy alone has been shown to produce otoscopic clearance of the middle ear effusion, alteration of tympanometric status and improvement of hearing loss. There has also been a reduction of the overall duration of the condition.

The studies show some differences in relation to the duration of the effect, which in some has been short term, only 6 months, and in others, longer term, that is, for up to 3–4 years. There has been a gender effect in only one study, which indicated better improvement in girls than in boys. These trials have also shown some conflict over the benefit of adenoidectomy alone compared with ventilation tube insertion alone. Dempster *et al.*[13]

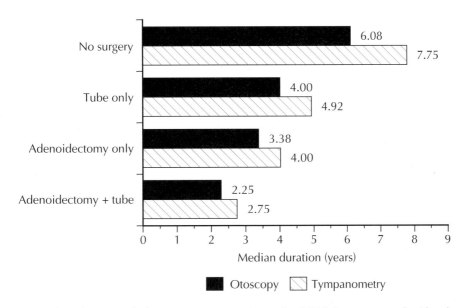

Fig 26.7 Median duration of chronic secretory otitis media (SOM) in ears treated with adenoidectomy and ventilation tube; with adenoidectomy only; with a tube only and in ears not receiving any treatment, demonstrated by otoscopy and tympanometry.

showed no difference at 6–12 months but Maw and Bawden[7] showed a differential effect in the overall duration of the effusion in terms of otoscopic clearance and tympanometric status change (Fig 26.7). Without any treatment the overall duration of the condition was shown to be 6.1 years by otoscopy and 7.8 years tympanometrically. Ventilation tube treatment alone reduced this to 3.5 and 4.9 years, respectively. Adenoidectomy reduced it to 3.4 and 4.0 years, respectively. The combination of the two procedures produced the best overall reduction in duration of the disease to 2.3 and 2.8 years, respectively.[7] Further long-term multicentre studies are in progress to evaluate the possible additional benefit of adenoidectomy.

There may be significant complications as a result of adenoid removal, but it can now be carried out as a daycase procedure. There is the possibility of reactionary and secondary haemorrhage and there is a fatality rate that has been estimated in the order of 1:25 000 to 1:50 000. Velopharyngeal insufficiency may develop and clearly the operation is more hazardous in younger children. Tonsillectomy has not been shown to be of any benefit.

The trials of surgical treatment methods that have been reported during the past few decades have generally suffered from significant methodological flaws. Small numbers of patients have been studied without sufficient power to demonstrate any effect. There have been high or unknown 'dry tap' rates at operation. The period of follow-up has often been too short, particularly to demonstrate any requirement for re-treatment. There has been loss of patients at follow-up and studies have not been designed on an intention-to-treat basis. There has been lack of uniformity of clinical material, with unilateral and bilateral cases considered together, and there has frequently been failure to control for a wide variety of risk factors. Changes in treatment have been recorded during the trials and observations have often not been made blind. Frequently the most severely affected patients have been excluded. Finally, not every trial has assessed all of the potential outcome measures in relation to inclusion criteria.

Prognostic factors for outcome

In untreated patients the spontaneous resolution of chronic secretory otitis media is related to age and gender and also to middle ear and mastoid volumes. After surgery with either ventilation tubes or adenoidectomy, the outcome is again dependent on the age at operation, parental smoking and to some extent on adenoid and nasopharyngeal airway size.

There is some relationship with a preceding history of acute suppurative otitis media before surgery. The reported effect of atopy has been variable in terms of outcome.

Guidelines for treatment

In 1992 in the UK the Effective Health Care Bulletin was published by the University of Leeds.[14] This was funded in part by the Department of Health and the Royal College of Physicians. It investigated the surgical treatment methods for persistent chronic secretory otitis media. It suggested a period of watchful waiting before surgery, with placement of the patient on a provisional waiting list from which assessment could be made immediately before operation. In 1993 in Australia, guidelines very similar to those produced in draft in the USA were recommended. These were advocated by the New South Wales Health Department Working Party to produce a simplified algorithm that recommended primary antibiotic treatment with amoxycillin for 10–28 days. In 1994 in the USA the final publication of the Clinical Practice Guideline on otitis media with effusion in young children was made by a consortium of the American Academy of Pediatrics, Otolaryngologists, Head and Neck surgeons and family physicians.[15] The report was made under contract to the agency for Health Care Policy and Research. It addressed only children aged 1–3 years and recommended the use of antibiotics at diagnosis and at 6 weeks and 3 months after diagnosis. Ventilation tube insertion was recommended when the disease became chronic and when there was a hearing loss of 20 dB or more. There have been reports of dissatisfaction with all of these guidelines. In the USA there are problems concerning the significance of such a hearing loss in a child of the prescribed age group. There is also concern that there is no scientific evidence or clinical trial to support the recommendation that adenoidectomy should not be undertaken before the age of 3 years for this condition. Until such trials are performed there is the possibility of an improvement in some of these patients after adenoid removal.

Sequelae

Sequelae seen in relation to chronic secretory otitis media may be due to the disease itself or to the treatment. They may be structural, in the middle or inner ear, or functional due to the hearing loss. The main concern is the possibility that the long-standing effects of the hearing loss associated with the middle ear effusion may impair subsequent development of speech, language, cognition and behaviour. There is also a possible effect on familial and, in particular, maternal responsiveness.

STRUCTURAL EFFECTS

Middle ear

The potential sequelae relate to the disease and to the insertion of ventilation tubes. There may be tympanic membrane scarring, segmental atrophy, tympanosclerosis or perforation. Atelectasis may develop and attic retraction with erosion of the outer attic wall may occur. Finally, there is a possibility of cholesteatoma formation. Structural abnormalities may occur as an extension of the inflammatory disease from the middle to the inner ear with hair cell damage and changes in the vestibular labyrinth.

Segmental scarring occurs at the site of placement of the ventilation tube and is due to the tube and not the effusion. By contrast, other tympanic membrane scarring appears equally in the untreated condition and in those treated with tubes. Tympanosclerosis or, more correctly, myringosclerosis is seen in 40 per cent of ears treated with ventilation tubes but in 3–10 per cent of untreated ears. Ears with only a myringotomy show a much lower incidence than those in which a tube is inserted. The sclerotic changes increase during the first 3 years after placement of the tube and then stabilize. Resolution has not been demonstrated. Insertion of one tube produces much the same incidence and degree of sclerosis as does insertion of several tubes on different occasions into the same tympanic membrane. The cause of the sclerotic change is multifactorial. Haemorrhage at the site of placement of the tube has been implicated together with the effect of mechanical strain and sheer stresses caused by tube insertion. It is interesting that the sclerotic changes occur away from the site of placement of the tube. It has been suggested that a hyperoxic effect initiates the sclerosis after the introduction of air with an increased partial pressure of oxygen into the middle ear, where there is a lower partial pressure of oxygen. The sclerotic change has only a minimal effect on hearing ability, resulting in a 3–4 dB deficit. However, in certain patients very severe myringosclerosis can occur with fixation of the malleus handle and in these few patients the hearing loss may be greater. Why some cases progress to this severe extent is unknown.

Attic retraction has been graded by Tos and Poulson and pars tensa retraction by Sadé, both on a four-point scale (see Chapter 24). Both these conditions have been shown to be related to longer duration of chronic secretory otitis media. Whether this is causal is unknown, but there is no evidence to suggest that tube insertion either causes or affects the later development of these complications. Some degree of atelectasis occurs in 15–17 per cent of ears, with a similar rate in untreated ears and in those treated with ventilation tube insertion. Thirty-five to forty per cent of treated and untreated ears develop some degree of attic retraction. The severity of the attic retraction is similar whether the ears are treated with tubes or untreated. However, only 1–2 per cent of ears develop severe attic retraction. In most mild to moderate cases, both complications are associated with only a minor hearing loss of less than 5 dB. There is no relationship between the development of the conditions and age at operation; duration of preoperative hearing loss or otalgia; adenoid size; nasal obstruction; allergy or parental smoking. Thus at present we have no means of detecting preoperatively those children in whom these complications might be anticipated.[10]

In their mild to moderate forms the complications are probably not of great significance, but in severe forms atelectasis will lead to myringoincudostapediopexy, erosion of the long process of the incus and a significant conductive hearing loss. There is the potential for very severe cases of attic retraction with outer attic wall erosion to progress to cholesteatoma formation. Very large multicentre studies would be required to confirm the suspicion of this type of development (Figs 26.8 and 26.9).

Inner ear

Studies with conventional pure tone audiometry have not shown high frequency hearing loss as a consequence of either chronic secretory otitis media or treatment with ventilation tubes. However, recent studies using high frequency testing have shown an ultra-high frequency hearing loss with chronic secretory otitis media. Inflammatory mediators and neurotoxins have been found in middle ear effusions. Using body sway studies, abnormalities of balance have been shown to be associated with chronic secretory otitis media and these improve after ventilation tube insertion.

FUNCTIONAL EFFECTS

Hearing acuity

Direct effects of hearing loss are often very obvious and well described by parents who react to them. The effects of ultra-high frequency hearing loss or of interaural asymmetry and listening difficulties

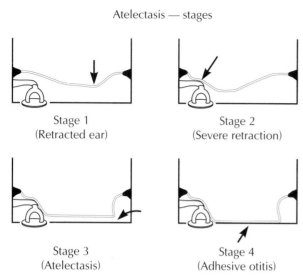

Atelectasis — stages

Stage 1
(Retracted ear)

Stage 2
(Severe retraction)

Stage 3
(Atelectasis)

Stage 4
(Adhesive otitis)

Fig 26.8 Stages of atelectasis: stage 1, retracted tympanic membrane; stage 2, severe retraction; stage 3, atelectasis and stage 4, adhesive otitis media.

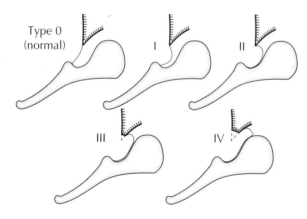

Type 0
(normal)

I

II

III

IV

Fig 26.9 Four types of attic retraction and outer attic wall erosion.

within a background noise are not known. A major obstacle has been to define the effects, consequent upon the hearing loss, on speech, language, cognition and behaviour. It is a difficult and complex problem to prove and relates to the time with the disease and also to its severity. It also relates to the age at onset of chronic secretory otitis media and the time at which the effects are assessed. There are obvious problems with the assessment of these variables in young children and reliable tests have not been developed by which significant standard deviation shifts may be anticipated. Mostly, however, the problem relates to the difficulty in separating the effects of the hearing loss on these

variables from those of the confounding factors, which are known also to affect speech and language, learning and behaviour. These confounding variables include gender and ethnic background, environment and, in particular, daycare management, maternal education and IQ together with socioeconomic status. There may also be particular problems for high IQ children and there is a so-called 'middle class effect'. Here the effects of socioeconomic grouping on these factors overshadow those due to the conductive hearing loss. There is now increasing evidence of a small but significant effect of hearing loss on speech, language, learning and behaviour, but it is synergistic with environmental factors and especially with the increasing frequency of daycare management of young children.

In 3- to 8-years-olds after confirmation of recurrent acute suppurative otitis media or chronic secretory otitis media in the first 3 years of life, an adverse effect has been shown with minor behavioural changes at age 5 years that are reported by teacher and parent. These include impairment of task orientation and distractability, short-term attention spans; and goal orientation together with restlessness, fidgetiness, destructive behaviour and disobedience.

Adverse effects have also been reported on expressive verbal vocabulary, speech perception, language cognition tests and phonological representation. Receptive language abilities have been affected. Later, at 10 and 11 years of age, there have been reports of adverse effects on picture language, articulation, attention and social behaviour together with a slight effect, reported by teachers, on reading ability. Very recently a study from Dunedin, New Zealand[16] has reported longer term adverse sequelae on verbal full scale IQ and reading and spelling in 13-year-olds, and also on reading in 15-year-olds.

However, other studies report that the mild association of chronic secretory otitis media with expressive language and communication problems at the age of 5 years is due to socioeconomic grouping and ethnic background, maternal IQ and smoking. In small studies, although some adverse effects such as speech perception in noise are noted, other functions, for example, dichotic filtered speech, auditory memory and binaural fusion, assessed in 7- to 8-years-olds are unaffected. Similarly, although task orientation and distractability can be shown in 3-year-olds, overall intellectual development seems unaffected. Some studies fail to show significant adverse effects on cognition and language development at 2 years of age and any defects that may present initially are not apparent by the age of 4 years.

This important aspect of chronic secretory otitis media is a difficult problem that requires further research, and prospective studies are in progress in the UK and in the USA.

References

1. Zielhuis GH, Rach GH, van den Bosch AV, van den Broek P. The prevalence of otitis media with effusion: a critical review of the literature. *Clinical Otolaryngology* 1990; **15**:283–8.
2. Maw AR, Counsell A. International perspectives and future directions. In: Roberts JE, Wallace I, Henderson F eds. *Otitis media in young children: medical, developmental and educational considerations*. Baltimore: Brookes, 1997:267–86.
3. Maw AR, Smith IM, Lance GN. lateral cephalometric analysis of children with otitis media with effusion: a comparison with age and sex matched controls. *Journal of Laryngology and Otology* 1991; **105**:71–7.
4. Sade J, Luntz M. Middle ear as a gas pocket. *Annals of Otology, Rhinology and Laryngology* 1990; **99**:529–34.
5. Fiellau-Nikolajsen M. Tympanometry and secretory otitis media. Observations on diagnosis, epidemiology, treatment and prevention in prospective cohort studies of three year old children. *Acta Oto-laryngologica (Stockholm)* 1983; **Suppl 394**:1–73.
6. Haggard M, Hughes G. Screening children's hearing: a review of the literature and the implications of otitis media. London: HMSO, 1991.
7. Maw AR, Bawden R. Spontaneous resolution of severe chronic glue ear in children and the effect of adenoidectomy, tonsillectomy, and insertion of ventilation tubes (grommets). *British Medical Journal* 1993; **306**:756–60.
8. Armstrong BW. A new treatment for chronic secretory otitis media. *Archives of Otolaryngology* 1954; **59**:653–4.
9. Maw AR, Bawden R. Does adenoidectomy have an adjuvant effect on ventilation tube insertion and thus reduce the need for treatment? *Clinical Otolaryngology* 1994; **19**:340–3.
10. Maw A. Glue ear in childhood. *Clinics in Developmental Medicine* 135. MacKeith Press, 1995.
11. Gates GA, Avery CA, Prihoda TJ, Cooper JC. Effectiveness of adenoidectomy and tympanostomy tubes in the treatment of chronic media with effusion. *New England Journal of Medicine* 1987; **317**:1444–51.
12. Paradise JL, Bluestone CD, Rogers KD, *et al*. Efficacy of adenoidectomy for recurrent otitis media in children previously treated with tympanostomy tube placement. Results of parallel randomized and nonrandomized trials. *Journal of the American Medical Association* 1990; **263**:2066–73.
13. Dempster JH, Browning CG, Gatehouse SG. A randomized study of the surgical management of children with persistent otitis media with effusion associated with a hearing impairment. *Journal of Laryngology and Otology* 1993; **107**:284–9.
14. *Effective Health Care Bulletin no 4*. The treatment of persistent glue ear in children. Leeds: University of Leeds, 1992.
15. *Otitis media with effusion in young children*. US Department Health and Human Services; 1994; AHCPR publication no 94-0622. (Clinical practice guideline; no 12).
16. Chalmer D, Stewart I, Silva P, Mulvena A. Otitis media with effusion in children – the Dunedin Study. Oxford: MacKeith Press, 1989.

CHAPTER 27

Chronic suppurative otitis media – mucosal disease

ROBIN YOUNGS

Definitions and terminology

Otologists for many years have attempted to establish a uniform terminology to describe the clinical and pathological features of chronic middle ear disease (see Chapter 23). The lack of universally accepted definitions is testimony to the difficulty involved in this process.

The basic feature common to all cases of chronic suppurative otitis media is the presence of a non-intact tympanic membrane. With this in mind a relatively simple working definition of these conditions is 'chronic or intermittent otorrhoea through a persistent non-intact tympanic membrane'. The reference to a non-intact tympanic membrane in most cases denotes a perforation, but can also include discharge through a ventilation tube.

Perforations in the tympanic membrane are described according to their anatomical location. Central perforations are in the pars tensa and are surrounded by some residual tympanic membrane or at

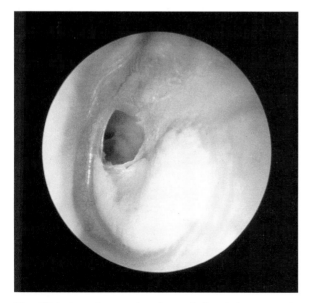

Fig 27.1 Anterior perforation of the left tympanic membrane.

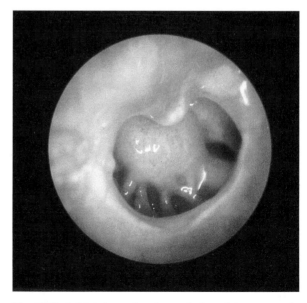

Fig 27.2 Subtotal perforation of the right tympanic membrane.

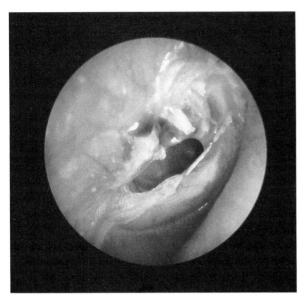

Fig 27.3 Marginal perforation of the right tympanic membrane.

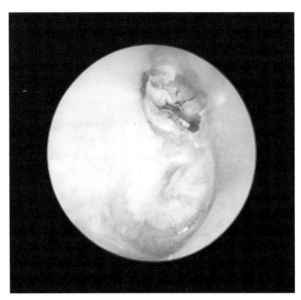

Fig 27.4 Attic perforation of the right tympanic membrane.

least the annulus. The location of central perforations is denoted by their relationship to the handle of the malleus. These defects can hence be termed as anterior (Fig 27.1 and Plate section), posterior, inferior or subtotal. A subtotal perforation is a large defect surrounded by a completely intact annulus (Fig 27.2 and Plate section). Marginal perforations usually occur in the posterior part of the tympanic membrane with pathological loss of the annulus allowing direct exposure of the bony canal wall (Fig 27.3 and Plate section). Attic perforations occur as defects of the pars flaccida (Fig 27.4 and Plate section).

Central perforations are only rarely associated with cholesteatoma. As the presence of cholesteatoma has traditionally been associated with the complications of chronic suppurative otitis media, central perforations are often referred to as 'safe'. Marginal and attic perforations are commonly associated with cholesteatoma and are often termed 'unsafe'. A fuller discussion of cholesteatoma and the concept of the 'unsafe' ear will be found in subsequent chapters.

As central perforations expose the mucosa of the middle ear and Eustachian tube orifice, their presence is often denoted by the term 'tubotympanic disease' (Fig 27.5).

Marginal and attic defects expose the anatomical structures of the attic, antrum and mastoid cell system and are referred to as 'attico-antral disease' (Fig 27.6). It should be emphasized however, that

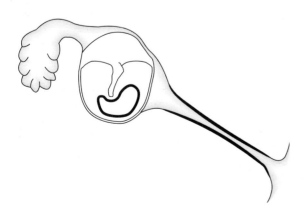

Fig 27.5 Tubotympanic chronic suppurative otitis media.

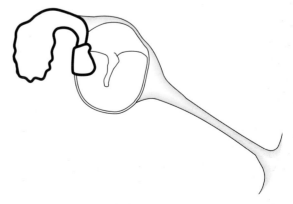

Fig 27.6 Attico-antral chronic suppurative otitis media.

not all cases fit conveniently into these categories and there is often considerable overlap in pathological terms. In individual cases there is no substitute for an accurate anatomical description of the tympanic membrane defect and associated macroscopic middle ear pathology.

Aetiology

Traditionally the pathogenesis of chronic suppurative otitis media is considered to be the chronic stage that follows an attack of acute otitis media in which a perforation has developed, followed by continuous otorrhoea. In the past necrotizing streptococcal otitis media and the otitis media complicating acute exanthemata led to large residual tympanic membrane perforations. These severe infections are now, however, much less common. In addition, the vast majority of perforations complicating acute suppurative otitis media heal spontaneously. In most cases the development of chronic suppurative otitis media is insidious, patients often presenting with no previous history of acute suppurative otitis media. These factors indicate that the link between acute and chronic otitis media is frequently tenuous.

Many otologists consider there to be more of a relationship between chronic suppurative otitis media and persistent middle ear effusions. It has been shown that in patients with chronic secretory otitis media with effusion there is histological degeneration of the lamina propria of the tympanic membrane, with a decrease in thickness of the fibrous layers.[1] This weakness of the tympanic membrane could predispose to breakdown and perforation formation, with less possibility of spontaneous healing.

There are certain anatomical features that are associated with chronic suppurative otitis media. Abnormal Eustachian tube function is a predisposing factor seen in children with cleft palate and Down's syndrome. The presence of a patulous Eustachian tube, allowing reflux of nasopharyngeal contents, may account for the high incidence of chronic suppurative otitis media in North American Inuits. An additional host factor associated with a relatively high incidence of chronic suppurative otitis media is systemic immune deficiency. Abnormalities of humoral (e.g. hypogammaglobulinaemia) and cell-mediated (e.g. HIV infection, lazy leucocyte syndrome) can manifest as a chronically discharging ear.

It is known that chronic middle ear disease is often associated with poor mastoid pneumatization. Although mastoid 'pneumatization' begins in the latter half of embryonic development, the greater part of this process takes place in the first five years of life. Complete pneumatization is not present until adult life. There are several possible explanations for the association between chronic middle ear disease and poor mastoid pneumatization:

- infection in infancy or early childhood prevents normal cellular development
- infection within a pneumatized cleft provokes sclerosis, with obliteration of the cells
- failure of air-cell development predisposes to all varieties of the disease.

There is evidence to support each of these three hypotheses. Particularly strong evidence is found in the study of temporal bone histopathology, which shows new bone formation and sclerosis to be an important part of the overall disease process.

In addition to perforations occurring as part of the natural history of chronic suppurative otitis media, a large number of iatrogenic perforations are created by the insertion of ventilation tubes in the surgical treatment of chronic secretory otitis media with effusion. Various studies have shown that up to 50 per cent of ears with ventilation tubes will suffer with at least one episode of otorrhoea, and that up to 3 per cent will have persistent discharge lasting for more than 6 weeks.[2] It is likely that the pathogenesis of chronic infection in the middle ear cleft when a ventilation tube is *in situ* is similar to that found when a perforation is present. After spontaneous extrusion of ventilation tubes most tympanic membrane defects heal spontaneously. A proportion of ears, however, will have residual tympanic membrane defects (Fig 27.7 and Plate section).

With simple short-term ventilation tubes the residual perforation rate is approximately 2–3 per cent.[3] With long-stay ventilation tubes such as the Goode T-tube the residual perforation rate is much higher; 47.5 per cent has been reported.[4]

The development of chronic suppurative otitis media depends on the persistence of the tympanic membrane defect, which provides a pathway for bacterial contamination of the middle ear cleft from the external auditory canal. The tympanic membrane possesses remarkable properties of regeneration which are seen best after traumatic perforations (Fig 27.8 and Plate section). The healing of tympanic membrane defects depends on the proliferation of connective tissue and squamous epithelium at the margins of the defect. The defect is closed by an acceleration of the normal process of epithelial migration that takes place on the surface of the tympanic membrane.

There are a number of factors responsible for the persistence of tympanic membrane perforations in chronic suppurative otitis media.

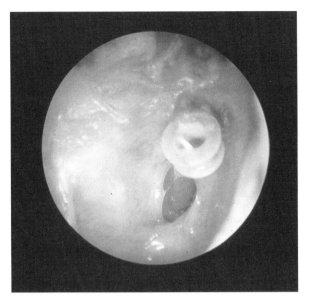

Fig 27.7 An extruding ventilation tube with a residual perforation of the right tympanic membrane.

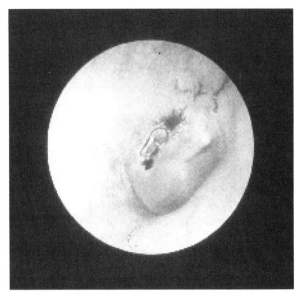

Fig 27.8 Healing traumatic perforation of the right tympanic membrane.

- Persistent infection in the middle ear and mastoid results in continued production of purulent otorrhoea. The perforation acts as a continuous drainage pathway from the middle ear to the external canal.
- Continued Eustachian tube obstruction retards spontaneous closure of the perforation.
- Some perforations are too large to undergo spontaneous closure through the mechanisms of epithelial migration.
- At the margins of a perforation the squamous epithelium can overgrow and impinge on the medial side of the tympanic membrane. This process also prevents spontaneous closure of the perforation.

Epidemiology

The prevalence of chronic suppurative otitis media varies between racial and socioeconomic groups. But many epidemiological studies of chronic middle ear disease fail to distinguish between ears with and without cholesteatoma. In the UK a prevalence of active chronic suppurative otitis media of 0.6 per cent in the adult population was reported by Browning.[5] A study from Israel[6] estimated the yearly incidence of chronic suppurative otitis media to be 39 per 100 000 children from birth to 15 years of age. This study identified a number of risk factors for the development of chronic middle ear disease, including a history of recurrent acute suppurative otitis media, parental history of chronic suppurative otitis media and overcrowding, at home and in large daycare nurseries.

Chronic suppurative otitis media without cholesteatoma is extremely common in certain racial groups, including native American Indians, Canadian and Alaskan Inuits, Australian Aborigines and New Zealand Maoris. The ear disease in these ethnic groups usually has an early onset, often under 2 years of age. A study of the prevalence of chronic middle ear disease in Maori children aged 4–13 years showed a rate of 9 per cent in 1978, which had dropped to 4 per cent when the study was repeated in 1987.[7] The high prevalence in the initial study was attributed to adverse socioeconomic status, poor housing with damp and overcrowded living quarters and limited access to medical care. The subsequent decrease in prevalence was thought to be due to an overall improvement in living conditions, along with the availability of specialized otological, diagnostic and treatment facilities. The incidence of cholesteatoma in these communities with a high overall rate of chronic suppurative otitis media tends to be low. A study of ear disease in Canadian Inuits found a higher incidence of chronic suppurative otitis media, but a lower incidence of cholesteatoma than the white population in the same area.

Histopathology

The histopathological changes seen in chronic suppurative otitis media vary with the degree and extent of disease. The degree of inflammation seen is related to clinical activity, with the most intense changes seen in ears with continuous otorrhoea.

The middle ear cleft is lined by a single layer of cuboidal or columnar epithelium, which may bear cilia. Goblet cells are a feature of the hypotympanum and the region below the horizontal course of the facial nerve, whereas above and behind this region the lining cells are flat and devoid of glandular structures. The changes occurring in chronic otitis media without cholesteatoma are as follows.

1. A chronic inflammatory infiltrate consisting of lymphocytes, plasma cells and histiocytes develops. Associated with this is increased capillary permeability of the lamina propria of the middle ear mucosa, with mucosal oedema.
2. The middle ear epithelium undergoes transformation to resemble respiratory epithelium found in other sites. This consists of an increase in the number of goblet cells and ciliated cells. In addition the epithelium becomes glandular. This change in character of the epithelium may take place in the mastoid air cells as well as in the middle ear cavity. The secretion from newly formed glands is an important part of the discharge seen in chronic suppurative otitis media.

3. An inflammatory granulation tissue develops during the early stages of healing after destruction of tissue. In some cases florid granulation tissue results in the gross appearance of an aural polyp. The polyp is usually covered by ciliated columnar epithelium (Fig 27.9). Occasionally polyps are covered with squamous epithelium, which may occur by metaplastic change. Although aural polyps can occur in all types of chronic suppurative otitis media, their histological features can be used as a predictor of underlying cholesteatoma, as is discussed in the next chapter. Another chronic inflammatory change seen in some diseased ears is the cholesterol granuloma, which is discussed in more detail below.
4. The late stages of the disease are characterized by a decrease in vascularity and fibrosis. These changes are particularly well seen in the mastoid air cells, in which sclerosis and new bone formation can occur. Tympanosclerosis is a special form of fibrosis often occurring in chronic suppurative otitis media, which also is discussed in more detail below.

OSSICULAR CHANGES IN CHRONIC SUPPURATIVE OTITIS MEDIA WITHOUT CHOLESTEATOMA

The main ossicular lesion is bony resorption. This occurs either as a result of osteoclastic activity in

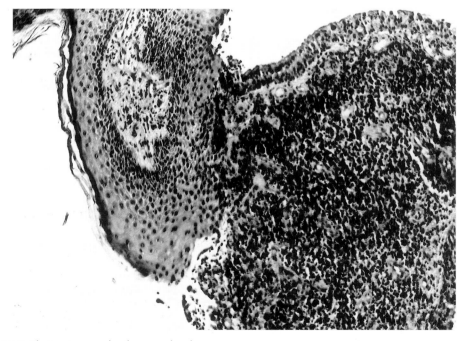

Fig 27.9 Photomicrograph of an aural polyp.

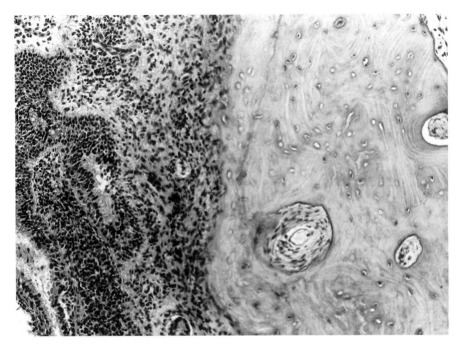

Fig 27.10 Photomicrograph showing ossicular bony erosion adjacent to granulation tissue.

relation to granulation tissue (Fig 27.10) or by avascular necrosis. The parts of the ossicular chain most prone to bony loss by avascular necrosis are the long process of the incus and the stapes superstructure (Fig 27.11). Occasionally, new bone formation can occur, which can have the effect of fixing the heads of the malleus and incus in the attic.

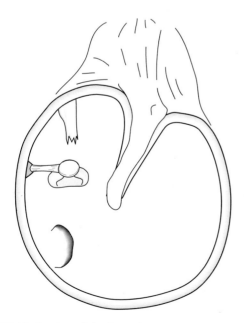

Fig 27.11 Erosion of the incus long process.

CHOLESTEROL GRANULOMA

The cholesterol granuloma is a foreign body granulomatous response to cholesterol crystals, which are frequently formed in the submucosal tissues of patients with chronic suppurative otitis media. The main aetiological factor is thought to be haemorrhage into the middle ear mucosa. Macroscopically cholesterol granuloma appears as yellow-brown semi-solid material that can fill the middle ear and mastoid air-cell system. Microscopically there is a characteristic appearance of cholesterol crystals surrounded by foreign body giant cells and other chronic inflammatory cells (Fig 27.12).

TYMPANOSCLEROSIS

Tympanosclerosis is often associated with chronic suppurative otitis media. It also occurs in the absence of tympanic membrane defects, especially in ears that have suffered with recurrent acute suppurative otitis media. Multiple ventilation tube insertions are a particular risk factor in the development of tympanosclerosis. The macroscopic appearance is of dense white deposits laid down in the tympanic membrane and within the tympanomastoid cavity (Fig 27.13 and Plate section). In the middle ear cleft these deposits may be related to the ossicular chain, particularly the stapes crura

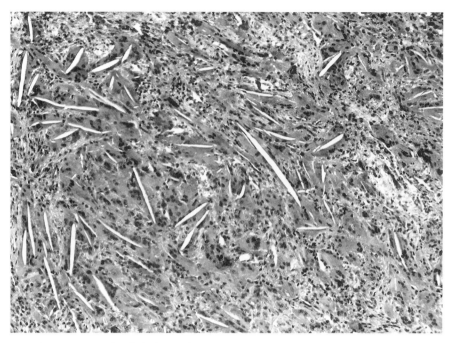

Fig 27.12 Photomicrograph of cholesterol granuloma.

and footplate. Microscopically there is hyalinization of collagen and calcium deposition, with a characteristic lamellar structure. In advanced cases bony change (heterotopic ossification) can occur.

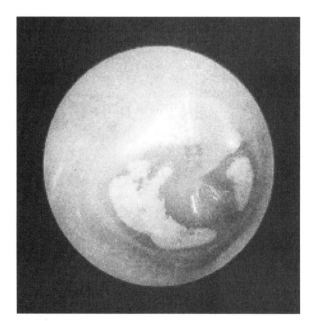

Fig 27.13 Tympanosclerosis of the right tympanic membrane.

Tympanosclerosis is thought to be the result of a specific autoimmune reaction against the lamina propria of the tympanic membrane or the basement membrane of the middle ear mucosa.

Microbiology

Although the development of chronic suppurative otitis media may follow an initial acute infection, the type of micro-organisms found in chronic discharge differ from those found in acute suppurative otitis media. Many studies have investigated the bacterial flora in chronic suppurative otitis media. The commonest organisms isolated are *Pseudomonas aeruginosa*, *Proteus* species (*P. mirabilis* and *P. vulgaris*) and *Staphylococcus aureus*. These organisms are most likely to gain access to the middle ear from the external auditory canal through the tympanic membrane defect. Other organisms found less commonly in chronically discharging ears include *Escherichia coli*, *Streptococcus pneumoniae*, diphtheroids, *Klebsiella* species and the anaerobic *Bacteroides* species.

An additional group of organisms that can cause chronic suppurative otitis media are the *Mycobacterium* species. Tuberculous otitis media, although uncommon in affluent societies, is increasing in worldwide incidence.

Clinical features

SYMPTOMATOLOGY

The two classic symptoms of chronic suppurative otitis media are otorrhoea and deafness, which can affect one or both ears. The discharge can be continuous or intermittent, and varies in character from serous or mucoid to frankly purulent. An increase in the amount of discharge can be precipitated by upper respiratory tract infections or by contamination from the external canal after bathing or swimming. Bloodstained discharge is found in association with florid granulation tissue and aural polyps and is a frequent indicator of underlying cholesteatoma. Persistent otorrhoea unresponsive to medical treatment can indicate a so-called 'mastoid reservoir' of disease with inflammation throughout the middle ear cleft.

The predominant deafness in chronic middle ear disease is conductive in nature. Factors that influence the degree of conductive deafness are as follows.

- The size and position of the tympanic membrane defect: large perforations will reduce the efficiency of the tympanic membrane to a greater degree. Perforations exposing the posterior mesotympanum produce a more severe deafness owing to a reduction of the 'baffle' effect on the round window. Small anterior defects often produce no deafness.
- Impairment of the ossicular chain: this occurs through bony loss, most commonly of the incus long process or stapes superstructure. Ossicular fixation either by new bone formation or tympanosclerosis can also increase the degree of deafness.
- The presence of middle ear pathology such as oedema and granulation tissue can also influence the sound conducting mechanism.

More recently the occurrence of sensorineural deafness in chronically discharging ears has been recognized. A study by Paparella *et al.*[8] found a definite increase in the incidence of sensorineural loss in patients of all ages with chronic suppurative otitis media, ranging from mild to severe. This loss is mainly in the high frequencies and is thought to result from the passage of bacterial toxins across the round window membrane to the cochlea.

EXAMINATION FINDINGS

The principal examination finding in chronic suppurative otitis media is the tympanic membrane defect. As previously mentioned, in ears without cholesteatoma the perforation is almost always of the central type. Perforations can vary in size from a pinhole-type defect to the large subtotal defect. The activity of the disease will be indicated by the degree of discharge. In inactive cases there is no discharge and the middle ear is dry. In active cases the discharge can be mucoid or purulent. Pulsatile purulent discharge occurs in heavily infected cases with capillary engorgement of middle ear mucosa (Fig 27.14 and Plate section).

Depending on the size of the perforation, various middle ear structures may be seen. The middle ear mucosa may be normal or oedematous. In ears with florid inflammation an aural polyp may be present, arising from the middle ear mucosa or the margins of the perforation. In some cases the aural polyp may be large enough to fill the external auditory canal and may manifest at the lateral meatus (Fig 27.15 and Plate section).

The integrity of the ossicular chain can often be observed through the perforation. Ossicular abnormalities most commonly seen are disruption of the incudostapedial joint, necrosis of the incus long process and medial retraction and shortening of the malleus handle. Other middle ear structures visible through perforations are the Eustachian tube orifice, the promontory (with the tympanic plexus) and the niches of the oval and round windows. The actual round window membrane is usually hidden from view and protected by mucosal folds.

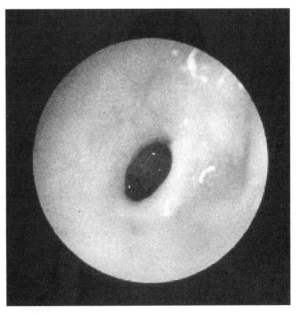

Fig 27.14 Discharging right tympanic membrane perforation.

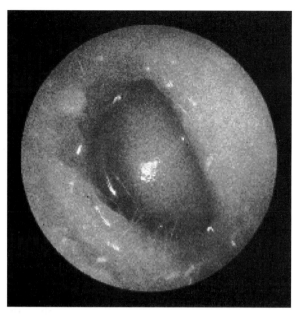

Fig 27.15 Aural polyp manifesting in the external auditory canal.

Other features sometimes observed are secondary otitis externa in ears with profuse discharge and scars in patients with previous otological surgery. The history and examination findings discussed are found in the uncomplicated case. The symptoms and signs of complicated chronic suppurative middle ear disease are discussed in a subsequent chapter.

The diagnosis of tuberculous otitis media should be considered when a chronic perforation and discharge is associated with a progressive and profound hearing loss, particularly when there is no response to routine therapy. In some patients there may be evidence of tuberculosis elsewhere, but often the ear disease is the only manifestation. Tuberculous otitis media is frequently complicated by facial paralysis.

Clinical management

INITIAL ASSESSMENT

When a patient with chronic suppurative otitis media first presents to an otologist a number of diagnostic steps are essential. The most important manoeuvre involves accurate documentation of the tympanic membrane defect. To this end examination with an operating microscope and adequate suction equipment is required. In adults microscopic examination can be carried out as an outpatient or 'office' procedure. In young children, however, a short general anaesthetic is sometimes required, particularly if suction is needed. The nature of the tympanic membrane defect and any associated middle ear or external canal pathology should be noted. A drawing of the tympanic membrane should be made in the case records. The disadvantage of the subjective assessment of ears by

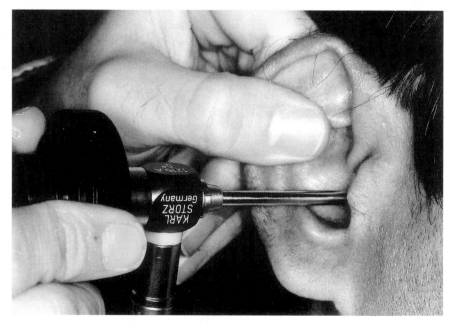

Fig 27.16 Use of the tele-otoscope for examination and documentation.

otoscopy and drawing is the significant inter-observer error found.[9] If available, examination with a rigid lens tele-otoscope is to be preferred. The use of a 4 mm 0° rigid tele-otoscope allows accurate photographic documentation (Fig 27.16). Smaller bore endoscopes with angles of view of 30° and 70° are particularly useful for inspecting the recesses of the middle ear when the presence of cholesteatoma is suspected.[10]

During microscopic examination of the ear, if there is discharge a microbiology swab should be taken. Microbiological investigation should aim to identify aerobic and anaerobic pathogens. The laboratory should be informed of any prior treatment with topical or systemic antimicrobial drugs and of any intention to treat with particular agents so that sensitivity studies can be undertaken.

An assessment of hearing loss should be made, initially by standard Rinne and Weber tuning fork tests (see Chapter 4). Pure tone audiometry with air and bone conduction threshold estimation should be performed. Adequate masking is essential, particularly in patients with bilateral conductive or mixed hearing loss. Speech audiometry is often helpful, and is required for any patient in whom surgical reconstruction is being considered.

Radiological examination is not necessary in uncomplicated cases of chronic suppurative otitis media without cholesteatoma.

MEDICAL TREATMENT

The aim of medical treatment in uncomplicated cases of chronic suppurative otitis media is to eliminate infection and hence control otorrhoea. Correction of hearing loss and re-establishment of an intact tympanic membrane may require a surgical procedure. The successful treatment of chronically discharging ears requires close otological supervision. The treatments available have been somewhat controversial, largely because of the potential risks of topical agents. The various modalities available are described below.

Aural toilet

The removal of discharge from an ear with active chronic suppurative otitis media is an essential prerequisite for successful treatment. At the initial assessment examination with an operating microscope with suction apparatus would have been performed. This microscopic aural toilet may need to be repeated, sometimes daily, until resolution of discharge occurs. Aural toilet is particularly important when topical medication is used, as profuse discharge may prevent the topical agents from reaching the middle ear in sufficient concentration. The use of cotton-tipped applicators by patients, under supervision, can be useful in mopping up discharge from the lateral parts of the ear canal, as long as patients are aware of the trauma that can be caused by inserting the applicator too deeply. Some otologists perform gentle syringing of the ear with isotonic saline at body temperature to remove discharge; this method is not, however, practised widely in the UK or the USA. In patients who have severe canal narrowing due to secondary otitis externa the tympanic membrane may not be visible initially. In these patients attention to the canal skin, with the use of medicated wicks if necessary, is needed as a primary measure.

Topical medications

Topical agents used in the treatment of chronic middle ear disease are a combination of antibiotics, antifungals, antiseptics, solvents and steroids. Preparations are usually in liquid form and should be administered by the displacement method. In this method the ear to be treated is placed uppermost and ear drops instilled. Pressure on the tragal cartilage forces the drops through the perforation into the middle ear. The controversy surrounding topical therapy centres on potential ototoxicity. The commonest antibiotics to be used topically for chronic suppurative otitis media are aminoglycosides, with gentamicin, framycetin and neomycin being common constituents of aural preparations. Aminoglycosides administered systemically are potent cochleovestibular toxins when their serum concentration exceeds known levels. In the UK the 'data sheets' produced by pharmaceutical companies for topical aminoglycoside preparations contraindicate their use in the presence of a tympanic membrane perforation. Nevertheless ear drops containing aminoglycosides are widely used by otologists in treating chronic middle ear disease. Theoretically, topical agents can gain access to the inner ear through the round window membrane. Most studies of the ototoxicity of topical preparations have been performed in laboratory animals in whom the anatomy of the round window niche differs substantially from that of the human. The scientific literature contains sporadic reports of sensorineural deafness associated with the use of topical agents. However, planned clinical studies in humans have failed to show significant sensorineural deafness attributable to their use.[11] In a 1992 survey of US otolaryngologists, 80 per cent believed that the risk of sensorineural deafness due to chronic suppurative otitis media was greater than the risk with ototopical therapy. A common adverse effect of topical aminoglycosides is the development of allergic sensitivity, which is found particularly with neomycin and framycetin. Sensitivity should be suspected when the clinical response is poor, and it may be confirmed by patch testing. Antibiotics other than aminoglycosides have been used topically. Polymyxin B has a broad-spectrum bactericidal activity that includes *P. aeruginosa*, but like aminoglycosides causes hair cell damage in experimental animals. Chloramphenicol otic preparations have a high incidence of local sensitivity reactions. At the time of writing there is optimism that antibiotics of the quinolone group such as ciprofloxacin and ofloxacin may have useful topical activity in chronic ear disease. Topical ciprofloxacin has been used successfully in humans with chronic suppurative otitis media and discharging mastoidectomy cavities without any adverse effects.[12] Ofloxacin has been shown to be a useful systemic agent, and in animal studies has been shown to have no ototoxicity when used topically.[13]

Antiseptics are used in topical preparations partly to create an acidic solution, as most microbes prefer an alkaline environment. Corticosteroids such as hydrocortisone and dexamethasone in topical preparations impart an anti-inflammatory action, which is useful when there is florid oedema of middle ear mucosa.

Systemic antibiotics

The use of systemic antibiotics in chronic suppurative otitis media is limited by a number of factors. In the presence of diffuse mucosal disease there may be poor antibiotic penetration into the middle ear. Aminoglycosides given systemically have to be administered parenterally, with close monitoring of serum levels to avoid ototoxicity; this usually involves in-patient treatment. In the past the use of systemic antibiotics in chronic middle ear disease has been limited by the lack of suitable oral preparations with activity against Gram-negative organisms, particularly *P. aeruginosa*. This situation has changed with the development of quinolone derivatives such as ciprofloxacin and ofloxacin, which have excellent antipseudomonal activity. Ciprofloxacin has been shown to be effective in chronic suppurative otitis media as a sole agent in bacteriologically documented cases.[14]

In children and adolescents the choice of antibiotic is complicated by the fact that quinolone derivatives are contraindicated because of potential side effects. Thus appropriate antibiotics for children must be administered parenterally. This limits the choice in children to broad-spectrum penicillins

(e.g. piperacillin), cephalosporins (e.g. ceftazidime) and aminoglycosides.

The failure of a discharging ear to respond to topical or systemic antibiotic treatment can be due to a number of factors, which often require surgical intervention. There may be poor drainage of inflammatory exudate from the middle ear, particularly with a pinhole perforation or discharging ventilation tube. The presence of persistent osteitis with mastoid granulation will often indicate a poor response to medical treatment. Microbiological factors, including virulent and resistant organisms, may be responsible for failure, and antibiotic penetration may be inadequate. In some patients repeated reinfection via the Eustachian tube may be due to chronic infection in the nasopharynx, palatine tonsils or sinuses, which will require surgical attention.

Additional measures

The application of substances to the margins of a tympanic membrane perforation in order to promote closure has been advocated. A trial of the application of 1 per cent sodium hyaluronate to the margins of central perforations produced a reduction in size in 75 per cent of defects, of which 37.5 per cent showed complete tympanic membrane healing.[15] It seems reasonable that a trial of this type of treatment should be considered before resorting to formal surgical tympanic membrane reconstruction. Another substance used in this way is a dilute solution of trichloroacetic acid, which clearly has to be used with extreme care, administered under microscopic control in suitable patients.

Patients with tympanic membrane perforations should take precautions to avoid the passage of liquid into the middle ear. During hair washing, bathing or showering an effective method is to plug the ear with cotton wool moistened with petroleum jelly. Patients may have to avoid swimming, although the use of ear plugs and a swimming cap may prevent infection in many cases.

The auditory rehabilitation of patients with chronic suppurative otitis media is complicated by the fact that occlusion of the ear canal by a hearing aid mould often causes an exacerbation of middle ear infection. This is a particular problem in patients with bilateral infection who are significantly disabled by conductive deafness. Surgical tympanic membrane reconstruction, if successful, will produce a dry ear with improved hearing and the ability to tolerate a meatal appliance. In the bilateral case if tympanoplasty is not desired or indicated the use of a bone conductor hearing aid will be have to be considered. Osseo-integrated bone-anchored hearing aids (BAHA) (see Chapter 8) are highly successful in patients with bilateral otorrhoea, but require careful patient selection and strong patient motivation.

References

1. Sano S, Kamide Y, Schachern PA, Paparella MM. Micropathalogic changes of pars tensa in children with otitis media with effusion. *Archives of Otolaryngology – Head and Neck Surgery* 1994; **120**:815–9.

2. McClelland CA. Incidence of complications from use of tympanostomy tubes. *Archives of Otolaryngology – Head and Neck Surgery* 1980; **106**:97–9.

3. Larsen PL, Tos M, Stangerup SE. Progression of drum pathology following secretory otitis media. In: Lim DJ, ed. *Recent advances in otitis media*. Philadelphia: BC Decker, 1988:34–8.

4. Von Schoenberg M, Wengraf CL, Gleeson M. Results of middle ear ventilation with Goode's tubes. *Clinical Otolaryngology* 1989; **14**:503–8.

5. Browning GG. Medical management of chronic mucosal otitis media. *Clinical Otolaryngology* 1983; **9**:141–4.

6. Fliss DM, Shoham I, Leiberman A, Dagan R. Chronic suppurative otitis media without cholesteatoma in children in Southern Israel: incidence and risk factors. *Pediatric Infectious Diseases Journal* 1991; **10**:895–9.

7. Giles M, Asher I. Prevalence and natural history of otitis media with perforation in Maori school children. *Journal of Laryngology and Otology* 1991; **105**:257–60.

8. Paparella MM, Morizono T, Le CT, Mancini F, Sipilla P, Choo YB. Sensorineural hearing loss in otitis media. *Annals of Otology, Rhinology and Laryngology* 1984; **93**:623–9.

9. Hampal S, Padgham N, Bunt S, Wright A. Errors in the assessment of tympanic membrane perforations. *Clinical Otolaryngology* 1993; **18**:58–62.

10. Poe DS, Rebeiz EE, Pankratov MM, Shapshay SM. Transtympanic endoscopy of the middle ear. *Laryngoscope* 1992; **102**:993–6.

11. Merifield DO, Parker NJ, Nicholson NC. Therapeutic management of chronic suppurative otitis media with otic drops. *Otolaryngology – Head and Neck Surgery* 1993; **109**:77–82.

12. Esposito S, D'Errico G, Montanaro C. Topical and oral treatment of chronic otitis media with ciprofloxacin. *Archives of Otolaryngology – Head and Neck Surgery* 1990; **116**:557–9.

13. Nobori T, Hanamure Y, Matuzaki T. A study of the influence of ofloxacin on the cochlea after topical administration into the middle ear cavity. *Otologica Fukuoka* 1988; **34**:1028–34.

14. Fombeur JP, Barrault S, Koubbi G, *et al*. Study of the efficacy and safety of ciproflocacin in the treatment of chronic otitis. *Chemotherapy* 1994; **40(suppl 1)**:29–34.

15. Rivas Lacarte MP, Casasin T, Alonso A. Effects of sodium hyaluronate on tympanic membrane perforations. *Journal of International Medical Research* 1992; **20**:353–9.

CHAPTER 28

Chronic suppurative otitis media – cholesteatoma

ROBIN YOUNGS

Definitions and terminology

The term 'cholesteatoma' was first used by the anatomist, Johannes Muller, in 1838. Although Muller meant to describe a neoplasm, the term is actually a misnomer as cholesteatoma is not a true neoplasm, nor does it contain cholesterol. There have been many attempts to replace the term cholesteatoma with a more pathologically appropriate one; none have been successful, however, and cholesteatoma remains the term used by the vast majority of otologists. A simple definition of cholesteatoma as 'skin in the wrong place' is correct on gross microscopic grounds. A more thorough definition of aural cholesteatoma has, however, been provided by Abramson *et al.*[1]

> Cholesteatoma is a three dimensional epidermal and connective tissue structure, usually in the form of a sac and frequently conforming to the architecture of the various spaces of the middle ear, attic and mastoid. This structure has the capacity for progressive and independent growth at the expense of underlying bone and has a tendency to recur after removal.

Traditionally, cholesteatoma has been classified as being congenital or acquired. Acquired cholesteatoma, seen in association with chronic suppurative otitis media, is described as being 'primary' or 'secondary'. Primary cholesteatoma refers to a lesion with no previous history of infection, whereas secondary cholesteatoma is said to follow active middle ear infection. In practice the distinction between primary and secondary

acquired cholesteatoma is often difficult, and the terms are not in common clinical use.

As mentioned in the previous chapter, cholesteatoma is a frequent feature of the so-called 'attico-antral' type of chronic suppurative otitis media. As ears with cholesteatoma are traditionally associated with the complications of chronic ear disease, they are termed 'unsafe' (see Chapter 23).

A useful working classification of cholesteatoma is based on the anatomical site of the disease, with reference to tympanic membrane pathology. This classification is valuable because the different types of cholesteatoma are often distinct from pathological, clinical and therapeutic standpoints. Three

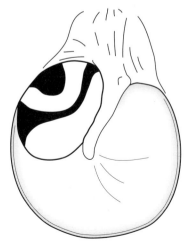

Fig 28.1 Marginal perforation or retraction of the pars tensa with accumulating keratin.

types of cholesteatoma are recognized: pars tensa cholesteatoma, pars flaccida cholesteatoma and occult cholesteatoma.

Pars tensa cholesteatoma results from a retraction pocket or perforation in the posterosuperior quadrant of the pars tensa (Fig 28.1). Granulations and osteitis are found in association in the deep meatus and annulus region. Conductive deafness occurs because of destruction of the ossicular chain, usually the incudostapedial joint.

Pars flaccida cholesteatoma results from a retraction pocket or perforation in the pars flaccida (Fig 28.2). Associated with this type of cholesteatoma is osteitis and destruction of the outer attic wall.

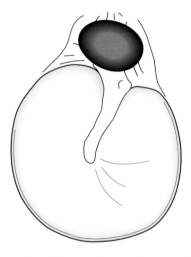

Fig 28.2 Pars flaccida retraction pocket or perforation.

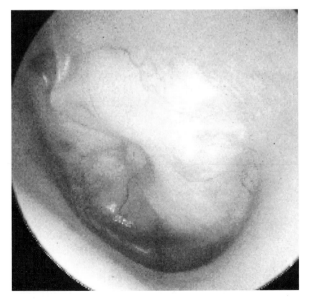

Fig 28.3 Occult cholesteatoma of the left middle ear.

Occult cholesteatoma occurs deep to an intact tympanic membrane and is often congenital (Fig 28.3 and Plate section).

Aetiology

The aetiology of acquired middle ear cholesteatoma has been the subject of long-standing debate in the otological literature. The definition of cholesteatoma as 'skin within the middle ear cleft' is pathologically correct. The difficulty has been, however, ascribing a cellular and anatomical origin to the squamous epithelium in cholesteatoma.

Four main theories have been used to explain the development of cholesteatoma: the presence of congenital cell rests, metaplasia of middle ear epithelium, papillary ingrowth through an intact tympanic membrane, and invagination of epithelium into a pre-existing retraction pocket or through a perforation of the tympanic membrane. Each of these possibilities is considered in more detail below.

CONGENITAL CELL RESTS

Although congenital cell rests are known to account for certain congenital cholesteatomas of the temporal bone, their role in the pathogenesis of the common type of acquired cholesteatoma is doubtful. Recent interest in such a possibility has been heightened, however, with the discovery by Michaels[2] of an epidermoid formation in the anterior epitympanic area of developing fetal middle ears (Fig 28.4 and Plate section). Persistence and

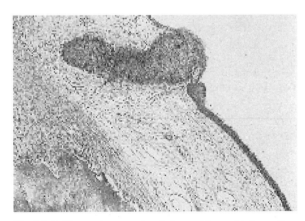

Fig 28.4 Photomicrograph of the epidermoid formation in the developing middle ear. (Reproduced with permission of Professor L. Michaels.)

growth of this structure may account for some true congenital cholesteatomas, particularly as the majority of these lesions are found anatomically to correspond with the location of the epidermoid formation. A relationship of the epidermoid formation to acquired cholesteatoma, which is located primarily in the posterior epitympanic and marginal regions, is unlikely, however.

METAPLASIA OF MIDDLE EAR EPITHELIUM

Sadé *et al.*,[3] in a histopathological study, observed squamous metaplasia of middle ear epithelium in patients with cholesteatoma, particularly when granulation tissue was a prominent feature. They considered this finding as analogous with squamous metaplasia of the lower respiratory tract. Whether purely metaplastic changes can produce a disease process with the clinical features of cholesteatoma is highly questionable, given the common anatomical location of cholesteatoma in the attic and posterior marginal regions. As a result the metaplastic theory of cholesteatoma origin has attracted little in the way of popular support.

PAPILLARY INGROWTH THROUGH AN INTACT TYMPANIC MEMBRANE

Production of a cholesteatoma by papillary ingrowth of epithelium through its own basement membrane has been proposed by Ruedi.[4] Papillary ingrowth, in the proper sense of the term, refers to the development of cholesteatoma arising from the pars flaccida (Fig 28.5). Ruedi demonstrated that in experimental animals cholesteatomas could be generated by the application of foreign material onto the medial aspect of the pars flaccida, with the active proliferation of basal cells breaking through the basement membrane. Extrapolating this finding to humans, Ruedi postulated that cholesteatoma could be generated by an inflammatory reaction in Prussack's space, usually due to poor ventilation in this area.

INVAGINATION OF EPITHELIUM THROUGH A PRE–EXISTING RETRACTION POCKET OR PERFORATION

This theory is the most widely supported mechanism for the formation of the majority of acquired

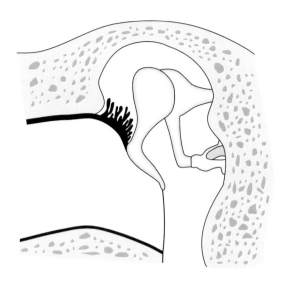

Fig 28.5 Papillary ingrowth through the pars flaccida.

cholesteatomas. The initiating factor in the production of cholesteatoma is functional obstruction of the Eustachian tube, leading to impaired middle ear and mastoid ventilation. Under the influence of fluctuating or sustained negative middle ear pressure the tympanic membrane becomes flaccid and prone to retraction, particularly in the attic and posterior marginal regions (Fig 28.6).

As retraction occurs, associated middle ear inflammation may lead to adhesive otitis media. The posterior marginal and attic 'perforations' associated with cholesteatomas are usually the openings of retraction pockets rather than true perforations. As the retraction pocket enlarges medially and posteriorly, continued desquamation leads to the accumulation of keratin debris and cholesteatoma formation. Although this explanation for the origin of cholesteatoma is attractive, there are almost certainly aetiological factors involved other than Eustachian tube obstruction. Support for the existence of other factors is suggested by the fact that only a small proportion of retraction pockets develop into frank cholesteatomas. Other factors postulated to encourage cholesteatoma formation from a pre-existing retraction pocket include impaired epithelial migration, sudden changes in middle ear pressure and changes in the underlying middle ear space, including oedema, granulation tissue and adhesive otitis media. The relationship between cholesteatoma and chronic secretory otitis media is an interesting one. The two conditions may share a common aetiological factor in Eustachian tube

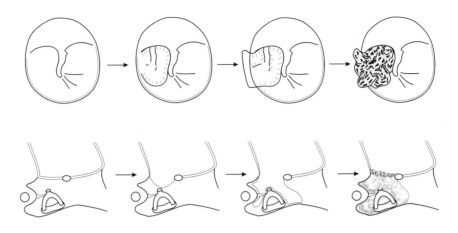

Fig 28.6 Stages in the development of cholesteatoma from the posterior marginal pars tensa.

obstruction. However, whereas chronic secretory otitis media is very common, cholesteatoma is comparatively uncommon. Persistent chronic secretory otitis media, however, has been shown to be associated with a greater inflammatory reaction in the posterior quadrant of the pars tensa and pars flaccida,[5] which may partially explain the development of retraction and cholesteatoma in these sites.

If the invagination–retraction theory were true, the epithelium in cholesteatoma would be identical to that surrounding posterior marginal and attic retractions (i.e. deep ear canal skin and pars flaccida). The most convincing evidence for this notion comes from the study of cytokeratin profiles. Cytokeratins are cellular proteins found in all epithelial cells. Many different cytokeratins have been identified through the use of monoclonal antibody techniques. Each type of epithelium has a unique cytokeratin profile. The cytokeratin profile in cholesteatoma has been found to be identical to that of auditory canal skin.[6] In contrast, middle ear mucosa has a cytokeratin profile different from that of cholesteatoma, suggesting that metaplasia of middle ear epithelium is not the source of cholesteatoma. In addition other ultrastructural studies have shown a close similarity between cholesteatoma, ear canal skin and pars flaccida.[7]

Epidemiology

A study of cholesteatoma in the USA[8] revealed a prevalence in the general population of 6 per 100 000. Within this population cholesteatoma was most common in children aged 10–19 years, with a prevalence of 9.2 per 100 000.

Cholesteatoma is particularly common in children with cleft palate; one study indicated a prevalence of 7.1 per cent.[9] The frequent association of cleft palate with cholesteatoma is thought to be due to functional Eustachian tube obstruction. In racial groups with a high incidence of central tympanic membrane perforations, such as North American Inuits and Australian Aborigines, cholesteatoma is relatively uncommon.

The experience of most otologists in the UK over the past 20 years has been of an apparent decrease in the incidence of cholesteatoma. Over the same period there has been a marked increase in the diagnosis and surgical treatment of chronic secretory otitis media. The relationship between cholesteatoma and chronic secretory otitis media is complex, with many factors involved. The effect of ventilation tube insertion on the development of cholesteatoma is controversial. At one end of the spectrum is the notion that tube insertion is implicated in the causation of cholesteatoma by implantation of epithelium at the time of surgery. Certainly a relatively high proportion of patients with cholesteatoma have a history of previous ventilation tube insertion. This association, however, probably reflects the severity of disease in a high risk group. At the other end of the spectrum, some otologists consider the insertion of ventilation tubes a measure to prevent the development of cholesteatoma. A study from Liverpool[10] has shown that between 1963 and 1990 there was a marked rise in ventilation tube insertion and a decrease in the incidence of surgery for cholesteatoma. Although insertion of a ventilation tube can result in lateralization of an atelectatic, retracted tympanic membrane, this effect is only apparent while the tube is *in situ*. It is unlikely that ventilation tube insertion alters the eventual outcome in ears that develop cholesteatoma.

Histopathology

Macroscopically cholesteatoma appears as a cyst-like structure in the middle ear cleft that contains pale debris. Light microscopy reveals a number of component parts. The capsule of the cholesteatoma, or matrix, consists of fully differentiated stratified squamous epithelium resting on connective tissue (Fig 28.7).

The squamous epithelium differs from skin by the absence of appendages such as glands or hair follicles. The central pale core of cholesteatoma is composed of anucleate keratin squames. As in non-cholesteatomatous chronic suppurative otitis media other pathological features are found, including aural polyps, foreign body granulomas and granulation tissue. As mentioned in the previous chapter the histological nature of aural polyps can be used to predict the presence of underlying cholesteatoma. Milroy *et al.*[11] concluded that the finding of a combination of raw granulation tissue with keratin as masses or flakes in an aural polyp made the presence of an underlying cholesteatoma

highly likely, with a probability of between 70 and 80 per cent. Conversely the absence of these features, coupled with the presence of a covering epithelium, a connective tissue core, glands and lymphoid aggregates, provides a 70–80 per cent probability of there being no underlying cholesteatoma. A particular type of foreign body granuloma found in association with cholesteatoma is caused by an inflammatory reaction to keratin squames, which become surrounded by foreign body giant cells (Fig 28.8).

The subepithelial connective tissue of cholesteatoma is of varying thickness and contains inflammatory infiltrate and fibroblasts. The fibrous reaction can be intense and in extreme cases heterotopic ossification is found. One type of cell found in relatively high numbers in cholesteatoma is the epidermal Langerhans cell, thought to be an epidermal macrophage important in the activation of the body's immune response to cholesteatoma.[12]

INTERACTION OF CHOLESTEATOMA WITH BONE

The principal clinical features of cholesteatoma are attributable to its interaction with the bone of the ossicular chain and the bony walls of the middle ear

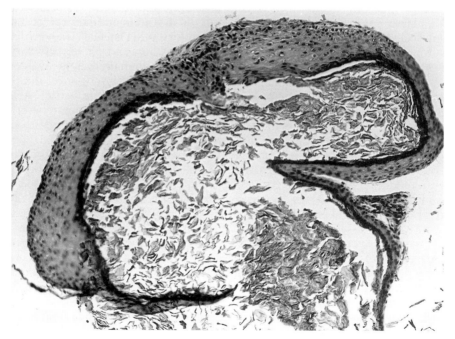

Fig 28.7 Photomicrograph of a cholesteatoma 'pearl' with squamous epithelium and a central core of keratin squames.

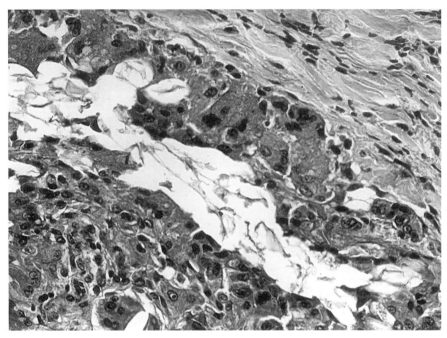

Fig 28.8 Photomicrograph of a keratin foreign body granuloma.

and mastoid. This feature of cholesteatoma is dependent on its ability to erode any bone in contact with the squamous epithelium. The parts of the ossicular chain most susceptible to erosion are the incus long process and the stapes superstructure. Potential complications of cholesteatoma occur with erosion of bone covering the lateral semicircular canal, Fallopian canal (VIIth nerve) and the dura of the middle and posterior cranial fossae.

The mechanisms of bony erosion in cholesteatoma are not completely understood. For many years it was thought that the physical pressure of cholesteatoma caused bony loss; it is likely, however, that other factors are responsible. At a cellular level the chief factor in bony erosion is activation of osteoclasts. Recent research has implicated the release of inflammatory mediators such as the cytokine interleukin-1α from macrophages and epidermal keratinocytes as being important in osteoclast activation.[13] Other humoral factors that have been suggested are prostaglandins, cathepsin D and a parathyroid hormone-like protein. In addition to bony erosion, new bone formation (osteoneogenesis) can occur in association with cholesteatoma. This phenomenon has been found mostly in the attic and mastoid antrum regions and is thought to be a response to infection in the early stages of the disease.[14]

Microbiology

Organisms cultured from the discharge in an infected cholesteatoma are similar to those found in chronic suppurative otitis media without cholesteatoma. The most common organisms found are the Gram-negative *Pseudomonas aeruginosa* and *Proteus* species. In approximately 50 per cent of infected cholesteatomas a mixture of aerobic and anaerobic organisms can be identified.[15]

Clinical features

The cardinal symptoms of chronic suppurative otitis media are purulent otorrhoea and progressive conductive deafness. These symptoms apply regardless of the presence of underlying cholesteatoma, and it is doubtful whether a diagnosis of cholesteatoma can be made purely on symptomatic grounds. A study of 99 patients with cholesteatoma compared symptoms at presentation with those of a similar number of patients who had chronic suppurative otitis media without cholesteatoma and found no significant difference between the two groups.[16] The discharge from an ear with cholesteatoma is often said to be offensive, probably because of infection within accumulations of keratin debris. The advent of a bloodstained discharge indicates the presence of granulation tissue and underlying osteitis. The presence of otalgia, headache or vertigo suggests the possibility of serious complications and merits further investigation.

The natural history of untreated cholesteatoma is progressive expansion at the expense of the bony structures and confines of the middle ear cleft. The rate of growth of cholesteatoma varies markedly from patient to patient. Small slow-growing cholesteatomas can often be relatively asymptomatic, only discovered as an incidental finding, whereas extensive cholesteatomas in well pneumatized mastoids can undergo rampant growth. The factors determining the rate of growth of cholesteatoma are poorly understood. Progressive growth in some cases will lead to the development of complications, intratemporal and intracranial. The complications of otitis media will be discussed in detail in the next chapter. In some cases erosion of the outer attic wall and posterior ear canal wall can result in the production of large cavities, similar to those created surgically. These spontaneous cavities, often known as autoatticotomy and automastoidectomy, can eventually achieve a stable epithelial lining and be relatively free of symptoms.

The clinical features of acquired cholesteatoma vary to some extent with the anatomical site of the disease; pars tensa and pars flaccida cholesteatomas differ slightly in their manifestations.

PARS TENSA CHOLESTEATOMA

Development of a pars tensa cholesteatoma follows chronic impairment of middle ear ventilation in association with recurrent acute suppurative otitis media and chronic secretory otitis media. Loss of the fibrous middle layer of the tympanic membrane occurs preferentially in the posterosuperior quadrant of the tympanic membrane and leads to retraction onto the incus long process, incudostapedial joint and the promontory. Repeated inflammation in the middle ear cleft leads to adhesions between the drum and the medial wall of the middle ear, and the development of a fixed retraction pocket. Retention of squamous epithelium in the retraction pocket heralds the production of cholesteatoma. In this site cholesteatoma tends to envelop and invaginate the structures in the posterior mesotympanum (Fig 28.9).

The ossicular chain is involved at a relatively early stage; marked conductive deafness is caused by loss of the incus long process and stapes superstructure. Occasionally the hearing is relatively well preserved, however, by a retraction directly

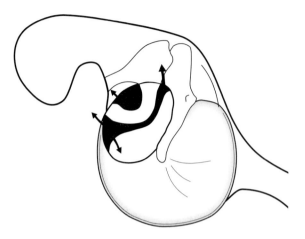

Fig 28.9 Extension of pars tensa cholesteatoma.

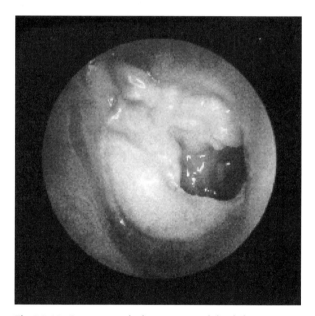

Fig 28.10 Pars tensa cholesteatoma of the left ear.

onto the stapes head or bridging of an ossicular chain defect by cholesteatoma. Invagination of the cholesteatoma into the facial recess, sinus tympani and round window niche occurs. Involvement of these less accessible sites account for the frequent difficulty in surgical eradication of this type of cholesteatoma. Examination of a pars tensa cholesteatoma reveals the cholesteatoma sac to be in continuity with the skin of the deep ear canal. In the region of the posterior annulus there is often exposed bone that can be the site of osteitis and granulation tissue (Fig 28.10 and Plate section).

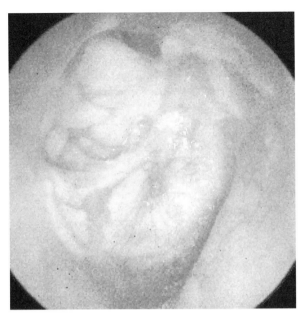

Fig 28.11 Pars flaccida cholesteatoma of the right ear.

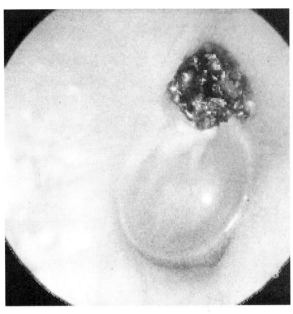

Fig 28.13 Crust in the right attic overlying a cholesteatoma.

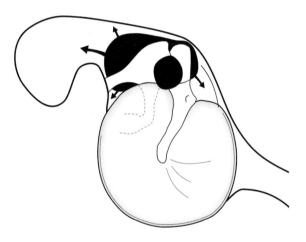

Fig 28.12 Extension of pars flaccida cholesteatoma.

PARS FLACCIDA CHOLESTEATOMA (ATTIC CHOLESTEATOMA)

The epithelium of the cholesteatoma sac is continuous with that of the pars flaccida and, viewed from the ear canal, the accumulation of white keratin debris indicative of cholesteatoma is often visible (Fig 28.11 and Plate section).

Cholesteatoma in this site is thought to occur by progressive enlargement of an attic retraction pocket, with eventual retention of desquamated keratin. Pars flaccida cholesteatoma is frequently associated with osteitis, granulation tissue and erosion of the outer attic wall, or scutum. As the cholesteatoma expands, the ossicular heads of the malleus and incus become surrounded by squamous epithelium. Erosion of the ossicular heads occurs relatively late in the disease process, and it is not uncommon to encounter a large pars flaccida cholesteatoma with an intact ossicular chain and a relatively minor degree of conductive deafness. Further progression of disease occurs anteriorly into the anterior epitympanum and posteriorly into the mastoid antrum and air-cell system (Fig 28.12).

In some pars flaccida cholesteatomas a relatively small external defect can be covered by a crust that overlies an extensive cholesteatoma (Fig 28.13 and Plate section). Only after removal of the attic crust is the epithelial debris typical of cholesteatoma apparent.

Clinical assessment

INITIAL ASSESSMENT

As in all cases of chronic suppurative otitis media, accurate documentation of tympanic membrane pathology is essential when cholesteatoma is suspected. To this end examination with an operating microscope with the availability of adequate suction equipment is required. A general anaesthetic may be necessary to achieve this in children. Particular note should be made of the site and extent of the

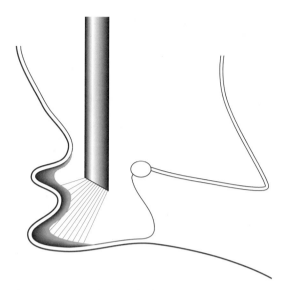

Fig 28.14 Use of an angled tele-otoscope in the examination of the facial recess and sinus tympani.

tympanic membrane defect, the presence and extent of squamous epithelium and keratin debris, the involvement of the ossicular chain and the presence of inflammatory polyps, granulation tissue or osteitis. If possible, examination with a rigid lens otoscope and otophotography should be undertaken. Rigid endoscopes are particularly useful in assessing the extent of cholesteatoma. The use of angled endoscopes permit examination of the facial recess and sinus tympani, which are frequently involved in pars tensa cholesteatoma (Fig 28.14). At the time of initial examination a microbiology swab should be taken of discharge present.

Assessment of auditory function should be made initially with standard Rinne and Weber tuning fork tests. Pure tone audiometry with air and bone conduction thresholds is essential. If surgical treatment is contemplated a speech audiogram is required.

RADIOLOGY

Most cholesteatomas will eventually be treated surgically and the requirements for radiology have to be considered with this in mind. In general terms radiological documentation of chronic ears with cholesteatoma serves two functions: first, the demonstration of underlying anatomical variation and second, the diagnosis of the extent and nature of pathological change. The most important anatomical variation when considering the surgical treatment of cholesteatoma is the extent of mastoid pneumatization, as this may influence the surgical approach undertaken. The surgical creation of a large open cavity in the treatment of cholesteatoma is often associated with poor outcome in terms of persistent otorrhoea, and faced with a cellular mastoid some surgeons would adopt an intact canal wall approach. Other anatomical variations important surgically are the positions of the sigmoid sinus and the tegmen covering the middle fossa dura. For a full discussion on surgical decision-making in the treatment of cholesteatoma the reader is referred to Chapter 30. In order to be useful in diagnosing pathological change, the ideal radiological investigation in cholesteatoma has to be able to detect the characteristic bony erosion, and also to distinguish cholesteatoma from associated lesions such as cholesterol granuloma and inflammatory granulation tissue. It should also be noted that in the interpretation of any radiological investigation for cholesteatoma the comparison between the diseased and normal ear in unilateral cases is of prime importance.

In terms of diagnostic quality the use of plain X-rays in the management of cholesteatoma have been superseded by computed tomography (CT) and magnetic resonance imaging (MRI). However, if surgical landmarks are required, a single plain lateral oblique radiograph will provide useful information on mastoid cellularity and the positions of the sigmoid sinus and tegmen. CT is generally the imaging modality of choice in the assessment of cholesteatoma. CT images can be provided in the coronal or axial planes, with most centres recording slices at 2 mm increments. High resolution CT can demonstrate bony erosion of the tegmen, the lateral semicircular canal and the bony covering of the facial nerve. Ossicular erosion of the malleus and incus is often visible on CT, although stapes erosion is frequently not demonstrated. Cholesteatoma on CT appears as an abnormal mass of soft-tissue density in the middle ear and mastoid, and is impossible to differentiate from fluid, inflammatory granulation tissue and cholesterol granuloma (Fig 28.15).

MRI is inferior to CT in the demonstration of the bony abnormalities associated with cholesteatoma. The primary advantage of MRI over CT lies in the ability of the former to distinguish between differing pathological processes causing soft tissue accumulation in the mastoid and middle ear spaces. Thus cholesteatoma on MRI usually appears as hypointense on T1-weighted and hyperintense on T2-weighted images. The administration of intravenous gadolinium DTPA contrast produces only a thin peripheral ring of enhancement in most cholesteatoma. In contrast cholesterol granulomas and inflammatory granulation tissue nearly always appear uniformly hyperintense on T1- and T2-weighted images and demonstrate intense

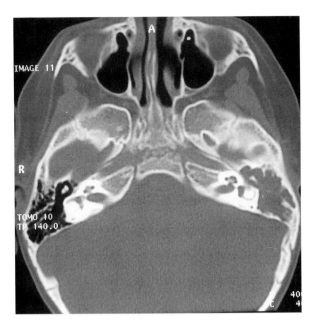

Fig 28.15 CT scan showing extensive cholesteatoma in the well pneumatized mastoid of a child (left ear).

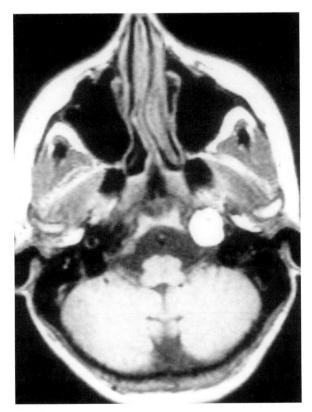

Fig 28.16 MR scan (T1-weighted) showing a cholesterol granuloma of the petrous apex. (Reproduced with permission of Dr Peter Phelps.)

enhancement with gadolinium.[17] This ability to distinguish between cholesteatoma, cholesterol granuloma and inflammatory granulation tissue makes MRI particularly useful in the assessment of petrous apex lesions (Fig 28.16) and when intracranial complications are suspected.

Although CT and MRI can provide useful information on the extent of cholesteatoma, there is considerable debate among otologists regarding the indications for imaging for individual patients. Given that most cholesteatomas are treated surgically, some otologists would argue that preoperative CT should be a standard requirement in all cases of cholesteatoma. Preoperative imaging can be justified if it can conclusively be shown to influence the surgical approach or result in a decrease in postoperative morbidity. This has not been shown to be the case. Leighton *et al.*[18] suggested that CT scanning should not be used in every case of cholesteatoma, but should be reserved for routine use in children to exclude petrous apex disease; medically unfit patients; only or better hearing ears; patients in whom the tympanic membrane cannot be seen; some patients with previous mastoid surgery and patients with intratemporal or intracranial complications, such as a facial palsy. Most cases of cholesteatoma in developed countries do not fulfil these criteria, and probably the only reason for performing preoperative radiology in adults with uncomplicated cholesteatoma is to plan the surgical approach.

Treatment

The principal aims of treating cholesteatoma are to remove the disease and eliminate the risk of major complications, thereby producing a safe ear, dry if possible. An additional objective is to restore the hearing mechanism if this has been compromised by cholesteatoma. The effective treatment of cholesteatoma requires a surgical approach in the vast majority of patients. The surgery of cholesteatoma is considered in Chapter 30.

In addition to surgery, medical treatment has a role to play in the treatment of many cases of cholesteatoma. In patients who are medically unfit for surgery or in some patients with cholesteatoma in an only-hearing ear conservative medical treatment may be the only therapeutic option. On initial presentation many ears with cholesteatoma have active discharge with the presence of granulation tissue and inflamed middle ear mucosa. As in chronically diseased ears without cholesteatoma treatment with a topical agent containing antibiotic and a steroid will often reduce discharge and oedema, facilitating a more thorough microscopic assessment before surgical exploration. The same considerations regarding the potential ototoxicity of topical agents as discussed in the previous chapter apply in the treatment of cholesteatoma. In heavily infected ears with cholesteatoma a course of systemic antibiotic treatment based on microbiological culture of discharge can often produce significant reduction in otorrhoea. As in noncholesteatomatous chronically diseased ears the most frequent organism is *Pseudomonas* species for which the availability of quinolone antibiotics such as ciprofloxacin has been an important advance.

In patients in whom surgery is contraindicated conservative treatment includes attempts to remove accumulation of keratin debris from within the cholesteatoma sac. This is achieved by the application of suction under microscopic control to the mouth of the sac, the so-called 'suction clearance' method of treatment. In addition to suction clearance some degree of symptomatic control can also be obtained by the removal of aural polyps and the application of caustic material such as silver nitrate to florid granulation tissue. When conservative measures for treating cholesteatoma are adopted regular outpatient review is essential. It must be stressed, however, that these non-surgical measures seldom produce long-term symptomatic relief and surgery remains the mainstay of treatment.

The ideal medical treatment for cholesteatoma would be a topical agent that had the potential for either eliminating squamous epithelium or reducing its activity in order to curtail the production of desquamated keratin debris. Recent studies have suggested that the antimetabolite 5-fluorouracil (5FU) may have some useful activity in this respect. The cellular rationale for the use of this agent is the demonstration of intense DNA turnover in the germinal layer of cholesteatoma matrix and an immune response in the subepithelial layers. Initial clinical studies by Sala[19] in which 5FU was applied to the cyst wall in initial cholesteatoma, relapsing cholesteatoma and in large discharging cavities showed inhibition of keratin formation and reduction in otorrhoea.

CHOLESTEATOMA IN CHILDREN

The management of cholesteatoma in childhood presents particular problems, partly because the disease in this group appears to behave in a more aggressive fashion. It is unlikely at a purely cellular level that cholesteatoma behaves any differently from the disease that is manifest in adulthood. There are, however, anatomical reasons for the different clinical features. The chief feature of paediatric cholesteatoma is the frequent association with extensive mastoid pneumatization. In these cases very large cholesteatomas extending throughout the pneumatized spaces of the temporal bone can be encountered. The surgical management of extensive cholesteatomas in well pneumatized mastoids is frequently difficult, accounting for the relatively high postoperative recurrence rate of paediatric cholesteatoma. In cases treated with open cavity mastoidectomy a large unlined cavity in a young child often occurs with troublesome otorrhoea and difficulty with microscopic cleaning. The complications of cholesteatoma such as facial nerve paralysis and lateral semicircular canal fistula are in fact more common in adults than in children, probably because of the longer duration of the disease process in adults. Conversely complications of acute suppurative otitis media are more common in the young.

The discharging open mastoidectomy cavity

The surgical creation of an open mastoid cavity (radical and modified radical mastoidectomy, canal wall down procedure, open-cavity technique) remains the principal method of treatment of cholesteatoma among most otologists. For details of the surgical technique involved the reader is referred to Chapter 30. The management of many patients with mastoid cavities continues on a long-term basis in the outpatient clinic. Despite regular aural toilet and topical medication a significant proportion of patients continue to have symptoms reminiscent of their primary disease, chiefly troublesome otorrhoea. The reported prevalence of intermittent or persistent otorrhoea after open cavity mastoidectomy varies from 20 to 60 per cent.

The occurrence of otorrhoea in mastoid cavities appears to depend upon a combination of mechanical and mucosal factors. Sadé *et al.*[20] identified four factors that determine a dry cavity postoperatively. Small and medium-sized cavities were likely to be dry, as were those with a low facial ridge, a large meatal opening and an air containing middle ear space excluding the Eustachian tube orifice from the cavity. Other authors, although they acknowledge the importance of these mechanical factors, have implicated the lining of the cavity in producing otorrhoea. Rambo[21] attributed the majority of discharging cavities to retained infected mucosa in the mastoid bowl and stressed the need to exenterate all cells that do not drain into the middle ear, particularly cells of the zygomatic root, sinodural angle and mastoid tip.

From a histopathological standpoint the lining of mastoid cavities is predominantly stratified squamous epithelium, with subepithelial fibrosis similar to that observed in middle ear cholesteatoma. A large study of specimens removed from 159 patients undergoing revision surgery[22] revealed a variety of histological features, almost all of which can be found as part of the pathological processes involved in the original cholesteatomatous disease. Of particular significance was the very infrequent finding of discharging cavities with a lining consisting of respiratory epithelium. This suggests that retained mucosa in mastoid air cells is not a common cause of persistent otorrhoea. Some otologists have equated the macroscopic appearances of red, weeping tissue in mastoid cavities with residual 'mucosal' disease, whereas microscopic examination of these areas reveals inflammatory granulation tissue, usually in association with ulceration of squamous epithelium or foreign body granulomas.

The production of a trouble-free 'self-cleaning' mastoid cavity has been assumed to rely on the re-establishment of the process of epithelial migration within the squamous epithelium of the mastoid bowl. The fact that this assumption is correct has only recently been confirmed in a study investigating the migratory pathways in established mastoid cavities.[23]

References

1. Abramson M, Gantz BJ, Asarch RG, Litton WB. Cholesteatoma pathogenesis: evidence for the migration theory. In: McCabe B, Sadé J, Abramson M eds. *Cholesteatoma. First International Conference*. Aesculapius: Birmingham, 1977:176–86.
2. Michaels L. An epidermoid formation in the developing middle ear: possible source of cholesteatoma. *Journal of Otolaryngology* 1986; **15**:169–74.
3. Sadé J, Babiacki A, Pinkus G. The metaplastic and congenital origin of cholesteatoma. *Acta Otolaryngologica (Stockholm)* 1983; **96**:119–29.
4. Ruedi L. Pathogenesis and surgical treatment of the middle ear cholesteatoma. *Acta Otolaryngologica (Stockholm)* 1978; **361 (suppl)**:1–45.
5. Ruah CB, Schachern PA, Paparella MM, Zelterman D. Mechanisms of retraction pocket formation in the pediatric tympanic membrane. *Archives of Otolaryngology – Head and Neck Surgery* 1992; **118**:1298–305.
6. Lee RJ, Mackenzie IC, Hall BK, Gantz BJ. The nature of the epithelium in acquired cholesteatoma. *Clinical Otolaryngology* 1991; **16**:168–73.
7. Youngs RP, Rowles PM. The spatial organisation of keratinocytes in acquired middle ear cholesteatoma resembles that of external auditory canal skin and pars flaccida. *Acta Otolaryngologica (Stockholm)* 19990; **110**:115–9.
8. Harker LA, Koontz FP. The bacteriology of cholesteatoma. In: McCabe BF, Sadé J, Abramson M, eds. *Cholesteatoma: First International Conference*. Aesculapius: Birmingham, 1977:264–7.
9. Severeid LR. Development of cholesteatoma in children with cleft palate. In: McCabe BF, Sadé J, Abramson M eds. *Cholesteatoma: First International Conference*. Aesculapius: Birmingham, 1977:287–92.
10. Roland NJ, Phillips DE, Rogers JH, Singh SD. The use of ventilation tubes and the incidence of cholesteatoma surgery in the paediatric population of Liverpool. *Clinical Otolaryngology* 1992; **17**:437–9.
11. Milroy CM, Slack RWT, Maw AR, Bradfield JWB. Aural polyps as predictors of underlying cholesteatoma. *Journal of Clinical Pathology* 1989; **42**:460–5.
12. Gantz B. Epidermal Langerhans cells in cholesteatoma. *Annals of Otology, Rhinology and Laryngology* 1984; **93**:150–6.
13. Kurihara A, Toshima M, Yuasa R, Takasaka T. Bone destruction mechanisms in chronic otitis media with cholesteatoma: specific production by cholesteatoma in culture of bone-resorbing activity attributable to interleukin-1 alpha. *Annals of Otology, Rhinology and Laryngology* 1991; **100**:989–98.
14. Hoshino T, Ishisaki H, Iwasaki S, Sakai T. Osteoplastic changes in attic cholesteatoma. *Journal of Laryngology and Otology* 1995; **109**:703–6.
15. Karma P, Jokipii L, Ojala K, Jokipii AMM. Bacteriology of the chronically discharging middle ear. *Acta Otolaryngologica (Stockholm)* 1978; **86**:110–14.
16. Aberg A, Westin T, Tjellstrom A, Edstrom S. Clinical characteristics of cholesteatoma. *American Journal of Otolaryngology* 1991; **12**:254–8.
17. Mahmood F, Mafee MD. MRI and CT in the evaluation of acquired and congenital cholesteatomas of the temporal bone. *Journal of Otolaryngology* 1993; **22**:239–248.
18. Leighton SEJ, Robson AK, Anslow P, Milford CA. The role of CT imaging in the management of chronic suppurative otitis media. *Clinical Otolaryngology* 1993; **18**:23–9.
19. Sala DT. Topical applications of 5-fluorouracil in the medical treatment of cholesteatoma of the middle ear. *Ear, Nose and Throat Journal* 1994; **73**:412–4.
20. Sadé J, Weinberg J, Berco E, Brown M, Halvey A. The marsupialised (radical) mastoid. *Journal of Larynogology and Otology* 1982; **96**:869–75.
21. Rambo JH. The use of musculoplasty: advantages and disadvantages. *Annals of Otology, Rhinology and Laryngology* 1965; **74**:535–54.
22. Youngs RP. The histopathology of mastoidectomy cavities with particular reference to persistent otorrhoea. *Clinical Otolaryngology* 1992; **17**:505–10.
23. Youngs RP. Epithelial migration in open mastoidectomy cavities. *Journal of Laryngology and Otology* 1995; **109**:286–90.

CHAPTER 29

Complications of suppurative otitis media

ROBIN YOUNGS

Introduction

Complications of suppurative otitis media occur when infection spreads outside the confines of the bony walls of the middle ear and mastoid spaces. Spread can occur to intracranial structures or can involve structures within the temporal bone itself. Complications are hence known as intracranial or intratemporal and may be classified as in Table 29.1.

The concept of the unsafe ear

Spread of infection outside the confines of the middle ear space can occur in association with acute and chronic suppurative otitis media, and no infected ear can be regarded as completely free from the risk of life-threatening complications. The incidence of complications after acute suppurative otitis media has declined substantially with the availability of antibiotics. However, in parts of the world where acute suppurative otitis media manifests late on in its development or is neglected intracranial complications are a persisting problem. Samuel et al.[1] presented a series of 335 patients with complicated suppurative otitis media from South Africa, 224 of whom had intracranial complications. The majority of complications followed acute infection, with 74 per cent of patients being under 15 years of age. For unknown reasons, otogenic intracranial complications occur predominantly in males.

Table 29.1 Complications of suppurative otitis media

Intracranial complications	Intratemporal complications
Extradural abscess	Facial nerve paralysis
Subdural abscess	Suppurative
Lateral sinus	labyrinthitis
thrombophlebitis	Labyrinthine fistula
Meningitis	Acute mastoiditis
Brain abscess	Subperiosteal abscess
Otitic hydrocephalus	Postauricular fistula
	Petrositis

The traditional view in chronic suppurative otitis media has been to regard ears harbouring cholesteatoma as unsafe. However, the validity of this assumption has been seriously challenged in recent years. There have been reports of large numbers of patients with otogenic complications in whom ears traditionally regarded as 'safe' predominated. Rupa and Raman[2] carried out a retrospective analysis of patients with chronic suppurative otitis media who underwent mastoid surgery between the years 1981 and 1989. The overall prevalence of complications was high, with 122 out of 360 patients having either an intratemporal or an intracranial complication. They found that patients with complications had a short history of ear disease and were more likely to have central perforations rather than pars tensa or pars flaccida retraction pockets, and that cholesteatoma occurred equally in complicated and uncomplicated cases.

The risk of a patient with chronic suppurative otitis media developing an otogenic brain abscess has been evaluated by Browning,[3] in an epidemiological study of the population of the west of Scotland. Browning reviewed the cases of 26 consecutive brain abscesses considered secondary to active chronic suppurative otitis media occurring in the 7-year period from 1973 to 1980. A cholesteatoma was present in 12 (46 per cent) of these patients, mucosal disease without cholesteatoma was present in 10 (38 per cent) and a modified radical mastoidectomy had been performed in four (15 per cent). Browning concluded that chronic ears without cholesteatoma or modified radical mastoidectomy cavities should no longer be considered 'safe'. In a further report Nunez and Browning[4] calculated that the annual risk of an adult with active chronic suppurative otitis media developing a brain abscess was about one in 10 000. They also estimated that the lifetime risk of an individual aged 30 years with active chronic suppurative otitis media developing an abscess was one in 200, commenting that, as yet, there was no evidence that surgery reduced this risk.

From a pathological standpoint many authors have emphasized the almost universal finding of granulation tissue in the middle ears and mastoids of patients with complicated chronic suppurative otitis media regardless of the presence of cholesteatoma. In the 26 patients with otogenic brain abscesses studied by Browning[3] all had active granulation tissue in the middle ear and mastoid. Samuel *et al.*[1] also commented that granulation tissue seemed to play a bigger role in the spread of disease than cholesteatoma in complicated cases. As granulation tissue is usually associated with purulent exudate it seems pertinent to avoid complacency in any ear with active discharge regardless of the site of the tympanic membrane defect.

Routes of spread of infection from the middle ear

There are a number of pathways for infection to spread outside the confines of the middle ear and mastoid and hence give rise to complications of otitis media. The various routes of spread are as follows (Fig 29.1):

- extension through pathological bony defects caused by demineralization in acute suppurative otitis media or bony erosion by cholesteatoma and granulation tissue in chronic suppurative otitis media.
- spread of infected thrombus within small veins through bone and dura to adjacent venous

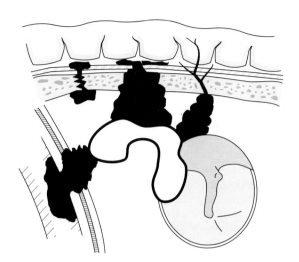

Fig 29.1 Routes of spread of infection from the middle ear space.

sinuses and thence to intracranial structures. Involvement of the lateral sinus is particularly associated with the development of cerebellar abscesses, whereas superior petrosal sinus involvement can lead to temporal lobe abscess formation.
- spread through normal anatomical pathways. These include the oval and round windows, and the cochlear and vestibular aqueducts. In addition anatomical dehiscence of bone covering the jugular bulb, middle fossa dura and the intratympanic facial nerve can facilitate spread of infection to these structures.
- through non-anatomical bony defects caused by trauma, either accidental or surgical, or neoplastic erosion. Iatrogenic defects include the oval window after stapedectomy and lateral semicircular canal fistulae following the fenestration operation. During open-cavity mastoidectomy surgery the middle fossa dura is frequently exposed, leaving in theory a possible route for intracranial spread should the subsequent cavity be the site of persisting granulation tissue or cholesteatoma.
- once into brain tissue infection can spread via the periarteriolar spaces of Virchow–Robin. This spread avoids the cortical vasculature and explains the frequent abscess development in the white matter with no apparent continuity to the brain surface.

In general the spread of infection from the middle ear to adjacent structures occurs in a progressive way from the middle ear cleft to the extradural space and venous sinuses. Passage through the dura leads to meningeal infection and eventually to brain tissue involvement. In keeping with this steady progression in many patients multiple complications are found and should be actively sought.

In addition to anatomical considerations there are other host factors that influence the susceptibility of individuals to developing complications of suppurative otitis media. Decreased immunity from whatever cause can increase the risk of complications. Microbiological considerations also influence the course of suppurative otitis media; particular, virulent strains of organisms (see below) are associated with complications. Another important factor influencing the course of middle ear infection is the availability of treatment for the original suppurative otitis media, whether acute or chronic. Thus economic and cultural factors undoubtedly account for the considerable difference in the prevalence of complicated suppurative otitis media in various parts of the world,[1,5] In populations in which suppurative otitis media is neglected and chronic otorrhoea common, it is frequently the catastrophic development of one or more complications that leads to the seeking of medical advice.

Intracranial complications

GENERAL PRINCIPLES

There are certain features common to the majority of cases of otogenic intracranial suppuration that will be discussed in general terms before individual complications are described in detail.

Symptoms

Once a patient has developed an otogenic intracranial complication there is a significant risk of death as a result. Although the mortality rate has decreased over the years, rates as high as 18.6 per cent have recently been reported.[6] A critical factor in the management of intracranial complications is early diagnosis, hence an awareness of the sometimes subtle initial symptoms is vital. The association of aural discharge with fever and headache should particularly alert the otologist to the presence of intracranial involvement.[7] In addition otalgia and vertigo are frequent early symptoms of ensuing complications.[6] Decreasing levels of consciousness and the onset of convulsions are late features associated with a less favourable outcome.

Microbiology

The infecting organisms in complicated suppurative otitis media will vary depending on whether the initial ear infection is acute or chronic. In complicated acute suppurative otitis media *Haemophilus influenzae* and *Streptococcus pneumoniae* are the commonest pathogens. Organisms from chronically discharging ears are more frequently Gram-negative or anaerobic (*Pseudomonas aeruginosa*, *Proteus* species, *Streptococcus milleri* and *Bacteroides* species). In a study of 75 patients with cerebral abscesses of differing aetiology Pit *et al.*[8] found *Proteus* species, *Pseudomonas* species, and *Bacteroides* species to be almost exclusively associated with abscesses secondary to chronic suppurative otitis media.

Investigations

The availability of high quality diagnostic imaging has been a major advance in the management of otogenic intracranial complications. In particular high resolution CT scanning in axial and coronal planes facilitates accurate diagnosis, and should be urgently requested as soon as intracranial complications are suspected. The administration of intravenous contrast adds to the diagnostic capability and is useful in the diagnosis of brain abscesses and subdural abscesses. Serial CT scanning can be used to follow the response to treatment in individual patients. MRI scanning has a lesser, complementary role compared with CT. The ability of MRI to demonstrate soft-tissue pathology has been shown to be of value in the early diagnosis of brain abscesses.[10] The administration of intravenous gadolinium DTPA can be used to show evidence of meningeal infection.

If meningitis is suspected, a lumbar puncture will be required for examination of cerebrospinal fluid. It must be remembered that lumbar puncture in the presence of raised intracranial pressure carries the risk of 'coning', which has a potentially fatal outcome. For this reason a lumbar puncture should only be performed after a space-occupying intracranial lesion has been excluded by CT scanning.

Microbiological investigation should include microscopy, culture of aural discharge and blood culture. Treatment should not be delayed while waiting for the results of cultures.

Treatment

The successful treatment of otogenic intracranial infection depends first on early diagnosis and then on combined management by neurosurgeon and otologist. In general terms treatment involves the administration of antibiotics, neurosurgical attention and treatment of the underlying ear condition.

The exact choice of antibiotics will depend on local microbiological policy. Suitable agents are given in high doses, intravenously and in combination. Most drugs have been shown to cross the blood–brain barrier if given in sufficient doses, especially in the presence of meningeal inflammation. The pus in cerebral abscesses has been shown to absorb significant amounts of chloramphenicol, penicillin, ampicillin, metronidazole, rifampicin and some cephalosporins. It is routine practice to include an agent active against anaerobes, such as metronidazole, in all otogenic intracranial infections. For the complications of acute suppurative otitis media an example of a suitable initial combination would be chloramphenicol, flucloxacillin and metronidazole, until specific sensitivies are known. In the presence of chronic suppurative otitis media when Gram-negative organisms predominate a combination of gentamicin, ampicillin and metronidazole might be used. Antibiotics are in a constant state of development and it is impossible to be dogmatic about the choice of drugs in this type of publication. It is likely that newer agents, such as new generation penicillins and cephalosporins, and quinolone derivatives such as ciprofloxacin may also play a part in treatment.

The type of neurosurgical attention required will depend on the individual case, and will be mentioned in the discussion of each complication. Needless to say optimum care will involve the active participation of an experienced neurosurgeon with the facilities of a specialist unit at hand.

The treatment of the underlying ear disease will also depend on the individual case and is always secondary to neurosurgical treatment. In acute suppurative otitis media antibiotics alone will often resolve middle ear infection, although occasionally a myringotomy or a cortical mastoidectomy will be required. In cases of chronic suppurative otitis media with intracranial complications definitive surgical treatment is usually delayed until the patient's neurological condition has stabilized. Traditional teaching has recommended the performance of open-cavity radical or modified radical mastoidectomy in all cases of chronic suppurative otitis media with intracranial complications, whether cholesteatoma is present or not. This view has recently been challenged with the proposal to tailor the ear surgery to the underlying ear pathology. In a prospective study of 268 patients with complicated chronic suppurative otitis media Singh and Maharaj[10] performed cortical mastoidectomy in non-cholesteatomatous ears and radical mastoidectomy when cholesteatoma was present. In total they had a mortality rate of 8 per cent, which was unrelated to the type of ear pathology or surgery. They concluded that open-cavity mastoidectomy is only warranted in cases secondary to cholesteatoma.

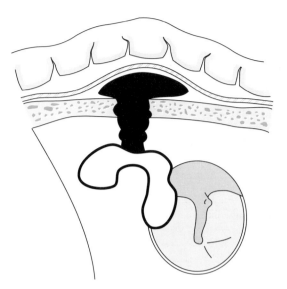

Fig 29.2 Formation of a middle fossa extradural abscess.

EXTRADURAL ABSCESS

Extradural abcess is the most common intracranial complication and occurs after bone demineralization or erosion adjacent to the middle or posterior fossa dura. The size and rate of enlargement depend on the exact location. A middle fossa extradural abscess caused by erosion of the tegmen tympani can strip a large area of dura from the inner surface of the squamous temporal bone, whereas medial extension is prevented by the firm attachment of the dura to the arcuate eminence (Fig 29.2).

Spread of infection from the petrous apex can cause a middle fossa extradural abscess medial to the arcuate eminence and result in irritation of the trigeminal ganglion and VIth cranial nerve producing the triad of symptoms (otorrhoea, facial pain and diplopia) known as the Gradenigo syndrome (Fig 29.3).

A posterior fossa abscess occurs in close association with the lateral sinus and is frequently associated with lateral sinus thrombophlebitis. The spread of posterior fossa abscesses is limited medially by the internal auditory meatus (Fig 29.4).

Apart from the characteristic Gradenigo syndrome, the clinical features of an extradural abscess are often non-specific. As in all intracranial complications the presence of unilateral headache and pyrexia should raise suspicion. If there is free communication with the middle ear there may be relief of pain during periods of otorrhoea.

If any intracranial complication is suspected, a CT scan is mandatory and may demonstrate an

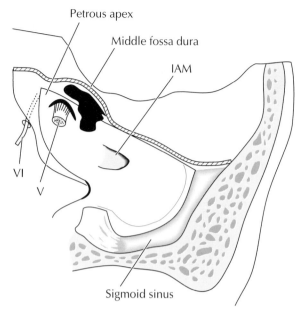

Fig 29.3 Anatomical relations of a petrous apex extradural abscess.

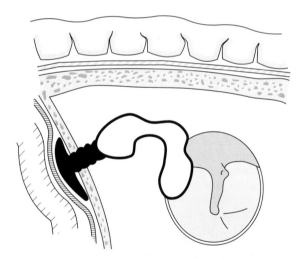

Fig 29.4 Formation of a perisinus posterior fossa extradural abscess.

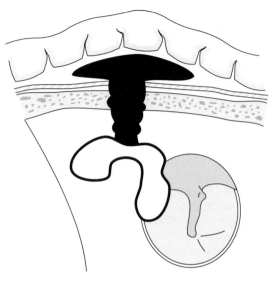

Fig 29.5 Formation of a subdural abscess.

extradural abscess. The diagnosis is confirmed by surgical exploration.

Treatment is by a combination of high-dose antibiotics and surgical drainage. The abscess should be exposed via a mastoidectomy approach, with the most common finding being granulation tissue adjacent to the dura. The bone over the dura should be removed, allowing evacuation of pus, until normal dura is exposed. It is prudent not to remove granulation tissue attached to the dura for fear of creating a passage to the subdural space.

SUBDURAL ABSCESS

Spread of infection through the dura with the formation of granulation tissue in the subdural space heralds the formation of a subdural abscess (Fig 29.5).

Once established, pus spreads over the surface of the cerebral hemispheres and between the hemispheres along the falx cerebri. Some limitation of spread can be provided by obliteration of the space by granulation tissue, and in such cases a multiloculated abscess can occur.

The prime clinical feature of a subdural abscess is the rapidity of neurological deterioration. The onset of headache and drowsiness can be followed within hours by the development of coma and, if untreated, death. Sometimes localizing signs such as hemiplegia and Jacksonian convulsions occur, and signs of meningeal irritation may be present.

The diagnosis of subdural empyema is often difficult, but should always be suspected in the presence of rapid neurological deterioration. Diagnosis is by enhanced CT scanning, although the radiological changes are often subtle (Fig 29.6). MRI may prove a useful adjunct to CT scanning.

The treatment of an otogenic subdural abscess involves a combination of high-dose antibiotics and neurosurgical drainage. The operative measures involved may include multiple burr holes or formal craniotomy and abscess excision, depending on local practice. Postoperative anticonvulsant medication is often required. Surgical exploration of the middle ear is usually delayed until the patient's general condition has improved.

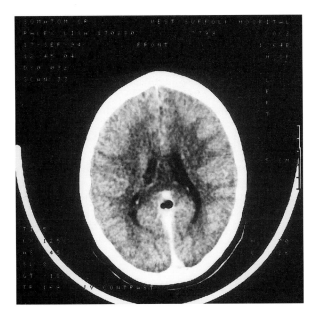

Fig 29.6 Enhanced CT scan showing pus and air between the cerebral hemispheres in an otogenic subdural abscess.

LATERAL SINUS THROMBOPHLEBITIS

In the pre-antibiotic era thrombosis of the sigmoid and transverse sinuses, together forming the lateral sinus, was a common complication of acute ear infections. In recent times this complication has become much less common, and more frequently follows chronic suppurative otitis media. Thrombophlebitis of the lateral sinus is often associated with a perisinus extradural abscess. Development of infected clot in the lumen of the sinus may cause release of organisms into the circulation resulting in bacteraemia, septicaemia and septic embolization. Cranial extension of the thrombus may lead to sagittal sinus thrombosis or may spread to the cavernous sinus via the petrosal sinuses. Caudal extension can occur to the internal jugular and subclavian veins.

The typical presentation of lateral sinus thrombophlebitis is now often masked by antibiotic therapy. Untreated the clinical picture is of a wasting illness with fluctuating pyrexia, rigors and headache developing over several weeks in a patient with chronic suppurative otitis media. Extension of the thrombus leads to additional symptoms and signs. Spread to the neck results in tenderness along the internal jugular vein. Sagittal sinus thrombosis manifests as papilloedema and visual loss, whereas cavernous sinus thrombosis causes proptosis and chemosis. Septic embolization occurs to the lungs and joints. Modification with antibiotics results in a more subtle presentation with fever, otalgia, neck pain and tenderness along the sternomastoid muscle. A rare finding is pitting oedema around the occiput caused by thrombosis in a large mastoid emissary vein – Griesinger's sign. Lateral sinus thrombophlebitis is frequently accompanied by other intracranial complications, particularly meningitis and cerebellar abscess.

The diagnosis of lateral sinus thrombus is now largely based on radiological investigation. CT scanning with intravenous enhancement may show the increased density of fresh clot and filling defects within the sinus. Septic thrombosis shows as intense inflammatory enhancement of the sinus walls and dura, with non-enhancement of the lumen, constituting the 'delta' sign.[11] CT scanning may also demonstrate associated multiple complications. MRI will demonstrate established thrombus with increased signal intensity in T1- and T2-weighted

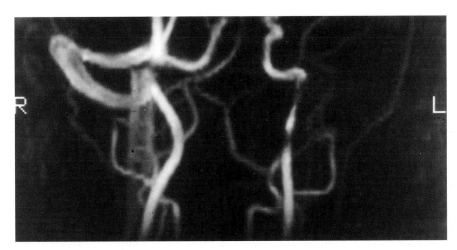

Fig 29.7 MR angiogram showing enhancement in the right sigmoid sinus caused by thrombosis. (Reproduced with permission of Dr Peter Phelps.)

images. Confirmation of diagnosis comes from vascular studies, with MR angiography (Fig 29.7) being the preferred imaging technique. In addition digital subtraction venography can be used, with contrast being administered intravenously without the risk of clot detachment associated with arteriography.

Before the advent of sophisticated imaging the diagnosis of lateral sinus thrombosis was based on blood culture and lumbar puncture, with confirmation by surgical exploration. Although blood cultures should always be performed if the diagnosis is suspected, in recent times cultures have frequently been negative, particularly when the clinical picture is masked by prior antibiotic therapy.

In the past, changes in the cerebrospinal fluid pressures measured by lumbar puncture, constituting the Queckenstedt or Tobey–Ayer test, were thought to be diagnostic of lateral sinus thrombosis. The test entails observing changes in cerebrospinal fluid pressure produced by compression of one or both internal jugular veins. In the normal subject, compression of each internal jugular vein in turn is followed by a rapid rise in cerebrospinal fluid pressure of 50–100 mmHg above the normal level. In a case of lateral sinus thrombosis, pressure over the vein on the affected side causes either no rise or a very slow one of 10–20 mmHg. Compression of the normal internal jugular vein produces a rise of 2–3 times the normal level. The diagnostic value of this test, however, is small owing to frequent false-negative and false-positive results.

Treatment of lateral sinus thrombosis consists of a combination of high-dose antibiotics and surgical exploration through an otological approach. In the past anticoagulation was also recommended. However, there is now general agreement that anticoagulation is only required in the rare patient in whom thrombosis spreads to the cavernous sinus. Internal jugular vein ligation, which in the past was routinely performed, is now thought to be necessary only in patients in whom septicaemia fails to respond to antibiotics, or for septic embolization in children. Once the patient's general condition has been stabilized with antibiotics, surgical exploration needs to be undertaken early in order to expose and remove the infected lesion. In acute suppurative otitis media a cortical mastoidectomy approach is necessary, whereas in chronic suppurative otitis media, an open-cavity mastoidectomy will be required depending on the otological findings. In some patients there will be obvious disease macroscopically associated with the sigmoid sinus, which may include a perisinus extradural abscess. In these instances necrotic bone can be lifted off the sinus walls with blunt probes and curettes. In other patients the bone over the sinus may appear normal and will have to be removed by drilling the sinus

plate until this is thin enough to be gently lifted off the sinus wall. Once the sinus is exposed the diagnosis should be confirmed by inserting a needle through the wall into the lumen. If there is free flow of venous blood the diagnosis of thrombophlebitis was incorrect and no further action is required apart from placing either a small piece of soft tissue or a pack over the sinus. If the sinus appears white and opaque or has a firm feeling on palpation, it should be opened with a sharp instrument and the necrotic tissue, pus and clot removed. It is no longer thought essential to follow an organized clot until the free flow of blood is achieved. If profuse bleeding is encountered the mastoid should be packed with ribbon gauze impregnated with antibacterial material.

MENINGITIS

Meningitis remains the most common complication of suppurative otitis media.[12] Spread of infection to the meninges usually occurs directly through necrotic bone from the middle ear. Another route of spread is as a complication of suppurative labyrinthitis, through the internal auditory meatus or vestibular and cochlear aqueducts.

When the pia-arachnoid becomes inflamed the initial response is an outpouring of fluid into the subarachnoid space, with an increase in cerebrospinal fluid pressure. This is followed by the presence of white blood cells and multiplying organisms, causing the cerebrospinal fluid to change from clear to turbid and finally to purulent. Irritation of upper cervical nerve roots by inflammatory exudate produces the typical features of neck pain and stiffness.

The early symptoms and signs of meningitis are headache, neck stiffness and photophobia. Alternating restlessness and drowsiness occur in adults, with initial hyperactivity in children. Progression causes the neck stiffness to intensify with a positive Kernig's sign. There is usually a high pyrexia and there may be vomiting due to raised intracranial pressure. With further deterioration the level of consciousness steadily decreases with passage into coma. The presence of focal neurological signs or convulsions should raise suspicion of other intracranial complications such as subdural or cerebral abscess.

As in all cases of suspected intracranial complications of suppurative otitis media the primary investigation is radiological, with CT scanning being most frequently used. In pure meningitis the CT scan is normal, although MR images with gadolinium enhancement may show abnormality in the basal cisterns. If a CT scan fails to reveal evidence of raised intracranial pressure, a lumbar puncture should be performed to allow examination of the cerebrospinal fluid should meningitis be suspected. In the early stages there is a rise in cerebrospinal fluid pressure and the appearance of the fluid passes from cloudy to turbid. Polymorphonuclear leucocytes not normally present appear on cerebrospinal fluid microscopy. Biochemical analysis of cerebrospinal fluid reveals a decrease in the glucose level from the normal value of 1.7–3.0 mmol/l to zero, with the appearance of free bacteria. There is also an increase in the protein content. Microbiological examination entails Gram stain and microscopy followed by culture and is often negative, particularly when previous antibiotic treatment has been administered. The mainstay of treatment for otogenic meningitis is the administration of large doses of antibiotics. The choice of drugs depends on the nature of the ear infection, and has been discussed previously. In addition steroid therapy with dexamethasone has been shown to reduce the incidence of neurological sequelae, including deafness, in bacterial meningitis.[13] Repeated lumbar puncture also has a role in management in the early stages to reduce cerebrospinal fluid pressure, and to monitor the response to treatment. Surgical attention to the diseased ear will be necessary once the neurological condition has been stabilized medically.

BRAIN ABSCESS

The incidence of otogenic brain abscess has fallen along with other intracranial complications. Complicated suppurative otitis media remains the principal cause of brain abscesses, particularly in adults. In children brain abscesses secondary to other causes such as congenital heart disease have increased in relative terms but remain less common than otogenic infection.[14] Before the advent of antibiotics the mortality of otogenic brain abscesses was 60–70 per cent. Even today with modern radiological diagnosis and expert neurosurgical management mortality rates of 10–20 per cent are typical.[14]

Otogenic brain abscesses develop either in the temporal lobe or the cerebellum. Temporal lobe abscesses usually follow direct spread of infection through the tegmen tympani, whereas cerebellar abscesses are often found in association with lateral sinus thrombosis. The development of an otogenic brain abscess takes place over a variable period of 1–3 weeks. Initial encephalitis is followed and contained by capsule formation. The brain within the abscess liquifies and the abscess may enlarge to produce features of a space-occupying lesion. If the

capsule formation is slow a multiloculated abscess may form. Untreated the abscess enlarges producing progressively more mass effect. Rupture into the ventricles or subarachnoid space is frequently a terminal event.

The clinical features reflect the stages of abscess development. The initial period of encephalitis is associated with headache, fever and vomiting. With encapsulation a latent asymptomatic period follows, which may last for several weeks. As the abscess enlarges the mass effect and interference with cerebrospinal fluid circulation cause raised intracranial pressure with decreasing conscious level, vomiting, papilloedema, bradycardia and hypopyrexia. The location of the abscess determines the type of localizing signs present. Temporal lobe abscesses are characterized by nominal aphasia, quadrantic homonymous hemianopia and, in the late stages, motor paralysis. Cerebellar abscesses are characterized by muscular incoordination with ataxia, and sometimes coarse spontaneous nystagmus.

Diagnosis of brain abscess is radiological, with enhanced CT scanning being the modality of choice. The typical appearance demonstrates the abscess with an enhancing capsule and surrounding cerebral oedema. As in all cases the scans must be carefully inspected for the presence of multiple complications (Fig 29.8).

The treatment of brain abscess involves a combination of medical and neurosurgical therapy. High

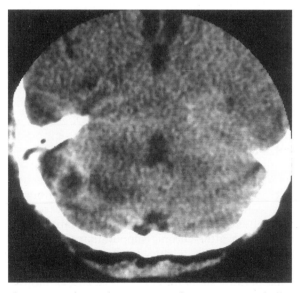

Fig 29.8 Enhanced CT scan showing a cerebellar intracranial abscess in association with a posterior fossa extradural abscess. (Reproduced with permission of Dr Peter Phelps.)

doses of antibiotics are given intravenously and in combination. If there is raised intracranial pressure intravenous dexamethasone and mannitol may be used to reduce cerebral oedema. Neurosurgical treatment involves either repeated burr hole aspiration or abscess excision via a craniotomy. The advent of stereotactic methods to locate the abscess accurately seems to suggest that stereotactic aspiration is the treatment of choice.[15] Aspiration, as well as being therapeutic, produces a specimen for microbiological examination and culture. The high incidence of epilepsy after temporal lobe abscess makes the use of long-term anticonvulsant medication necessary.

OTITIC HYDROCEPHALUS

Otitic hydrocephalus is a rare complication of otitis media, and is most frequently found in adolescents and children. The condition is also known as benign intracranial hypertension and refers to the finding of raised intracranial pressure in association with middle ear infection. The name of the condition is misleading as the ventricular size remains normal. The aetiology of the condition is poorly understood and is thought to be due to impairment of cerebrospinal fluid resorption consequent on superior sagittal sinus thrombosis often after lateral sinus thrombosis.

Clinically the illness follows a chronic course over many weeks, and the original suppurative otitis media may have resolved. The common features are headache, decreased visual acuity, drowsiness, nausea and vomiting. CT scanning will reveal normal ventricular size. Treatment is aimed at reducing intracranial pressure and includes steroids and mannitol. The prognosis for survival is good, although the condition can recur.

Intratemporal complications

FACIAL NERVE PARALYSIS

Facial nerve paralysis may occur as a result of acute or chronic suppuration within the temporal bone. This complication, although uncommon, occurs more often in children after acute suppurative otitis media than after chronic suppuration. The exact pathophysiological changes affecting the facial nerve in suppurative otitis media are poorly understood because of an understandable lack of biopsy or cadaver temporal bone material. The detailed management of facial paralysis is discussed in Chapter 17. There now follows a discussion of facial nerve involvement in middle ear infection.

Acute suppurative otitis media

Involvement of the facial nerve in acute suppurative otitis media results from spread of infection from the middle ear into the Fallopian canal presumably via congenital dehiscences in the canal. The prognosis for nerve recovery is usually excellent providing the acute infection is treated promptly with intravenous antibiotics. Myringotomy and occasionally cortical mastoidectomy may also be required.

Chronic suppurative otitis media

As in all complicated chronic suppurative otitis media, involvement of the facial nerve can occur in cases with and without cholesteatoma. However, facial paralysis occurs much more commonly in the presence of cholesteatoma. The exact pathological processes are uncertain but facial nerve involvement is thought to be the result of infectious processes causing a combination of osteitis, bony erosion, compression resulting from oedema and direct infection of the nerve. As in all complicated chronic suppurative otitis media it seems likely that inflammatory granulation tissue plays an important role. In cases without cholesteatoma there is evidence that a dehiscent Fallopian canal is a frequent finding.[16] Facial nerve involvement is a particular feature of tuberculous otitis media.

The clinical presentation of facial paralysis is variable in its speed of onset. Relatively uninfected attic cholesteatomas can undergo progressive expansion over a long period and can manifest as slowly progressive paralysis, with scant or absent otorrhoea. At the other end of the spectrum a chronically diseased ear with gross infection and florid granulation tissue can manifest with a more rapid onset of paralysis within the space of a few hours. The investigation of choice in facial paralysis complicating chronic suppurative otitis media is the high resolution CT scan. Direct axial and coronal cuts of slices not greater than 2 mm thick will demonstrate the tympanic cavity and facial nerve canal adequately, although expert radiological interpretation will be necessary.

In cases of facial paralysis complicating chronic suppurative otitis media urgent surgical exploration via mastoidectomy is mandatory. There is some debate over the type of mastoidectomy required, with the majority of otologists using a canal wall down, modified radical type of operation. In patients with extensive pneumatization some surgeons advocate a canal wall up approach with posterior tympanotomy to facilitate nerve exposure.[16] Whatever the surgical approach, the middle ear and mastoid should be cleared of disease before attention is focused on the facial nerve. In decompressing the nerve the use of broad flat instruments to allow gentle blunt dissection of disease from the epineurium is essential. If prompt surgical decompression is carried out, the prognosis for facial nerve recovery is good.

SUPPURATIVE LABYRINTHITIS AND LABYRINTHINE FISTULA

In acute suppurative otitis media spread of infection from the middle ear to the labyrinth usually occurs through the round window membrane. Spread can also occur through the oval window niche, particularly if the stapes footplate has been modified by disease or stapedectomy surgery. In chronic suppurative otitis media spread of infection to the labyrinth usually occurs as a result of bony erosion of the otic capsule. The bony covering of the lateral semicircular canal is the most common site of erosion leading to labyrinthine complications.

Suppurative labyrinthitis

Spread of pyogenic organisms into the labyrinth causes a severe insult to the sensitive vestibular and cochlear neuro-epithelium that almost invariably results in permanent vestibular and cochlear failure. Very rarely, with prompt treatment of an early case, the inner ear deficit may be reversible, in which case a retrospective diagnosis of 'serous labyrinthitis' may be made. The clinical features of sudden vestibular failure are prominent, with severe rotatory vertigo and vomiting in association with profound unilateral deafness. The principal clinical sign is spontaneous horizontal nystagmus. In the initial stages an irritative nystagmus with the fast component towards the affected ear is occasionally seen. This is soon replaced by a paralytic nystagmus, usually of third degree, with the fast component away from the affected ear. As in other types of sudden vestibular failure, recovery takes place by contralateral compensation over a period of days and weeks. Poor balance in the dark and in the absence of visual fixation and positional vertigo may persist for longer periods. Infection is usually confined to the ear, and constitutional signs such as pyrexia are usually absent. Otoscopic examination will reveal the underlying otological pathology.

Investigation should include a CT scan to locate possible sites of labyrinthine erosion and to exclude other complications. Cerebellar abscess can manifest with disequilibrium and, although the distinction from suppurative labyrinthitis can usually be made on clinical grounds, radiological back-up is essential.

The treatment of suppurative labyrinthitis in the initial stages is predominantly medical, although vestibular and cochlear failure are usually permanent. Intravenous antibiotics are given in combination in order to treat the middle ear infection and to prevent meningitis. It is doubtful whether antibiotics can alter the course of the labyrinthine damage itself. Vestibular symptoms are suppressed by parenteral administration of sedatives such as prochlorperazine while complete bedrest is observed. Surgical treatment of the underlying middle ear disease may be required and should be delayed until the initial vertigo has subsided. In the long term the symptoms of vestibular deficit can often be alleviated by vestibular rehabilitation exercises of the Cawthorne–Cooksey type.

Labyrinthine fistula

Erosion of the bony covering of the labyrinth and exposure of the underlying endosteum occurs as a complication of chronic suppurative otitis media, usually with cholesteatoma. This places the ear at risk from suppurative labyrinthitis. The arch of the lateral semicircular canal is the most common site, although the other semicircular canals and the vestibule can also be exposed.

The most common symptom of a labyrinthine fistula is short-lived episodic vertigo. The vestibular symptoms are often non-specific, however, and the diagnosis must be suspected in any vertiginous patient with chronic middle ear disease. The principal diagnostic indicator of labyrinthine erosion is a positive fistula sign (see Chapter 3). This test depends on the production of eye movement and vertigo by increasing the pressure in the external auditory canal, thereby causing stimulation of the exposed membranous labyrinth. Although this sign can be elicited by tragal pressure, it is best provoked by the use of a pneumatic otoscope with a well fitting speculum. With a fistula of the arch of the lateral semicircular canal an increase in pressure causes an immediate conjugate deviation of the eyes away from the affected side. Maintenance of pressure causes an irritative nystagmus towards the affected ear. As the pressure is released the eyes return to the midline. The nystagmus is accompanied by the sensation of vertigo. If other parts of the labyrinth are affected the ocular deviation may differ. A lateral canal fistula anterior to the ampulla causes deviation of the eyes towards the affected ear. A superior canal fistula causes rotatory deviation away from the affected ear, whereas a posterior canal fistula causes vertical deviation. Finally, erosion of the vestibule cause rotatory horizontal deviation towards the affected ear. A false-negative fistula sign can occur if the seal of the speculum in the external canal is inadequate, or if the fistula is 'cushioned' by a collection of epithelial debris. A false-positive fistula sign in the presence of an intact tympanic membrane is known as Hennebert's sign. At one time Hennebert's sign was thought to be diagnostic of labyrinthine syphilis, although this is almost certainly not the case. More recently a positive fistula sign has been equivocally related to the presence of a perilymph fistula.

Extensive erosion of the labyrinth by cholesteatoma with loss of vestibular function can occur without the development of suppurative labyrinthitis. In rare cases with extensive erosion of the semicircular canals cochlear function may be preserved.

Definitive confirmation of a labyrinthine fistula is made by surgical exploration, although the diagnosis may be suspected on CT scans, with 30° tilted axial scans being the preferred CT technique.[17]

Suspicion of a labyrinthine fistula in an ear with chronic middle ear disease demands surgical exploration via a mastoidectomy approach. Most otologists would utilize an open-cavity approach, although an intact canal wall technique can be used. The mastoid is cleared of cholesteatoma and granulation tissue leaving inspection of the lateral semicircular canal until the final stages of the procedure. Exposure of the lateral semicircular canal is performed delicately under high magnification. There is some debate surrounding surgical technique concerning the fate of squamous epithelium overlying a fistula. Some otologists advocate preservation of the epithelium, whereas others advocate gentle removal and repair of the defect with connective tissue such as temporalis fascia.[18] If an intact canal wall approach is undertaken, a 'second look' operation after approximately 1 year will be required.

ACUTE MASTOIDITIS

The proximity of the mastoid system to the middle ear ensures that most cases of suppurative otitis media are to some degree associated with mastoid air-cell inflammation. In acute suppurative otitis media, because of the widespread availability of antibiotics, clinical mastoid involvement is now uncommon. The significance of mastoiditis depends largely on the anatomical relations of the mastoid, with spread of infection to the middle and posterior cranial fossae, semicircular canals, facial nerve, sigmoid sinus and petrous apex being possible sequelae.

The commonest form of mastoiditis is that complicating acute suppurative otitis media in children. Pneumatization of the mastoid bone extends from the mastoid antrum after birth and is usually well

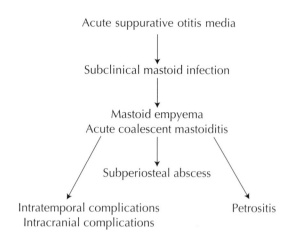

Fig 29.9 The progression of acute mastoiditis.

developed by 2 years of age. Consequently, acute mastoiditis is predominantly a disease of childhood, most prevalent at 6 years of age. Infecting organisms in acute mastoiditis are similar to those found in most cases of acute suppurative otitis media, with *Streptococcus pneumoniae* and *Haemophilus influenzae* being most commonly isolated. Occasionally, particularly in subacute cases, Gram-negative organisms such as *Pseudomonas aeruginosa*, *Proteus* species and *Escherichia coli* are found.

The features of acute mastoiditis are best understood by consideration of the pathological changes in the untreated patient. There is a progression of stages from simple acute suppurative otitis media through to life-threatening complications (Fig 29.9).

As previously mentioned, most cases of acute suppurative otitis media are associated with subclinical mastoid inflammation. Usually resolution occurs either spontaneously or after tympanic membrane rupture. Continued infection and mastoid inflammation leads to serous and then purulent exudation in the mastoid. The presence of pus under pressure produces demineralization of the bony air-cell walls, leading to **coalescence** of air cells and the formation of an empyema in the mastoid (acute coalescent mastoiditis). This process usually takes 2 weeks or more from the onset of the acute suppurative otitis media. Empyema formation is followed by escape of pus into adjacent areas. The development of mastoid periostitis and subsequently a subperiosteal abscess is the most common outcome, although medial spread can give rise to more serious intratemporal and intracranial complications. The speed of development of the untreated case depends on the infecting organism, host resistance and mastoid anatomy, with most cases developing within 7–10 days of the onset of acute suppurative otitis media. In advanced cases the presence of inflammatory granulation tissue in the mastoid is a prominent feature, particularly associated with the development of serious complications. At any stage in the development of acute suppurative mastoiditis the clinical course may be arrested or modified by antibiotic treatment.

Clinical features

Pain over the mastoid is a common symptom in acute suppurative otitis media, usually occurring over MacEwen's triangle (the surface marking of the mastoid antrum). The development of acute mastoiditis may be suspected in untreated patients when mastoid pain worsens. In treated patients the persistence of pain despite antibiotic therapy or the recurrence of pain may indicate acute mastoiditis. Rupture of the tympanic membrane and mucopurulent discharge is a frequent event in acute suppurative otitis media and often leads to resolution of infection. An increase in the volume and purulence of the discharge may suggest mastoiditis and reflects the increased surface area of infected mucosa. Persistent discharge unresponsive to medical treatment is a feature of the so-called 'mastoid reservoir' of infection and may herald the development of a chronic perforation. Deafness as a result of middle ear involvement is almost always a feature, but in many patients may be overshadowed by pain and discharge. Fever and systemic upset are often features of acute mastoiditis, but may be suppressed by antibiotic therapy.

The signs of acute mastoiditis vary with the stage and extent of disease. Otoscopy in acute mastoid infection never reveals a normal tympanic membrane. If the tympanic membrane is intact there may be signs of acute middle ear infection with a red, bulging drum or opacity due to a middle ear effusion. There may be a perforation of the tympanic membrane of the central type, with purulent otorrhoea. The most important otoscopic indicator of acute mastoiditis is sagging of the posterosuperior deep meatal wall due to underlying osteitis, and this sign in combination with purulent discharge is almost diagnostic of acute mastoiditis.

Tenderness over the mastoid cortex, particularly the mastoid tip, postauricular groove and zygomatic root is a significant sign. Swelling of the soft tissues behind the ear does not occur until the mastoid cortex is involved. Oedema and erythema of the postaural tissues occurs with loss of the normal postauricular crease. The pinna is pushed forwards and inferiorly, becoming much more prominent than the normal, contralateral side (Fig 29.10).

The development of a subperiosteal abscess causes an increase in postaural swelling, and in

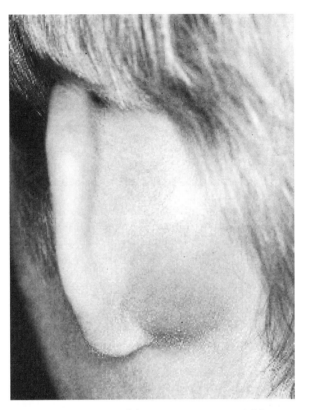

Fig 29.10 Protrusion of the ear in acute mastoiditis.

advanced cases spontaneous rupture may occur usually midway between the mastoid tip and MacEwen's triangle.

Masked mastoiditis

This variant of mastoiditis occurs when progression of acute mastoiditis has been modified by antibiotic therapy. The typical picture is of a case of acute suppurative otitis media initially subsiding with antibiotics. However, the tympanic membrane fails to return to normal and there may be persistent tenderness over the mastoid in association with low-grade fever and general malaise.

Radiology

Once the diagnosis of acute mastoiditis is suspected, confirmation should be sought by radiology. As in the radiological investigation of any otological condition comparison of the diseased and the normal temporal bone is of prime importance. In the past plain radiographs were commonly used (lateral oblique, 35° fronto-occipital and submentovertical views) and demonstrated haziness or opacity of the air cells. CT is now the imaging modality of choice. In addition to opacity of mastoid air cells, CT can demonstrate the underlying middle ear pathology and the presence of complications.

Differential diagnosis

Children frequently present with severe otalgia with pain and tenderness behind the ear. However, only rarely are such cases due to acute mastoiditis. The conditions that are most often misdiagnosed as acute mastoiditis are acute suppurative otitis externa, meatal furunculosis and suppuration of postauricular lymph nodes. The differentiation of these conditions from mastoiditis, although sometimes difficult, can usually be made on clinical grounds. The features strongly suggestive of acute mastoiditis are a recent history of acute otitis media, deafness, mucopurulent discharge and an abnormal tympanic membrane with sagging of the posterosuperior meatal wall. Difficulty can arise in cases of acute otitis externa and furunculosis with secondary postauricular lymphadenitis, particularly when canal oedema prevents a view of the tympanic membrane. In these latter conditions acute pain is often exacerbated by traction of the pinna, and there may be tenderness over the tragus. In these difficult cases the diagnosis of acute mastoiditis can be confirmed or ruled out by the appearance of opaque mastoid air cells on CT.

Treatment

Treatment of acute mastoiditis involves a combination of intensive antibiotic therapy and surgery. Some early cases will resolve with antibiotic therapy alone and it is the timing of surgical drainage that remains the principal challenge in the management of these patients. In cases with radiological evidence of mastoiditis but without subperiosteal abscess formation a trial of intravenous antibiotic therapy for a period of 24 hours is justified. The choice of antibiotic will reflect the likely pathogens (*Haemophilus influenzae, Streptococcus pneumoniae*). In the presence of purulent discharge, antibiotic therapy may be based on the results of microbiological examination. Some otologists have advocated the routine use of myringotomy, aspiration and ventilation tube insertion in all cases of acute mastoiditis with an intact tympanic membrane. Myringotomy in children, however, requires a general anaesthetic, and many early cases of mastoiditis will resolve with empirical antibiotic therapy alone.

If after initial intravenous antibiotic therapy there is no improvement or worsening of symptoms and signs, a drainage operation should be performed as a surgical emergency. In addition urgent surgery is required when a subperiosteal abscess is present. The operation of choice is a cortical mastoidectomy with the combined aims of draining pus, exenterating mastoid air cells and opening the mastoid antrum to produce a widely pneumatized tract from the middle ear to the mastoid. The surgical principles of cortical mastoidectomy are described at the end of this chapter. Under the same anaesthetic the tympanic membrane should be examined with an operating microscope and if intact a myringotomy performed and a ventilation tube inserted in order to facilitate middle ear ventilation.

SUBPERIOSTEAL ABSCESS AND POSTAURICULAR FISTULA

Acute and chronic suppurative otitis media can be complicated by spread of infection through the mastoid air cells into the soft tissues around the ear. This lateral spread of infection is usually a relatively late feature of untreated or inadequately treated suppurative otitis media. Although these complications are now rare in many parts of the world, they remain common in areas where access to health care is poor.

In acute mastoiditis the presence of an empyema or florid granulation tissue in the mastoid may cause necrosis of the overlying bone, most commonly over the suprameatal triangle. In chronic suppurative otitis media the onset is more insidious and can be the presenting feature of a large cholesteatoma. Spread of infection to the soft tissues results in subperiosteal abscess formation. Clinically there is swelling and erythema behind the ear with protrusion of the pinna and loss of the postauricular crease. Although the commonest site for a subperiosteal abscess is in the postauricular area, other sites can be involved. Escape of pus from the anteriorly placed zygomatic cells can give rise to an abscess presenting above and in front of the ear, in the parotid region. Tracking of infection through bony erosion of the external canal can lead to Luc's abscess in the subtemporal position. Perforation of the bone over the mastoid tip can lead to von Bezold's abscess in the sternomastoid muscle. Lastly, a pharyngeal abscess can occasionally occur with pus tracking from peritubal air cells.

The treatment for subperiosteal abscess is surgical drainage (Fig 29.11). At the same time the underlying ear disease should be explored and dealt with according to its nature and extent. Hence an abscess complicating acute mastoiditis will require a cortical mastoidectomy. In chronic suppurative otitis media a mastoidectomy will also be required,

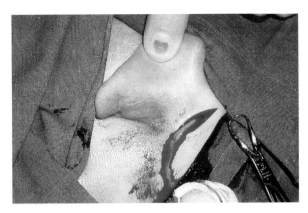

Fig 29.11 Surgical drainage of a postauricular subperiosteal abscess. The incision swings backwards to avoid risk to the facial nerve in a child (see Fig 29.13).

the extent of surgery depending on the tympanic membrane defect, presence of cholesteatoma and mastoid pathology. In any case of subperiosteal abscess the possibility of simultaneous medial spread with intracranial complications should be borne in mind and positively excluded by CT scanning.

If it remains untreated, the eventual fate of a subperiosteal abscess is spontaneous rupture. In acute cases this spontaneous drainage will release pressure and may cause a resolution of symptoms. In cases of complicating chronic suppurative otitis media rupture of a subperiosteal abscess may lead to the formation of a postauricular fistula between the mastoid and the exterior. These fistulae can be a source of intermittent discharge from the direct communication with infected middle ear mucosa and cholesteatoma. Treatment involves surgical excision of the fistulous tract with mastoidectomy to deal with the underlying chronic suppurative otitis media.

PETROSITIS

Spread of infection to the petrous apex can occur as a complication of acute and chronic suppurative otitis media. Pneumatization of the petrous bone is present in about 30 per cent of individuals and occurs after 3 years of age. Two principal pneumatized chains to the petrous apex are recognized: the posterosuperior chain extends from the attic and antrum, around the semicircular canals and into the apex, and the anteroinferior chain from the hypotympanum and Eustachian tube around the cochlea into the apex. The characteristic clinical signs of petrositis occur by virtue of close anatomical relationships to the trigeminal ganglion and the VIth

cranial nerve. The proximity of the petrous apex to intracranial structures renders petrositis a potentially lethal development in suppurative otitis media.

Acute petrositis

Acute petrositis is a rare complication that occurs as an extension of acute suppurative otitis media and mastoiditis into the pneumatized petrous air cells. As with acute mastoiditis the condition can be self-limiting, however, obstruction to drainage either because of mucosal swelling or granulation tissue can lead to the development of acute osteomyelitis of the petrous bone.[19] As in acute mastoiditis, petrositis can be 'masked' by prior antibiotic therapy.

The typical clinical features of petrositis are pain in the distribution of the Vth cranial nerve (particularly behind the eye) and diplopia due to VIth nerve paralysis (Fig 29.12). These two features in combination with evidence of middle ear disease (usually otorrhoea) form the triad known as Gradenigo's syndrome, which, as previously mentioned, can also indicate the development of a petrous apex extradural abscess. In addition the patient is likely to be systemically unwell with pyrexia, malaise and vomiting. Petrous apex infection can also occur as persistent discharge that apparently follows adequate cortical mastoidectomy for acute mastoiditis, with residual disease in petrous cells. The diagnosis once suspected clinically should be confirmed by CT, which is also required to exclude intracranial complications.

The development of Gradenigo's syndrome during the course of acute suppurative otitis media demands urgent treatment. Initially a trial of high-dose intravenous antibiotic therapy may be administered. In most cases rapid improvement in the

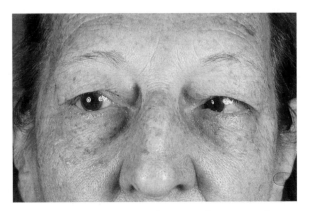

Fig 29.12 Right VIth nerve palsy in Gradenigo's syndrome.

patient's general condition will result with antibiotics, although Vth and VIth nerve symptoms may resolve over a matter of days. When there is no improvement or a worsening of the patient's condition, surgical exploration should be undertaken. The operation of choice is a complete cortical mastoidectomy, with skeletonization of the semicircular canals, and any pneumatized tracts should be followed along the posterosuperior route to the petrous apex.

Chronic petrositis

Petrositis complicating chronic suppurative otitis media is more common than the acute type and can occur with or without cholesteatoma. Pneumatization of the petrous apex is not a prerequisite as the infection can spread by thrombophlebitis, osteitis or along fascial planes.[20] This type of infection is often fairly indolent, usually manifesting as persistent discharge in the presence of chronic suppurative otitis media, which can include a discharging open mastoid cavity. The development of Gradenigo's syndrome in association with long-standing otorrhoea raises the suspicion of a petrous apex extradural abscess.

When persistent discharge from a petrous apex tract is suspected, surgical exploration is necessary. A complete exenteration of all mastoid cells is performed first, usually with an open-cavity technique. If a discharging tract to the petrous apex can be found it should be carefully followed and diseased bone curetted. The posterosuperior route to the petrous apex is usually followed, which may pass through the arch of the superior semicircular canal (Frenckner's approach). More major approaches to the petrous apex include the Ramadier–Lempert approach between the internal carotid artery and the cochlea and the Thornval approach under the middle fossa dura. These latter approaches are required only very rarely.

Cortical mastoidectomy

Cortical mastoidectomy, or simple mastoidectomy or Schwartze mastoidectomy, is a procedure of fundamental importance in otology. It was developed for the management of acute suppurative mastoiditis, but the technique has far wider applications, so its careful and correct performance is an essential part of the otological armamentarium, and every otologist must become competent to perform it, with preliminary extensive practice on the cadaver temporal bone.

USES

Cortical mastoidectomy is used clinically in a wide range of operations, for which the approach requires exposure of the otic capsule and the bony plates covering intratemporal structures. Among other numerous applications, the following may be listed:

- the treatment of suppurative mastoiditis
- exposure of the mastoid segment of the facial nerve
- exposure of the mastoid region in combined approach (canal wall up) tympanoplasty, to delineate the descending portion of the facial nerve and to provide the access for opening the posterior tympanotomy into the middle ear
- saccus decompression surgery, to offer the safest and widest access to the posterior fossa dura
- translabyrinthine operations, to provide the exposure of the bony labyrinth needed for its exenteration to allow access to the internal auditory meatus
- retrolabyrinthine approaches to the vestibular nerve
- exposure of the sigmoid sinus for obliteration before petrosectomy
- exposure of the otic capsule for cochlear implantation

In suppurative mastoiditis

In suppurative mastoiditis the purpose of cortical mastoidectomy is to provide free drainage of pus from the multioculated mastoid air-cell system and to remove the infected and diseased mucosa that is producing the pus. The tortuous anatomical confines of the air-cell system are converted by this procedure into as smooth and continuous a cavity as anatomical constraints will allow.

TECHNIQUE

The patient lies on the operating table with the head turned away from the operator. The foot of the table should be lowered by about 20°, and the head lowered to the horizontal to dispose the plane of the middle fossa dura as near to vertical as possible. The incision is postural, sited about 1 cm behind the postauricular fold. If the mastoid process in an adult is well developed, the incision should extend down to its limit. In the infant, before development of the tip, the facial nerve is superficial at this position and, for safety, the incision must be placed higher and more horizontally (Fig 29.13).

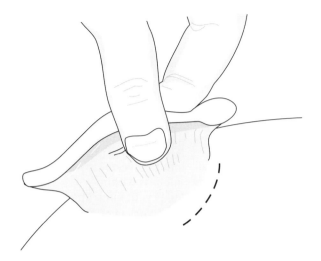

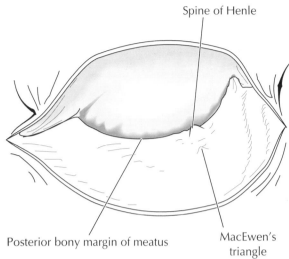

Fig 29.14 Exposure of mastoid cortex.

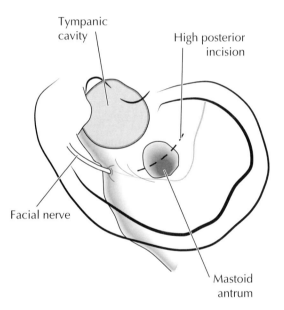

Fig 29.13 High posterior incision in the infant.

The incision is deepened through the periosteum to the bone. At this stage a subperiosteal abscess will discharge pus. Periosteum is lifted off underlying bone with a periosteal elevator to expose the spine of Henle, MacEwen's triangle and the posterior bony margin of the meatus. The tip should be cleaned of fibromuscular insertions. A self-retaining retractor is inserted to hold the soft tissues away from the underlying exposed bone.

The mastoid cortex is now removed over MacEwen's triangle (Fig 29.14), which is a rough guide to the position of the underlying mastoid antrum, using a drill fitted with a large (5–6 mm diameter) cutting burr. The antrum will be encountered at a depth of about 1.5 cm in the adult, but

approach to it can be seriously misled by deviations in direction of the drilling. To be safe the approach should be wide externally, so that the access is through a funnel-shaped passageway. The work should err, if it must, on drilling high and posteriorly, so that any error will be more likely to expose the middle fossa dura than damage the facial nerve. An experienced otologist may be able to drill straight down into the antrum through a tunnel little wider than the burr, but this bravado is not for the neophyte.

Identification of the antrum is usually apparent when it is opened by the drill and can be confirmed by gently probing anteriorly with a Dundas Grant probe, which will slip into the aditus. At this point care is needed to avoid displacement of the short process of the incus.

The antral exposure is enlarged, opening adjacent cells until the lateral semicircular canal, which is the important landmark at this stage, can be identified. Next, all air cells in all directions are opened by drilling gently through their separating trabeculae. If the region is filled with necrotic mucosa, it may be safer to scoop out the material with a curette, sweeping always away from the position of the vertical part of the facial nerve as it descends just below the back of the lateral semicircular canal. Ultimately a cavity is created, bounded above by the bony tegmen separating the region from the dura of the middle cranial fossa, behind the bony plate over the sigmoid sinus and in front by the posterior meatal wall and the aditus ad antrum. In front of the bulge of the sigmoid sinus plate, removal of cells will uncover the bone of Trautmann's triangle, protecting the dura of the posterior cranial fossa and leading anteriorly and medially to the so-called solid

(a)

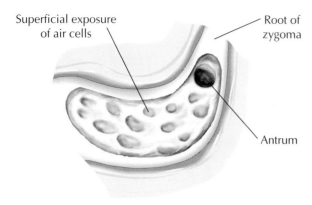

Superficial exposure
of air cells

Root of
zygoma

Antrum

(b)

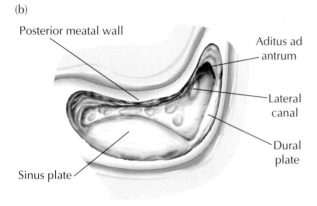

Posterior meatal wall

Aditus ad
antrum

Lateral
canal

Dural
plate

Sinus plate

(c)

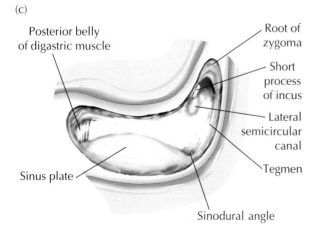

Posterior belly
of digastric muscle

Root of
zygoma

Short
process
of incus

Lateral
semicircular
canal

Tegmen

Sinus plate

Sinodural angle

Fig 29.15 Continuation of cortical mastoidectomy. (a) Mastoid cortex removed; (b) initial cell clearance; (c) final cell clearance and tip removed.

angle, where the dense bone of the otic capsule protects the posterior semicircular canal. Anteriorly, and much more superficially, cells should be opened, as far as they extend, into the root of the zygoma, whereas inferiorly, cell pursuit will lead to the bone covering the digastric muscle as it passes forwards, deep to the inferior part of the facial nerve at the stylomastoid foramen (Fig 29.15).

Removal of the mastoid tip is advocated to allow soft tissue to fall in and partly obliterate the remaining cavity.

Whenever this operation is performed for proved suppurative mastoiditis, the bone over the sigmoid sinus should be removed sufficiently to allow insertion of a fine needle into that vessel to confirm that there is no thrombophlebitis within.

Closure of the wound is with interrupted sutures, and most otologists will leave a soft drain in the lower part of the cavity for a day or two. A firm pressure dressing will control bleeding.

COMPLICATIONS

This is not an easy operation in the presence of infection, despite its name, and there are risks of injury to the facial nerve; dislocation of the incus; penetration of the middle fossa (or even posterior fossa) dura; rupture of the sigmoid sinus and labyrinthine transgression and destruction.

Otologists nowadays gain much less experience of the procedure for infection than did their forebears; therefore, they should always err on the side of conservatism and caution in cell exenteration, particularly to avoid the facial nerve.

References

1. Samuel J, Fernandes CMC, Steinberg JL. Intracranial otogenic complications: a persisting problem. *Laryngoscope* 1986; **96**:272–8.
2. Rupa V, Raman R. Chronic suppurative otitis media: complicated versus uncomplicated disease. *Acta Otolaryngologica (Stockholm)* 1991; **111**:530–5.
3. Browning GG. The unsafeness of 'safe' ears. *Journal of Laryngology and Otology* 1984; **98**:23–6.
4. Nunez DA, Browning GG. Risks of developing an otogenic intracranial abscess. *Journal of Laryngology and Otology* 1990; **104**:468–72.
5. Palva T, Virtanen H, Makinen J. Acute and latent mastoiditis in children. *Journal of Laryngology and Otology* 1985; **99**:127–36.
6. Kangsanarak J, Fooanant S, Ruckphaopunt K, Navacharoen N, Teotrakul S. Extracranial and intracranial complications of suppurative otitis media. report of 102 cases. *Journal of Laryngology and Otology* 1993; **107**:999–1004.
7. Schwaber MK, Pensak ML, Bartels LJ. The early signs and symptoms of neurotologic complications of chronic suppurative otitis media. *Laryngoscope* 1989; **99**:373–5.

8. Pit S, Jamal F, Cheah FK. Microbiology of cerebral abscesses: a four year study in Malaysia. *Journal of Tropical Medicine and Hygiene* 1993; **96**:191–6.

9. Haimes AB, Zimmerman RD, Morgello S, Weingarten K, Becker RD, Jennis R *et al*. MR imaging of brain abscesses. *American Journal of Roentgenology* 1989; **152**:1073–85.

10. Singh B, Maharaj TJ. Radical mastoidectomy: its place in otitic intracranial complications. *Journal of Laryngology and Otology* 1993; **107**:1113–8.

11. Irving RM, Jones NS, Hall-Craggs MA, Kendall B. CT and MR imaging in lateral sinus sinus thrombosis. *Journal of Laryngology and Otology* 1991; **105**:693–5.

12. Maksimovic Z, Rukovanjski M. Intracranial complications of cholesteatoma. *Acta Oto Rhino Laryngologica Belgica* 1993; **47**:33–6.

13. Lebel MH, Hoyt MJ, Waagner DC, Rollins NK, Finitzo,T. McCracken GJ. Magnetic resonance imaging and dexamethasone therapy for bacterial meningitis. *American Journal of Diseases in Childhood* 1989; **143**:301–6.

14. Nunez DA. Aetiological role of otolaryngological disease in paediatric intracranial abscess. *Journal of the Royal College of Surgeons of Edinburgh* 1992; **37**:80–2.

15. Stapleton SR, Bell BA, Uttley D. Stereotactic aspiration of brain abscesses: is this the treatment of choice? *Acta Neurochirurgica* 1993; **121**:15–9.

16. Harker LA, Pignatari SSN. Facial nerve paralysis secondary to chronic otitis media without cholesteatoma. *American Journal of Otolaryngology* 1992; **13**:372–4.

17. Jackler RK, Dillon WP, Schindler RA. Computer tomography in suppurative ear disease: a correlation of surgical and radiographic findings. *Laryngoscope* 1984; **94**:746–52.

18. Parisier SC, Edelstein DR, Han JC, Weiss MH. Management of labyrinthine fistulas caused by cholesteatoma. *Otolaryngology – Head and Neck Surgery* 1991; **104**:110–5.

19. Chole RA, Donald P. Petrous apicitis; clinical considerations. *Annals of Otology, Rhinology and Laryngology* 1983; **92**:544–51.

20. Allam AF, Schuknecht HF. Pathology of petrositis. *Laryngoscope* 1968; **78**:1813–32.

CHAPTER 30

Surgery of chronic suppurative otitis media

JAMES ROBINSON

Introduction

The aim of surgery for chronic ear disease is to eliminate the disease processes and to perform such reconstruction as is necessary to ensure that the patient is left with a dry, safe and trouble-free ear. This process may also result in the maintenance of existing hearing, or provide a surgical environment suitable for reconstruction of the sound transformer mechanism.

The elimination of disease must, however, always take precedence to ensure the patient's safety and it should always be realized that however sophisticated an ossicular repair may be, it will not survive if the ear is not stable. There is no place today for mastoid surgery that exteriorizes the disease process without achieving a dry, stable ear in the long term.

There are numerous techniques available to the otologist to line, reconstruct or obliterate bony cavities, and there are techniques to preserve anatomical structures so that cavity formation is avoided in the first place. The surgeon should therefore be familiar with a range of techniques in order to be able to deal with the multiplicity of presentations that characterize middle ear and mastoid disease.

Early cholesteatoma

Retraction pockets may become so deep that desquamating epithelium cannot clear and therefore debris collects, which causes extension of the pocket. Early diagnosis allows the potential for limited surgery by elimination of the pocket.

Initial insertion of a ventilation tube into the undamaged area of the tympanic remnant allows air to enter and facilitate dissection. The pocket is carefully freed from the adjacent structures and then dissected out and removed (Fig 30.1). Sometimes a pocket will come away intact, but often piecemeal removal is required.

The ossicular chain may still be intact, therefore care is needed not to overstimulate the cochlea by excessive movement of the stapes. Not infrequently erosion may have already occurred to the long

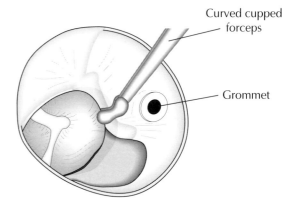

Curved cupped forceps

Grommet

Fig 30.1 Excision of retraction pocket. Deep retraction pocket 'vacuum packed' over incus and stapedius tendon. Curved forceps grasping atrophic membrane and pulling it out and away, leaving a perforation in the posterior part of the tympanic membrane.

process of the incus and more rarely some of the bony Fallopian canal may also have been eroded exposing the facial nerve. During the elevation and dissection of these pockets it is important to remember that the chorda tympani runs along the posterosuperior margins of the area of dissection and is at risk.

The traumatic perforation that results from this technique frequently closes spontaneously. However, if desired, reinforcement can be carried out using fascia, perichondrium or cartilage.

The risk of squamous epithelium being retained appears to be overemphasized. However, epithelial pearls do occur but these are readily visible and accessible by simple tympanotomy. If cartilage is used as part of the reinforcing technique then such pearls are not visible and only appear once they have reached a reasonable size; thus they can be more difficult to control.

This technique achieves excellent disease control and when the ossicular chain is intact normal hearing can be expected. Where the long process of the incus has been eroded there is a reasonable chance of success using ossiculoplasty techniques; these are discussed in Chapter 31.

Attic cholesteatoma

History and examination give little or no information as to the extent of the disease. But an attic defect with minimal infection and inflammatory response may contain cholesteatoma limited to the attic and be amenable to confined resection. Infection and associated inflammation make intact dissection of the sac more difficult. A mild conductive hearing loss may suggest some ossicular involvement, but sometimes the disease is bridging the gap.

Initial inspection and manipulation of the attic defect will indicate whether an atticotomy is worth attempting. Slight enlargement of the defect anteriorly and superiorly may allow a sight of the margins of the sac and so encourage perseverance to see whether further exposure will bring the whole sac into view (Fig 30.2).

These sacs can frequently be dissected out intact with preservation of the ossicular chain, which, if it is still intact, will preserve hearing at preoperative levels or better. These patients can benefit from the closing of the attic defect with autograft cartilage, bone or hydroxylapatite (Fig 30.3).

When disease is more extensive, anteriorly or posteriorly, removal is likely to be piecemeal. A decision is then required as to whether to proceed with a more extensive atticotomy or attico-antrostomy, to perform an open mastoid exploration or convert to a closed-cavity approach.

If an atticotomy or attico-antrostomy approach is favoured further bone is removed anteriorly or posteriorly, or in both directions, to expose all diseased areas. If the middle war is free of disease the tympanic membrane only needs to be elevated to allow inspection and provide a flap to place over the graft that will be needed at the end of the procedure.

If there is disease in the middle ear further elevation will be needed and attention to the ossicular chain may indicate erosion or involvement with disease.

All diseased areas must be exposed to view and all diseased tissue removed. On occasion this means

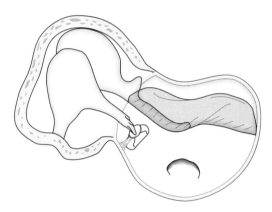

Fig 30.2 Atticotomy. The posterior tympanic membrane has been elevated forwards using the malleus handle as a hinge. The outer attic wall has been drilled away to expose the bodies of incus and malleus. There is early erosion of the tip of the incus.

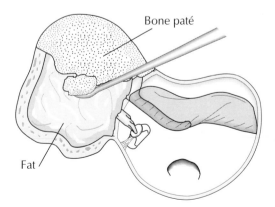

Fig 30.3 Atticotomy with bone paté repair. The same procedure as in Figure 30.2. The atticotomy has been plugged with some fat followed by bone paté (moist bone dust) to fill the atticotomy completely and reconstruct the canal wall.

that an initially small atticotomy extends into a large open cavity. However, most chronically diseased ears are acellular and if healthy tissue is not interfered with these cavities can be quite limited in extent, particularly in those cases in which good postoperative ventilation occurs.

The atticotomy or attico-antrostomy approach does risk incomplete disease eradication and poor ventilation postoperatively, which results in retraction of the attic graft with consequent recurrence of cholesteatoma in the mastoid segment. The approach logically extends as far as the disease extends; it spares uninvolved tissue but risks leaving a large cavity when disease is unexpectedly extensive.

Some atticotomies and attico-antrostomies can be lined by using a large fascia or connective tissue graft to repair any tympanic membrane defect, laying the remainder of the graft into the attic. This will have one of two effects: either the attic ventilates – there is then no cavity but a membranous canal wall results – or the graft retracts into the cavity and lines it. Healthy squamous epithelium then grows over the graft.

More extensive cholesteatoma

Larger cholesteatomas extending into the mastoid antrum and beyond require more aggressive surgery. Historically these, and also smaller cholesteatomas, were dealt with by exteriorizing the disease by open-cavity mastoidectomy. This is still the routine method in many parts of the world and is considered by many to be the only truly safe approach to this disease.

The radical mastoidectomy of the nineteenth century is rarely justified today. This opened up the mastoid cavity by removing the canal wall posteriorly and superiorly and exteriorized the disease by removing the mastoid air-cell system as far as the lateral sinus posteriorly and the dura of the middle cranial fossa superiorly (Fig 30.4). The ossicular remnants and remains of the tympanic membrane were also eliminated and the Eustachian tube was obliterated to prevent any further contact between the middle ear and the postnasal space. This is the only operation that can truly claim to exteriorize all the disease, many otologists feel that it can rarely be justified today.

In the early years of the twentieth century the modified radical mastoidectomy sought to exteriorize disease by performing an open procedure on the mastoid portion of the ear, but leaving the ossicles and tympanic membrane or their remnants if they were not involved with disease (Fig 30.5).

Today the term 'modified radical' is used to describe a further modification of the open-cavity procedure. The ability to graft the tympanic membrane and reconstruct the ossicular chain has broadened the scope of this type of surgery and today's procedure should better be described as 'an open mastoidectomy with tympanoplasty'.

There are two approaches to the procedure: from within outwards, as in the atticotomy mentioned

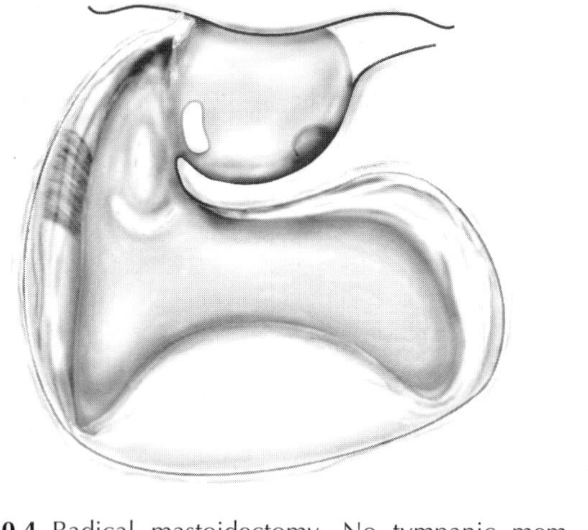

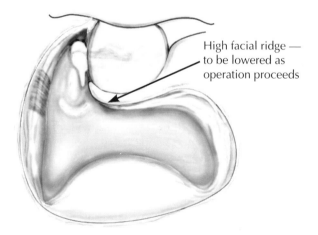

High facial ridge — to be lowered as operation proceeds

Fig 30.4 Radical mastoidectomy. No tympanic membrane. No ossicles. Stump of tensor and footplate of stapes present. Lateral and posterior semicircular canals skeletonized. Lateral sinus and middle fossa dura exposed or skeletonized. In all these open-cavity operations the facial ridge must be lowered as far as is safely possible.

Fig 30.5 'Classic' modified radical mastoidectomy. As Figure 30.4 but the tympanic membrane and ossicles have been preserved.

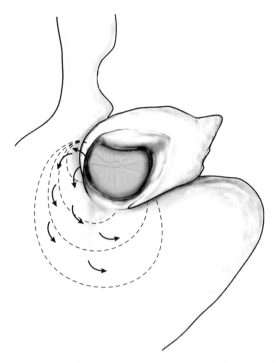

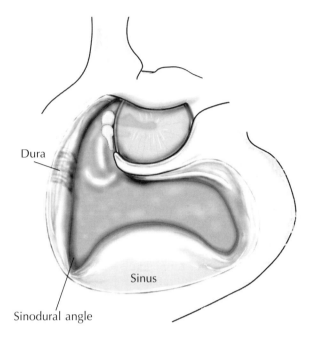

Fig 30.6 Inside–out mastoid exploration. The mastoid is opened up progressively starting with an atticotomy and progressing as far as the disease requires.

Fig 30.7 Outside–in approach. This approach starts from the surgical limits and proceeds inwards from the dura, lateral sinus and sinodural angle towards the antrum and the seat of the disease. Again, the facial ridge must be lowered.

above (Fig 30.6), or starting from the mastoid antrum and working forwards towards the attic and middle ear, that is, the outside–in approach (Fig 30.7).

The inside–out procedure has the advantage of limiting the operation strictly to the diseased tissues and sparing healthy tissue, but the surgical approach may be restricted and there is some increased risk of damage to vulnerable structures in the middle ear especially in less experienced hands.

The outside–in approach ensures total disease removal with a wider approach and a gentler exposure of the important middle ear structures. However, healthy tissue is sacrificed to obtain access and care must be taken not to create an excessively large cavity.

Cavity management

All the open-cavity procedures previously mentioned suffer from one disadvantage – the resulting cavity.

The defect that follows these operations is formed in bone and therefore has bony walls. Skin does not readily grow on the surface of bare bone and when it does it tends to be of poor quality, with a tendency to break down and ulcerate and sometimes to become eczematous.

In addition the external auditory meatus is designed to ventilate a normal-sized canal. The volume of a mastoid cavity is significantly greater and therefore ventilation tends to be inadequate.

Under normal conditions the squamous epithelium of the tympanic membrane and canal has migratory properties and the external ear is therefore self-cleansing. The surgery itself and the irregular nature of the remaining mastoid cavity interfers with this natural migration so that debris, desquamated epithelium and wax tend to collect in the cavity; this eventually becomes infected, thus causing further deterioration in the state of the mastoid lining. When no attempt has been made to deal with this problem a high incidence of persistent and recurrent aural discharge will occur. It is no longer acceptable to leave bare open cavities postoperatively in the vain hope that the development of granulomatous tissue will eventually provide a suitable environment for epithelial ingrowth.

Numerous grafting procedures have been developed over the years and these can substantially modify the end result.

Free grafts of fascia taken locally from the temporalis muscle or imported from the fascia lata have been used. Muscle and periosteal grafts can be obtained locally, and abdominal fat has also been used. Initially these grafts can largely obliterate the cavity but later atrophy is inevitable. Despite this, however, these cavities are often rendered much smoother, with a healthier epithelial lining and a better chance of some useful migration.

Thin free skin grafts have been used, but when applied at the time of surgery they have proved disappointing. Better results have been achieved when grafting has been delayed until a healthy granular reaction has developed. Migration in these grafted ears has, however, been disappointing, presumably because the grafted skin does not possess the migratory properties of skin from the external ear canal.

Pedicle grafts are more likely to remain viable and have better obliterative properties. Muscular periosteal flaps from the temporalis muscle, sternomastoid, or even occipitalis muscles can be used, and large temporalis fascia grafts can be obtained and turned into the cavity (Fig 30.8). These grafts, because they retain a blood and nerve supply, are more likely to reduce the size of the cavity on a long-term basis, and they also provide excellent nutrition for epithelial ingrowth.

Primary obliteration with more solid material can also be used, provided the surgeon is confident that all disease has been eliminated; this, of course, applies to all obliteration or lining techniques.

Autogenous cartilage from the chondral part of the pinna can be laid into the mastoid bowl. Bone chips or dust can similarly be used. These have the advantage of being strongly osteogenic and result in bony obliteration of the cavity. Pedicle muscle flaps can be used in conjunction with these filling materials to hold them in place and provide them with a blood supply.

Artificial materials have also been used in the past. Currently, inorganic bony analogues such as hydroxylapatite are sometimes used, as is bioglass, but these materials probably have no advantage over bone dust in this situation and are expensive.

The size of the cavity is dictated to a large extent by the surgical technique used in removing the disease. If the procedure is carried out with the minimal amount of bone removal, the side walls of the cavity will tend to be vertical and, therefore, the cavity will have maximum depth. If the surrounding bone is removed and the edges of the cavity are saucerized, when the pinna and scalp are replaced at the end of the procedure the tissues will be allowed to fall inwards and largely obliterate the cavity. Therefore, during the procedure the outer table of the skull can be drilled away around the cavity, the mastoid tip should be removed and bone

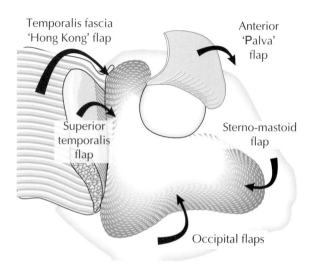

Fig 30.8 Flaps for cavities. Various flaps from all directions that can be used to line the mastoid cavity.

should be drilled away to the level of the vertical part of the facial nerve. All bony buttresses must be eliminated to present a smooth, shallow bowl in which the skin flaps can lie. When this is carried out well the operated ear should come to lie significantly more medial than the unoperated ear, leaving very little additional obliteration to be carried out.

In order to cope with the increased volume caused by the creation of the cavity, the diameter of the external auditory meatus should be widened by performing a meatoplasty. The size of the opening should be in proportion to the cavity, but care needs to be taken not to be too enthusiastic. A very large meatus is cosmetically unacceptable and can result in vertigo as a result of thermal stimulation of the exposed lateral semicircular canal, in cold wind or water, or in hot air blasts during the use of a hairdryer.

Techniques for meatoplasty are numerous but it is usually necessary to remove some conchal cartilage to ensure an adequate opening, and flaps cut in the posterior meatal skin need to be sutured to ensure permanence (Fig 30.9). It is not sufficient to rely on packing to hold the meatus in position.

In younger patients there is a tendency over the years for the ear to move anteriorly, causing the cartilage to override the canal opening. This may be prevented by using firm well placed sutures to pull the meatal skin backwards before closing the incision. The middle postauricular muscle should be resutured if it has been cut during the approach.

The above techniques all rely on exteriorization to deal with the disease, and they leave a cavity.

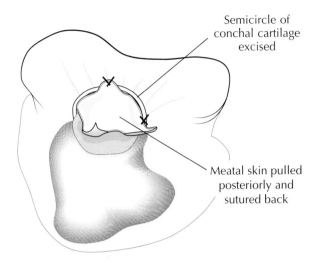

Fig 30.9 Meatoplasty.

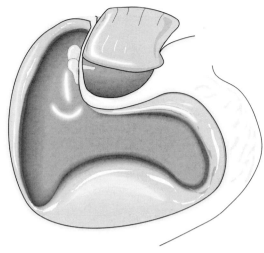

Fig 30.10 Closed-cavity mastoid exploration: saucerization of bony margins; wide development of sinodural angle and wide exposure towards root of zygoma. It is important not to make the attic part of the canal wall too thin.

This needs to be dealt with by lining or obliterating to avoid long-term postoperative problems with recurrent discharge, which can in the worst cases lead to further destruction and cholesteatoma recurrence.

Closed-cavity techniques

The alternative to open-cavity procedures is to leave the bony canal wall intact and rely on improvements in surgical techniques to eliminate the disease.

In the late 1950s Jansen, in Germany, developed the posterior tympanotomy approach to allow access from the closed mastoid into the middle ear by removing bone between the tympanic annulus and chorda tympani laterally, and the second genu and first part of the descending facial nerve medially. This leaves a triangular space, variable in extent, which in many cases can expose the long process of the incus and stapes superstructure, if these are present; if these are not present then it provides good access to the oval window and can be extended inferiorly to give access as far as the hypotympanum. When the mastoid air-cell system is well developed there is usually excellent exposure of the attic and dissection can be carried beyond the ossicular bodies, if they are present, allowing removal of anterior attic disease as well as providing a superior ventilation route when the ear heals postoperatively.

Acellular mastoids with a low middle fossa dura or a forward lateral sinus, or both, provide a greater surgical challenge, but with suitable retraction and good surgical experience there are few patients who cannot be managed this way if desired (Fig 30.10).

The combined approach tympanoplasty, or closed-cavity mastoidectomy, offers an intact canal and a tympanic membrane in the normal anatomical position. This favours middle ear and mastoid ventilation and there is no postoperative cavity. This may provide a better environment for ossicular reconstruction, and the more normal anatomy and physiology should result in long-lasting stability.

Unfortunately the method has its problems and there is a price to pay. Because the bony canal is retained, the attic, antrum and mastoid are not open to postoperative inspection. Should the surgical clearance have been incomplete and the retained squamous epithelium survive, cholesteatoma will reform as residual disease. Similarly, any mucosal disease that is not removed or that does not resolve after surgery will result in the persistence of the preoperative state.

It has been found clinically that cholesteatoma known to have been left at primary surgery has disappeared by the time a second stage procedure has been carried out. This, however, cannot be relied upon and many surgeons who use this technique routinely perform a second look 6–18 months after the first procedure. The prevalence of residual disease at second stage varies greatly, but most occur as discrete epithelial pearls that can easily be removed intact. Ears once free of disease rarely seem to cause further problems.

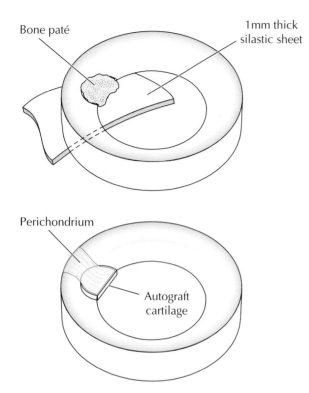

Bone paté

1mm thick silastic sheet

Perichondrium

Autograft cartilage

Fig 30.11 Repair of outer attic wall in closed-cavity surgery.

The closed procedure, however, presents its own special difficulty. Because the anatomy of the ear is retained, disease can recur. In non-cholesteatomatous cases mucosal disease can become re-established and the ear break down and discharge once more. Further retraction of the tympanic membrane and outer attic wall erosion with retraction can also occur and proceed to a recurrence of cholesteatomatous disease.

Prevention of mucosal disease relies on the establishment and maintenance of good middle ear and mastoid ventilation, which can be helped by good initial surgical technique, encouragement of autoventilation and maintenance of a healthy upper respiratory tract.

Cholesteatoma recurrence may also be affected by the above factors. In addition the repair of any bony defect in the outer attic wall is essential to long-term stability (Fig 30.11). The material used for such repair must be chosen with longevity in mind and it seems likely that autologous bone or cartilage are likely to behave best in this respect. Bone was the original natural material and this is probably the best choice.

Non-cholesteatomatous middle ear and mastoid disease

Chronic suppurative otitis media without cholesteatoma results from chronic inflammatory disease of the mucosal lining of the middle ear cleft and mastoid. The disease can vary from relatively mild oedematous changes to severe mucosal disease with granulation tissue and polyp formation and the presence of cholesterol granuloma. These chronic changes can also result in the formation of tympanosclerosis involving the tympanic membrane or its remnants and the mucosa of the middle ear and adjacent spaces. Many of these changes are irreversible and there may be very little, if any, normal mucosa, although there may be some mucosa that is reversibly damaged.

The absence of cholesteatoma prompts surgeons to be more conservative and to consider closed surgical procedures as being more appropriate. It is true that there is no risk of residual or recurrent cholesteatoma unless it be iatrogenic. However, these cases can prove difficult to control. The presence of so much irreversibly damaged tissue and the very limited areas of reversibly damaged mucosa do not allow the ear to regenerate a satisfactory lining for the air spaces within the middle ear and mastoid easily.

Surgery in these severely damaged ears can be complicated by excessive bleeding, poor visibility and difficulty of access. Ossicular damage and erosion of the Fallopian canal or vestibule are at least as frequent as in the cholesteatomatous cases. The surgery needs to be meticulous to eliminate all disease, entailing considerable bone removal. A well grafted tympanic membrane, good ventilation – if necessary using thin silastic sheeting – and drainage through the Eustachian tube are all prerequisites of a well healed ear postoperatively.

Cases of chronic suppurative otitis media without cholesteatoma have a reputation for postoperative instability and there is a tendency to underestimate their severity because of the absence of cholesteatoma. Therefore all the techniques appropriate for cholesteatomatous diseases are just as relevant to non-cholesteatomatous disease.

Chronic suppurative otitis media in children

Chronic ear disease in children has a reputation for being more aggressive and more difficult to control than in adults. Mucosal disease is complicated by the frequency of secretory otitis media secondary to a greater tendency to upper airway problems. Natural ventilation is poor in childhood and therefore, once established, chronic ear disease is difficult to control and may not resolve fully until the child grows up.

Cholesteatoma also has a bad reputation in children. This is partly linked to the factors affecting non-cholesteatomatous disease. However, there is clear clinical evidence that cholesteatoma in children tends to be more extensive and the mastoid air-cell system better developed. On the basis of this evidence a significant number of these children may have congenital or primary cholesteatoma rather than acquired disease, which would explain the extent of the spread as it would have had the whole of the child's lifetime to grow. It also explains the well developed mastoid which has originally not been infected. It is difficult to prove this hypothesis as most of these cases of cholesteatoma are well advanced and the tympanic membrane has been perforated, allowing infection to enter so that the patient presents with signs and symptoms similar to those of the acquired disease.

The higher prevalence of residual disease can be explained by the extent of the spread, which makes primary total removal technically difficult. Once under control, however, these ears behave much like their adult counterparts, suggesting that there is no fundamental difference between the disease in children and in adults.

Surgical approach

Now that the various surgical techniques available have been described, it is appropriate to discuss the surgical access briefly. There are three surgical approaches: permeatal, endaural and postaural. The permeatal approach is through the ear canal using incisions in the meatal skin to obtain access to the middle ear and bony ear canal (Fig 30.12). This approach has been used for elimination and excision of early middle ear and attic cholesteatoma. It has also been used in atticotomy and attico-antrostomy, but the limited access has caused problems and most surgeons who have tried this approach have eventually found it easier to provide wider access.

The endaural incision starts in the superior meatus, passes through the cartilaginous gap just posterior to the tragus and extends superiorly and posteriorly around the root of the helix (Fig 30.13). It was popularized by Lempert originally in order to avoid creating postaural fistulae but became popular for atticotomy and attico-antrostomy work.

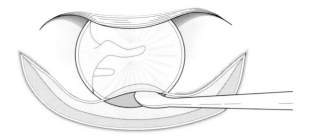

Fig 30.12 Permeatal incision. The incision should run from one o'clock to five o'clock and is about 2 mm from the annulus of the tympanic membrane.

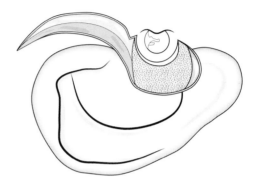

Fig 30.13 Endaural incision.

It is also used by extending the incision for wider mastoid exploration. It gives good access to the middle ear, attic and antrum, and also for work in the anterior part of the middle ear. There have been reports of meatal stenosis occurring in relation to the meatal part of the incision.

The postaural incision goes back into history. For mastoid work the incision should extend just beyond the superior root of the helix and well below the pinna to allow the cartilaginous part of the pinna to be retracted anteriorly to give access to the root of the zygoma (Fig 30.14). Provided good anterior retraction is used, access to the posterior part of the middle ear is very little different from the endaural approach. Access into the anterior part of the middle ear is excellent and the whole of the mastoid, including the tip, is easily explored.

In 1967 Jako showed that the postaural approach provides a 20 per cent greater viewing angle than the endaural incision. However, one possible disadvantage of the postaural over the endaural approach is greater sensory disturbance of the skin of the pinna. This loss of sensations can last for several months but is rarely permanent. The endaural approach is less likely to result in this side effect.

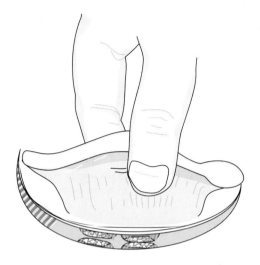

Fig 30.14 Postaural incision. The superior end of the incision is carried well forwards towards the zygoma and extends just anterior to the root of the top of the pinna. Temporalis muscle fascia is exposed in the superior part of the incision. Postauricular muscles are divided in the mid part of the incision. The incision stops at the periosteum and its overlying connective tissue.

A range of surgical procedures is available for the management of chronic ear disease and surgeons should be familiar with all of them, as there is no single correct procedure for a disease that manifests in so many very different ways and at different stages in its development. There is no place for a dogmatic approach. The important consideration is that the patient needs a dry, safe and trouble-free ear. All the techniques described in this chapter have well documented series showing results that comply with the above requirements. There is no longer any justification for the following situation: the patient presents with a discharging ear, is subjected to an operative procedure that exteriorizes the disease, but is left with the ear still unstable and liable to discharge.

In summary, early, middle ear and attic disease responds well to excision of the pocket, with or without repair. Somewhat more extensive disease extending into the attic is suitable for atticotomy, with or without reconstruction of the attic defect at the same time. This technique can be extended into an attico-antrostomy or small cavity mastoidectomy.

More extensive disease can be dealt with by a range of techniques from the open mastoid procedure, with various flap techniques for lining or obliterating the space, to obliterative techniques that exteriorize the disease and then reconstruct the canal by filling in the mastoid bowl or repairing the canal wall with bone or cartilage. Finally there is the closed-cavity technique and its variations, which rely on eliminating the disease and preserving the anatomy of the ear.

All modern techniques involve closing the tympanic membrane defect. There is therefore a risk of burying disease in the middle ear. The prevalence of residual disease in these areas is much the same in all techniques and must be allowed for by suitable follow-up. Obliterative, reconstructive and closed techniques also risk burying disease in the attic and antrum; open techniques in which a graft is carried into the areas run the same risk. Residual disease will occur in these areas with much the same frequency in most techniques.

The obliteration, reconstruction and closed-cavity techniques also fill in the mastoid and risk residual disease in this area, but fortunately leaving squamous material in this area is uncommon.

Residual disease can occur in all techniques with similar frequency. Only the true radical procedure can be expected to exteriorize all disease, but it has such a high incidence of long-term discharge and instability because of exposed middle ear and unhealed mastoid bowl that it is now virtually obsolete.

The closed techniques all have a potential problem that the open procedures lack, namely possible recurrent cholesteatoma from the formation of a new retraction pocket. The prevalence of this varies greatly depending on the techniques used to provide long-term middle ear and mastoid ventilation, and the method used to repair the outer attic wall, with or without reinforcement of the posterosuperior quadrant of the tympanic membrane.

All patients undergoing surgery for chronic ear disease require long-term expert and detailed follow-up. This should include the routine use of microscopy, and must be carried out by an experienced clinician. In this way the early signs of disease can be identified and appropriate remedial surgery be performed before further extensive damage occurs.

Revision surgery

It is clear from the above that chronic ear disease does not always respond to surgery as might be wished and consequently revision surgery is required from time to time. These operations can vary from relatively simple re-excision of retraction pockets and tympanic membrane reinforcement to major reconstruction. The more complex of these can be extremely difficult and require considerable experience if revision surgery is to prove successful and avoid major complications.

A combination of long-term extensive disease and previous surgery can eliminate many of the normal surgical landmarks and make orientation difficult. Disease can be extensive and unexpected with the risk of incomplete surgery, surgical damage and no improvement in the patient's symptoms.

The temptation in open procedures is to remove yet more tissue and make the surgical defect even larger, whereas what is required is reconstruction and reduction in the volume of the cavity to reduce the ratio between the volume of the cavity and the available ventilation through the meatus. Meatoplasty can help this ratio but there are limits as to how far this principle can be applied.

Persistent discharge after mastoid surgery may arise from a defect in the tympanic membrane or non-healing of the squamous lining of the mastoid bowl, or both.

Tympanic membrane defects can be corrected by myringoplasty using one of the techniques described in Chapter 31. A larger than usual graft is required when the canal wall has been removed so that the graft can be laid over the facial ridge and can receive adequate support and blood supply.

Mastoid bowl problems may be due to inadequate initial surgery. If so, completing the procedure may be effective. Extensive saucerization and removal of all bony overhangs and lowering the posterior bony wall as far as the level of the facial nerve will allow the superficial tissues to fill most of the defect, and any potential cavities can be filled in with pedicled flaps or solid material such as bone dust, chips or cartilage. The success rate of this procedure is high but the surgery itself can be challenging and prolonged. Obliterative techniques without removal of so much bone can also be employed. Pedicle flaps of fascia, periosteum or muscle work well. Free grafts of these materials and of abdominal fat are also used but have a much greater tendency to atrophy over time, leading to reappearance of the cavity.

Solid materials can also be used to obliterate cavities (Fig 30.15). Cartilage strips and chips may be used and bone dust and bone chips are also effective, having a powerful osteogenic effect.

Artificial materials have been used extensively in the past but have been found to extrude. The most commonly used today is hydroxylapatite, either in granular form or as a shaped canal wall replacement.

Bearing in mind that all these patients will have had a persistently discharging ear before revision surgery, the success rate of most of these methods is high. The impression from reviewing the litera-

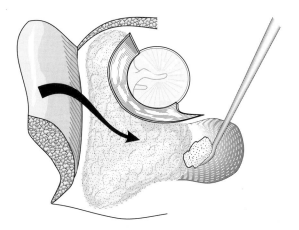

Fig 30.15 Mastoid obliteration. The posterosuperior canal wall is reconstructed with a sheet of connective tissue. The attic and mastoid are filled with bone dust or other suitable material. The superior flap is turned down on top of the obliterated space.

ture is that the more solid the obliterating material, the longer lasting its benefit. Eliminating or substantially reducing the volume of the cavity appears to be the key to success.

For patients who have no hearing in the operated ear, obliteration can be carried into the middle ear with advantage. There are several series of such patients with nearly 100 per cent success in eliminating discharge.

Complications and complicating factors

The level of the middle fossa dura and the position of the lateral venous sinus vary greatly, largely depending upon the degree of pneumatization of the mastoid system. In open-cavity surgery this may be beneficial as it limits the size of the postoperative cavity. In closed-cavity surgery, however, the operative field can be severely restricted and make exposure of the attic difficult. The problem can usually be overcome by performing a limited excision of the outer attic wall and reconstructing at the end, by elevating the dura, or by decompressing the sinus. When a lateral sinus is unusually prominent thought should be given to the possibility that the sinus on the opposite side may be underdeveloped.

The next most common problem is dehiscence of the facial nerve, which usually occurs in the horizontal portion. This can be a natural anatomical occurrence, or the Fallopian canal may have been eroded by the disease process. Provided the anatomy is well understood and the possibility of such an abnormality is known, the risk of damage to the nerve is small. The problem may be compounded, however, by the presence of granulation tissue over the Fallopian canal. Careful dissection is needed in such a case and is better carried out from superior to inferior. A facial nerve monitor can be reassuring in such circumstances, but should never be allowed to substitute for good anatomical knowledge and surgical technique.

Fistulae into the vestibular system, and more rarely into the cochlea, can be created by advanced disease. These patients often present with vertigo, which is otherwise unusual in chronic ear disease. Sensorineural deafness is also likely and may be total in severe cases.

As with facial nerve dehiscence the secret to successful management is to be aware of the possibility that a defect might exist. Dissection in the region of the semicircular canals and promontory should be slow and careful. Any sign of tethering or unexpected change in contour should be treated with suspicion. Opinion concerning management varies; the matrix can be carefully removed and the fistula repaired using fascia, with or without bone dust. This is much more difficult with large fistulae but it is essential that no cholesteatoma be left in a position from which it can erode into the vestibule or cochlea. Alternatively the matrix can be left, provided it is not becoming invaginated.

If the operative procedure is an open one there is a risk of persistent postoperative vertigo due to the exposure of the fistula to caloric stimulation through the meatus. The closed-cavity technique protects the vestibule from temperature variation but a second stage is mandatory. When matrix has been left on the fistula it has been found to have disappeared in up to 50 per cent of such cases and the fistula not infrequently closes with new bone formation.

The majority of cases of significant sensorineural loss are in large fistulae and in fistulae not recognized by the surgeon until damage has already been done.

The jugular bulb runs in close proximity to the floor of the middle ear. On occasion it is superiorly placed and encroaches on the posterior hypotympanum, sometimes rising as high as the round window and on rare occasions causing hearing loss by interference with round window function. It is important to recognize the possibility of this anomaly, as the bulb can be entered when dissecting the posteroinferior part of the tympanic membrane out of its tympanic annulus. Fortunately there is usually complete bony covering to a high jugular bulb, but this is not always the case.

Some of these anomalies may be predicted by preoperative examination and by radiological imaging. However, this cannot be relied upon and it is always safer to assume that all anomalies are present until proven otherwise.

Postoperative complications mostly relate to the function of the mechanisms that are subject to surgery. A conductive hearing loss may result from the need to disarticulate an intact ossicular chain, or because hearing was being maintained through the disease itself and in removing it contact between tympanic membrane and cochlea has been lost. Cochlear damage can occur because of excessive manipulation of the stapes footplate or as a result of surgical manipulation of a fistula.

It is as well to remember that topical medications can be ototoxic, and antiseptics, antibiotics and vasoconstrictors should be chosen carefully.

Vertigo can result from surgical stimulation in the same way that damage can occur to the cochlea.

Tinnitus is a highly unpredictable phenomenon and is particularly liable to occur in patients whose hearing is impaired.

The chorda tympani is frequently lost in the dissection required for the removal of chronic ear disease. When the nerve is cut cleanly the patient rarely notices much inconvenience but stretching the nerve may result in unpleasant symptoms affecting the tip of the tongue on the operated side.

Haemorrhage at the time of surgery can pose a problem, especially in an infected ear.

Hypotensive anaesthesia provided by a skilled anaesthetist can be very helpful, but in less skilled hands can make the situation worse. The surgeon needs to take care to control bleeding vessels at an early stage and infiltration with adrenaline postaurally and permeatally has a considerable beneficial effect. Perioperative bleeding can be controlled to some extent by irrigation and topical adrenaline application.

Postoperative haemorrhage can be a risk especially after hypotensive anaesthesia. The surgeon should be aware of this risk and take particular care not to miss potential bleeding areas before closing a wound.

Postoperative infections seem to be an unusual complication. If the surgery has been carried out thoroughly the ear should be sterile by the end of the procedure. The disease process should have been removed and the drilling procedures will have necessitated copious irrigation, which will have diluted the bacterial count considerably. Non-ototoxic biocidal solutions can also be employed as extra security.

The need for prophylactic or perioperative antibiotics has been much discussed. Some surgeons always use them and some do not, without any apparent difference. This would suggest that their role is doubtful. It is clear, however, that swabbing the external ear canal does not provide a representative culture of the organisms within the middle ear or mastoid, as these superficial bacteria are largely adventitious.

Summary

The preceding part of this chapter has attempted to demonstrate the range of procedures available to the otologist to deal with chronic ear disease, whether the disease be mucosal, cholesteatomatous or a combination of the two. Only complete eradication of tissues that have undergone irreversible change can ensure success.

The type of disease and its extent, and the preference and experience of the surgeon will influence the choice of technique to be employed. The choice of technique, however, does not alter the need for meticulous attention to detail to ensure identification and elimination of all irreversibly diseased tissue.

The end result should be an ear that is permanently dry and trouble-free, it should be checked annually for any sign of instability and for the removal of wax or debris.

Part of the surgical process should include a consideration of function. Details of ossiculoplasty techniques are discussed in Chapter 31, but it is appropriate to include some thoughts on the middle ear transformer mechanism at this stage.

If the chain is intact and disease can be removed without risk to the cochlea an excellent postoperative hearing state can usually be achieved; however, great care needs to be exercised in deciding whether an intact chain should be sacrificed in order to ensure disease eradication. This requires experience and skill, which can only be learnt with time and practice.

When the ossicular chain is deficient appropriate surgical management can help to create a situation in which the processes of healing can maximize the chances of a hearing gain, either naturally or by an ossicular reconstruction. It is necessary to bear in mind that the auditory function of the ear can only be expected to work when there is a ventilated middle ear space lined by healthy mucosa and closed by a vibrating membrane.

The principles of physiological preservation or restoration, or both, should be constantly borne in mind. The Eustachian tube orifice needs to be unobstructed, healthy mucosa should be preserved and, when necessary, silastic sheeting used to prevent adhesions obliterating the middle ear space. An adequate middle ear cleft should be preserved or created and the tympanic membrane should always be repaired.

The need for staging in the management of chronic ear disease requires careful consideration. It provides security in ensuring disease eradication and allows time for healing and stabilization before further reconstruction is carried out.

The original aims of the operation should never be forgotten. Eradication of the disease takes precedence over function and the state of the opposite ear should be borne in mind. A perfectly functioning ear on the other side will always remain dominant, however good the result of the surgery. If the opposite side is functionally inadequate, a dry stable ear with a hearing aid is preferable to risking the remaining cochlea function with overambitious surgery.

Suggested reading

Albera R, Cesarani A, Fagnani E, Disani P, Gedda F. Surgical approach to the sinus tympani. *Proceedings of the Third International Conference on Cholesteatoma and Mastoid Surgery*. Amsterdam: Kugler and Ghedini, 1989:781–5.

Anson BJ, Donaldson JA. *Surgical anatomy of the temporal bone and ear*. Philadelphia: WB Saunders, 1973.

Ars B. Typamic membrne retraction pockets. *Acta Oto-Rhino-Laryngologica Belgica* 1995; **49**:163–71.

Black B. Prevention of recurrent cholesteatoma: use of hydroxyapatite plates and composite grafts. *American Journal of Otology* 1992; **13**:273–8.

Brookers DS, Smyth GDL. Management of posterior mesotympanic cholesteatoma. *Journal of Laryngology and Otology* 1992; **106**:496–9.

Harner SG. Management of posterior tympanic membrane retraction. *Laryngscope* 1995; **105**:326–8.

Donald P, McCabe BF, Loevy SS. Atticotomy: a neglected otosurgical technique. *Annals of Otology* 1974; **83**:652–62.

Glasscock ME, Miller GW. Intact canal wall tympanoplasty in the management of cholesteatoma. *Laryngoscope* 1976; **86**:1639–57.

Jackson CG, Glasscock ME, Nissen AJ. Open mastoid procedures: contemporary indications and surgical techniques. *Laryngoscope* 1985; **95**:1037–43.

Jahn AF. Chronic otitis media: diagnosis and treatment. *Medical Clinics of North America* 1991; **75**:1277–91.

Jako GJ. The posterior bony ear canal wall and the antrum threshold angle in conservative middle ear surgery. *Laryngoscope* 1966; **76**:1260–76.

Jansen C. Cartilage tympanoplasty. *Laryngoscope* 1963; **77**:2022–31.

Jansen C. The combined approach for tympanoplasty. *Journal of Laryngology and Otology* 1968; **82**:779–93.

Jansen C. Posterior tympanotomy: experiences and surgical details. *Otolaryngologic Clinics of North America* 1972; **5**:79–96.

Marquet J. My current cholesteatoma techniques. *American Journal of Otology* 1989; **10**:124–30.

Nadol JB Jr, Schuknecht HF. *Surgery of the ear and temporal bone*. New York: Raven, 1993.

Palva T, Makinen J. The meatally based musculoperiosteal flap in cavity obliteration. *Archives of Otolaryngology* 1979; **105**:377–80.

Robinson JM. Closed cavity tympano-mastoidectomy: a continuing study. *Proceedings of the Third International Conference on Cholesteatoma and Mastoid Surgery*. Amsterdam: Kugler and Ghedini, 1989:839–41.

Shambaugh G. *Surgery of the ear, 2nd ed*. Philadelphia: WB Saunders, 1967.

Smyth GDL. Postoperative cholesteatoma in combined approach tympanoplasty. *Journal of Laryngology and Otology* 1976; **90**:597–621.

Smyth GDL, Brooker DS. Small cavity mastoidectomy. *Clinical Otolaryngology* 1992; **17**:280–3.

Toner JG, Smyth GDL. Surgical treatment of cholesteatoma: a comparison of three techniques. *American Journal of Otology* 1990; **11**:247–9.

Tos M. Volume 1: approaches, myringoplasty, ossiculoplasty and tympanoplasty. In: *Manual of middle ear surgery*. Stuttgart: Thieme, 1993.

Tos, M. Volume 2: mastoid surgery and reconstructive procedures. In: *Manual of middle ear surgery*. Stuttgart: Thieme, 1993.

CHAPTER 31

Reconstruction of the middle ear

JAMES ROBINSON

Introduction

Destruction of the middle ear is usually the result of chronic ear disease, discussed in Chapter 30. However, damage can also occur from various forms of trauma.

Direct physical injury, burns, scalds or pressure effects and head injuries can disrupt the tympanic membrane and may fracture or dislocate the ossicular chain. Acute infections may result in the perforation of the tympanic membrane, but these usually heal spontaneously. Iatrogenic damage to the middle ear also occurs, most commonly after insertion of ventilation tubes, especially the long-term variety.

In considering reconstruction of the middle ear the integrity of the whole mechanism must be considered: the tympanic ring to support the tympanic membrane, the membrane itself, the mucosa that lines the middle ear cleft and finally the ossicles themselves. If any one of these items is deficient a good result cannot be expected.

Reconstruction of the middle ear involves not only the restoration of the anatomical or mechanical components but also of the physiology or function of the ear. It is frequently the difficulty in achieving the latter part of this process that leads to unsatisfactory results. Zollner and Wullstein laid down the requirements for a functioning middle ear in the 1950s: an intact elastic tympanic membrane, a ventilated middle ear space, a mobile and unobstructed oval and round window, and a mechanism to link the tympanic membrane to the oval window.

Perforation of the pars tensa can involve any part of the membrane and can be of any size from a pinhole to total loss. Loss of the annulus can occur but is unusual.

The principles of the various techniques can apply to most sizes and positions of defect but there are detailed modifications for certain specific problems. Large perforations are more difficult to close as they are more difficult to stabilize and have a smaller recipient site to provide a blood supply to the graft. Very small perforations may be providing ventilation to a naturally poorly ventilated ear; closing these can result in the collapse of the membrane or persistent recurrence of the perforation.

Minor outpatient procedures for closing tympanic membrane perforations have a long history and rely on the natural tendency of traumatic perforations to heal themselves. Once the edges of the perforations have epithelialized, further closure is unlikely. Occasionally, especially in children, a minor ear infection will stimulate the perforation to close, so that a period of delay in an asymptomatic patient is quite acceptable and may save the need for surgery.

The rim of the perforation may be carefully dissected off to create a fresh margin. In a stoical patient this may require no anaesthesia, but local injections are highly effective. Similarly the rim can be treated with tricholoracetic acid to destroy the epithelial margin. This needs to be applied sparingly and with care. The procedure can be uncomfortable and is not suitable for children. It has been suggested that after either of these procedures the application of a small piece of fine silastic sheet, oiled silk, or tissue paper to cover the defect will increase the success rate. It is certainly a technique

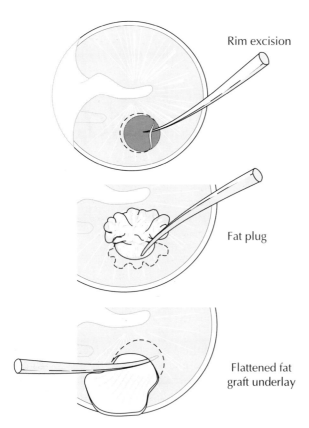

Rim excision

Fat plug

Flattened fat graft underlay

Fig 31.1 Simple procedures for repair of tympanic membrane defects.

that can indicate whether closing the perforation will result in a hearing gain.

The above methods are well worth trying for small perforations for which a high success rate can be achieved (Fig 31.1), although repeated procedures may be needed. Large defects are less likely to respond but it is worth trying in patients in whom surgery is contraindicated or not acceptable.

A slightly more aggressive approach that can be employed under either local or general anaesthetic is to excise the rim of the perforation as described above, and then to fill the gap with some bio-acceptable material. Fat taken from the ear lobe is simple and effective and can be placed as a plug or flattened into a sheet and inserted through the perforation to lie on the inside of the tympanic membrane remnant. Fibrin glue and gelfoam have also been used but fat probably has a higher take rate.

Myringoplasty

Myringoplasty is the operation specifically designed to close tympanic membrane defects. The approach to the ear can be permeatal (transcanal), endaural or postaural.

APPROACHES

A permeatal approach has the advantage of least disturbance to the patient but gives limited access and can be difficult in narrow ear canals, which may require drilling of the bone to achieve a satisfactory view. Depending on technique an external incision will usually be needed to harvest graft material.

The endaural incision gives good access to posterior perforations and also to the oval window area. Fascia can be taken through the upper extension of the incision. Anterior perforations can, however, be a problem because of lack of access. Bone can be removed from the anterior canal wall but there is a risk of exposure of the temporomandibular joint and also of stenosis.

A postaural incision gives excellent anterior access. The posterior view may be slightly restricted but can be improved quite easily by drilling bone away posteriorly from an area already denuded of meatal skin. Fascia is also easily accessible.

GRAFT MATERIALS

The materials available for grafting are numerous: temporalis fascia, connective tissue, perichondrium cartilage or vein. Temporalis fascia is the most commonly employed as it is effective and easily harvested through the same incision as is used to gain access to the ear.

Homograft materials have been used widely in the past but are less commonly used today because of the perceived risk of the transmission of viral disease. Collecting and preparing these grafts involves considerable organization and is expensive. Some surgeons have also found the results disappointing compared with autologous fascia. Homograft dura was also used in the past but is probably rarely used today because of the possible risk of transmission of Creutzfeldt–Jakob disease (CJD).

A number of xenografts have also been proposed and some are available commercially. Such materials avoid the problems inherent in the homografts but still suffer from the problem of cost and efficacy.

The original technique for myringoplasty was to separate the squamous epithelium carefully from the drum remnant and elevate it, leaving the fibrous layer in position. The graft material was then laid onto the fibrous layer and the elevated epithelium was replaced on top. The technique is still used in

(a)

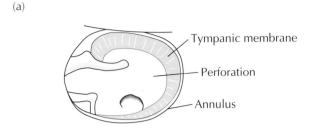

Tympanic membrane

Perforation

Annulus

(b)

Anterior remnant of
TM lifted forwards

Slit to wrap
round malleus handle

Graft

Tympanomeatal flap
lifted forwards

(c)

Anterior part of graft under
malleus handle and under
annulus anteriorly

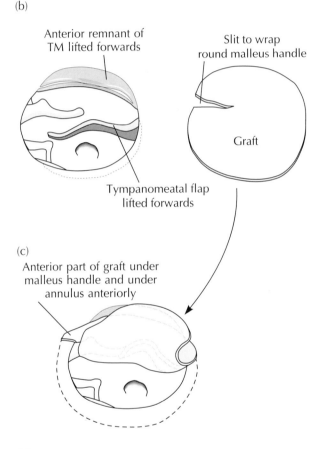

(d)

Annulus and residual TM
replaced over graft

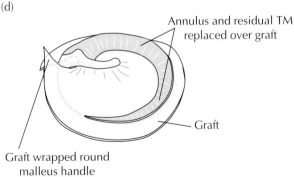

Graft

Graft wrapped round
malleus handle

Fig 31.2 Underlay myringoplasty.

many centres throughout the world. It has a good success rate but can be technically difficult and risks leaving squamous epithelium under the graft, which results in iatrogenic cholesteatoma pearls forming in the new tympanic membrane. There is also the risk that the new membrane may become lateralized due to inadequate location, especially anteriorly.

The more commonly used technique is to elevate the whole of the tympanic remnant by dissecting the fibrous annulus out of its groove in the bone. The graft can then be placed under the tympanic membrane remnant (Fig 31.2). This considerably reduces the risk of burying squamous epithelium and provides a more secure location for the graft and virtually eliminates lateralization or blunting.

To reduce the risk of iatrogenic cholesteatoma further it is wise to excise the rim of the perforation. The squamous epithelium frequently grows around the edge of the perforation onto the medial surface for a short distance. If it is not excised before elevating the tympanic membrane remnants, this squamous epithelium can be buried.

The placement of the graft in relation to the malleus is a matter of some debate. If placed lateral to the handle the new drum may become lateralized. It is probably wise therefore to place the graft deep to the malleus handle to ensure a proper relationship of graft to malleus.

The graft, epithelial remnants and meatal skin are all carefully repositioned to ensure a correct anatomical alignment. The meatus is then usually packed, but the range of materials used is very wide: various ointments, ribbon gauze impregnated with a range of pharmaceutical products, sponges and foams, sometimes with protective strips of plastic sheet or oiled silk. The length of time they are left in the ear also varies greatly, from days to weeks. This would all suggest that the packing of the meatus may not be a very important part of the procedure.

This basic technique has numerous variations depending on the site and size of the perforation.

Posterior perforations can be closed by simply raising the posterior half of the drum remnant and sliding the graft underneath. Similarly an inferior perforation can be dealt with using a limited approach. Anterior perforations and reniform perforations, or subtotal perforations, usually require more extensive elevation. It is wise to carry the dissection of the annulus well forward, superiorly and inferiorly, when performing an underlay graft. This makes positioning much easier later.

Whether the remnants need to be dissected off the malleus handle is a matter of opinion, but it needs to be done with care to avoid cochlear trauma. It would, however, appear that the more the tissues are elevated and the wider the graft bed, the higher the take rate.

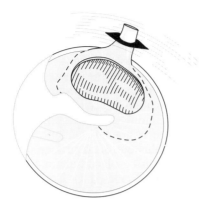

Fig 31.3 Anterior locating flap for anterior or subtotal perforations with inadequate rim. This flap will be tucked under the annulus before final insertion into tunnel in anterior meatal wall skin.

In cases in which there is no anterior rim, location of the anterior part of the graft is a problem. An overlay technique taking the dissection up the anterior canal wall provides location but with loss of the angle by blunting. A similar problem sometimes arises if the anterior annulus is raised and the graft tucked underneath. However, a limited tunnel, 1–2 mm wide, under the anterior annulus can be used to pull a small tag of graft material through the tunnel and so locate the unstable segment (Fig 31.3).

There is also disagreement as the need or otherwise to support the graft material in the middle ear. The concern is that the graft will collapse at the edge, especially anteriorly. Overlay grafting reduces this risk by using the fibrous layer to support the graft. Many surgeons who use the underlay technique fill the middle ear with gel foam to support the graft. However, if a good location technique is used with anterior tagging, if necessary, and the patient is encouraged to autoinflate a day or two after surgery, then gel foam does not seem to be necessary.

The use of nitrous oxide during general anaesthesia for myringoplasty is also in question. The concern is that the nitrous oxide diffuses into the middle ear and mastoid across the epithelium and raises the pressure slightly within the tympanomastoid space. Overlay grafts can be dislodged by this pressure and surgeons who use this technique usually try to avoid the use of this anaesthetic agent.

In underlay grafts, especially when the graft is placed deep to the malleus handle, a positive pressure is helpful as it pushes the graft up into contact with the graft bed, making final adjustments to the graft easier and providing a check that the position is good with no leaks or inadequate location.

Results of tympanic membrane repair vary according to technique, but more importantly are affected by the experience of the surgeon.

Most outpatient methods have a success rate of between 30 and 80 per cent depending on pathology, technique and operator patience. Minor surgery for small defects can be successful in 80 per cent or more. Myringoplasty can be expected to close 90 per cent of perforations with a follow-up of 12 months in experienced hands.

Whether these results are maintained is debateable. Late reperforations occur, particularly in children. Poor ventilation leads to retraction or atrophy, or both, and fibrosis in the middle ear may develop. All of these can result in redevelopment of hearing loss and discharge. The reoperation rates for myringoplasty certainly underestimate the size of the problem.

COMPLICATING FACTORS

Complicating factors in the management of tympanic membrane perforations are numerous. The age of the patient is a contentious issue. The consensus seems to be that children have a poorer success rate; however, some authors find no difference and others suggest that myringoplasty should be delayed until the age of anything up to 13 years. The suggestion is that the greater tendency to upper respiratory tract infection and consequent middle ear infection in children affects the graft take rate and survival. On the other hand, there does not appear to be any suggestion that elderly patients have a higher failure rate. The limitation here is their ability to cope with surgery and anaesthesia.

The preoperative state of the ear is of great importance. A narrow meatus may require widening to allow access. The presence of otitis externa can make surgery difficult because of excessive bleeding and poor skin quality.

Abnormalities of the tympanic membrane are rarely much of a problem as they can be eliminated and replaced by the graft. Severe tympanosclerosis, however, may need to be dissected out to allow the graft to lie well, but moderate amounts within the layers of the tympanic membrane can be left without jeopardizing the survival of the graft.

Squamous epithelium on the medial side of the tympanic membrane must always be eliminated, if necessary by resecting the affected part of the drum remnant. Adhesions need to be divided to allow proper graft positioning but this must be performed with as little damage to the middle ear mucosa as possible.

When severe middle ear fibrosis has occurred silastic sheeting may be needed to prevent refibrosis and adherence of the graft to the medial wall. Whether such sheeting should be allowed to remain *in situ* is debatable, but extrusion does occur on occasions and silastic is certainly not inert.

When there is serious doubt about the patency of the Eustachian tube a fine epidural catheter can be passed to confirm patency. This does not, of course, imply physiological function, but it does exclude total obliteration of the tube. Routine catheterization should be avoided as there is always the risk of causing more harm to the tubal mucosa.

The presence of infection can be a problem as some ears will not settle until the tympanic membrane is repaired, despite vigorous preoperative therapy. A mild degree of inflammation is not a contraindication to surgery. On the contrary, it may encourage vascularization of the graft. Frank infection with discharge, however, is a different matter and these cases should be considered for a combined myringoplasty and cortical mastoidectomy with or without a posterior tympanotomy to eliminate mastoid disease and open up ventilation pathways from the middle ear through the attic and into the antrum.

The presence, or otherwise, of the ossicles is obviously of importance from the point of view of auditory function, but the presence of the malleus handle is helpful in locating the graft and preventing lateralization.

A ventilated middle ear space is an essential component of a functioning middle ear transformer mechanism. An intact tympanic membrane protects the middle ear from the outside world and in so doing makes the normal functioning of the middle ear ventilation mechanism essential. This is provided by the Eustachian tube and the middle ear and mastoid mucosa. At present there is much debate about the relative importance of these two mechanisms and new research methods seem likely to change our views on this important aspect of middle ear physiology.

Gaseous diffusion across the epithelium that lines the middle ear and mastoid is undoubtedly of great importance in maintaining the gas pressure, but how much the Eustachian tube is involved in this regulation is now a matter of much interesting research. What seems clear is that the tube acts as a drain and when functioning well can cope effectively with sudden major changes of pressure.

Numerous attempts have been made in the past to improve inadequate Eustachian tube function, by insufflation, catheterization and various surgical manipulations at the middle ear end of the structure. These do not seem to have achieved success and some, undoubtedly, seem to have done more harm than good. Left to its own devices the Eustachian tube usually remains patent; total obstruction is very rare. However, impaired active function during swallowing movements may be another matter.

Similarly attempts to improve upon the state of the epithelium by grafting nasal or buccal mucosa seems to have been disappointing. The best course of action would seem to avoid inflicting damage on normal or salvageable mucosa in the middle ear or mastoid, to eliminate irreversible disease, to open up good ventilation pathways and when necessary to use silastic sheeting to prevent reformation of adhesions.

Postoperative ventilation by politzerization or autoinflation or nasal balloons should also be used to re-establish ventilation as soon as possible after surgery. The risk of displacing a well positioned graft has been overemphasized.

Mobility of the round and the oval windows is essential if the cochlea is to function. Experience from surgery of otosclerosis has shown that rigid fixation of the round window is better not disturbed as there is a high risk of cochlear damage. Tympanosclerosis in the round window is unusual but probably carries the same risk as otosclerosis. Soft-tissue obstruction can, however, reasonably be removed provided it is done with great care. The membrane is usually well hidden under the overhanging lip of the window, but there are anatomical variations. The discrete use of the surgical laser should avoid overmanipulation of the membrane, but it must be directed tangentially to avoid damage.

Similar caution needs to be applied to the oval window. It is tempting to assume that a stapedectomy or stapedotomy should be as effective in dealing with stapes fixation due to chronic ear disease as it is when it is employed to deal with otosclerosis. Unfortunately this has not been the experience of many surgeons who have employed this approach for tympanosclerosis. Initial results may be good but in the long term the hearing has been found to deteriorate. Similarly in cases of coexisting otosclerosis the results of stapedectomy can be disappointing. It may also be that the surgical laser has the advantage of allowing the performance of surgery on an already traumatized oval window without any additional damage to the cochlea.

Ossicular repair

If all the above factors have been satisfactorily dealt with, the next problem that arises is to bridge the gap between the tympanic membrane and the cochlea. It is easy to assume that a conductive hearing loss due to chronic ear disease should respond to surgery with the same degree of success as an otosclerotic ear. However, there is a fundamental difference. The otosclerotic ear only has fixation of the stapes footplate; the rest of the ear is anatomically and physiologically normal. This is not the case in the chronically diseased ear and despite the best endeavours of the surgeon the ear can only be improved, it cannot be returned to normal.

Over the past 35–40 years much of the emphasis has been on designing more and more sophisticated ossicular prostheses and the development of many materials designed to be bio-inert or bioactive together with techniques to reuse the patient's own components. There are now more than enough techniques, but if a satisfactory environment is not provided for them, they will not work. It is therefore essential that the surgeon, as a number one priority, provides a working environment for the ossicular repair and this may require the operation to be staged.

The problem faced by the surgeon in reconstructing the ossicular chain varies depending on the damage caused by the disease process. The replacements required and the results of the surgery are dependent on how much of the chain is missing. The degrees of damage encountered can be conveniently divided into four groups:

1 (a) loss of part of the long process of the incus
  (b) total loss of the incus, or at least all of the long process
2 loss of the incus and the stapes superstructure, but with the malleus handle still present
3 loss of the incus and malleus, or at least the malleus handle, with the stapes superstructure still present
4 loss of the incus, malleus and stapes, but with a mobile footplate remaining

In addition to these lost ossicular components, fixation of parts of the chain also needs to be considered. The incus, or malleus, or both, may be fixed in the attic by bony ankylosis or tympanosclerosis. The stapes may be fixed by tympanosclerosis in the oval window niche or perhaps by coexisting otosclerosis.

Fixation of the malleus or incus can be corrected by performing an atticotomy or closed-cavity mastoidectomy and obtaining access to the area of fixation and removing it. The closed-cavity technique or repair of the atticotomy ensures an intact outer attic wall. If there is no incus but a remaining malleus that is fixed in the attic, it is simple to divide the malleus neck, leaving a mobile handle in the tympanic membrane to help in any subsequent ossicular reconstruction. The malleus head must be removed or adequately separated from the neck otherwise it may become re-ankylosed.

Fixation of the stapes by tympanosclerotic infiltration of the oval window niche should be correctable by dissecting out the tympanosclerosis.

This, however, is often technically difficult and the bone in contact with the tympanosclerosis may be found to be eroded. There is therefore a risk of entering the cochlear or vestibule if such erosion is present and, even if it is not, the dissection may cause undue movement of the stapes footplate, resulting in cochlear damage.

Fixation of the footplate by tympanosclerosis or otosclerosis should respond well to stapedectomy, but experience has shown that although initial results may be good there is a tendency to progressive sensorineural deterioration. It may be that small fenestra stapedotomy and the use of the surgical laser will improve the prognosis in this otherwise disappointing procedure.

If the defect in the mechanism is a more straightforward loss of mechanical structure, a wide range of possibilities exist for their reconstruction.

Autografts make use of the patient's own tissues and this avoids the problems of rejection and can result in a living repair.

Homografts can be harvested from human cadavers. Rejection is a theoretical possibility but in practice rarely occurs. If severe damage has occurred and autografts do not exist, homografts can be equally effective. Unfortunately there is the possibility of transmission of viral disease and, although this has been shown to be statistically nearly insignificant, few surgeons still use these materials. A number of homograft banks still exist in various parts of the world.

Xenografts have also been used; transmission of disease is not a problem but rejection and extrusion is more common.

Non-biological prostheses are numerous and have been available since the earliest days of tympanoplasty. These prostheses have been made from plastics, metals, glass and inorganic bone analogues. They exhibit varying degrees of biocompatibility and bioreactivity. There have been problems with rejection, extrusion and instability but, in their favour, prostheses are readily available and relatively simple to use. To aid in the use of these various prostheses additional products such as gelatin sponges and film, inorganic, and organic adhesives have also been developed.

The non-autograft materials have the advantage of being available off the shelf but have the disadvantage of costing money.

The four degrees of ossicular disruption mentioned above require somewhat different approaches. The first is the eroded incus. The amount of damage may be only 1 mm or less, leaving some contact with the stapes, or the damage may be greater with total loss of contact. Provided some of the long process is still available, reconnection may be achieved. Autologous bone dust

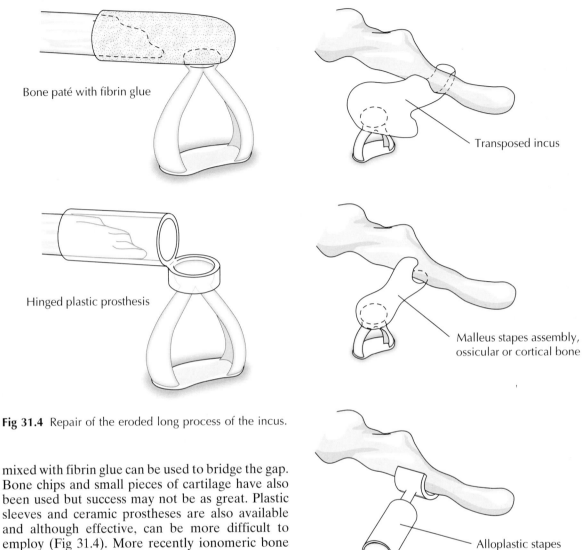

Bone paté with fibrin glue

Hinged plastic prosthesis

Transposed incus

Malleus stapes assembly, ossicular or cortical bone

Alloplastic stapes to malleus prosthesis

Fig 31.4 Repair of the eroded long process of the incus.

Fig 31.5 Malleus to stapes assembly.

mixed with fibrin glue can be used to bridge the gap. Bone chips and small pieces of cartilage have also been used but success may not be as great. Plastic sleeves and ceramic prostheses are also available and although effective, can be more difficult to employ (Fig 31.4). More recently ionomeric bone cement has been used to good effect. It is not as easy to use as bone dust and its longevity is, as yet, unknown.

The more severe version of this group, in which the long process of the incus is no longer available, may lend itself to re-establishing a link between the stapes head and the malleus handle. If the body of the incus is still present this can be sculpted into a strut to bridge between the incus head and the malleus handle. If not, a piece of cortical bone can be used. Homograft ossicles can similarly be employed. Artificial prostheses are also available to perform the same task (Fig 31.5).

The limiting factor here is the relationship of the stapes to the malleus. The potential benefit from the strut is related to the angle it makes between the stapes and the malleus, the more vertical the better. If the malleus is particularly anteriorly placed, the angle may be more than 45° in which case the chances of hearing gain are minimal.

On the benefit side this arrangement relies on linking bone to bone. There is no direct contact with the tympanic membrane so that extrusion is unusual. The presence of the stapes also allows a more stable assembly, the head of the stapes providing a fixed point over which an acetabular connection can be placed.

In Group 2 a mobile malleus handle remains but there is no incus or stapes superstructure. Provided the angle between the malleus and the stapes footplate is less than 45° a strut may be inserted with its medial end on the mobile footplate and the

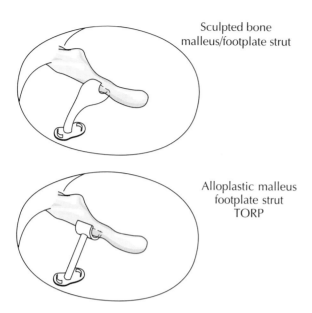

Sculpted bone
malleus/footplate strut

Alloplastic malleus
footplate strut
TORP

Fig 31.6 Footplate to malleus strut. TORP, total ossicular replacement prosthesis.

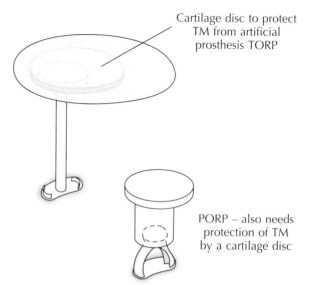

Cartilage disc to protect
TM from artificial
prosthesis TORP

PORP – also needs
protection of TM
by a cartilage disc

Fig 31.8 Artificial footplate to tympanic membrane prosthesis – TORP (total ossicular replacement prosthesis), and artificial footplate to stapes prosthesis – PORP (partial ossicular replacement prosthesis).

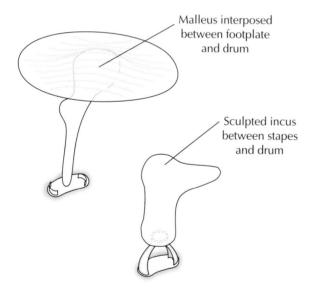

Malleus interposed
between footplate
and drum

Sculpted incus
between stapes
and drum

Fig 31.7 Tympanic membrane to footplate or stapes assembly, autograft or homograft.

lateral end hooked under the malleus handle, or encircling it (Fig 31.6). Autologous or homologous bone can be used by suitable sculpting. Purpose-made prostheses in synthetic materials are also available. The advantage of a bone-to-bone assembly still applies but the stability of the

medial end is poor, especially if there is no stump of the posterior crus present to prevent posterior dislocation.

In Groups 3 and 4 the malleus handle is missing, and in Group 4 the stapes superstructure is also gone, leaving only a mobile footplate.

Sculpted autograft or homograft bone can be employed to bridge the gap between the under surface of the tympanic membrane and the head of the stapes, or the footplate (Fig 31.7). The assembly tends to be more unstable, especially in the Group 4 patients with no stapes arch. Extrusion through the tympanic membrane is rare, especially with autologous grafts.

Artificial prostheses are also available to a similar design (Fig 31.8). In Group 3 patients, a tubular medial end fits over the head of the stapes with an expanded head situated under the tympanic membrane. In Group 4 patients, the medial end is a simple piston to make contact with the footplate. Sometimes a footplate shoe is provided to stabilize this part of the assembly.

MATERIALS FOR OSSICULOPLASTY

Early attempts to use artificial prostheses in this way failed because of a high rate of extrusion through the unprotected tympanic membrane. The use of autologous cartilage, usually from the tragus, virtually eliminated the problem. Later prostheses of inorganic bone analogues have shown a much reduced tendency to extrude but may be lost in the long run if middle ear ventilation is poor.

The reinforcement of the posterosuperior part of the tympanic membrane by the protecting cartilage probably confers some degree of protection in those patients in whom cartilage is used to cover the prostheses, especially if a relatively large piece is used.

In summary, in all cases of ossicular damage requiring reconstruction the middle ear environment must be rendered suitable for the insertion of the prosthesis. Without this the chances of success are poor, however sophisticated and expensive the device.

The range of materials and prostheses available is considerable and so far there appears to be no very clear leader in terms of functional success. Some are easier to use than others and there is a very definite cost implication. None of the artificial prostheses devised so far are immune from problems of rejection and extrusion, and biological processes can result in phagocytosis, remodelling, replacement and resorption. Good short-term results have been achieved with all methods and materials, but good long-term results have been much more elusive.

The posterior canal wall

One more aspect of middle ear reconstruction needs to be considered and this overlaps with the surgical management of chronic ear disease and with revision surgery. The bony canal wall is an essential part of the middle ear mechanism as it supports the tympanic membrane at a level that allows for an adequate middle ear space. In open-cavity surgery the tympanic membrane is more medially placed and the middle ear cleft is therefore reduced in depth. In favourable cases this area may ventilate well and when a stapes superstructure is present the tympanic membrane may come naturally into contact with it (Fig 31.9), resulting in a satisfactory hearing level. On other occasions, however, this space is inadequate and the canal wall may need to be rebuilt to deepen the middle ear space (Fig 31.10). This can be done at the time of primary surgery, or later at a further stage, or as part of a revision procedure. Autologous material such as bone dust and chips, cortical bone grafts and tragal or scaphoid cartilage are all used, and have the advantage or providing a living repair. Inorganic bone analogues such as hydroxylapatite can also be employed and have been shown to integrate and develop bony ingrowth and remodelling. They

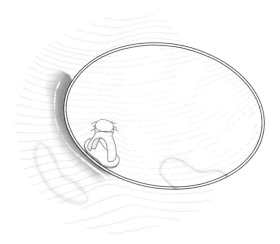

Fig 31.9 Natural myringostapediopexy in well ventilated open cavity.

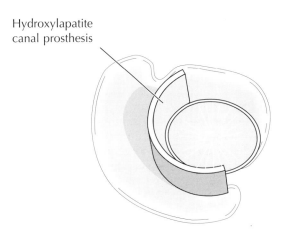

Hydroxylapatite canal prosthesis

Fig 31.10 Reconstruction of the posterosuperior canal wall.

are, however, more sensitive to infection and may be more difficult to handle. Homograft bone canal repairs have also been employed but suffer from the same disadvantages as tympanic membrane and ossicle homograft repairs.

It may be considered that in a patient undergoing mastoid surgery the intact canal wall technique overcomes this problem by preserving the canal wall initially. Reports in the literature of long-term results in ossiculoplasty are not consistent in showing any advantage over open techniques, although several authors are convinced that the technique does confer a benefit. The loss of the canal wall and consequent reduction in middle ear space is only one problem out of many faced by the surgeon attempting to reconstruct the middle ear and its function. Perhaps when more of the other factors have been solved, the benefits of retaining or repairing the canal wall will become more apparent.

Summary

The foregoing pages have illustrated the complexity of the problem of middle ear reconstruction. Repair of the tympanic membrane itself can be achieved in several different ways, and the multiplicity of techniques available for ossicular reconstruction can easily lead to confusion.

Each case must be considered on its merits and the appropriate methods and materials chosen from the wide range available. The trainee otologist will do well to observe as many experienced surgeons as possible and to gain first- or second-hand experience of as many of the variations in surgical techniques as they can. In this way they will be able to select wisely from an otherwise bewildering array of possibilities.

Every case is different and the otologist needs to be highly flexible, with a wide range of techniques at their disposal, to provide the best chance of success in a difficult surgical field. Most of these ears have a long history of disease and despite the best endeavours of the surgeon to reverse the disease processes, the surgical field tends to remain hostile to the micro-engineering that is needed to reconstruct a functioning sound transformer mechanism.

Suggested reading

Ars B, Miled I, Ars P. Allograft myringoplasy. *Acta Oto-Rhino-Laryngologica Belgica* 1995; **49**:207–18.

Black B. Prognisis: the spite method of assessment. *American Journal of Otology* 1992; **13**:544–51.

Bojrab DI, Causse JB, Battista R, Vincent R, Gratacap B, Vandeventer G. Ossucloplasty with composite P prostheses. *Otolaryngology Clinics of North America* 1994; **27**:759–76.

Deddens AE, Muntz H, Lusk R. Adipose myringoplasty in children. *Laryngoscope* 1993; **103**:216–9.

Donaldson I, Snow DG. A five year follow-up of incus transposition in relation to the first stage tympanoplasty technique. *Journal of Laryngology and Otology* 1992; **106**:607–9.

Dormer KJ, Bryce GE, Hough JVD. Selection of biomaterials for middle and inner ear implants. *Otolaryngology Clinics of North America* 1995; **28**:17–27.

El Seifa A, Fouad B. Autograft ossiculoplasty in cholesteatoma. *Otorhinolaryngology* 1992; **54**:324–7.

Emmett JR. Plasti-pore implants in middle ear surgery. *Otolaryngology Clinics of North America* 1995; **28**:265–72.

Geyer G, Helms J. Ionomer-based bone substitute in otologic surgery. *European Archives of Otorhinolaryngology* 1993; **250**:253–6.

Gersdorff M, Decat M. Ossiculoplasty: some physical and physiological considerations. *Acta Oto-Rhino-Laryngology* 1991; **45**:105–9.

Gimenez F, Marco-Algarra J, Carbonell R. Prognostic factors in tympanoplasty: a statistical evaluation. *Revue de Laryngologie, Otologie et Rhinologie,* 1993; **144**:335–7.

Jackler RK, Schindler RA. Myringoplasty with simple mastoidectomy: results in eighty-two consecutive patients. *Otolaryngology – Head and Neck Surgery* 1983; **91**:14–17.

Komune S, Hisashi K, Wakizono S. Importance of atticotomy in chronic otitis media with fixation of ossicles. *Auris Nases Larynx (Tokyo)* 1992; **19**:23–8.

Mills RP. Ossicular geometry and the choice of technique for ossiculoplasty. *Clinical Otolaryngology* 1991; **16**:476–9.

Ossiculoplasty. *The Otolaryngologic Clinic of North America* 1994; **24(4)**.

Shih L, Detar T, Crabtree JA. Myringoplasty in children. *Otolaryngology – Head and Neck Surgery* 1991; **105**:74–7.

Snow DG, Robinson JM, Peters J. Bone paté repair of the erodid incus – five years on. *Journal of Laryngology and Otology* 1995; **109**:1048–50.

Toner JG, Smyth GDL, Kerr AG. Realities in ossiculoplasty. *Journal of Laryngology and Otology* 1991; **105**:529–33.

Vartianen E, Nuutinen J. Success and pitfalls in myringoplasty: follow-up study of 404 cases. *American Journal of Otology* 1993; **14**:301–5.

Vartianen E. Findings in revision myringoplasty. *Ear, Nose and Throat Journal* 1993; **72**:201–4.

CHAPTER 32

Temporal bone trauma

DAVID A MOFFAT

In the late twentieth century trauma remains a significant cause of morbidity and mortality. Head injury is one of the most frequently suffered traumatic events; over 500 000 head injuries occur annually in the UK, in a population of about 60 000 000.

Symptoms of an injury to the temporal bone and its contents occur in 25–30 per cent of head injuries.[1] The male to female ratio is 3 : 1 because the male group is more prone to overall traumatic injuries.[2] The most common cause of temporal bone injury is motor vehicle accidents.

Traumatic injuries to the temporal bone are common and mostly occur in children and young people. A classification of temporal bone trauma is given in Table 32.1.

Table 32.1 Classification of temporal bone trauma

Blunt trauma
    Fracture injuries
    Non-fracture injuries
        Blast injuries
        Injuries caused by water under pressure

Penetrating trauma
    Foreign bodies
    Surgical trauma
    Stab and gunshot wounds

Whiplash trauma

Barotrauma
    Injuries caused by water pressure
    Injuries caused by air pressure

Thermal trauma

Radiation injury

Acoustic trauma

Blunt trauma

FRACTURE INJURIES

A fracture of the skull base is the result of sudden intense contact between a solid object and the head. The middle cranial fossa is involved in 60–80 per cent of basal skull fractures. The temporal bone forms two-thirds of the floor of the middle cranial fossa, and it is therefore not surprising that it is the most commonly injured bone in the base of the skull. The temporal bone is made up largely of dense bone, and intense mechanical forces must be present to distort it. The presence of numerous foramina, an irregular surface and numerous thin osseous panels explains the frequency with which this otherwise solid bone is prone to fracture. The air-containing spaces of the temporal bone are surrounded and strengthened by bony buttresses, the anatomy of which are relatively constant. Consequently, it is not surprising that there are predictable patterns of temporal bone fracture. Types of temporal bone fracture include longitudinal, transverse, mixed, oblique and unusual.

Longitudinal temporal bone fracture

The 'longitudinal' temporal bone fracture is one whose lines run parallel to the petrous ridge, that is, the longitudinal axis of the bone (Fig 32.1). According to most standard textbooks, the longitudinal type constitutes approximately 85 per cent of temporal bone fractures. Twenty-three per cent are bilateral.

The blow that results in a longitudinal temporal bone fracture usually originates lateral to the skull, with the impact directly onto the temporal

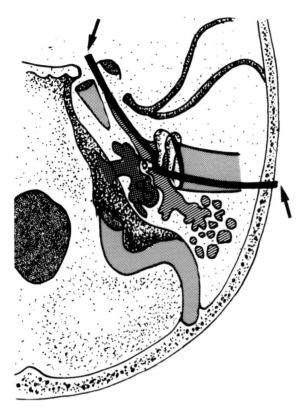

Fig 32.1 A longitudinal fracture of the temporal bone. The fracture line is along the longitudinal axis of the petrous bone (heavy line indicated by black arrows).

or parietal region. To understand the injury, consider the fracture to begin in the squamous temporal bone and continue towards the petrous apex, coursing around the dense otic capsule bone. The 'classic' longitudinal fracture is described as beginning in the superior temporal squamosa, passing anteroinferiorly to reach the posterosuperior roof of the external auditory canal, then spreading medially across the roof of the middle ear, disrupting the tegmen tympani and possibly dislocating the incudomalleolar joint. The fracture then disrupts the medial wall of the middle ear in the region of the geniculate ganglion. It bypasses the otic capsule and runs anterior to the carotid canal. The fracture plane then courses anteromedially towards the clivus, between the carotid artery and the foramen spinosum (i.e. between the petrous and sphenoid bones).

A posterior variant originates in the posterior parietal region of the area of the transverse dural venous sinus and sigmoid sinus and extends medially from the tegmen to involve the otic capsule or the jugular foramen.

The structures that are most commonly disrupted in these fractures are the tympanic membrane, the roof of the middle ear and the structures contained in the petrous apex. Hearing loss is common after the injury; it is usually a conductive or mixed hearing loss. Sensorineural hearing loss is relatively uncommon, and if it does occur it is usually a mild high-frequency loss, maximal at 3000–4000 Hz. This hearing loss is thought to arise from the effect of labyrinthine concussion and not from the disruption of the inner ear by the fracture.

The conductive hearing loss is often temporary, arising from blood in the external and middle ear and from soft-tissue swelling. Persistent conductive hearing loss is usually the result of ossicular disruption, and the most common type is an isolated incus or incudostapedial dislocation. Ossicular dislocation may also resolve spontaneously, because of minimal displacement of the incus.

These fractures invariably result in laceration of the roof of the external auditory canal and, often, the tympanic membrane. Blood from the middle ear will appear in the external auditory canal, leading to the dictum that bloody otorrhoea after head injury represents a longitudinal temporal bone fracture until proved otherwise. If the dura is disrupted, cerebrospinal fluid (CSF) may leak through a disrupted tegmen tympani, resulting in CSF otorrhoea or otorhinorrhoea.

Vestibular disorders are unusual after longitudinal fracture and, when present, are usually mild and temporary. Spontaneous nystagmus is rare.

The facial nerve is usually spared in fractures of this type, with a prevalence of facial paralysis of 20 per cent. Most fractures extend along the Fallopian canal rather than across it. When the nerve is injured, the fracture line usually involves the Fallopian canal in its tympanic portion, in the region of the geniculate ganglion or, less commonly, in the mastoid portion.[3] Facial weakness after these fractures is usually incomplete and is most often delayed, secondary to oedema rather than disruption of the nerve.

Transverse temporal bone fracture

The 'transverse' temporal bone fracture is one that runs at right angles to the longitudinal axis of the petrous bone (Fig 32.2). This pattern represents 15–30 per cent of temporal bone fractures. Such fractures are caused by a blow to the occiput or, less commonly, a direct frontal blow. Those transverse fractures caused by a frontal blow will most often be accompanied by a fracture of the floor of the anterior cranial fossa. Transverse fractures have a higher immediate mortality than longitudinal fractures and a greater force is required to generate them.

The 'classic' transverse temporal bone fracture begins in the posterior cranial fossa, usually in the

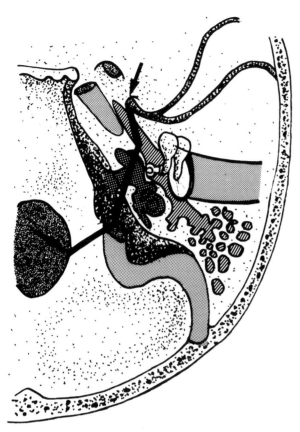

Fig 32.2 A transverse fracture of the temporal bone. The fracture line is perpendicular to the longitudinal axis of the petrous bone (heavy line indicated by black arrows).

region of the foramen magnum. It then extends through the jugular foramen and courses across the petrous pyramid and the floor of the middle cranial fossa to the region of the foramen lacerum or foramen spinosum. This fracture traverses the otic capsule or the internal auditory canal.

The hearing loss associated with transverse fractures is usually sensorineural, caused by disruption of the integrity of the labyrinth or the neurovascular bundle in the internal auditory canal. The fracture may disrupt the lateral wall of the otic capsule and extend to the medial wall of the middle ear, occasionally through the oval or round windows, resulting in middle ear haemorrhage and the clinical finding of haemotympanum.

Vertigo with spontaneous nystagmus and posttraumatic dysequilibrium is common after transverse temporal bone fracture. Facial nerve paralysis is also common (50 per cent), and is more often immediate and of greater severity than that seen in longitudinal fracture. This is because the orientation of the fracture line is perpendicular to the

course of the facial nerve and the nerve is therefore more vulnerable to complete transection.

Mixed

Severe crushing injuries to the skull base can result in multiple fractures, involving a combination of several of the routes described for classic longitudinal and transverse injuries.

Oblique temporal bone fracture

Recently, the advent of high resolution CT scanning of the skull base has resulted in a reinvestigation of the patterns of temporal bone fractures. Ghorayeb and Yeakley[4] reported a study of 150 temporal bone fractures and found that the oblique temporal bone fracture was actually the most common pattern of fracture, occurring in 75 per cent.

Other fractures of the temporal bone

Fractures of the anterior wall of the external auditory canal can occur in conjunction with injuries to the mandible. Unrecognized injuries in this area can result in the late complication of external auditory canal stenosis, whereas early recognition often results in easily accomplished reduction of the fracture. Late recognition of this lesion presents the otologist with a difficult reconstruction, often requiring the use of local skin flaps or split-thickness skin grafts.

An unusual type of temporal bone fracture involves the mastoid process alone. Such a fracture may open into the external canal and middle ear and may involve the mastoid segment of the facial nerve.[5]

CLINICAL ASSESSMENT OF TEMPORAL BONE FRACTURES

Wherever possible, given the patient's other injuries and neurological status, a full clinical evaluation of the injury should be undertaken at the earliest opportunity. Concomitant neurological injury is a bad prognostic factor and should be excluded as quickly as possible.

Hearing loss is a common complaint after blunt trauma to the temporal bone. An accurate history may reveal potential risk factors for significant injury to the hearing apparatus. These risk factors include unconsciousness, bleeding from the ear and subjective hearing loss; the combination of all three has been called the 'traumatic conductive triad'.[6]

Unconsciousness occurs in the vast majority of patients who suffer temporal bone fractures.[6] Bleeding from the ear is the hallmark of the longitudinal fracture and is usually brief in duration and mild in severity. Persistent bloody otorrhoea should alert the physician to the possibility of a vascular injury or CSF leak. Bleeding from the ear is unusual in transverse fractures, as the tympanic membrane is commonly left intact. Severe bleeding occurs in only 15 per cent of temporal bone fractures and, by draining down the Eustachian tube, can compromise the airway. Death caused by temporal bone fracture is unusual, but when it occurs it is most frequently the result of exsanguination. Laceration of the internal carotid artery with bleeding through the fracture to the middle ear is the pathological mechanism of these catastrophic events.

Vertigo and dysequilibrium occur as sequelae of head injury, with or without a fracture of the temporal bone. Seventeen per cent of children suffering a temporal bone fracture will have vestibular symptoms.[7] The head-injured patient should have thorough evaluation of their history and a full neurotological examination when the neurological status allows. This should include an examination for spontaneous and positional nystagmus, including the Dix–Hallpike manoeuvre. This examination is considerably enhanced by the use of Frenzel's lenses (see Chapter 3).

Every patient with a head injury should have an otoscopic examination as soon as possible after the injury. The status of the external canal wall and tympanic membrane should be determined, and removal of debris under the microscope should be undertaken. This debris may be an external source of bacterial contamination and acts as a culture medium for bacterial multiplication. Irrigation of the external auditory canal is absolutely contraindicated, as this greatly increases the likelihood of ascending infection and contamination of the central nervous system. Any fluid emanating from the external auditory canal should be considered possible CSF, and an attempt should be made to collect some for analysis. This is often difficult because of the small quantities available for sampling, but even a drop of bloody otorrhoea on a tissue may demonstrate a 'halo' sign, or central red blood patch surrounded by a clear ring of watery fluid, heralding the presence of CSF in the otorrhoea. Ecchymosis over the mastoid region, or 'Battle's sign' is often indicative of blood in the air-filled spaces of the temporal bone. Tuning fork testing should be performed in all head-injured patients, and this may give important clues as to the nature of any hearing loss.

A full examination of the cranial nerves should be conducted as soon as the patient's condition permits it. The most critical of these is the evaluation and documentation of the function of the VIIth nerve.

RADIOLOGICAL ASSESSMENT

When the patient is stable enough for the test, a high resolution CT scan of the head should be undertaken. Fracture lines may be seen and the nature of the fracture identified (Fig 32.3). Unless there is suspected intracranial or vascular involvement, there is no need for the use of contrast. Temporal bone fractures can be difficult to detect and describe, even in the presence of good CT equipment and competent appraisal.[8] One clue to such cryptic injuries may be the presence of air in the temporomandibular joint and this finding is seen in 20 per cent of temporal bone fractures.[9] The finding of free air in the labyrinth, or a 'pneumolabyrinth', has been described in transverse fractures.[10]

In severe blunt and penetrating trauma an assessment of the vascular structures of the temporal bone may be necessary. The most common vascular lesion of the skull base after trauma is occlusion of the jugular bulb and transverse sinus, which may be identified by lack of contrast enhancement on CT scan, or by an absence of 'flow-void' on MRI. Impingement on or injury to the carotid artery can be identified using carotid arteriography or digital subtraction angiography. Traumatic carotid aneurysms and arteriovenous malformations are identified in this way. An unusual complication of skull base trauma is a caroticocavernous fistula, which requires carotid angiography for diagnosis and can be treated with transarterial balloon occlusion.

AUDIOMETRY

All patients suspected of having sustained a significant trauma to the temporal region should undergo thorough audiometric testing, including an assessment of pure-tone thresholds, speech discrimination and impedance for both ears. This is particularly relevant for patients with immediate, total facial nerve weakness in whom facial nerve decompression surgery is being considered, as hearing loss is a common complication of this procedure.[11] Preoperative assessment of hearing is therefore imperative. Other more advanced audiological tests such as brainstem auditory evoked potentials (BAEPs) and electronystagmography (ENG) may also be indicated.

In one study, 60 per cent of patients with temporal bone fractures had a post-traumatic hearing loss; of these, 43 per cent were conductive, 52 per cent were sensorineural, and 5 per cent were mixed.[7]

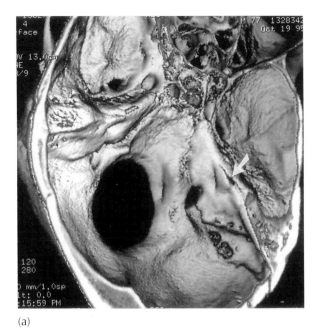

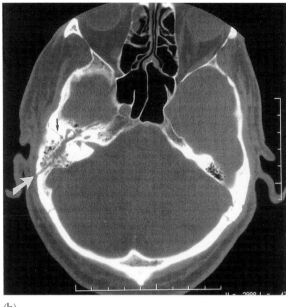

(a)   (b)

Fig 32.3 (a) Transaxial CT scan demonstrating a longitudinal fracture (white arrow) and a transverse fracture (black arrow) of the right temporal bone. (b) Three-dimensional CT reconstruction of the same patient demonstrating the longitudinal fracture (white arrow).

INJURIES TO THE CONDUCTIVE HEARING APPARATUS

External auditory canal and tympanic membrane injuries

Careful debridement of the ear is carried out under the microscope and an inspection of the external auditory canal and tympanic membrane is undertaken. The ear canal may be narrowed by fracture of the anterior canal wall associated with trauma to the mandible. Fracture lines, lacerations, protruding bone or displaced ossicles may be seen in the external auditory canal. Abnormalities of the external auditory canal are almost always associated with further, deeper temporal bone injuries. The most frequent finding in a longitudinal fracture is a laceration of the meatal skin and bony disruption of the posterosuperior external auditory canal in the region of the notch of Rivinus. Because many of these patients are referred to the otolaryngologist late, months or even years after the injury, careful examination may reveal healed fracture lines that are often visible as step deformities in the region of the notch of Rivinus. The tympanic membrane is frequently torn in the posterosuperior quadrant and a paper patch may be placed over this to aid healing, even at the time of the original examination under the microscope. Most perforations have healed spontaneously within 3 weeks and all have healed within 3 months.

The presence of a haemotympanum without rupture of the tympanic membrane or laceration of the external auditory canal is suggestive of a transverse temporal bone fracture.

Middle ear injuries

In those patients with a conductive hearing loss as a result of trauma to the temporal bone, the most common injury is incudostapedial joint separation, which occurred in 82 per cent of patients in one study.[6] The incus may be massively dislocated and the stapedial arch may be fractured in these patients. Fractures of the malleus are uncommon. Multiple sites of ossicular disruption are observed in one-third of patients. Late post-traumatic ankylosis and tympanosclerosis are common, occurring in up to 25 per cent of these injuries. Cholesteatoma is another late complication in 9 per cent, presumably caused by the entrapment of squamous epithelium through a tympanic membrane perforation, behind a healed tympanic membrane perforation or within a fracture line itself.

The incudostapedial joint

The incudostapedial joint is the area of the ossicular chain most vulnerable to damage by traumatic forces, regardless of the direction or origin of that force. Such damage may result from foreign body insertion into the ear canal or forces transmitted during skull fractures. The possible forces that can be exerted in this region include severe transmitted vibratory energy from the impact itself, torsional forces resulting in twisting of the incudostapedial joint by momentary movement of the attached regional bone masses, inertial forces inherent in the ossicular chain and the action of the tympanic muscles when sudden tetanic contraction occurs during trauma.

Massive dislocation of the incus

The incus has the weakest ligamentous and soft-tissue attachments of the three ossicles. It is therefore not surprising, given all the potential forces exerted on it during skull base trauma, that it may become completely detached. The dislocated incus has been observed in remote parts of the middle ear and mastoid, trapped within a fracture line, and may even be extruded through a fracture line to be discovered in the external auditory canal.[6] McHugh[12] discovered an incus in the middle cranial fossa and a malleus jammed into the Eustachian tube orifice. For this to occur there must be a brief moment during the traumatic incident when the fracture is at least as wide as the body of the incus, demonstrating the massive forces that must have been necessary for such a derangement to occur. This is confirmed by experimental work, which has demonstrated that a fracture line opens widely at the moment of injury at a site distant from the site of impact.

Other ossicular abnormalities

The same forces involved at the level of the incudo-stapedial joint may be transmitted to the arch of the stapes and result in fractures in this area. This is particularly true of mixed longitudinal–transverse fractures, in which forces are maximal in the region of the medial wall of the middle ear.[13] Injuries to the stapes are four times less common than injuries to the incus. Malleus abnormalities are rare, given the well secured location of the malleus as part of the tympanic membrane and its firm ligamentous attachments to the anterior and superior walls of the epitympanum. Injuries to the malleus are usually associated with massive trauma, and other ossicular abnormalities are almost always present.[2]

Treatment

The treatment for ossicular disruption is exploratory tympanotomy and repair of the ossicu-

lar defect. It is often possible to replace the displaced incus in its original position and to stabilize it with gelfoam and fibrin glue. This is the most satisfying result surgically and usually renders the best hearing result but, unfortunately, late adhesion formation may draw the replaced incus away from its anatomical position months after the repositioning procedure and this may account for the redevelopment of late conductive hearing losses.

If the incus or the head of the stapes is damaged by the fracture, it may be necessary to perform an ossiculoplasty. The body of the incus is often the best raw material for such a reconstruction, as it can be sculpted to appropriate size microscopically and replaced into the ear of the patient by means of a Wullstein type-IIb tympanoplasty over the stapedial head or a Wullstein type-IIc technique in the case of the stapedial arch fracture. In one clinical series of patients presenting with conductive hearing loss after temporal bone fracture, closure of the air–bone gap to 10 dB or less was achieved in 78 per cent,[6] and was equal to or better than the pretrauma hearing in 45 per cent.

Ossicular fixation as a late sequel of skull base trauma is relatively common and is due to the extensive scarring and new regional bone formation involved in healing temporal bone fractures. Hyperostosis may result in the fusion of the head of the malleus and incus and the fixation of these to the tegmen tympani. Tympanosclerosis may cause a similar fixation of the ossicular chain, particularly in the region of the attic. These lesions are treated by mobilization or ossicular replacement. Occasionally, stapedectomy is necessary for lesions that cause significant footplate immobilization.

Prognosis of traumatic conductive hearing loss

In one series 75 per cent of patients suffering a mild conductive hearing impairment after a temporal bone fracture regained normal hearing.[7] Of those with a moderate conductive loss, 43 per cent resolved completely with no intervention. A conductive hearing loss persisting longer than 6 weeks after trauma and exceeding 30 dB may indicate ossicular disruption and surgical exploration is then an option.

INJURIES TO THE SENSORINEURAL HEARING APPARATUS

Inner ear injuries

The pathological basis for inner ear injuries in patients in whom temporal bone fracture is absent is thought to be 'labyrinthine concussion' – neuro-epithelial damage in the inner ear caused by the force of a head injury. Auditory impairment may result from hair cell damage in the organ of Corti due to the transmission of high-energy vibration.[14] The spectrum of sensorineural hearing loss after such concussive injuries is similar to that seen in noise exposure and is centred around 4000 Hz. The severity of the hearing loss is related to the severity of the traumatic injury and the concussive forces at work during the event.

Treatment

Aural rehabilitation in the form of hearing aid fitting may be appropriate for those patients suffering a permanent incomplete loss of sensorineural hearing. The indications for this are the same as for stable sensorineural hearing loss of any aetiology.

The advent of cochlear implantation has provided an additional means of possible rehabilitation for those rare patients who suffer bilateral complete audiovestibular injuries in skull base fractures and has been successfully employed in several of these individuals.[15] Successful aural rehabilitation is not always achieved, however, which has led several authors to advocate strict patient selection criteria for cochlear implantation after skull base fracture.[16]

Prognosis of traumatic sensorineural hearing loss

All patients in one large series who suffered a transverse temporal bone fracture had complete and permanent sensorineural hearing loss in the affected ear.[17] In the same series, 59 per cent of patients suffering a longitudinal temporal bone fracture had a conductive hearing loss, 4 per cent had a pure sensorineural hearing loss and 4 per cent had a mixed loss. The hearing returned to normal in the majority of these, with 63 per cent doing so in the first 6 weeks. Over the long term, 80 per cent of patients had a complete return to normal hearing, 13 per cent had ossicular disruptions amenable to surgical repair, 4 per cent had a mixed loss and 4 per cent had a persisting sensorineural hearing loss.

DURAL DEFECTS

Concomitant fracture of the floor of the middle cranial fossa and its associated dura can result in a CSF leak into the middle ear. The incidence of CSF otorrhoea in one large series of 1800 patients was 1.4 per cent,[18] although it has been reported to be as high as 11.5 per cent. Purulent inflammation of the middle ear is a common sequel of temporal bone trauma,[6] and it is important to be vigilant for the early signs of meningitis. The incidence of meningitis in patients with CSF otorrhoea is relatively high, 20 per cent in the series of Canniff,[18] which represented all ages and 24 per cent in a similar series of children.[19] Most authors now agree that the use of antibiotics prophylactically is not helpful in these injuries.

The diagnosis of CSF leakage can be difficult to confirm. Intrathecal injection of fluorescein or a radioactive carrier substance may be useful when CSF is suspected to be leaking from the external auditory canal. Fluorescein is visible under an ultraviolet light and, for a radioactive carrier, packing can be placed in the ear canal to be analysed under a gamma camera for radioactive activity. If CSF otorhinorrhoea is suspected, these same procedures can be performed using intranasal inspection for fluorescein or pledget placement for analysis in the department of nuclear medicine to confirm the diagnosis.

Most CSF leaks close spontaneously within 7–10 days of the injury. If CSF drainage persists beyond this point, active intervention is usually required. A lumbar drain is the first step in management in the otherwise healthy patient. If the leak is profuse, or if it fails to close with these conservative measures, surgical exploration should be undertaken.[13] The floor of the middle fossa is the most likely site of leakage in temporal bone fractures. The choice of transmastoid or intracranial middle fossa repair depends upon the personal preference of the surgical team. If an intracranial exploration is planned, the repair may be intradural or extradural.

Many temporal bone fractures heal with a fibrous union only, and this may break down and lead to the late complication of intracranial infection.[20]

Large dural defects in association with loss of the osseous integrity of the temporal bone may result in encephalocoele or meningoencephalocoele formation. These are usually the late sequelae of temporal bone fractures or subsequent infection with loss of bone. Surgical repair with reconstitution of the barrier between the central nervous system and respiratory mucosa of the middle ear and mastoid may be necessary. Obliteration of the mastoid is one option in the surgical treatment of these lesions.[21]

VERTIGO AND DYSEQUILIBRIUM

Injuries to the temporal bone may be associated with mechanical disruption of any or all parts of the vestibular system, from the labyrinth to the vestibular nuclei of the brainstem. These disruptions may be partial or total, immediate or delayed, short-lived or permanent. This provides for a spectrum of symptoms that can be a challenge to diagnosis and treatment. Moreover, these injuries are often compounded by concomitant injuries to those elements of the central nervous system involved in balance and eye movement coordination, such as the cerebellum and higher cortical centres.

Benign paroxysmal positional vertigo is a relatively common complaint after severe head trauma, and may be the most common post-traumatic syndrome of labyrinthine injury. Schuknecht[14] believes that free-floating particles become dislodged within the endolymph of the vestibule during the violent events of labyrinthine concussion. These free-floating particles, which have mass and move under the influence of gravity, will therefore stimulate the affected inner ear in response to positional changes. This theory is strongly supported by the findings of Parnes and Price-Jones.[22] They have suggested that the aetiology of the majority of cases of benign paroxysmal positional vertigo may be free-floating particles in the posterior semicircular canal, and that the repositioning of these particles into the utricle results in resolution of the vertigo in 68 per cent of patients. This represents an improvement over the natural history of this disorder as described by Berman and Fredrickson.[23]

Spontaneous nystagmus after head injury is always significant and is almost always the result of an acute injury to the labyrinth. ENG recording with the eyes closed or with the use of Frenzel's lenses greatly enhances the ability of the clinician to detect a spontaneous nystagmus. Nystagmus is usually paralytic soon after the injury, beating away from the affected side, but may beat towards the affected side weeks to months after the injury as recovery of peripheral vestibular function occurs after central compensation.

Thirteen per cent of people remember vertigo after a longitudinal fracture of the temporal bone,[6] but few suffer long-term vertiginous symptoms. A transverse fracture of the temporal bone may result in disruption of the integrity of the labyrinth itself and is usually associated with a sudden and complete loss of vestibular function on the involved side. The patient experiences a period of severe vertigo until central compensation occurs. Bilateral vestibular injury is an unusual outcome in temporal bone trauma and is almost always the result of bilateral transverse fractures, which result in permanent oscillopsia and long-term disability in the majority of patients.[24]

Central vestibular compensation may be delayed by the patient's other bodily or central nervous system injuries (see Chapter 15). Visual disturbance or proprioceptive impairments will further impede the process of central compensation. Vestibular rehabilitation has been shown to enhance central compensation and reduce the number of chronic balance disorders that result from head injuries. Attention tends to be focused on auditory rehabilitation and only a few centres concentrate on the vestibular rehabilitation of patients with inner ear disorders.

Fluctuating vestibular symptoms may be the result of a perilymphatic fistula, that is, an abnormal leakage of perilymph from the inner ear into the middle ear. Although some authors dispute this entity as a cause of spontaneous hearing loss and vertigo, most would argue that mechanical trauma and barotrauma are recognized causes of this lesion (see Chapter 38). The diagnosis is a clinical one, made on the basis of a history of fluctuating vertigo, fluctuating hearing loss and possibly tinnitus. The treatment for this is exploratory tympanotomy and soft-tissue plugging of the round or oval windows or both.

Endolymphatic hydrops is an unusual outcome of temporal bone trauma that may also result in fluctuating vestibular symptoms.[25] When the vestibular aqueduct is involved in the traumatic injury, secondary endolymphatic hydrops may occur.

'Acute' endolymphatic hydrops has been seen in the cochlea of a patient who died shortly after a blunt traumatic temporal bone injury that did not result in fracture.[26] Delayed endolymphatic hydrops occurs when Ménière-like symptoms develop in an ear that has been previously deafened.[27] This disorder has been described in ears deafened by temporal bone fracture.[28] One interesting report implicates heavy noise exposure and acoustic trauma in the development of delayed endolymphatic hydrops in a group of professional soldiers.[29]

FACIAL NERVE PARALYSIS

The facial nerve, with its important somatic motor function and its lesser functions of taste, secretomotor and somatic sensation, is at great risk during head injury. Of the cranial nerves, the facial nerve travels the greatest distance through a confined bony canal and is therefore particularly vulnerable to injury during skull fracture. It is the second most commonly injured cranial nerve in trauma.

Complete paralysis of the facial nerve after head injury is pathognomonic of a temporal bone fracture. Facial nerve injuries are seen in 15 per cent of adults and in 6–21 per cent of children with temporal bone fractures. Although unilateral facial nerve weakness is a major concern, 0.8–1 per cent of these patients will present with bilateral weakness,[30] a devastating problem that presents particular difficulties in prognostic electrodiagnostic testing and management.

According to one series, longitudinal temporal bone fracture was associated with complete facial paralysis in 19.3 per cent of patients.[6] One-third of these recovered spontaneously without surgical intervention. The remaining two-thirds experienced incomplete return of facial function, with most suffering noticeable facial weakness during movement, synkinesis, facial tics and mass movement. A longitudinal fracture rarely causes total lysis of the facial nerve because the fracture is orientated parallel to the path of the nerve, which results in a sudden stretching force being applied to it. Transverse temporal bone fractures are associated with a far greater incidence of facial nerve injury, approximately 50 per cent. This is because the fracture is perpendicular to the path of the VIIth nerve, which results in the shearing of the connective tissue elements of the nerve. There is greater likelihood of the nerve being completely transected in transverse fractures.

Decisions about the management and prognosis of facial nerve injuries in temporal bone fractures are influenced by several factors. The most important of these is the nature and timing of the onset of facial paralysis. In those head-injured patients who develop facial palsy, approximately one-half will have immediate-onset paralysis. In those patients in whom it is difficult to determine when the onset of facial paralysis occurred, it is best to treat them as though they had immediate-onset paralysis.[12] Immediate-onset facial paralysis has a greater chance of resulting in long-term disruption of facial nerve function and permanent weakness than delayed-onset paralyses.

Facial paralysis that is delayed in onset is usually the result of local post-traumatic phenomena in the region of the fracture such as oedema, haemorrhage and ischaemia. Most injuries will manifest within 5 days of the head trauma, and in up to 94 per cent of patients facial nerve function will recover fully within 6–8 weeks of the injury.[31] If recovery does not become apparent after 3 weeks, the chance of complete recovery diminishes.

Site of injury

A CT scan can be helpful in determining the orientation of a temporal bone fracture, but most authors caution against relying solely on this in diagnosing the site of facial nerve injury or in planning surgical decompression of the nerve. Gadolinium DTPA-enhanced MRI is useful in demonstrating enhancement of the injured segment of the facial nerve in many patients.

Topognostic testing is sometimes helpful in determining the site of a facial nerve injury. The Schirmer test of lachrymation and the stapedial reflex test are recommended by some authors as a means of preoperative localization of the site of a VIIth nerve injury but electrogustometric measurement of taste and submandibular gland flow testing are of less diagnostic value.[13] Please refer to Chapter 16.

The Maximal Stimulation Test (MST) may be more accurate than the Minimal Excitability Test in predicting facial nerve outcome after injury.[32] Interestingly, the MST is of no value up to 72 hours after injury. Normal values are obtained before this time, even in facial nerves that have been completely transected.

Electroneuronography (ENoG) was popularized by Fisch[33] and records the actual compound action potential of the facial nerve after stimulation. May[34] recommended surgery when the amplitude of the affected side was 25 per cent of that of the normal side. The majority of patients, however, with less than 90 per cent degeneration will have complete recovery of facial nerve function, prompting most authors to advocate the figure of 10 per cent or less amplitude of the affected side compared with the normal as a more appropriate indicator for surgical decompression. Fisch[3,35] has recommended surgical intervention within 3 weeks in patients in whom a traumatic injury has resulted in 90 per cent amplitude reduction by ENoG testing within 6 days of the injury. Current recommendations are for operative exploration as soon as the patient's condition permits in cases of immediate paralysis with greater than 90 per cent degeneration.

Like MST, ENoG is not useful for at least 72 hours after the injury, and most authors advocate that testing begin on the third or fourth day after the trauma.

Electromyography (EMG) is not helpful in the evaluation of facial paralysis of recent onset as it does not demonstrate denervation potentials until 8–10 days after denervation has occurred. All electrical testing is therefore limited by the fact that it cannot provide an indication of the status of the facial nerve immediately after the injury.

Surgery for traumatic facial nerve paralysis

The facial nerve may be compressed by impinging bone fragments or by local haematoma. It may be partially or totally disrupted by a fracture. The surgeon should be prepared for any of these possibilities when exploring such a patient, and should be skilled in microsurgical techniques of nerve decompression, nerve grafting and nerve rerouting and transposition.

Immediate-onset facial paralysis after traumatic injury is an indication for surgical exploration and surgical decompression as soon as the patient's condition permits, especially if ENoG evidence indicates greater than 90 per cent neuronal degeneration.[36] Early surgical intervention will improve the final facial nerve outcome in immediate-onset facial palsy from temporal bone trauma.

Delayed-onset facial paralysis after traumatic injury should be followed clinically and electrodiagnostically at regular intervals. If more than 90 per cent neuronal degeneration occurs, facial nerve decompression may be indicated.

Another form of facial nerve injury due to temporal bone trauma is observed in the neonatal period. The majority of such injuries are caused by blunt trauma to the nerve during delivery, and this injury is thought to be due either to the shearing effect of forceps on the nerve as it exits the stylomastoid foramen (which is quite laterally placed and vulnerable in the skull base of a neonate), or compressive injury by forceps on the bone surrounding the vertical or mastoid portion of the Fallopian canal. The prognosis of these injuries is very good, with approximately 90 per cent of all acquired paralyses resolving spontaneously given time.[37]

NON-FRACTURE BLUNT INJURIES

Blast injuries

The sudden massive pressure changes that result from explosions may have devastating effects on the ear. In an explosion there is a short positive pressure phase, lasting milliseconds, followed by a longer-lived negative phase. The energy of the blast wave of each phase is equal but the force vector is opposite.[38]

Tympanic membrane injury in the pars tensa is common in blast injury, but chronic suppuration after this is less common than with perforations caused by pressurized water or welding trauma.[13] The majority heal spontaneously. Kerr and Byrne[39] reported that 83 per cent of 66 perforated tympanic membranes from one explosion healed spontaneously. The implantation of squamous epithelium deep to the tympanic membrane results in the late complication of cholesteatoma formation in up to 12 per cent.

Ossicular chain injuries are unusual after an explosion. Inner ear injuries, however, are common, and sensorineural hearing loss and vertigo are frequent complaints. Most patients sustaining a significant blast injury will have a temporary hearing loss, known as a 'temporary threshold shift'. This phenomenon may result in quite severe hearing loss and is most marked immediately after the explosion, but usually resolves spontaneously within 24 hours.[39]

Hearing loss lasting longer than 24 hours is likely to be permanent. Tinnitus is also a sequel of blast injury and mirrors the severity and duration of the sensorineural hearing loss. Vertigo is usually temporary and resolves spontaneously in the majority of patients, and those who do not improve should be suspected of having a perilymph fistula.

Injuries caused by water under pressure

The effects of water entering the ear under pressure can be devastating in certain cases. Diving is the commonest cause of these injuries (48 per cent) followed closely by water-skiing (30 per cent).[13] Damage to the ear can also be iatrogenic. Syringing of the ear may cause tympanic membrane perforation, especially when the full force of the jet of water is directed onto the tympanic membrane. Caloric testing in patients with atrophic tympanic membranes can result in the same lesion. This trauma can be easily prevented by directing the water jet against the posterior external auditory canal during irrigation.

Acute injuries from a sudden rush of pressurized water into the ear include tympanic membrane perforation (pars tensa), which is the commonest such injury, ossicular disruption and rupture of the oval window annular ligament or round window membrane. The late complications of this include otitis media and cholesteatoma.

Prevention is easily accomplished with occlusive ear plugs. Treatment of the actual injury is conservative. Even large perforations may heal given time, appropriate otomicroscopic toilet and medical treatment. Surgical repair is indicated in those perforations that fail to close spontaneously in 3–6 months.

Penetrating temporal bone trauma

FOREIGN BODIES

The external auditory canal has several features that are protective against accidental foreign body insertion. These include its location deep in the conchal bowl, its protective coarse hairs and cerumen at its meatus, its narrow width and tortuosity and its sensitive sensory innervation. Despite this, foreign body trauma via the ear canal remains one of the commonest presenting complaints in our speciality.

This is a large paediatric problem and 73 per cent of patients with foreign body trauma are children.

Tympanic membrane perforations are very common, usually occurring posteriorly and often involving a large portion of the surface area of the drum. Ossicular injuries are also common, with more than 50 per cent of ear explorations demonstrating significant ossicular disruption. The spectrum of these injuries is similar to that of temporal bone fractures. Occasionally a foreign body can cause inner ear damage, either through subluxation of the stapes and disruption of oval window integrity or through trauma to the round window region.

SURGICAL TRAUMA

The chorda tympani nerve is frequently disrupted during middle ear surgery, sometimes resulting in a disorder of taste and salivary secretion on the affected side, although such complaints are uncommon even after significant trauma to the nerve.[38]

The jugular bulb is occasionally injured during transcanal tympanotomy procedures as its bony covering in the floor of the middle ear may be deficient. Packing the area is frequently all that is required to alleviate the situation. Less frequently a dehiscent carotid artery may be injured during middle ear surgery, an injury that may on occasions lead to disruption of the blood supply to the central nervous system, stroke or death.

The facial nerve is at risk during surgery almost anywhere in the temporal bone and parotid regions. A thorough knowledge of the anatomy of the temporal bone and facial nerve and its variations is essential before the junior surgeon is allowed to undertake even the most simple of middle ear procedures.

STAB AND GUNSHOT WOUNDS

Other penetrating injuries in the temporal bone region include stabbing injuries and gunshot wounds.

Gunshot wounds are probably the commonest cause of penetrating injury to the temporal bone. The effect depends upon the mass and velocity of the bullet, the direction from which the missile comes when it makes contact with the skull and the course the projectile takes after it enters the temporal bone or the soft tissue of the skull base region. The ipsilateral infraorbital region is the most common entrance site for gunshot wounds involving the temporal bone.[40]

As many as one-third of gunshot wounds to the temporal bone will result in significant, life-threatening injuries to the vascular structures contained within it and to the underlying central nervous system.[40] Arteriography and CT or MRI scanning are mandatory investigations once the patient has been stabilized. Wounds should then be explored by the otoneurosurgical team and undergo debridement; exploration of the facial nerve and middle ear and soft-tissue and bone reconstruction should be undertaken as for gunshot wounds elsewhere in the head.

Whiplash

The term whiplash injury refers to a sudden extension or flexion, or both, of the neck resulting from rapid acceleration or deceleration.[41] Aural symptoms after whiplash include deafness, tinnitus, vertigo and dysequilibrium. The most common of these are vertigo and dysequilibrium. They are usually associated with neck pain, and the symptoms may be elicited by certain head positions or neck movements, leading to the term 'cervical vertigo'.

Treatment is conservative, including bedrest, anti-inflammatory drugs and splinting for early injuries. Patients with chronic symptoms should receive instruction in proper posture, neck exercises and physiotherapy, cervical traction, neck immobilization with a collar and local heat and massage.

Barotrauma

Barotrauma is defined as the pathophysiological effects of changes in ambient pressure affecting the air-containing spaces of the temporal bone.

INJURIES CAUSED BY WATER PRESSURE

The majority of barotrauma injuries are related to scuba diving.

Ear canal

If air is trapped in the ear canal and the ambient pressure is changed, external auditory canal barotrauma can occur. This is most commonly the result of using occlusive ear plugs, but may also occur with cerumen or foreign body impaction. Conditions that narrow the ear canal, such as external auditory canal exostoses, which occur commonly in divers, will predispose the patient to this problem.

If air is trapped in the ear canal and the ambient pressure is increased, the relative pressure of the trapped air drops. This results in a 'reverse ear squeeze', which causes intense otalgia, haemorrhage into the skin of the ear canal, which can coalesce and expand into subepithelial blebs, and tympanic membrane rupture.

Middle ear

Barotrauma of the middle ear, called a 'middle ear squeeze', is experienced on descent while diving and occurs because of failure to equalize the middle ear pressure with the increasing ambient pressure. This is the most common diving-related aural barotrauma, and is also the most common diving-related injury.[42,43] Middle ear mucosal haemorrhage and bleb formation is common and tympanic membrane rupture may occur. A pressure differential of 90 mmHg or more between the ambient pressure and the middle ear can result in the Eustachian tube locking, in which case it cannot be opened by Valsalva's manoeuvre. A pressure differential of 500 mmHg will result in tympanic membrane rupture, which is experienced at a depth of 5.4 m (17.4 feet) in salt water, although such ruptures can occur in depths as little as 1.3 m (4.3 feet) of water. If the tympanic membrane ruptures, a caloric response stimulating the labyrinth can result in vertigo. This can be a distressing and life-threatening event, but usually abates after several minutes and does not recur on ascent.

Inner ear

Vertigo has been experienced by as many as 50 per cent of divers at some point in their lives. In 'alternobaric vertigo' hearing loss and tinnitus do not occur, but the patient is suddenly seized by vertigo, which lasts minutes to hours. This phenomenon results from relative overpressure of the middle ear and the diver's inability to equalize pressure in the middle ear, which causes a change in the pressure of the inner ear fluids.

Perilymph fistula (see Chapter 38) is a recognized entity that causes fluctuating dizziness and deafness after otic barotrauma. The initial treatment of a patient with a perilymph fistula is bedrest. The fistula should be explored and repaired as soon as possible to preserve sensorineural hearing and stabilize vestibular function.[45]

AIR PRESSURE INJURIES

Most aural barotrauma resulting from air travel occurs during descent, as the pressure of the air in a pressurized aeroplane is less than atmospheric pressure at ground level. Alternobaric vertigo may occur on ascent. The vertical distances travelled in air must be greater than in water to experience the same pressure changes. For example, vertical change in altitude of 6000 m (18 000 feet) accomplishes the same change in pressure as a vertical move of only 5 m (16.5 feet) in salt water.

Thermal trauma

WELDING INJURIES

The external auditory canal is a protective structure that prevents the migration of hot slag to the tympanic membrane and middle ear in the majority of cases. The most common injury is therefore an external auditory canal burn and otitis externa, and usually no permanent damage is caused.

Tympanic membrane perforation is, however, an uncommon but recognized complication of welding activity. These injuries are less likely to heal spontaneously than other traumatic tympanic membrane perforations because of ingrowth of avascular scar tissue. In the middle ear, ossicular chain damage is rare. Complications of aural slag injury include chronic otitis media, which occurs in up to 85 per cent of affected ears.[13]

Radiation injury

The ear is at risk during radiation exposure to the head and neck region. This is particularly true of therapeutic radiation for nasopharyngeal carcinoma and other skull base tumours. The most common clinical presentation is Eustachian tube dysfunction, which results in middle ear effusion and conductive hearing loss. A ventilating tube in the affected ear is often required.

Osteoradionecrosis of the temporal bone is claimed to be an unusual result of radiotherapy,[46] but otologists believe it to be more common than was once thought. Symptoms of this disorder include hearing loss (conductive, sensorineural or mixed), otalgia, otorrhoea and sequestration of bone. The complications of temporal bone osteoradionecrosis include cranial neuropathy and intracranial infection. Treatment includes systemic antibiotics, local wound care and debridement of devitalized tissue, including bony sequestra. Reconstruction of extensive debridement defects in the form of importation of vascularized tissue or mastoid obliteration are occasionally required. Hyperbaric oxygen has provided some limited benefit in the treatment of this entity.

Sensorineural hearing loss and vestibular injury have been reported, although some authors feel the association between inner ear dysfunction and radiotherapy is speculative.[38]

Acoustic trauma

The reader is referred to Chapter 35.

Conclusion

Trauma to the head is common, sudden and often devastating for the patient. It frequently has profound and lasting physical and psychological sequelae. The resulting deterioration in quality of life for the individual and their family can wreak havoc at home and in the work place, and has far reaching implications for society as a whole.

It is important to realize that more people are killed and injured in road traffic accidents than by any other cause and that the latter are the major risk to health between the ages of 1 and 34 years. Almost 75 per cent of these involve the head and when the head is severely injured, the ear is the most frequently damaged sensory organ because of its remarkable sensitivity. Direct trauma to the ear in closed-head injuries therefore constitutes an area of correctable aural pathology in which the injuries are numerous and complex and vary enormously depending on the type and degree of the physical forces involved.

The importance of these injuries is undeniable and the earlier misconception that any permanent hearing loss secondary to skull trauma must be due to sensorineural damage and must therefore be irreparable should be banished forever. In the past otologists were seldom consulted about head injuries that involved hearing loss and when they were it was usually at a later stage when life-threatening injuries had been treated. Otologists must be an integral part of the head injuries team and the benefit of their expertise sought at the outset if morbidity from head injury is to be reduced and the concomitant improvement in quality of life realized.

Acknowledgements

The author wishes to acknowledge the expert help of Mr Robert Ballagh, Fellow in Otoneurological and Skull Base Surgery, Addenbrooke's Hospital, Cambridge in the preparation of this chapter.

References

1. Gurdjian ES. Head injury exhibit at World Congress of Neurological Sciences. *Medical Post* 1969; **5**:2.
2. Wright JW, Taylor CE, Bizal JA. Tomography and the vulnerable incus. *Annals of Otology* 1969; **78**:263–79.
3. Fisch U. Facial paralysis in fractures of the petrous bone. *Laryngoscope* 1974; **84**:2141–54.
4. Ghorayeb BY, Yeakley JW. Temporal bone fractures: longitudinal or oblique? The case for oblique temporal bone fractures. *Laryngoscope* 1992; **102**:129–34.
5. McHugh HE. The surgical treatment of facial paralysis and traumatic conductive deafness in fractures of the temporal bone. *Annals of Otology* 1959; **68**:855–89.
6. Hough JVD, Stuart WD. Middle ear injuries in skull base trauma. *Laryngoscope* 1968; **78**:899–937.
7. McGuirt WF, Stool SE. Temporal bone fractures in children: a review with emphasis on long-term sequelae. *Clinical Paediatrics* 1992; **31**:12–8.
8. Goligher JE, Lloyd GAS. Fracture of the petrous temporal bone. *Journal of Laryngology and Otology* 1990; **104**:438–9.
9. Betz BW, Weiner MD. Air in the temporomandibular joint fossa: CT sign of temporal bone fracture. *Radiology* 1991; **180**:463–6.
10. Weissman JL, Curtain HD. Pneumolabyrinth: a computed tomographic sign of temporal bone fracture. *American Journal of Otolaryngology* 1992; **13**:113–4.
11. May M, Klein SR. Facial nerve decompression complications. *Laryngoscope* 1983; **93**:299–305.
12. McHugh HE. Facial paralysis in birth injury and skull fractures. *Archives of Otolaryngology* 1963; **78**:443–55.
13. Hough JVD, McGee M. Otologic trauma. In: Paparella MM, *et al.* eds. *Otolaryngology*. London: WB Saunders, 1991:1137–60.
14. Schuknecht HF. Mechanism of inner ear injury from blows to the head. *Annals of Otology* 1969; **78**:253–62.
15. Jenkins H, Chmeil R, Jerger J. Speech tracking in the evaluation of a multichannel cochlear prosthesis. *Laryngoscope* 1989; **99**:177–86.
16. Morgan WE, Coker NJ, Jenkins HA. Histopathology of temporal bone fractures: implications for cochlear implantation. *Laryngoscope* 1994; **104**:426–32.
17. Tos M. Prognosis for hearing in temporal bone fractures. *Journal of Laryngology and Otology* 1971; **85**:1147–55.
18. Canniff JP. Otorrhoea in head injuries. *British Journal of Oral Surgery* 1971; **8**:203–10.
19. MacGee EE, Cauthen JC, Brackett CE. Meningitis following acute traumatic ceerbrospinal fluid fistula. *Journal of Neurosurgery* 1970; **33**:312–7.
20. Ward PH. The histopathology of audiological and vestibular disorders in head trauma. *Annals of Otology* 1969; **78**:227–38.
21. Moffat DA, GRay RF, Irving RM. Mastoid obliteration using bone plate. *Clinical Otolaryngology* 1994; **19**:149–97.

22. Parnes LS, Price-Jones RG. Particle repositioning maneuver for benign positional vertigo. *Annals of Otology, Rhinology and Laryngology* 1993; **102**:325–31.

23. Berman JM, Fredrickson JM. Vertigo after head injury: five year follow-up. *Journal of Otolaryngology* 1978; **7**:237–45.

24. Hough JVD. Surgical aspects of temporal bone fractures. *Proceedings of the Royal Society of Medicine* 1970; **63**:245–2.

25. Pararella MM, Mancini F. Trauma and Menière's syndrome. *Laryngoscope* 1983; **93**:1004–12.

26. Murakami M, Ohtani I, Aikawa T. *Journal of Laryngology and Otology* 1990; **104**:986–9.

27. LeLiever WC, Barber HO. Delayed endolymphatic hydrops. *Journal of Otolaryngology* 1980; **9**:375–80.

28. Rizvi SS, Gibbin KP. Effect of transverse temporal bone fracture on the fluid compartment of the inner ear. *Annals of Otology, Rhinology and Laryngology* 1979; **87**:797–803.

29. Ylikoski J. Delayed endolymphatic hydrops syndrome after heavy exposure to impulse noise. *American Journal of Otology* 1988; **9**:282–5.

30. Wormald PJ, Sellars SL, DeVilliers JC. Bilateral facial nerve palsies: Groot Schuur Hospital experience. *Journal of Laryngology and Otology* 1991; **105**:625–7.

31. Griffin JE, Altenau MM, Schaefer SD. Bilateral longitudinal temporal bone fractures: a retrospective review of seventeen cases. *Laryngoscope* 1979; **89**:1432–5.

32. May M, Harvey JE, Marovitz WF, Stroud M. The prognostic accuracy of the maximal stimulation test compared with that of the nerve excitability test in Bell's palsy. *Laryngoscope* 1971; **81**:931–8.

33. Fisch U. Surgery for Bell's palsy. *Archives of Otolaryngology* 1981; **107**:1–11.

34. May M. Facial nerve paralysis. In: Paparella MM, Shumrick DA eds. *Otolaryngology, 2nd ed.* London: WB Saunders, 1980:1680–1704.

35. Fisch U. Management of intratemporal facial nerve injuries. *Journal of Laryngology and Otology* 1980; **94**:129–34.

36. Lieberherr U, Schwarzenbach D, Fisch U. Management of severe facial nerve paralysis in temporal bone fracture – a review of 82 cases. In: Castro D ed. *Facial nerve.* Amsterdam: Kugler and Ghedini, 1990:285–9.

37. Falco NA, Eriksson E. Facial nerve palsy in the newborn: incidence and outcome. *Plastic and Reconstructive Surgery* 1990; **85**:1–4.

38. Kerr AG, Smyth GDL. Ear trauma. In: *Scott-Brown's Otolaryngology, 5th ed.* Somerset: Butterworths, 1987.

39. Kerr AG, Byrne JET. Concussive effects of a bomb blast on the ear. *Journal of Laryngology and Otology* 1975; **89**:131–43.

40. Adkins WY, Osguthorpe JD. Management of trauma of the facial nerve. *Otolaryngologic Clinics of North America* 1991; **24**:587–611.

41. McNab I. The 'whiplash syndrome'. *Orthopedic Clinics of North America* 1971; **2**:389–403.

42. Farmer JC, Thomas WG. Ear and sinus problems in diving. In: Strauss RM ed. *Diving medicine.* New York: Grune and Stratton, 1976:109–33.

43. Dickey LS. Diving injuries. *Journal of Emergency Medicine* 1984; **1**:249–62.

44. Inglestedt S, Ivarsson A, Tjernstrom O. Vertigo due to relative overpressure in the middle ear. *Acta Otolaryngologica* 1974; **78**:1–14.

45. Becker GD, Parell GH. Otolaryngologic aspects of scuba-diving. *Otolaryngology – Head and Neck Surgery* 1979; **87**:569–72.

46. Guida RA, Finn DG, Buchalter IH, Brookler KH, Kimmelman CP. Radiation injury to the temporal bone. *American Journal of Otology* 1990; **11**:6–11.

CHAPTER 33

Otosclerosis

ALEC FITZGERALD O'CONNOR

Otosclerosis is a hereditary osseous dysplasia of the petrous temporal bone, confined to bone derived from the embryonic otic capsule. It has an autosomal dominant inheritance with incomplete manifestation and varying degrees of expressivity.[1]

The histopathological features are of a pleomorphic lesion consisting of spongy bone with increased cellularity and vascularity alongside areas of fibrous replacement and sclerosis. The terms otospongiosis and otosclerosis are both histologically correct but otosclerosis is the term used in clinical practice as it reflects the histopathological status at the time of surgical intervention. The most common clinical presentation is a conductive hearing loss resulting from ankylosis of the stapes.

History

It is generally accepted that Valsalva in 1701 was the first to describe stapes fixation at postmortem examination. The term 'otosclerosis' was coined by Politzer in 1894 based on histopathological findings. The surgical treatment of hearing loss due to otosclerosis was attempted by Kessel in 1878 although Prosper Menière had advocated stapes mobilization for hearing loss as early as 1842. At the end of the nineteenth century, without the operating microscope, many attempts either to mobilize or to remove the stapes were described but the good results were short-lived and many patients had no hearing after surgery. The surgical management switched to fenestrating the lateral semicircular canal in order to short-circuit the fixed ossicular chain and allow free movement of the inner ear fluids in response to sound. Lempert's fenestration operation in the 1930s became the first

commonly performed surgical procedure for otosclerosis.[2] The emphasis then returned to the stapes, with the stapes mobilization of Rosen and closure of the air–bone gap (which was never achieved by the fenestration procedure), but this was liable to short-term refixation and the consequent recurrence of hearing loss. However, the young enigmatic John Shea in 1956, against the accepted teaching of his time, removed the stapes, covered the oval window with a vein graft and interposed a polyethylene tube between the graft and the incus.[3] The results were such that the stapedectomy era exploded. John Shea had described an operation that would relieve the deafness disability in thousands of patients. During the 1960s and 1970s a great backlog of patients existed and it was not unusual for surgeons to have the experience of several hundred stapedectomies. Different techniques evolved based on the least invasive approach to the vestibule (small fenestra stapedotomy) and the biocompatibility of the prosthesis. At the present in the UK the prevalence of cases is in the order of 1 in 100 000 of the population and otosclerosis surgery is once again becoming the domain of the specialist otologist.

Pathology

During the embryonic ossification of the cochlea the area anterior to the oval window remains cartilaginous before degenerating to simple fibrous tissue and forming the fissula ante fenestram, which becomes the most common site for the otosclerotic focus (Fig 33.1 and Plate section). This vascular connective tissue is then replaced by the neo-osteogenesis associated with otospongiosis.

The characteristics of the otosclerotic process are perivascular bony resorption resulting in vascular lakes due to osteoclastic and giant cell activity. Fibroblasts are transformed into osteoblasts and immature bone is then laid down with a marked deficiency in collagen yet rich in ground substances. A continuous cycle of resorption and bone formation occurs and with time the ratio of collagen to ground substances inverts to produce avascular otosclerotic bone (Fig 33.2 and Plate section).

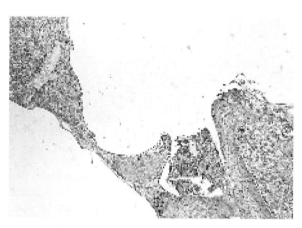

Fig 33.1 Stapes ankylosis by an otosclerotic focus (from an ear subject to a previous stapedectomy). Note anterior focus, area of new membrane over fenestra, remains of posterior crus and, posteriorly, the stapedius muscle in the pyramid. (Reproduced with permission of Professor AW Wright.)

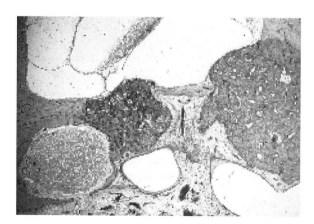

Fig 33.2 Active otospongiotic lesion and associated sclerotic lesion. (Reproduced with permission of Professor AW Wright.)

Clinical presentation

HISTORY

Gradual onset of hearing loss between 20 and 40 years of age, with active progression during pregnancy, is the predominant presenting symptom. The phenomenon of paracusis Willisii occurs whereby the patient perceives speech better in a noisy background (the opposite of what happens in sensorineural hearing loss) because of relatively good discrimination of speech when the stimulus is raised above the usual conversational level. Bilateral hearing loss is usual in 80–90 per cent of patients. Tinnitus is common and may be related to the middle ear pathology when it is low pitched and perhaps pulsatile; a high-pitched whistling noise may reflect cochlear dysfunction. The latter is infrequently abolished by stapedectomy whereas the former may resolve with the loss of the acoustic block to ambient sound.

Rotational vertigo can occur and suggests the presence of an otosclerotic focus in the labyrinth.[5] The attacks are transient and differ from those described with Menière's disease as they are not associated with fluctuations of the hearing, increase in tinnitus or a feeling of fullness in the ear. However, it should be remembered that otosclerosis and Menière's disease may coexist and stapedectomy is a relative contraindication in such circumstances. A family history of otosclerosis is obtained from approximately 50 per cent of patients. Hearing loss associated with long bone fractures would suggest osteogenesis imperfecta (Adair-Dighton syndrome).

EXAMINATION

Although otoscopic examination may reveal a 'flamingo flush' to the eardrum, the so-called Schwartz sign reflecting hypervascularity on the promontory, this is uncommon and in fact the tympanic membranes are usually unremarkable. Of course, stapes fixation may occur alongside other middle ear and Eustachian tube pathologies. The blue sclera, a feature of Adair-Dighton syndrome, may be present in otosclerotics without osteogenesis imperfecta.

Clinical examination of hearing may be achieved by using simple speech tests, with good speech discrimination a prominent feature. Tuning fork test with a 512 Hz or higher fork are mandatory, first to confirm the presence of a conductive hearing loss (Rinne negative) and second to confirm the presence of active cochlear function (Weber lateralized to the affected ear).

AUDIOMETRY

Pure tone audiometry

As the pathological process of stapedial otosclerosis primarily results in an increase in the stiffness component of the ossicular chain, elevated thresholds in the low frequencies are usually the first audiometric abnormality. As the process progresses with fixation of the footplate a mass effect is added to the total impedance, resulting in stabilization of the low frequencies and hearing loss in the mid and high frequencies with widening of the air–bone gap. When cochlear involvement occurs the sensorineural component becomes more prominent.

The measurement of bone conduction in patients with otosclerosis is of great importance. The recognition of the so-called Carhart notch is considered a diagnostic feature. The bone conduction threshold is essentially a measure of the cochlear reserve and thus an indicator of the potential hearing gain that can be achieved by stapedial surgery.

The Carhart notch (an elevation of the bone conduction threshold of 10 dB or more at one frequency) usually occurs at 2 kHz (Fig 33.3). The basis of this audiological phenomenon is not clear although the disruption of ossicular resonance, which is maximal at 2 kHz, and perilymph immobility have been suggested. The 'audiological' nature of the Carhart notch is reflected in its apparent disappearance after successful stapes surgery. An overclosure of the air–bone gap is defined as the postoperative air conduction threshold being better than the preoperative bone conduction threshold. Preoperative counselling should not overplay the potential gain from overclosure, which sometimes does not occur even after successful surgery.

Great care should be taken to obtain adequate masking of the non-test ear so that the cochlear reserve of the test ear is not overstated.

Speech audiometry

In patients in whom there is a significant elevation of the bone conduction threshold, speech audiometry should be performed. A masked speech audiogram in which the maximum speech discrimination score is below 70 per cent militates against operative intervention.

Tympanometry

Routine tympanometry is not considered helpful in the diagnosis or management of otosclerosis.

Stapedial reflex

The stapedial reflex, as measured by changes in acoustic compliance on the tympanometer in response to auditory stimulation, can be used to monitor progression of the otosclerotic process. In cases of clear footplate fixation the reflex is lost but during the development of the disease process subtle changes can be seen in the reflex pattern. In early disease the stimulus is followed by a paradoxically increased compliance, which is then followed by a marked decrease in compliance below that of the resting state; when the stimulus stops there is another increase in compliance before the return to the resting state. Later the decrease does not fall below the resting level, the so-called diphasic response or the 'on–off' effect. Such findings may precede an air–bone gap. The scientific basis for this phenomenon is not clear.

An important differential diagnosis to be made is between otosclerosis and the very rare perilymphatic hypertension. In both conditions a conductive hearing loss is evident but in the latter the stapedial reflex is present and on induction of the reflex the compliance falls, usually markedly, and stays depressed for the duration of the stimulus. Such cases may be misdiagnosed and at surgery be associated with stape gushers.[6]

Vestibulometry

Vestibular testing using caloric stimulation can show evidence of hypolabyrinthine function especially after stapedectomy; some clinicians feel that

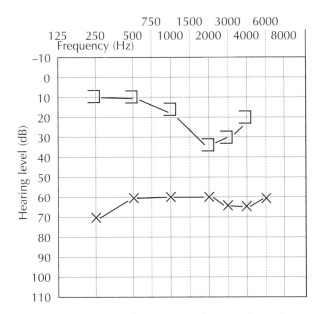

Fig 33.3 Pure tone audiogram – Carhart notch at 2 kHz.

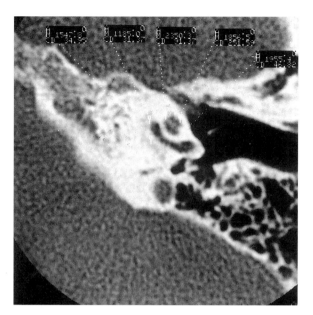

Fig 33.4 Axial CT scan with densitometry showing areas of demineralization of the labyrinthine capsule close to the basal turn of the cochlea.

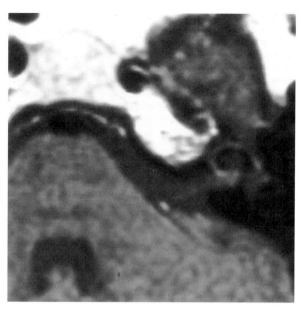

Fig 33.5 Axial MRI T1-weighted image with gadolinium enhancement. Hyperintense signal from vascular bone.

such testing is mandatory before second-side stapedectomy for fear of inducing bilateral vestibular hypofunction.

RADIOLOGICAL EXAMINATION

Otosclerotic involvement of the temporal bone is not demonstrated by plain X-rays although other pathologies in the differential diagnosis (e.g. Paget's disease) may be apparent.

The advent of computed tomography (CT) and magnetic resonance imaging (MRI) has introduced useful techniques for the diagnosis and clinical management of the disease.

Computed tomography

Using multiplanar spiral tomography the oval window may be seen on 20° coronal oblique sections. The clinical advantage of this technique is limited, but it may be of some use in recognizing obliterative otosclerosis preoperatively.

After stapedectomy CT scanning may be indicated when persistent vertiginous symptoms would suggest a prosthesis deep in the vestibule, or when there is a conductive hearing loss due to dislodgement of the prosthesis from the incus.

The characteristic otospongiotic foci in the cochlear capsule may be delineated by CT scanning because of changes in bone density. A quantitative assessment of such changes is compared with normative data and expressed in Hounsfield units (HU). Areas of the cochlear capsule with HU levels below 1400 are considered abnormally radiolucent. Similar findings occur in Paget's disease and otosyphilis (Fig 33.4).[7]

Magnetic resonance imaging

Although MRI is not the preferred imaging technique for otosclerosis, the features associated with the otospongiotic process (neovascularization) should be recognized when displayed as a result of an examination indicated for the diagnosis of a retrocochlear lesion (e.g. vestibular schwannoma).

The T1-weighted images may reveal an area of hyperintense signal in the pericochlear area that tends to enhancement with gadolinium (Fig 33.5).

Management

NON-SURGICAL TREATMENT

Hearing aid

Air conduction hearing aids, commencing when the hearing loss is moderate with an 'in the ear' aid and progressing to the stronger postaural aids, are the bedrock of non-surgical management. However, the good speech discrimination that can be achieved is sometimes dissipated by the unnatural sound perceived.

Sodium fluoride

Fluoride and otosclerosis have been linked since the work of Shambaugh and Scott in 1964.[8] Areas with low levels of natural fluoride in the water were found to have a high prevalence of otosclerosis and it was noted that fluoride reduced otosclerotic bone activity.

Therapeutic fluoride (excepting in the Public Health domain) has been subject to discussion for many years with no clear evidence as to its efficacy. Anecdotal data suggest that, at least, fluoride may prevent further hearing loss while not improving auditory thresholds. The recommended dose is 20 mg daily if there is evidence of an active foci as judged radiologically or surgically (including a positive Schwartze sign). Care should be taken to manage the side effects of the drug, notably gastric irritation, and appropriate anti-peptic acid therapy may be needed.

SURGICAL TREATMENT

Stapedectomy

Indications

A conductive hearing loss is associated with otosclerotic fixation of the footplate. For stapedectomy to be indicated there should be disability associated with the hearing loss and the maximum speech discrimination score should be in excess of 70 per cent. Patients with severe otosclerosis, in whom the hearing threshold is in excess of 100 dB and the bone conduction threshold is greater than that of the audiometer, may also benefit by becoming hearing aid users. There should be harmony between the tuning fork test and the pure tone audiogram. The tympanogram should be type A and the stapedial reflexes absent. Full and informed consent is mandatory and should be based on the operating surgeon's personal experience. I advise that, in my hands and considering my consecutive series of 316 stapedectomies with incomplete follow-up, the risk of profound sensorineural hearing loss is 2.5 per cent, with 91 per cert of patients having a good subjective hearing improvement. Complications such as tinnitus should be mentioned along with the possibility of postoperative vertigo. The decision to perform second-side stapedectomy is the subject of controversy. I am prepared to perform a second-side stapedectomy if I have performed the first procedure at least a year previously and it has not been associated with any intraoperative or postoperative complications. _Other otologists are more conservative and few will operate on unilateral otosclerosis as the results are poor, and the chances of obtaining nearly symmetrical hearing – necessary for benefit – are remote. [Eds.]_

Contraindications

Contraindications may be general and relate to the patient's medical condition, including pregnancy and the appropriateness for anaesthesia, or specific, such as active ear infection, poor Eustachian tube function, active otosclerosis with the Schwartze sign, absence of hearing in the other ear and Menière's disease. At operation if the surgical exposure is inadequate because of facial nerve or vascular anomalies proceeding to stapedectomy is not indicated.

Method of stapedectomy

Local anaesthesia

The operation may be performed under local or general anaesthesia and the choice is usually based on tradition, training and experience. Local anaesthesia averts the potential coughing and straining on reversal from general anaesthesia. However, the surgeon must be experienced and be able to complete the operation within 30–45 minutes. Confidence in managing the uncommon intraoperative problem, such as obliterative otosclerosis or an overhanging facial nerve, and a realization that on opening the vestibule and inserting the prosthesis the patient may experience vertigo is important. The local anaesthesic (1% lidocaine [lignocaine]/1 in 80 000 adrenaline) in a dental syringe may be injected into the ear canal at the level of the bony annulus by sliding the needle down the inside of an oversized aural speculum that delineates the cartilaginous bony junction. Four or five injections are made around the canal with care being taken to inject gently so that 'blisters' in the canal wall that make the tympanomeatal flap weak and difficult to incise are not formed. Excessive infiltration may lead to spreading of the anaesthetic through the parotid tissue and result in a transient facial palsy. Topical anaesthesia (10% cocaine) introduced on small cotton wool pledgets may be used in the middle ear cavity. Mild sedation may be induced with diazepam, and as with all operative procedures the patient's vital signs, including oxygen saturation, should be monitored.

General anaesthesia

If a general anaesthetic is used, hypotension is rarely indicated and may, by way of fluctuations in blood pressure and pulse rate, lead to reactive hyperaemia and be more trouble than it is worth. Reversal of the general anaesthetic should not be associated with coughing or straining that results in raised intercranial pressure and possible leakage of perilymph through the oval window. Local anaesthetic is used as above, for vasoconstricting purposes.

Surgical approach

The ear is prepared with a solution of aqueous hibitane (Hibitane 5% Zenela Pharma) and the operation is performed under aseptic conditions. In cases in which a size five speculum can easily be introduced into the ear canal, an endomeatal approach is adequate. If, however, the canal is small or there are osteomata present, an endural incision is required. A separate incision is made in the lobule for a fat graft or in the back of the hand for a vein graft. The graft is left in normal saline until needed. Surgical gloves without talc for all the surgical team are preferable. If they are not available, thorough washing is required as talc granulomas may occur in the middle ear.

The endomeatal incision is made by one cutting movement of the canal knife hard down onto bone, stretching from the annulus at about eight o'clock inferiorly on the right ear (or four o'clock on the left) creating a flap that is largest in the posterosuperior segment and passing back to the annulus at about eleven o'clock (one o'clock on the left ear) (Fig 33.6). A flap that is too small results in a defect when the posterior bony wall has been removed, and one too large is bulky and can compromise the introduction of the prosthesis into the middle ear. Ideally the flap should 'hinge' anteriorly on a line 2 mm anterior to the incudostapedial joint (Fig 33.7). Care is taken to use the double-ended Buckingham canal knife for the incision only, as using it as an elevator as well leads to premature blunting. A Hughes elevator than lifts the flap forward. Superiorly the rather thickened subcutaneous tissue has to be divided with microscissors. The use of the aspirator on the flap is to be avoided (if bleeding is a problem topical adrenaline 1:10 000 on a cotton wool ball can be used) as tears in the flap can easily occur. The fibrous annulus should be elevated from below using a curved needle. The chorda tympani is recognized but left *in situ* at this stage.

The preparation of the surgical field continues by curretting away the posterosuperior bony annulus. The amount differs from patient to patient but in general the bony ponticulus should be in vision; if the surgeon is right-handed it is important to be a little more generous in left ears (and vice versa) in order to facilitate instrumentation (Fig 33.8).

Preservation of the chorda tympani is achieved in almost all cases by first using a flat currette and thinning the bone from its lateral surface. An angled currette can then be used on the edge when accuracy is not tempered by the need for strength to remove the bone. If the chorda tympani is lying

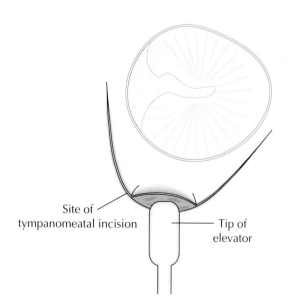

Fig 33.6 Tympanomeatal flap in the right ear.

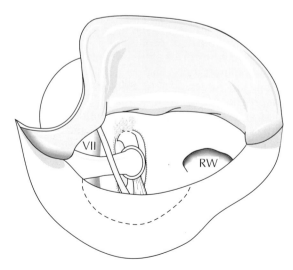

Fig 33.7 Tympanomeatal flap hinging anteriorly. RW, round window.

across the incus, more bone should be curretted inferiorly to release it and allow it to be retracted below the incudostapedial joint, otherwise it will impede the positioning of the prosthesis on the incus.

With a clear surgical field the footplate is exposed by removing any mucosal fold or adhesions, and any middle ear anomalies, such as a persistent stapedial artery or an overhanging facial nerve, are recognized. The finding of such anomalies may preclude continuation of the surgery. It is important to remove the mucosal folds early as resultant bleeding usually settles with time. Confirmation of a fixed footplate is obtained by gently palpating the stapes superstructure. The mobility of the rest of the ossicular chain is then displayed by gently rocking the malleus and noting movement at the incudostapedial joint. Poor results post-stapedectomy may reflect failure to recognize fixation of the malleoincudal joint. Mobility of the ossicular chain in the face of a conductive hearing loss and a normal tympanogram may suggest perilymph hypertension. Stapedectomy in such cases can result in profuse perilymph leakage and an ensuing sensorineural hearing loss.

The distance between the incus and the footplate or vestibule is measured. If a Schuknecht footplate measuring tool is used, care should be taken to see that it is aligned perpendicular to the footplate and close to the incudostapedial joint. The middle marker indicates a distance of 4.5 mm, the upper 5.0 mm and the lower 4.0 mm. In the majority of patients the distance is between 4.0 and 4.5 mm. An

alternative technique is by using a Teflon prosthesis with the loop cut off. A 4.5 mm prosthesis prepared in this way with about 0.2 mm paired off its extremity is the most common 'good fit' such that after footplate perforation a 4.5 mm piston would enter the vestibule by 0.1–0.2 mm.

Perforation of the footplate, which should be in its posterior third, is achieved by a hand-rotated drill or electrical microdrill. Perforation of the footplate while the superstructure is intact is advisable, for if the footplate becomes mobile a pick can be introduced into the vestibule to remove it. Uncommonly (<2 per cent of cases) fixation may be only fibrous and mobilization is all that is needed. The stapes tendon is then divided using the scissors or a sickle knife and the incudostapedial joint disarticulated with an angled joint knife. The stapes superstructure may then be down-fractured away from the facial nerve and removed. The footplate perforation is expanded to about 0.8 mm in diameter in order to accept a 0.6 mm prosthesis. If such a removal is not possible than the posterior third of the footplate can be extracted with a small right-angle hook. Blood in the oval window and vestibule does no harm but can be managed with gentle aspiration using the smallest gauge aspirator well away from the fenestra. In cases of obliterative otosclerosis, the electrical microdrill with a cutting burr of 0.8 mm is used. The angle of the burr to the footplate has to be 90° to allow the prosthesis to move freely in the vestibule when attached to the incus. The level of the vestibule may be difficult to gauge, the prevalence of sensorineural hearing loss in these cases is significantly greater (4 per cent) and an intraoperative decision not to continue with the procedure may have to be made.

The choice between a Teflon loop and a stainless steel loop is based on training and preference. The Teflon loop is expanded by running it down the tapered shaft of a microsurgical instrument. The 'memory' in the material allows it to self-crimp. If forceps are used to expand the loop the material memory may be overstretched and fail to return to its primary state. The design of the wire prosthesis is such that the loop needs no opening. The wire prosthesis may be conveniently removed from its package and introduced into the ear by using a suction aspirator. This technique stops the stainless steel wire or soft platinum wire from becoming bent if the prosthesis inadvertently touches the speculum or external meatus while being held rigid by forceps.

The length of the prosthesis indicated on the package most commonly relates to the distance between the lowest extent of the loop (i.e. the part lying in contact with the underside of the incus) and the tip.

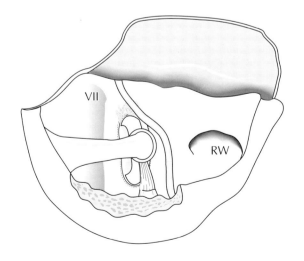

Fig 33.8 After bony resection of posterosuperior meatal wall.

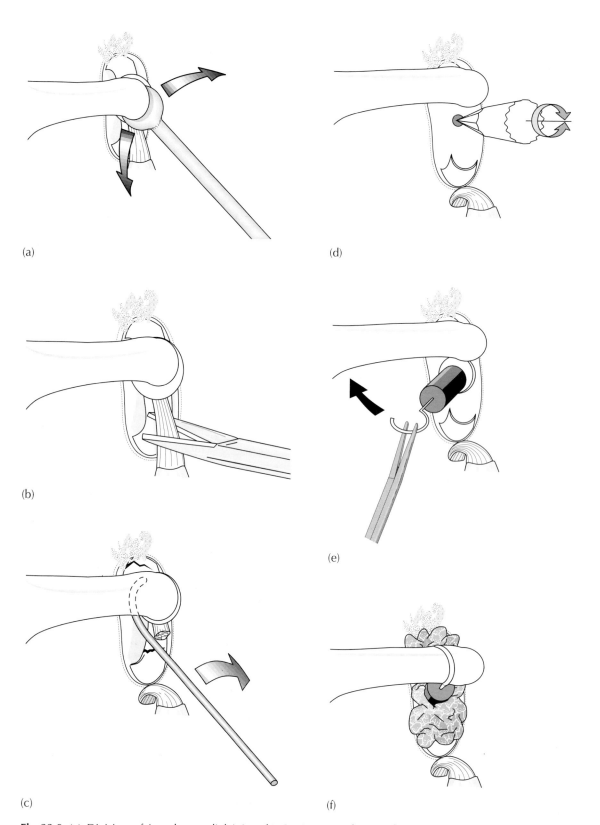

(a)

(b)

(c)

(d)

(e)

(f)

Fig 33.9 (a) Division of incudostapedial joint. (b) Cutting stapedius tendon. (c) Down fracture of stapes crura. (d) Trephining footplate. (e) Placing prosthesis. (f) Fat seal around prosthesis. Some surgeons, including the present author, trephine the footplate before breaking the crura.

Positioning of the prosthesis in the footplate fenestra and onto the long process of the incus is achieved by suspending the prosthesis on the aspirator and, when the correct position is achieved, opening the vacuum system (by means of a footswitch). A small right-angled instrument in the other hand may help to guide the prosthesis.

The wire loop has to be orientated at right angles to the shaft of the long process of the incus and crimped. Crimping should result in the prosthesis being firmly positioned. A loose prosthesis is likely to become detached and may also induce bone necrosis by continual movement. An overtightened prosthesis may also result in the avascular necrosis of the terminal long process of the incus. When crimping is complete the shaft is gently moved to check its stability in the vestibule. The oval window niche is sealed with a fat graft (Fig 33.9). If a total stapedectomy has occurred then a formal seal of the oval window using perichondrium or vein is mandatory.

A floating footplate (i.e. a freely mobile footplate after the stapes superstructure has been removed) presents a difficult surgical problem. There are several management options; one is for the operation to be aborted and the footplate allowed to refix. Reoperation can then take place at a later date. Other possibilities for the experienced stapes surgeon include careful and accurate placement of a prosthesis on the footplate, although the danger of depressing the bone into the vestibule is significant; alternatively, a small marginal burr hole can be made inferior to the oval window through which a microhook can be inserted to lift the footplate out of the fenestra. If possible the latter option is preferable.

Disarticulation of the incus may occur during the currettage of the posterosuperior meatal wall. If the incus remains in its original position, albeit excessively mobile, an incudovestibular reconstruction can continue; however, if it is subluxed medially its removal is necessary and the prosthesis has to be attached to the malleus. If misplaced or if excessive crimping results in a fracture of the long process of the incus, a longer wire prosthesis should then be used, crimping it further up the shaft of the incus or on the handle of the malleus.

A facial nerve overhanging the oval window niche has to be treated with the greatest caution. The surgeon needs to be confident not only that a prosthesis will fit into the vestibule without impinging on the nerve, but that instrumentation on the footplate (including the management of a floating footplate) is possible without trauma to the nerve. With these constraints it is sometimes possible to use a longer wire prosthesis than would be normally necessary and curve it inferiorly.

If a linear tear has occurred and is found after the tympanomeatal flap has been replaced, a gelfoam cover is all that is required. However, if there is tissue loss a silastic sheet should be placed over the flap or a formal underlay myringoplasty technique should be employed using perichondrium or temporalis fascia. Prophylactic antibiotics are not necessary.

The external auditory meatus is then packed with gelatine sponge with an outer packing of bismuth iodoform paraffin paste (BIPP).

Postoperative management

After a general anaesthetic the stapedectomy patient is normally kept in hospital for two nights although daycase stapedectomy is now possible. The patient is advised not to blow the nose and, if sneezing cannot be avoided, to let the pressure dissipate through the mouth. Normal activities can be resumed after 2 weeks, which includes commercial flying. Pain is not usually a problem but postoperative vertigo with nystagmus to the operated ear is not uncommon and is best treated with labyrinthine sedatives (prochlorperazine, 25 mg rectally). The BIPP pack can be removed 3–5 days after surgery along with any skin sutures.

Vertiginous symptoms beginning 3–7 days postoperatively may indicate an aseptic labyrinthitis, a diagnostic term that reflects the benign clinical outcome, characterized by marked vertigo, often positional in nature, transient sensorineural hearing loss and tinnitus. Operative intervention is not indicated as it may be associated with permanent hearing loss. Oral steroids have been suggested although their efficacy has not been proved in such circumstances. Acute otitis media and otitis externa should be considered as a medical emergency and treated with a broad spectrum of antibiotics; the current drug of choice is ciprofloxacin.

Dysequilibrium and fluctuating hearing loss may indicate a perilymphatic leak and can occur at any time after stapedectomy. Diagnosis relies on a high level of suspicion. Exploration of the ear should proceed cautiously and the prosthesis should not be displaced if it is in the vestibule as adhesion may well have formed with the membraneous labyrinth. If the fistula is seen it may be plugged with a fat graft; when no fistula is visible it is sensible to lay a graft around the prosthesis anteriorly – a blind spot that might be harbouring a fistula. Bedrest until symptoms subside is important.

Postoperative reparative granulomas are thankfully rare. They manifest with pain and swelling in the posterosuperior quadrant of the drum, which is discoloured a reddy-brown. The sensorineural hearing threshold falls and urgent surgery with the removal of the granuloma is indicated. The results of early surgical intervention may be excellent even if the speech discrimination scores have fallen to under 50 per cent.[9] A diagnostic dilemma may occur between serous labyrinthitis, perilymphatic leaks and reparative greanuloma.

Problems with the position of the prosthesis in relation to the oval window commonly arise between 6 and 18 months after surgery, although no closure of the air–bone gap after surgery suggests inappropriate placement of the prosthesis on the incus, insufficient bony footplate removal or a prosthesis that is too short. In patients in whom there has been immediate closure of the air–bone gap followed by fluctuations in hearing often associated with middle ear inflation, a 'loose wire' syndrome is likely.[10] The prosthesis may have just slipped off a normal incus or, as suggested previously, be associated with the necrosis of its long process. The surgical option for the former is simple recrimping; the latter is more difficult to manage as removal of the prosthesis from the oval window is hazardous. The use of ionomeric bone cements to reconstruct the long process may be a convenient option in this difficult situation. When the prosthesis has been extruded from the vestibule, careful dissection in the oval window niche with removal of fibrous tissue down to the level of the footplate but not into the vestibule allows repositioning of a new prosthesis with an intact oval window seal. If the incus is deficient then the prosthesis may be attached to the handle of the malleus, making sure that it passes medial to the tympanic membrane.[11]

Bone-anchored hearing aid

In patients with otosclerosis who have undergone the fenestration procedure, an air conduction hearing aid may result in a chronically discharging cavity resistant to surgical revision. A trial with a bone conduction hearing aid should be undertaken and, if the acoustic response is adequate, a bone-anchored hearing aid (BAHA) employed using the Branemark technqiue.

Cochlear implantation

End-stage otosclerosis and profound sensorineural deafness may, very rarely, be managed by multichannel cochlear implantation. The temporal bone histopathology studies indicate relatively good spiral ganglion populations. An accurate assessment of the intracochlear space using MRI and CT scanning is necessary in order to satisfy the surgeon that implantation is possible. Osteosclerotic are frequently cited as 'good responders' after cochlear implantation.

References

1. Morrison AW. Genetic factors in osteosclerosis. *Annals of the Royal College of Surgeons of England* 1967; **41**:202–37.
2. Lempert J. Improvement of hearing in cases of otosclerosis new one stage technique. *Archives of Otolaryngology* 1938; **28**:42–7.
3. Shea JJ Jr. Fenestration of the oval window. *Annals of Otology, Rhinology and Laryngology* 1938; **47**:932–51.
4. Schuknecht HF, Barber W. Histological variants in otosclerosis. *Laryngoscope* 1985; **95**:1307–17.
5. Causse J, Chevance LG, Bretlau P, Jorgensen MB, Uriel J, Berges J. Enzymatic concept of otospongiosis and cochlea otospongiosis. *Clinical Otolaryngology* 1977; **2**:23–32.
6. Cremers CWRJ, Hombergen GCJH, Wenteges RTT. Perilymphatic gusher and stapes surgery – a predictable complication? *Clinical Otolaryngology* 1983; **8**:235–40.
7. Valvassori GE. Imaging of otosclerosis. *Otolaryngological Clinics of North America* 1993; **26**:359–71.
8. Shambaugh GE, Scott A. Sodium fluoride for the arrest of otosclerosis. *Archives of Otolaryngology* 1964; **80**:263–70.
9. Gacek RR. The diagnosis and treatment of post-stapedectomy granuloma. *Annals of Otology, Rhinology and Laryngology* 1970; **79**:970–5.
10. McGee TM. The loose wire syndrome. *Laryngoscope* 1981; **91**:1478–83.
11. Mawson SR. Management of the complication of stapedectomy. *Journal of Laryngology and Otology* 1975; **89**:1445–9.

CHAPTER 34

Tumours of the middle ear and skull base

IAN S STORPER AND MICHAEL E GLASSCOCK

Introduction

Within the past 2 decades several reports have emerged describing approaches to the skull base, an area of the body in which tumours were previously considered unresectable.[1-4] At present, there exists a large body of literature describing the various lesions, diagnostic techniques and surgical appoaches that now make this area readily accessible to the subspecialist; nevertheless the postoperative course of the patient is often prolonged and occasionally complicated. Although the diagnosis of such lesions has become routine, management often remains a formidable challenge.

A number of tumour and tumour-like lesions are uncommon in the temporal bone. Although lesions that involve the auricle, external auditory canal and middle ear may be readily discovered on routine examination, lesions of the petrous apex, internal auditory canal and skull base may be characterized by insidious, occult growth. It is therefore imperative for the clinician to keep a high index of suspicion for such disease while obtaining a history and performing a physical examination. Fortunately, with increased awareness of clinicians and advanced diagnostic techniques, including axial computed tomography (CT) and magnetic resonance imaging (MRI) with gadolinium-DTPA, these lesions are being discovered earlier in their neoplastic history, thus decreasing surgical complexity and morbidity.

This chapter is devoted to the diagnosis and management of tumours of the middle ear and cranial base. Secondary to limitations on space and content, it is necessarily somewhat abbreviated. The interested reader should feel free to contact us regarding any quesions that may arise.

Tumour types

GLOMUS TUMOURS

Background

Non-chromaffin paragangliomas or glomus tumours, also known as chemodectomas, arise from glomus bodies distributed along parasympathetic nerves in the skull base, thorax and neck.[5] Glomus bodies are made up of chemoreceptor tissue capable of secreting hormonally active monoimmune peptides. They derive from cells of the neural crest and are believed to play a key role in the compensatory physiological response to hypoxia, hypercapnia and acidity.[6] Although Guild[7] is credited with renewing interest in this anatomical entity, it was Rosenwasser[8] who first reported the diagnosis of a glomus jugulare tumour correctly. Histologically, the glomus body consists of fibrous stromal septa that divide the gland into lobules. These tumours are hypervascular. Within the temporal bone, the glomus bodies may be found within the adventitia of the jugular bulb along any part of the glossopharyngeal or vagus nerves, including the tympanic canaliculus, retrofacial air cells, promontory and geniculate ganglion. In the neck, they are found at the nodose ganglion (vagal body), carotid body, along the superior and inferior laryngeal nerves and within the mediastinum.[8-12]

Glomus tumours are the most common benign tumours that arise within the temporal bone. They exhibit considerable variability in their behaviour; most commonly they manifest as indolent and protracted, with marked bone erosion and expansion along normally occurring tissue planes. Fewer than 5 per cent of tumours exhibit aggressive growth characteristics, with rapid erosion of bone and short survival periods. Fewer than 10 per cent of patients present with synchronous lesions; all patients with glomus tumours should be evaluated for multiple lesions.[13,14] All such tumours have the potential to secrete catecholamines, although few exhibit clinically evident hypersecretion. Hypersecretion of noradrenaline (norepinephrine), adrenaline (epinephrine), dopamine, serotonin, vasoactive intestinal polypeptide, glucagon, cholecystokinin-pancreozymin and other hormones have been described. All patients with glomus tumours should undergo evaluation by an endocrinologist for hormone secretion and for multiple endocrine neoplasia-type syndromes. These familial syndromes are present in approximately 10 per cent of patients.[14] If a tumour is found to be secreting catecholamine, the patient should be appropriately alpha- and beta-blocked preoperatively.

In fewer than 5 per cent of patients, metastasis may be found. This is the criterion for malignancy, as the histological appearance does not vary from benign to malignant disease. These patients tend to have a more aggressive course.

These tumours may arise in different regions of the skull base. When they are confined to the middle ear space, they are termed *glomus tympanicum*. When they arise in the region of the jugular foramen, regardless of their extent, they are termed *glomus jugulare*. When they arise high in the neck, extending towards the jugular foramen, they are termed *glomus vagale*. When they arise in the area of the carotid bifurcation, they are termed *carotid body tumours*. For the purposes of the scope of this chapter, only the first three of these lesions will be discussed.

Histology

Glomus tumours that involve the temporal bone most commonly have their origin at the jugular bulb. Both these types and glomus tympanicum types are consistent with the original description by Guild.[7] It is often impossible, however, to establish the exact site of origin. The usual site for the glomus body is the dome of the jugular bulb, near Jacobson's nerve. This entire body measures 0.25×0.5 mm. In 88 temporal bone, Guild[9] found a total of 248 glomus tumours, half in the dome of the jugular bulb and half equally distributed along Arnold's and Jacobson's nerves. He observed that the histological structure of this body was composed of precapillary or capillary blood vessels, lined by uniform, large epithelioid cells that failed to stain with chromium salts. The carotid body, which is similar in structure and composition, shares the blood supply of the ascending pharyngeal artery; they are both usually innervated by the glossopharyngeal nerve.

As stated above, glomus tumours may occur wherever glomus bodies are present. From the site of origin, the tumour grows insidiously, infiltrating adjacent structures. The tumour may compress the sigmoid sinus and jugular bulb from without, or protrude into the bulb and internal jugular vein. The rate of growth is usually slow; morbidity correlates directly with the particular site that is involved.

Microscopically, glomus tumours resemble glomus bodies, with a rich supply of vascular spaces lined by epithelioid cells. These cells are usually uniform in size and appearance.[4] Tumours that metastasize are usually more pleomorphic. As these tumours invade bone, the bone becomes soft and haemorrhagic, without a line of demarcation from normal bone. The hypervascular tumour bleeds profusely with minimal trauma. As the vascular spaces have no contractile elements, there is little tendency for the bleeding to stop. Tables 34.1 and 34.2 outline the most common staging classification for glomus tumours in the USA. The standard staging system proposed by Fisch is popular in Europe (Table 34.3).

Signs and symptoms

Presenting symptoms of these tumours often reflect their pathway of growth. Hearing loss, pulsatile tinnitus and aural fullness are frequent complaints. Bleeding, otalgia and aural suppuration may also be present. As the tumour mass invades the labyrinth, vertigo and profound hearing loss may occur. Encroachment within the Fallopian canal or direct

Table 34.1 Glasscock–Jackson classification system for glomus tympanicum tumours

Class I	Small mass confined to the promontory
Class II	Tumour completely filling middle ear space
Class III	Tumour filling middle ear and extending into mastoid process
Class IV	Tumour filling middle ear, extending into mastoid process or through tympanic membrane to fill external auditory canal; may also extend anterior to internal carotid artery

facial nerve invasion can cause facial paralysis, a finding reported as the index symptom in 10–40 per cent of patients.[15]

Other cranial nerve pareses may also occur. These result from tumour growth along the neurovascular planes of least resistance at the skull base, or from direct growth into the posterior and middle cranial fossae. Spector and Pensak have reported central nervous system invasion in 18 per cent of patients. These findings may include VIth, IXth, Xth, XIth and XIIth cranial nerve weaknesses, and are manifest as diplopia on lateral gaze, hoarseness, aspiration, inability to abduct the affected arm over the head and difficulty articulating, respectively.[15]

A red–blue retrotympanic mass may be seen in over 50 per cent of glomus tympanicum tumours and approximately 40 per cent of glomus jugulare tumours. Bleeding and a red mass, with or without an indistinct, poorly visualized tympanic membrane, are often encountered. Brown's sign, defined as a bluish middle ear mass that blanches in response to applied pneumatic pressure via the otoscope, is present in a significant number of vascular tumours of the middle ear.[16] There is a 3:1 female : male ratio in prevalence, with most tumours appearing in middle age. Glomus tumours are seen most frequently in Caucasians.

Table 34.2 Glasscock–Jackson classification system for glomus jugulare tumours

Class I	Small tumour involving jugular bulb, middle ear and mastoid process
Class II	Tumour extending under internal auditory canal; may have intracranial extension
Class III	Tumour extending into petrous apex; may have intracranial extension
Class IV	Tumour extending beyond petrous apex into clivus or infratemporal fossa; may have intracranial extension

Table 34.3 Fisch classification of glomus tumours

Type A	Tumours localized to the middle ear cleft
Type B	Tympanomastoid tumours with no destruction of bone in the infralabyrinthine compartment of the temporal bone
Type C	Tumours invading the bone of the infralabyrinthine compartment of the temporal bone
Type D	Tumours with intracranial extension

Diagnosis

The diagnosis of a glomus tumour begins with the initial history and physical examination. In all patients with pulsatile tinnitus, unilateral hearing loss, unexplained lower cranial nerve weakness, with or without a blue–red mass in the middle ear, further work-up is warranted. All otologic patients require a pure tone air and bone conduction audiogram with speech discrimination scores. Most patients with glomus tumours exhibit conductive hearing loss on the affected side; sensorineural loss may be present. Electronystagmography with caloric testing plays a very minor role in the diagnosis of these lesions, as there is usually a large amount of middle ear disease that could affect the outcome. In addition, all affected areas will be treated regardless of the vestibular function.

The diagnosis is established by radiographic studies. Equally important are MRI and CT. MRI should be performed with 1 mm sections, and axial, coronal and sagittal views should be obtained. This study should be performed before and after the administration of gadolinium-DTPA, extending superiorly from the affected area of the neck throughout the entire brain. Carotid bifurcations should be clearly visible. Characteristic of glomus tumours on MRI is a hypervascular lesion in the area of the jugular foramen, middle ear or neck (Fig 34.1) The administration of gadolinium-DTPA produces a characteristic 'salt and pepper' appearance. In addition to the known lesion, the presence of synchronous tumours should also be ruled out. As MRI does not image bone, CT scanning is also essential. CT should be performed in the axial and coronal planes, with images obtained at 1 mm intervals. Intravenous contrast dye should be used wherever safe, as the tumour is hypervascular. Using CT, the bone of the jugular foramen, mastoid, otic capsule, petrous apex, internal auditory canal and clivus may be investigated for extension of disease (Fig 34.2 and Plate section). Lastly, angiography is performed if the diagnosis is uncertain or before surgical resection so that the blood supply may be recognized and embolized. From angiography, the diagnosis is established without question. In addition, the feeding vessels (primary and secondary) may be readily recognized; contralateral filling may be appreciated, and the presence of additional masses may be ascertained. Flow status in the sigmoid sinus and jugular bulb may be assessed. The ability of the surgeon to remove the internal carotid artery, if necessary, may be evaluated by balloon occlusion testing.

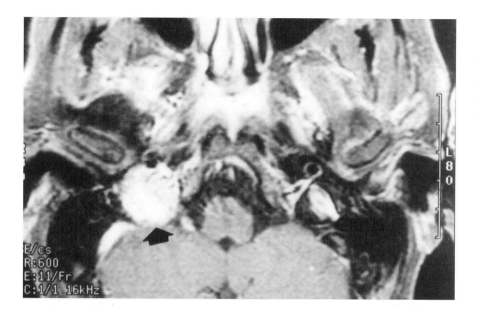

Fig 34.1 Axial gadolinium-enhanced T1-weighted MRI demonstrating glomus jugulare tumour. Arrow depicts hypervascular, non-uniform mass in the right jugular bulb.

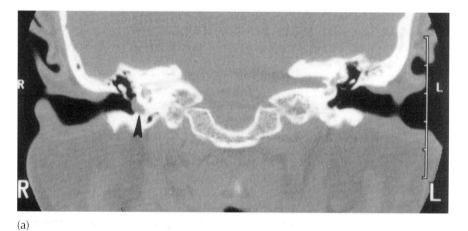

(a)

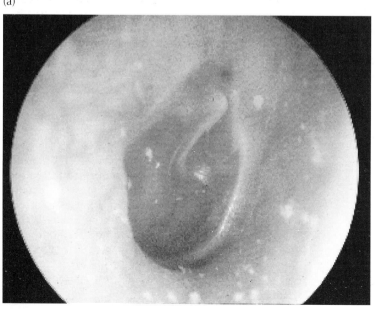

(b)

Fig 34.2 (a) Coronal unenhanced CT scan demonstrating a mass in the right middle ear and hypotympanum (arrow), which proved to be glomus tympanicum tumour at operation. (b) Otoscopic photograph of the tumour shown in the above scan.

Treatment

Treatment of glomus tumours is regarded as palliative or definitive; it is based on tumour size, tumour location and patient health. Surgery, irradiation, embolization and chemotherapy have been employed in the management of these tumours, either alone or in combination. At present the preferred method of management is surgical, but management strategies must be tailored to the individual patient. Using current surgical techniques, no glomus tumour is unresectable; but patient factors, including ability to tolerate an extended general anaesthetic with significant blood loss and willingness to undergo possible cranial nerve dysfunction, may make operation inadvisable.

In general, patients over the age of 75 years are regarded as poor candidates for neurological skull base surgery. This is secondary to the possible morbidities encountered; it should be remembered that slow growth of these tumours is the usual rule. Patients with chronic obstructive pulmonary disease are also poor candidates, secondary to the possible postoperative weakness of the vagus or hypoglossal, or both, nerves. As the usual presentation is in the fourth decade in otherwise healthy individuals, the morbidity associated with leaving a tumour in place greatly exceeds that of operation; surgery is the preferred method of treatment in these patients.[13]

In the asymptomatic patient who is not a surgical candidate, serial MRI imaging is an appropriate method of management. The symptomatic individual is treated with irradiation. If a patient can tolerate a brief general anaesthetic, palliative subtotal resection followed by irradiation offers an acceptable alternative and significant extension of life.[13]

If a healthy patient has multiple unilateral lesions, they are removed simultaneously. In a healthy patient with bilateral lesions, the more life-threatening one is the first to be addressed surgically. The method of treatment of the opposite side is tailored by the result of the primary surgery.

As a generalization, combination therapy is not necessary. It should be remembered that this lesion is usually benign; additional methods of therapy would be excessive. Irradiation complicates surgery by inhibiting nerve regeneration and wound healing. Preoperative embolization, however, is employed in all cases, and has been shown to decrease blood loss substantially. Addition of preoperative embolization is not regarded as combination therapy; it is currently considered part of appropriate surgical treatment. There has been no conclusive evidence of permanent benefit of chemotherapy, whether applied systematically or intra-arterially, for this tumour; rather, chemotherapy complicates a patient's medical condition and usual subsequent operative course.[13]

Radiation therapy for glomus tumours

The relative effectiveness of irradiation for glomus jugulare tumours remains controversial. Whereas a large body of literature confirms the effectiveness of surgery, there is no such convincing evidence for irradiation. This is because there is no large body of information available on long-term follow-up of patients who have been irradiated. This method has been employed, primarily, palliatively and as surgical salvage.

Part of the difficulty in examining the results of irradiation is that there is an extremely small number of studies that make tumour size and location evident. Some do not even distinguish between glomus tympanicum and glomus jugulare tumours. Therapeutic long-term outcome is rarely discussed.[17]

A wedge pair of radiation beams is used to administer 45 Gy over 4 weeks. This configuration minimizes brain necrosis; this dose has been found by Kim et al.[18] to be the minimum that will provide a failure rate of less than 2 per cent.

The difficulty with all of these studies is the post-irradiation histological appearance of the tumour tissue. Spector et al.[19] examined the histological effects of irradiation and noted perivascular fibrosis, endothelial hyperplasia, subendothelial hyaline degeneration and small vessel proliferative arteritis; there was, however, no overall decrease in vascularity. The authors concluded that proliferation of the fibrous stroma was the main effect. Gardner et al.[20] also noted no destruction of tumour in tissue exposed to irradiation; changes were limited to island formation and stromal proliferation. Many readers have concluded from these reports that radiation therapy is not curative. Subsequent examination of these studies has shown that some tumours were examined too early after irradiation to document a response adequately. At present, investigators are evaluating the efficacy of focused beam irradiation for glomus tumours. This technique offers the advantage of single-dose therapy.

In conclusion, the relative efficacy of irradiation in the treatment of glomus tumours remains controversial. What is universally agreed upon is that these lesions do not regress after treatment; it is unclear, at present, whether lesions actually cease to grow or just grow more slowly. It is for this reason that our current recommendation is for surgical therapy in patients who can tolerate it medically.

Surgical treatment of glomus tumours

As glomus jugulare and glomus tympanicum tumours originate from the jugular bulb and the hypotympanum, respectively, possible routes of spread are quite complex, as tumours grow along the pathway of least resistance (Fig 34.3). The approach to each tumour must therefore be individualized; there is no single operation for all of these lesions. Rather, a uniform approach has been developed that allows for adequate exposure of all margins, identification and preservation of all vital regional anatomy and access to intracranial extension. This approach allows for tumour removal while preserving as much normal anatomy and function as possible.

Neurotological skull base surgery is virtually always limited to the lateral, posterior skull base. Anterior access is only very rarely necessary. Table 34.4 describes our usual algorithm for removal of glomus tumours.

Essential to the proper neurotological removal of a glomus tumour is the respectful management of the facial nerve and major vessels. Whereas the facial nerve is considered a useful landmark in mastoid or acoustic neuroma surgery, it becomes a structure to be 'managed' in the removal of glomus tumours. Depending on the size and extent of a tumour, this implies that the facial nerve usually requires relocation. Although the extrinsic blood supply to the nerve is interrupted during translocation, the intrinsic supply is what allows the survival of the nerve. Facial nerve monitoring is considered an essential part of the surgery; glomus tumour removal should not be attempted without a nerve monitor.[21]

Tumour size and the exposure required to control the internal carotid artery dictate the amount of facial nerve mobilization that is necessary. When a tumour is confined to the jugular foramen, away from the internal carotid artery, simple exposure of the facial nerve is all that is necessary. More often, it is quite difficult to remove a tumour located between the facial nerve and the transverse process of C1, so that mobilization from the external genu is required. This is termed 'short' mobilization. Usually, postoperative facial nerve paralysis does not occur in this event.[21]

For larger tumours that involve the petrous carotid artery, anterior dislocation of the mandible is necessary for adequate proximal and distal vascular control. In this situation, mobilization from the internal genu (or 'long' mobilization) is required. Although postoperative paralysis of the face is common, the facial nerve usually regains acceptable levels of function over time.[21]

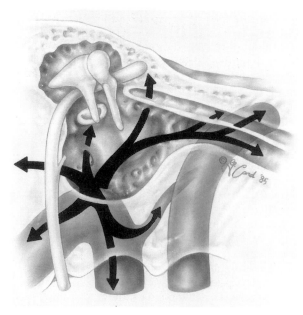

Fig 34.3 Possible routes of growth of glomus tumour from the hypotympanum. (Reproduced with permission.[21])

Table 34.4 Surgical approaches for glomus tumours

Glomus tympanicum	
Class I	Transcanal
Class II	Postauricular
Class III	Postauricular
Class IV	Postauricular
Glomus jugulare	
Class I	Lateral transtemporal
Class II	Lateral transtemporal
Class III	Modified infratemporal fossa
Class IV	Modified or extended infratemporal fossa

Paragangliomas characteristically encase and distort the facial nerve. Nevertheless, they often allow meticulous dissection of the nerve from the tumour. In patients in whom the nerve is actually invaded, who often present with a preoperative facial weakness, segmental resection and primary anastomosis or grafting is necessary. Ultimate facial function will necessarily be worse in these situations.

Virtually every glomus tumour will also relate to the internal carotid artery. The most meticulous portion of the surgical procedure is usually the dissection of the tumour from this artery in the subadventitial plane. The principles of proximal and distal exposure and control of the internal carotid artery must be respected. This implies necessary tympanic, petrous or intracranial exposure of this artery, in addition to exposure in the neck. The artery should be exposed over at least half of its circumference and mobilized, so that it may be instrumented if necessary. If the tumour cannot be removed from the internal carotid artery, carotid resection may be attempted if a patient has passed a preoperative balloon occlusion test. It should be remembered that there remains a finite risk of stroke, despite passing such a test.

Glomus tympanicum resection

Class I

If the margins of the lesion are clearly visible around the entire circumference of the lesion, transcanal removal may be attempted. In this approach, the middle ear is exposed via a tympanomeatal flap (Fig 34.4). Microbipolar cautery is applied to the feeding vessels and margins, and the tumour is avulsed (Fig 34.5). Haemostasis is achieved either with bipolar cautery or gelfoam soaked in adrenaline. The flap is then replaced.[21]

Classes II–IV

If the margins are indistinct, a postauricular incision is made and a complete mastoidectomy is performed (Fig 34.6). The facial recess is opened and extended inferiorly through the chorda tympani (Fig 34.7). Exposure of the hypotympanum is afforded between the facial nerve and tympanic annulus. Via this approach, the tumour may be removed from the ossicular chain, facial nerve, internal jugular vein and Eustachian tube (Fig 34.8). Tympanic membrane may be removed if it is involved with the tumour. Myringoplasty is performed once haemostasis has been achieved. If necessary, the posterior wall of the external auditory canal may be removed.[21]

Glomus jugulare resection

All glomus jugulare tumours are embolized preoperatively. In addition, a carotid balloon occlusion test is performed. To approach glomus jugulare tumours adequately, a team approach is necessary. This team includes a head and neck surgeon to perform the neck dissection and reconstruction, a neurotologist to perform the temporal bone and infratemporal fossa dissection, and a neurosurgeon to perform removal of intracranial extension. These resections should only be performed with an anaesthetist who is an expert in this field, as neurological and haemodynamic compromise may occur.

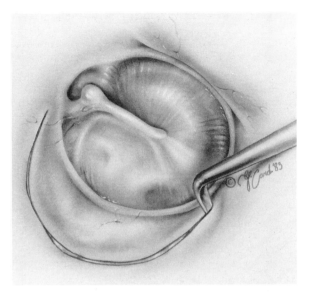

Fig 34.4 Right tympanomeatal flap being raised to expose small middle ear tumour. (Reproduced with permission.[21])

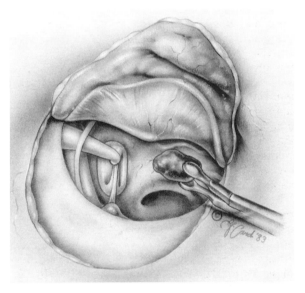

Fig 34.5 Tumour being removed after tympanomeatal flap is raised and haemostasis is achieved. (Reproduced with permission.[21])

Classes I and II

For Class I and II glomus jugulare tumours, the basic, lateral transtemporal approach is employed. This approach conserves the external auditory canal and ossicular anatomy. It is used in tumours that are confined to the jugular foramen and infralabyrinthine region, involving the internal carotid

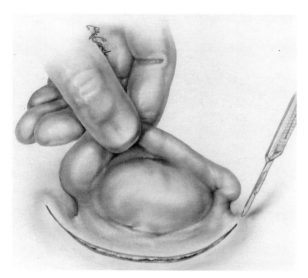

Fig 34.6 Exposure is begun with complete right mastoidectomy. (Reproduced with permission.[21])

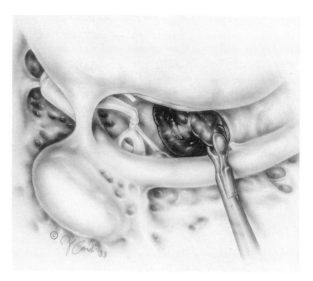

Fig 34.8 Once vital anatomy is secured and haemostasis is achieved tumour removal begins. (Reproduced with permission.[21])

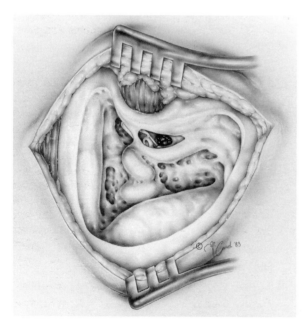

Fig 34.7 Extended facial recess approach affords access to right middle ear, Eustachian tube and hypotympanum. (Reproduced with permission.[21])

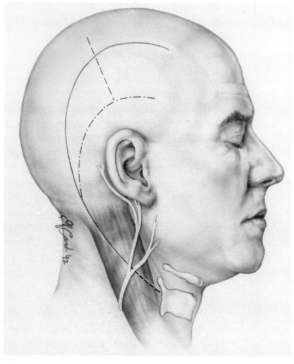

Fig 34.9 Surgical incision that provides adequate access for glomus jugulare resection. (Reproduced with permission.[21])

artery in the tympanic segment or more inferiorly. Here, an incision is made approximately 8 cm behind the postauricular crease (Fig 34.9), extending superiorly and inferiorly. The dissection begins in the neck, identifying the facial, glossopharyngeal, vagus, spinal accessory and hypoglossal nerves at the skull base. The major vessels of the neck are identified. The internal jugular vein is then divided. Proximal internal carotid control is obtained at the level of the bifurcation. Next, complete

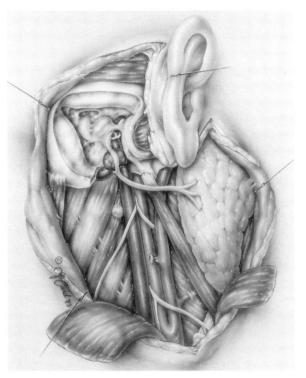

Fig 34.10 Facial nerve is involved with tumour and its course is distorted by this. (Reproduced with permission.[21])

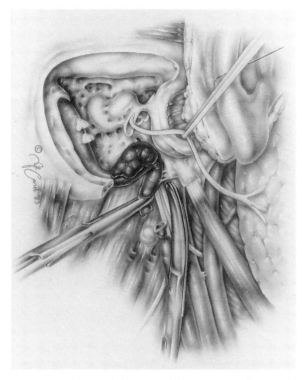

Fig 34.12 Short mobilization of facial nerve is frequently necessary to remove infralabyrinthine tumour extension. (Reproduced with permission.[21])

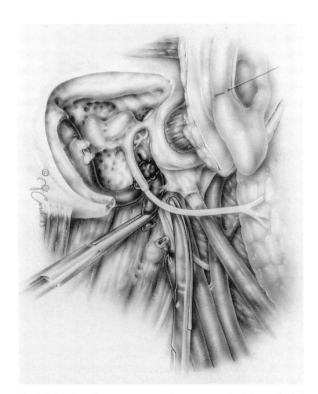

Fig 34.11 Small tumours may be removed without facial nerve mobilization. (Reproduced with permission.[21])

mastoidectomy, extended facial recess approach and mastoid tip removal is accomplished. After the facial nerve is identified in the mastoid, the styloid process is removed (Fig 34.10). The sigmoid sinus is then divided (Fig 34.11).[21]

On rare occasions, short mobilization of the facial nerve may be accomplished to remove the tumour (Fig 34.12). Small tumours allow dissection with minimal facial nerve vascular compromise. An extended facial recess approach will afford distal internal carotid exposure to the Eustachian tube. At this point, tumour removal may be begun, first from the carotid artery. Next, the tumour is removed in conjunction with the sigmoid sinus and internal jugular vein. Bleeding is controlled with Surgicel and Avitene packing. After the tumour is removed, the facial nerve is replaced and myringoplasty is performed.[21]

Classes III and IV

For class III and IV tumours, the modified infratemporal fossa approach is performed; it may be extended if necessary. This approach offers access to the infratemporal fossa, petrous carotid artery, nasopharynx, clivus and cavernous sinus. It may be extended intracranially.

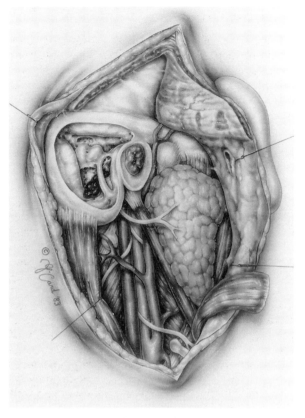

Fig 34.13 External auditory canal is transected and over-sewn. (Reproduced with permission.[21])

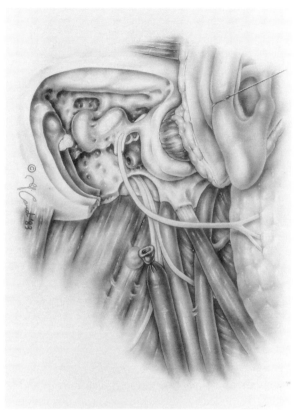

Fig 34.14 Ear structures lateral to stapes are removed. Long facial nerve mobilization is performed in order to mobilize mandible anteriorly. (Reproduced with permission.[21])

A large C-shaped incision is fashioned, forming an anteriorly based flap and transecting the external auditory canal. The latter is then oversewn (Fig 34.13). In addition to the initial exposure afforded as in Class I and II tumours, the tympanic ring and all middle ear contents lateral to the stapes are removed (Fig 34.14). To reach the petrous internal carotid artery, long mobilization of the facial nerve is accomplished, followed by anterior dislocation of the mandible. The temporomandibular joint is then removed. Next, the internal carotid artery is located distally and isolated. The pterygoid plates, foramen rotundum, clivus, cavernous sinus and nasopharynx may be reached after the middle meningeal artery is divided as it enters the foramen spinosum (Fig 34.15). The tumour is first removed from the carotid artery, followed by the infratemporal fossa and then the mastoid. The exposure may be extended to incorporate the transcochlear approach if the tumour extends anteromedially (Fig 34.16). Finally, intracranial extension is removed with the involved dura.

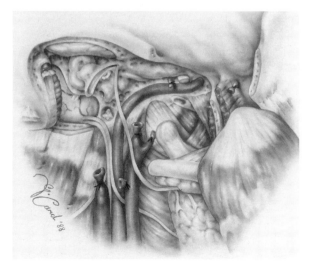

Fig 34.15 Eustachian tube and middle meningeal artery are sacrificed to expose petrous internal carotid artery to cavernous sinus. (Reproduced with permission.[21])

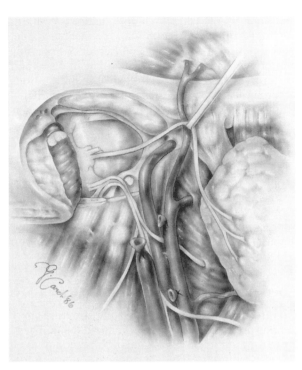

Fig 34.16 Transcochlear approach may be included. (Reproduced with permission.[21])

In general, dural defects are reconstructed with the deep temporalis flap; vascularized tissue provides the lowest risk of cerebrospinal fluid leak. If cerebrospinal fluid is encountered intraoperatively, a lumbar drain is placed and left for 5–7 days. Antibiotic prophylaxis is imperative in this situation. For a large defect that cannot be closed by a vascularized temporalis muscle flap, a microvascular free flap is employed. Two reasonable choices are rectus abdominis and latissimus dorsi. Rectus abdominis is preferred because the patient's position need not be altered.

If vocal cord weakness secondary to vagus nerve involvement is expected, an intraoperative vocal cord medialization procedure is recommended.[21]

Glomus vagale tumours

It is our opinion that a similar team approach should be used in the management of glomus vagale tumours. This type of approach will minimize the chance of partial resection, which could otherwise occur if the tumour were to invade the temporal bone or to extend intracranially. The neurotologist exposes the carotid artery in the temporal bone or more distally if proximal and distal control cannot be obtained in the neck.[21]

Negative outcomes

A discussion of the removal of glomus tumours would be incomplete if surgical negative outcomes were not covered. Although these tumours are often benign, their vascular nature and their location at the skull base afford certain risks. Unfortunately, in 1996, there appears to be no other mode of therapy that can achieve complete removal of disease. Although these tumours are embolized preoperatively, there remains a significant risk of haemorrhage, resulting in transfusion. This is because tertiary vessels cannot be embolized. A risk of cerebrospinal fluid leak exists, but is minimized by using vascularized tissue to close the dural defect. Other negative outcomes include facial paresis or paralysis (rarely), abducens weakness, hoarseness, aspiration, spinal accessory weakness, Horner's syndrome and difficulty articulating. The chance of a neurovascular event occurring is assessed preoperatively via balloon occlusion testing. Lastly, if intracranial extension is present, the risks include craniotomy and destabilization of the cervical spine or atlantoaxial joint (necessitating fusion) in addition to those already described. Needless to say, these procedures should only be performed by a surgical and anaesthesia team well experienced in this area.

OTHER TUMOUR TYPES

Numerous other lesions may exist in the middle ear and skull base. These lesions may be non-neoplastic, benign or malignant. Although the individual histology of each lesion varies, the general principles of diagnosis are similar to those of glomus tumours. It is not necessary to obtain an angiogram, however, unless a tumour appears vascular in nature on examination or by imaging study. Each specific lesion has its own appropriate plan of management. A fairly complete list of temporal bone tumours is given in Table 34.5.

Non-neoplastic lesions

Fibrous dysplasia

Fibrous dysplasia, a disorder of the bone with no known cause, is a non-neoplastic pathological condition resulting from an aberration of bone-forming mesenchyme.[22,23] Histologically, this lesion is characterized by poorly oriented osseous trabeculae and islands of cartilage. It may involve one bone (monostotic) or several bones (polyostotic). This lesion usually manifests clinically as a painless, asymmetric swelling in the temporal bone. Conductive

Table 34.5 Tumours of the temporal bone

Non-neoplastic
  Fibrous dysplasia
  Histiocytosis X
  Congenital cholesteatoma
  Aberrant vascular structures

Benign neoplasms
  Glomus jugulare
  Glomus tympanicum
  Adenoma
  Facial nerve neuroma
  Meningioma
  Haemangioma
  Dermoid
  Choristoma
  Chondroma
  Glioma

Malignant neoplasms
  Rhabdymyosarcoma
  Adenocarcinoma
  Chondrosarcoma
  Squamous cell carcinoma
  Basal cell carcinoma
  Nasopharyngeal carcinoma
  Metastasis

hearing loss secondary to involvement of the external auditory canal may occur. Entrapped tissue can result in infection. As the process grows, entrapment and compression of the VIIth and VIIIth cranial nerves can result in facial weakness or hearing loss, or both.[24] A strong suspicion for this lesion is generated by appearance on CT scan, on which fibrous dysplasia has a characteristic self-limited 'ground glass', expansile appearance. The differential diagnosis includes giant cell tumour, aneurysmal bone cyst and osseous fibroma. The diagnosis is established histologically; typically, a cyst-like mass of gritty, fibrous tissue beneath a thinned cortex is encountered. Appropriate treatment of fibrous dysplasia involves removal of all infected tissue and all tissue that is causing the patient's symptoms. Aggressive resection is rarely indicated; this lesion typically becomes quiescent after puberty. Radiation therapy is contraindicated; in rare instances it has resulted in malignant transformation.[25]

Histiocytosis X

The term histiocytosis refers to a group of interrelated, idiopathic clinical entities. These are characterized by the diffuse proliferation of mature histiocytes that are associated with tumour-like masses of foamy reticulo-endothelial cells containing lipid droplets, eosinophils and connective tissue. Three clinical forms are encountered: eosinophilic granuloma, Hand–Schüller–Christian disease, and Letterer–Siwe disease.[25] Otological manifestations occur in the first two of these ailments. Eosinophilic granuloma most often manifests with chronic ear discharge; CT scan may indicate a solid lytic lesion. Radiation therapy is the accepted method of treatment. Hand–Schüller–Christian disease appears with numerous possible symptoms, including exophthalmos and diabetes insipidus from osseous lesions, eczematoid dermatological changes, aural suppuration with granulation, fever, lymphadenopathy, hepatosplenomegaly and general malaise. In these patients, chemotherapy is often added if multiple sites are involved.[26,27]

Aberrant vascular structures

On rare occasions, aberrant vascular structures may be interpreted as tumours of the middle ear. These structures include a high jugular bulb and an aberrant carotid artery. The aberrant carotid artery frequently appears as a whitish mass located anteriorly, behind the tympanic membrane, mimicking a congenital cholesteatoma (Fig 34.17). A high jugular bulb appears as a bluish mass in the hypotympanum, mimicking a glomus tumour (Fig 34.18). Although either MRI or CT scan can diagnose these abnormalities, CT is the method of choice as it depicts the lesion in the bone clearly. Surgery is not contraindicated. Typical symptoms include conductive hearing loss and pulsatile tinnitus. The typical sign is a mass in the middle ear cavity. A high index of suspicion is therefore necessary when evaluating a middle ear mass, so that devastating vascular injury may be avoided.

Middle ear (congenital) cholesteatoma

Middle ear cholesteatomas are rare lesions that manifest with conductive hearing loss, most commonly in children. On examination, a white mass is seen behind the tympanic membrane (Fig 34.19). If not recognized and treated early, these lesions expand to erode the ossicles, encase the facial nerve and invade the promontory, producing a sensorineural hearing loss or perilymph fistula. CT scans of the temporal bones suggest the diagnosis. If the appearance is uncertain, MRI shows the characteristic appearance of low signal on T1 and high signal on T2-weighted scans. Treatment is with tympanoplasty, tympanomastoidectomy or canal wall down mastoidectomy as necessary to be sure the disease is eradicated or at least exteriorized. It should be remembered that these lesions are

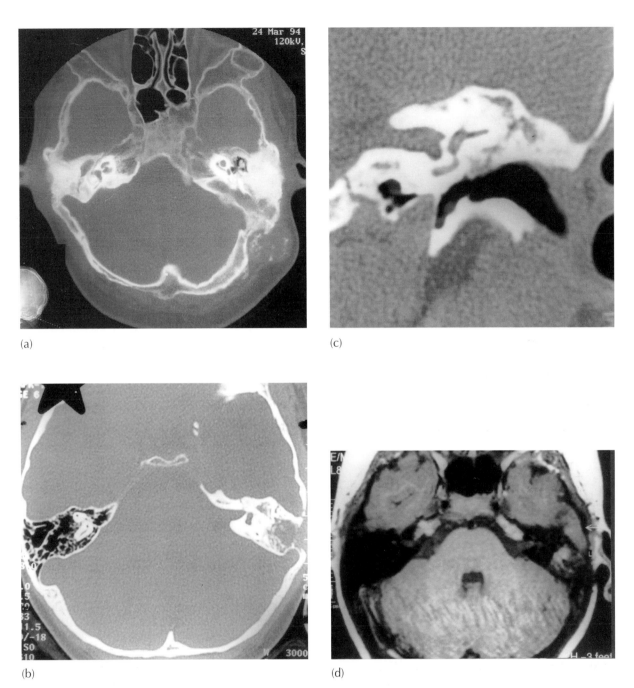

(a)

(c)

(b)

(d)

Fig 34.17 (a) Massive, polyostotic fibrous dysplasia involving the whole of the posterior skull base. There is the classic ground glass appearance affecting both temporal bones. (b) More limited disease involving the left temporal bone in a six-year-old girl. She presented with a progressive left-sided facial palsy that was complete when she was eventually seen by an ENT surgeon. An exploratory cortical mastoidectomy was performed and the surgeon came across firm but spongy 'bone' filling the aditus. This axial CT scan shows the cortical mastoid cavity and the mass of new 'bone' in the region of the geniculate ganglion. (c) In the coronal sections (compare with Fig 34.18) there is 'new bone' formation around the labyrinth, which has obliterated the facial nerve canal completely. (d) The T1 MRI shows only the soft tissue changes in the mastoid cavity and is completely unhelpful as far as the diagnosis of fibrous dysplasia is concerned. (Scans courtesy of Professor AW Wright.)

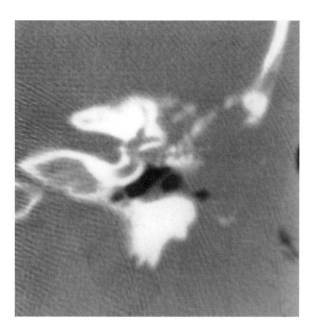

Fig 34.18 Histiocytosis-X of the temporal bone in the form of Hand–Shüller–Christian disease. The coronal CT scan, which is a cut at the level of the vestibule, shows the classic, 'punched out' lesion with extensive bone erosion, which has been replaced with a soft tissue mass. Compare with Fig 34.17 as both patients had a facial palsy. (Scans courtesy of Professor AW Wright.)

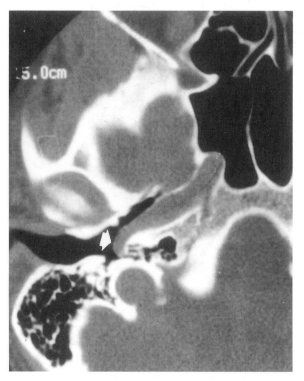

Fig 34.19 Aberrant, dehiscent right internal carotid artery seen on this axial CT scan (arrow).

impressively more aggressive than acquired cholesteatoma if they become infected. Diagnosis is confirmed by operative appearance and histological confirmation of a layer of squamous epithelium encasing a keratin matrix.

Benign tumours

Middle ear adenoma

Second to glomus tumours, adenomas are the most common primary tumours of the middle ear. These lesions usually appear with conductive hearing loss secondary to the growth against the ossicular chain. On examination, a mass is seen behind the tympanic membrane; colour may vary but the mass usually appears pink. Diagnosis is confirmed by preoperative CT scan to assess the extent of the disease (Fig 34.20); if intracranial invasion, a very rare occurrence, is present, MRI should also be performed. Treatment of these tumours is the same as for the corresponding approach to glomus tumours described above, that is, approaches are usually transcanal or transmastoid. Preoperative embolization is unnecessary.

Facial nerve schwannoma

Another benign, unusual tumour of the middle ear is the facial nerve schwannoma. These lesions can occur anywhere along the course of the facial nerve and can even mimic acoustic neuroma; the most common site, however, is in the region of the geniculate ganglion (Fig 34.21). The most common presentation for these tumours is a slowly progressive facial nerve paralysis. Hemifacial spasm and sudden-onset facial paralysis have, however, been reported. Sensorineural hearing loss and tinnitus are later symptoms. Diagnosis is established by CT scan, in which a large, expansile lesion is commonly seen replacing the geniculate ganglion. On occasion, MRI is necessary to evaluate intracranial extension. The recommended treatment for these lesions is complete excision of the tumour, together with the involved segment of the facial nerve. Primary grafting is performed if possible; if not, cable grafting is the procedure of choice. For a patient with a small facial neuroma with partial or complete function of the nerve, surgery is delayed until they are more symptomatic or the tumour grows, as resection virtually always causes initial complete unilateral facial paralysis.

Meningioma

In very rare instances, meningioma may be encountered in the middle ear, most often it is the result

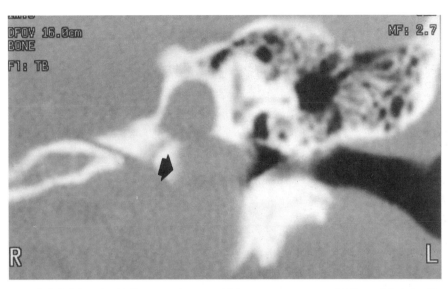

Fig 34.20 High left jugular bulb appearing as middle ear mass; coronal CT provided the diagnosis (arrow).

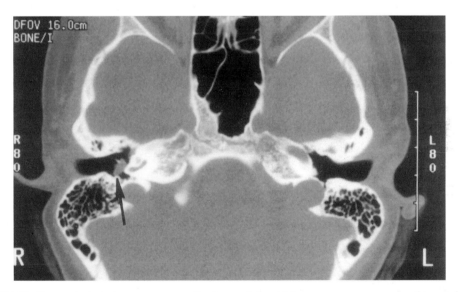

Fig 34.21 Congenital cholesteatoma manifesting as left middle ear mass, as seen on this axial CT scan (arrow).

of extension from a lesion located on the petrous ridge or in the cerebellopontine angle. In even rarer instances, these tumours may be malignant. These tumours frequently manifest with conductive hearing loss; in unusual circumstances, they can cause sensorineural hearing loss, tinnitus, vertigo or facial paralysis. The most appropriate diagnostic studies for these tumours are CT and MRI. On CT a mass is documented that continues into the bone of the middle ear and mastoid (Fig 34.22). On MRI, a uniform high signal mass is seen on T1-weighted imaging, which may posses a 'dural tail'. Treatment is complete excision; as these tumours frequently invade the bone, more aggressive excision is required than for the other benign tumours described above.

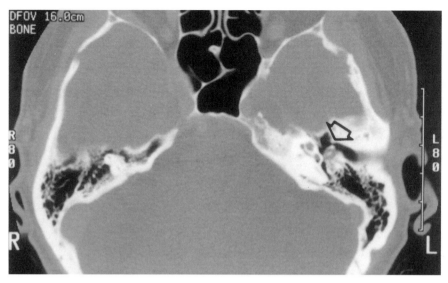

Fig 34.22 Left middle ear adenoma depicted by arrow on this axial CT scan.

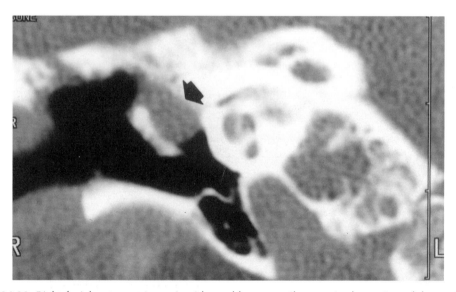

Fig 34.23 Right facial neuroma (arrow) evidenced by expansile mass in the region of the geniculate ganglion on coronal CT scan.

Malignant tumours

Rhabdomyosarcoma

Rhabdomyosarcoma is regarded as the most common temporal bone malignancy of childhood. Considerable controversy exists over its management. Overall, it is seen in the head and neck in 38 per cent of patients and in the temporal bone in 7 per cent.[25,28,29] Twenty per cent of patients have met-astasis at the time of diagnosis. This tumour appears with chronic otorrhoea and a friable polyp or infected granulation tissue, or both. Facial paralysis or extension into the infratemporal fossa is a particularly ominous sign. CT and MRI should be obtained. Surgery is only performed if it can be assured that the entire tumour may be removed *en bloc*; otherwise, biopsy is performed, followed by radiotherapy and chemotherapy as definitive treatment. The 4-year survival is 37.5 per cent.[30]

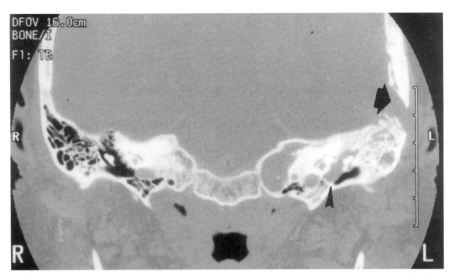

Fig 34.24 Small arrow depicts meningioma filling left middle ear, mastoid and petrous apex. Large arrow is site of prior craniotomy, as seen on coronal CT scan.

Squamous cell carcinoma

Primary temporal bone carcinoma is a particularly rare lesion, with a prevalence of less than 5 per cent of all temporal bone carcinoma. Much more commonly, it occurs via direct extension from the auricle or external auditory canal (see Chapter 22). In general, these tumours are best treated by combined therapy, namely surgery and irradiation. Either *en bloc* external auditory canal or temporal bone resections or 'drillouts' are performed, depending on the individual surgeon. We advocate lateral or subtotal temporal bone resection, followed by postoperative irradiation whenever possible; if not possible, complete 'drillout' followed by postoperative irradiation should be performed.

Adenocarcinoma

Adenocarcinoma of the middle ear or temporal bone, or both, is extremely rare, and is thought to arise from the respiratory epithelium of the Eustachian tube. Treatment is as for primary squamous cell carcinoma.

Metastasis

Metastases are also extremely rare. If the patient is otherwise disease-free and the lesion is self-contained, temporal bone resection may be performed. If there is primary disease in the patient or if other metastases are present, non-invasive techniques such as chemotherapy or radiotherapy may be considered.

Summary

Lesions of the middle ear and temporal bone are rare. Although they are usually histologically benign, their location, pattern of growth and frequently vascular nature makes their resection quite complex. By following the management plan described in this chapter, primary tumours of the middle ear and temporal bone may be approached logically. Negative, but sometimes unavoidable, outcomes include a haemorrhage and possible paralysis of cranial nerves V–XII. The surgical team should consist of a head and neck surgeon, a neurotologist, a neurosurgeon and a reconstructive surgeon to afford the lowest possible morbidity.

Acknowledgements

We wish to thank Mr George Card for his outstanding artwork. His drawings provide accurate descriptions for the surgical techniques which we attempt to convey verbally. Additional figures were provided by Pamela S. Bohrer, MD.

References

1. Graham MD, Sataloff RT, Kemink JL, Wolf GT, McGillicuddy JE. Total *en bloc* resection of the temporal bone and carotid artery for malignant tumours of the ear and temporal bone. *Laryngoscope* 1984; **94**:528–33.

2. Jackson CG, Glasscock ME III, Nissen AJ, Schwaber MK. Glomus tumour surgery; the approach results and problems. *Otolarygnological Clinics of North America* 1982; **15**:897–916.

3. Oldering D, Fisch U. Glomus tumours of the temporal region: surgical therapy. *American Journal of Otology* 1979; **1**:7–18.

4. Pensak ML. Skull base surgery. In: Glasscock ME III, Shambaugh GE Jr eds. *Surgery of the ear, 4th ed.* Philadelphia: WB Saunders, 1990:503–23.

5. Roland PS, Glasscock ME III. Surgery of the cranial base. In: Paparella MM, Shumrick DA, Gluckman JL, Meyerhoff WL eds. *Otolaryngology, 3rd ed.* Philadelphia: WB Saunders, 1991:1789–1807.

6. Pearse A. The cytochemistry and ultrastructure of polypeptide hormone-producing cells of the APUD series and the embryonic, physiologic, and pathologic implications of the concept. *Journal of Histochemistry and Cytochemistry* 1969; **17**:303–13.

7. Guild SR. A hitherto unrecognized structure, the glomus jugularis, in man. *Anatomical Record* 1941; **79(suppl 2)**:28–37.

8. Rosenwasser H. Carotid body tumour of the middle ear and mastoid. *Archives of Otolaryngology* 1945; **41**:64–7.

9. Guild SR. The glomus jugulare, a nonchromaffin paraganglion, in man. *Annals of Otology, Rhinology and Laryngology* 1953; **62**:1045–71.

10. Winship T, Klopp CT, Jenkins WH. Glomus jugularis tumours. *Cancer* 1948; **1**:441–8.

11. Gaffney JC. Carotid body-like tumours of the jugular bulb and middle ear. *Journal of Pathology and Bacteriology* 1953; **66**:157–70.

12. Fettergren L, Lindstrom J. Glomus tympanicum. *Acta Pathologica et Microbiologica Scandinavica* 1951; **28**:157–71.

13. Jackson CG. Section III. Diagnosis for treatment planning and treatment options. In: Glasscock ME III, Jackson CG eds. Neurotologic skull base surgery for glomus tumours. *Laryngscope* 1993; **103(suppl 60)**:17–22.

14. Jackson CG, Poe DS, Johnson GD. Lateral transtemporal approaches to the skull base. In: Jackson CG ed. *Surgery of skull base tumours.* New York: Churchill–Livingstone, 1991.

15. Pensak ML, Jackson CG, Glasscock ME III, Gulya AJ. Perioperative evaluation and care of patients with lesions involving the skull base. *Otolaryngology – Head and Neck Surgery* 1986; **94**:497–503.

16. Brown LA. Glomus jugulare tumour of the middle ear: clinical espects. *Laryngoscope* 1953; **63**:281–92.

17. Carrasco V, Rosenman J. Section IV. Radiation therapy of glomus jugulare tumours. In: Glasscock ME III, Jackson CG eds. Neurotologic surgery for skull base tumours. *Laryngoscope* 1993; **103(suppl 60)**:23–7.

18. Kim JA, Elkon D, Lim ML, Constable WC. Optimum dose of radiotherapy for cholesteatomas of the middle ear. *International Journal of Radiation, Oncology, Biology and Physics* 1980; **6**:815–9.

19. Spector GJ, Maisel RH, Ogura JH. Glomus jugulare tumours II. A clinicopathologic analysis of the effect of radiotherapy. *Annals of Otology, Rhinology and Laryngology* 1974; **83**:26–32.

20. Gardner G, Cocke EW, Robertson JT, Trumball ML, Palmer RE. Combined approach surgery for removal of glomus jugulare tumours. *Laryngoscope* 1977; **87**:665–8.

21. Jackson CG. Section V. Basic surgical principles of neurotologic skull base surgery. In: Glasscock ME III, Jackson CG eds. Neurotologic skull base surgery for glomus tumours. *Laryngoscope* 1993; **103(suppl 60)**:29–44.

22. Nager GT, Kennedy DW, Kopstein E. Fibrous dysplasia: a review of the disease and its manifestations in the temporal bone. *Annals of Otology, Rhinology and Laryngology* 1982; **101(suppl 92)**:1–52.

23. Stephenson RB, London MD, Hankin FM, Kaufer H. Fibrous dysplasia: an analysis of options for treatment. *Journal of Bone and Joint Surgery* 1987; **69(A)**:400–9.

24. Smouha EE, Edelstein DR, Parisier SC. Fibrous dysplasia involving the temporal bone: report of three new cases. *Amerian Journal of Otology* 1987; **8**:103–7.

25. Batsakis JG. *Tumours of the head and neck, 2nd ed.* Baltimore: Williams and Wilkins, 1979.

26. Esumi N, Hashida T, Matsumura T, *et al.* Malignant histiocytosis in childhood: clinical features and therapeutic results by combination chemotherapy. *American Journal of Pediatric Hematology and Oncology* 1986; **8**:300–7.

27. Lahey ME. Histiocytosis X: comparison of three treatment regimens. *Journal of Pediatric Surgery* 1975; **87**:179–211.

28. Feldman BA. Rhabdomyosarcomas of the head and neck. *Laryngoscope* 1982; **92**:424–40.

29. Maurer HM. The Intergroup Rhabdomyosarcoma Study: update November 1978. *National Cancer Institute Monographs* 1981; **56**:61–8.

30. Raney RB, Lawrence WJ, Maurer HM, Lindberg RD, Newton WA, Abdelsalam HR. Rhabdomyosarcoma of the ear in childhood: a report from the Intergroup Rhabdomyosarcoma Study – I. *Cancer* 1983; **51**:2356–61.

PART VI

Acquired inner ear disease

CHAPTER 35

Traumatic sensorineural hearing loss

PETER ALBERTI

ACOUSTIC TRAUMA

Introduction

Sound is a powerful means of distant communication. It is used to draw attention, to give warning and to communicate; a lullaby is soothing, a siren alerting and an explosion frightening. Each sound evokes a different physiological response. Thus there may be changes in heart rate, blood pressure and skin resistance in response to sound. These are normal physiological changes. However, excessive sound can be harmful.

It has long been known that extreme noise damages ears. The deafness of artillerymen was well known in the Napoleonic Wars and hearing loss was noted among industrial workers in the 1800s. Barr of Glasgow produced an excellent epidemiological study of 'Boiler Makers' Deafness' amongst shipyard workers in the 1880s and described rubber earplugs to protect hearing. Haberman described the histology of the cochlea in a deaf railway worker and putatively attributed it to noise. Thus the causes, pathology and epidemiology of noise-induced hearing loss (NIHL) were already known and techniques of hearing conservation were being applied by the beginning of the twentieth century.

Although sound may not be loud enough to damage hearing, it can still be intense enough to produce a hostile work environment. Warning signals may not be heard in high sound levels; even if they are heard they may not be localized and they may be confused. Think only of an intensive care unit or an operating room; the number of different acoustic signals that are used as warnings is great, perhaps eight on an anaesthetic machine and up to 30 in an intensive care unit. If there is much background noise, they may not be heard or they may not be immediately identified. Similarly, on a factory floor it may be difficult to distinguish between a reversing truck, a malfunctioning machine and a variety of other noises.

Noise-induced hearing loss

EFFECT OF SOUND ON THE EAR

Normal

Outer and middle ear

The external ear canal and middle ear act as an impedance matching mechanism for sound so that vibration in air is transmitted to the fluid of the cochlea with minimal reflective loss. The external canal is a resonating tube that enhances sound up to 20 dB at the tympanic membrane, particularly around 3 kHz. Thus broad band noise is differentially amplified by the external canal around this frequency. It has been known for many years that the cochlea is most damaged by sound about half an octave above the centre frequency of the intense sound. This mechanism may explain why the ear is most susceptible to damage around 4 kHz.

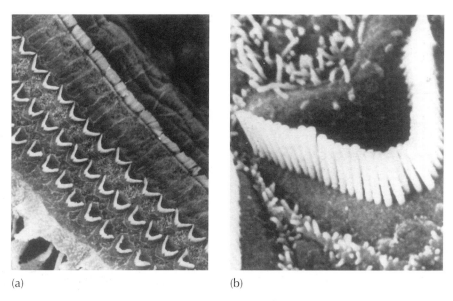

(a)   (b)

Fig 35.1 (a) Surface of the normal organ of Corti, guinea pig, ×1100 magnification. (b) Close-up view of the stereocilia of OHC, ×11 000 magnification. (From Gao *et al.*, with permission.)

Inner ear

When the footplate of the stapes vibrates, a travelling wave passes along the cochlea. The point of maximum excursion of the wave varies according to the frequency of the sound; high frequency vibration stimulates the basal end of the cochlea and low frequency the apex. This motion establishes a shear between the outer hair cells (OHCs) and Reissner's membrane because the tips of the cilia of the OHCs are attached to the membrane. Deforming the cilia opens or closes ionic channels in the hair cell wall, stimulating the cell to contract and amplify the movement of the basilar membrane. This enhances the stimulus provided to the inner hair cells (IHCs) which have over 90 per cent of the afferent innervation. The OHCs have very little afferent innervation but a plentiful efferent nerve supply and presumably this forms part of a feedback loop that modulates their activity and thus serves to tune and change the response of the IHCs to sound.

Abnormal

Cochlea

Exposure to excessive sound dulls hearing and may damage the ear. What does intense sound do to the cochlea? If moderate it produces a temporary threshold shift (TTS), which, if the ear is allowed to rest, recovers. Anyone who has visited a disco or been close to loud machinery has experienced this phenomenon. The mechanism is metabolic exhaustion and recovery. If the sound is sufficiently intense, it produces a much more severe TTS, which may go on to become a permanent threshold shift (PTS). There is a critical point at which moderate TTS changes to longer term PTS, which correlates well with anatomical damage to the OHCs, a process of damage and scarring or repair. The threshold for TTS is somewhere between 78 and 85 dB and the point at which it changes from mid-term to long-term is about 140 dB. The spectrum of the sound and the length of exposure are critical.

Cilia of the OHCs are attached to each other near their tips by linking filaments and each cilium has a little rootlet that passes through the ciliary plate (Fig 35.1). If the mechanical disturbance produced by sound is sufficient to fracture the rootlet or to disturb the linkages (these often happen together), the anatomical correlate of sound exposure is to produce a floppy cilium. These only partially recover and frequently the cilia are destroyed by phalangeal scarring. By contrast moderate sound excursion produces much less distortion of the cilia and they recover (Fig 35.2). Noise characteristically damages the OHCs of the basilar turn. If sound is intense enough, there is physical disruption of the cochlea and other structures such as the stria vascularis and the supporting cells may also be damaged. Some time after hair cell death there is also neural degeneration of the first order neurons. Very intense sound has been shown to produce damage to the vestibular epithelium of guinea pigs but this has not been convincingly demonstrated in humans.

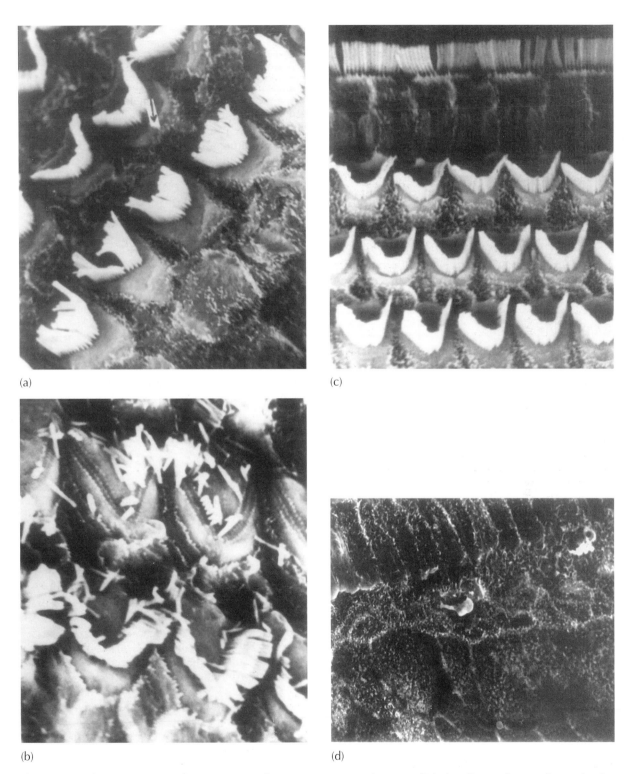

Fig 35.2 (a) Changes in stereocilia 30 minutes after exposure at 110 dB. Note slight bending and separation at the tips of the stereocilia. The ear had a 20–25 dB TTS. (b) Changes in the stereocilia after 30 minutes exposure at 120 dB. Note complete collapse at the bases of stereocilia. The ear showed a 45–50 dB TTS (×1700 magnification). (c) Changes in the stereocilia of the 110 dB group 80 days after exposure. The hearing was normal and so is the appearance of the stereocilia. (d) Changes in the apical surface of the organ of Corti of the 120 dB group 80 days after exposure. The surface is devoid of stereocilia and hair cells. (From Gao *et al.*, with permission.)

It has recently been shown that avian hair cells destroyed by noise regenerate, whereas those of mammals do not. What makes the avian cells recover is currently the subject of intense research (see Chapter 1).

Tuning curves

Each auditory nerve fibre is most responsive to a specific frequency but as the intensity of sound increases it becomes progressively sensitive to adjacent frequencies. With OHC loss the most sensitive finely tuned part of the response is lost. It is generally assumed that the sharp tuning of these curves at low intensity is the result of active mechanisms in the OHCs and associated efferent nerve pathways. Their loss may be correlated with the clinical finding of poor sound discrimination, a common complaint in NIHL.

Toughening

There is some evidence in animals that prior exposure to non-damaging levels of low frequency noise protects the cochlea from damage by subsequent high intensity sound. This may also be so in humans.

IMPACT ON HUMAN HEARING

Overview

What is the impact of sound on the human ear? Exposure up to 78 dBA is totally safe. Above this level TTS occurs, the amount depending upon the frequency of the sound and individual susceptibility. An asymptote is never quite reached under normal working conditions. TTS recovers after a period out of noise, with the speed of recovery depending upon the amount of the TTS: the greater the exposure, the longer the recovery time. This has importance in terms of administrative controls related to length of work shifts. If sound levels are high enough they produce long-term TTS and recovery takes much longer. For example people exposed to an explosion may partially lose their hearing and recovery may continue for several days or even weeks. Recovery in these circumstances is rarely complete. The threshold for long-term TTS marks the upper limit of safe working conditions. Zajtchuk *et al.* give an excellent review of blast injuries to hearing. Safe in this context means that only 15 per cent of individuals exposed to 90 dBA for 8 hours will develop a hearing loss. Reducing the work exposure to 85 dBA for 8 hours results in 3 per cent developing some loss.

Hazardous sounds

Occupational hearing loss

Occupational hearing loss is the dominant cause of preventable sensorineural hearing loss in adults. Noise is the most ubiquitous industrial pollutant. It is particularly a problem in heavy engineering, metal working, the construction industry, transportation and the resource industries such as mining and forestry. In the USA alone there are 31 million workers at risk from excessive workplace noise; in Europe at least 15 million industrial workers are at risk.

Any noise, all noise

All noise exposure is important. The ear does not distinguish between social, military or industrial noise; they are additive. The public should be cautioned about all. Thus the employee exposed to the equivalent of 90 dBA for 8 hours at work who then rides a motorcycle and uses power tools at home may well exceed the hazardous level even though work is deemed 'safe'. The critical value is the total sound exposure above 80 dBA in a 24-hour period, irrespective of the source, although this is not often recognized.

Military

Military noise is an order of magnitude louder than that found in industry. Soldiers are deafened on the way to the battlefield inside diesel-powered metal-armoured troop carriers and helicopters. A wide range of weapons inflict damage on their operators as well as on the targeted enemy. Even shooting on the range may produce hearing loss; up to 3 per cent of recruits will receive a permanent measurable hearing loss from their first exposure to rifle practice, whereas others with 'tough' ears can shoot with impunity virtually all their life. The US military pay over $300 million annually in hearing loss pensions and as a result has developed effective hearing conservation programmes.

Social

Social noise exposure is pervasive and increasing, particularly in the tropics where people tend to spend more time outdoors than in temperate climates. The two-stroke gasoline engine is a particular culprit, whether used in motorcycles as in Southeast Asia or to power gardening equipment such as edgers, leaf blowers and lawn mowers. Transportation noise is ubiquitous as diesel engines are used to power most buses throughout the world.

Music

Musicians are at risk from occupational noise exposure, although the amount of hearing loss is less than would be predicted from sound measurements. It is unlikely that personal cassette players are a major cause of trouble; repeated studies show only very small effects. Boom boxes and some rock concerts may be harmful. It is prudent, however, to warn those who develop tinnitus when listening to amplified music that their ears are at risk; they should either use hearing protection or turn down the volume. Instrumentalists should be provided with flat response ear plugs (see below).

Fireworks

There are well documented cases of permanent hearing loss from deliberate or inadvertent exposure to firecrackers, including good epidemiological studies of hearing loss from their use, for example, in the Norwegian national day and celebration of the Hindu festival of Dewali.

Equal energy hypothesis

The total amount of acoustic energy to which the ear is exposed is important because damage appears to be dose dependent: the 'equal energy' concept. This states that between the threshold of damage – about 80 dB – and an upper limit above which physical disruption takes place, similar total amounts of sound energy produce similar damage, no matter whether the sound is of high intensity for a short period or a low intensity for a longer period, that is, double the sound level, halve the safe time and vice versa. Remember that the decibel scale is logarithmic; the addition or subtraction of two identical decibel sums always changes the intensity by 3 dB. Thus if one knows the safe level of sound exposure for an 8-hour work day, one can compute the safe exposure time for differing intensities of sound. Therefore, if 85 dB is assumed to be safe for 8 hours then 88 dB is safe for 4 hours and 91 dB safe for 2 hours et cetera. If the intensity of a sound and the length of exposure is known, one can compute the equivalent intensity for 8 hours – the Leq_8.

The equal energy concept is valid if the individual is exposed to the sound continuously; if sound exposure is intermittent, as is the case with much industrial noise, this may be too severe a rule. As a result in North America a 5 dB trading relationship was adopted – $Losha_8$. The international standard ISO 1999 was established based on the equal energy concept. It also provided correction for ageing and other ear disease. As North Americans saw the sense of this and started changing their regulations,

the European advocates of the 3 dB rule recognized the protective effect of intermittent noise exposure and are now moving in the opposite direction (Robinson 1987). There appears to be no single correct figure – it depends upon the nature of the sound exposure. Leq_8 is a conservative approach as it protects more people; the truth in most industrial sound exposure probably lies near 4 dB halving and doubling. There is also controversy about the lower limit; some jurisdictions have adopted 85 dB, others 87 dB and most still stick with 90 dB. The upper limit above which no ear should be exposed appears to be about 115 dB Leq_8.

So far the discussion has dealt with steady-state noise; impact noise is a different matter. Impulse noise is difficult to measure and there are many types; think only of the difference between a nail being hammered and a rifle shot. Important features include the rise and decay times and the absolute peak level. It is suggested that when impulse noise is measured by standard sound pressure meters, it is rather more hazardous by about 5 dB than steady-state noise of the same intensity. Rules tend to limit the absolute number of impulses in a 24-hour period. Further discussion is outside the scope of this chapter.

Individual susceptibility

There is a huge individual variation in susceptibility to NIHL, also evident in well controlled animal experiments.

Biological factors

Many attempts have been made to determine why some ears are more sensitive to sound than others. It is now believed that women have slightly 'tougher' ears than men and that melanization is protective, fair-haired blue-eyed people being more sensitive to the harmful effect of intense sound than brown-haired, brown-eyed people and Caucasians being more sensitive than those of African descent. The effect is small, only a few decibels in a lifetime's exposure.

Predicting susceptibility

How to determine susceptibility to noise exposure before the event is elusive. Attempts to correlate TTS after 1 day's exposure to long-term loss have repeatedly failed. TTS at the end of a work shift does mark the upper limit of the PTS produced by the same sound exposure after 10 years. However, the PTS may be much less. A promising (and fashionable) test is based on changes in oto-acoustic emissions; some investigators have suggested that there is a reduction in these emissions before a change is evident in the pure tone threshold, giving an early warning of incipient damage.

Hearing loss

What sort of hearing loss is produced by noise? Classically it produces a notch based at 3, 4 or 6 kHz, most commonly at 4 kHz (Fig 35.3). With industrial noise exposure this begins in the first year or two but the loss continues to grow for about 10 years at these frequencies. Beyond 10 years the hearing loss may spread into lower frequencies and the high frequency recovery disappears; the loss at the initial frequencies may also continue to grow, but at a lesser rate. Thus after many years in noise there is no characteristic notch and the lower frequencies at 2 and 1 kHz are gradually involved. Later in life it is difficult to disentangle presbyacusis from NIHL (Fig 35.4).

Impact noise also produces a notched loss, but its shape may be more variable. A single impulse, as from a gunshot or a firecracker, may be enough to produce a permanent audiometric notch in a sensitive ear, although, usually, damaging exposure is repetitive.

COMPLEX INTERACTION: SYNERGISM

Noise exposure cannot be viewed in isolation. Workers may be exposed to a mixture of steady-state and impulse noise; they may be involved in heavy exercise, they may be exposed to vibration, to extremes of temperature and humidity and to a variety of atmospheric pollutants such as volatile chemicals. Above all, they age. How do these various factors interact?

Physical

Impulse and steady-state noise

Many workers function against a background of high level relatively steady-state noise, which is then interjected by higher level impulse sound. It appears that the two act synergistically and that the resultant hearing loss is greater than if the two were simply additive.

Vibration and exercise

Neither whole body vibration nor extensive exercise during noise exposure put ears at greater risk. Only those who suffer from vibration-induced white hand, such as forestry workers using chain saws, develop worse hearing loss than non-affected fellow workers.

Pressure

Divers may be exposed to extremely high sound levels under water and the ear may also be unduly susceptible to the effects of excessive sound while operating at high pressure.

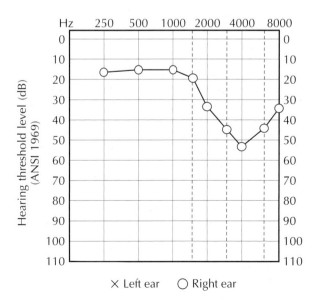

Fig 35.3 Typical audiogram in NIHL. Generating station mechanic, 20 years exposure.

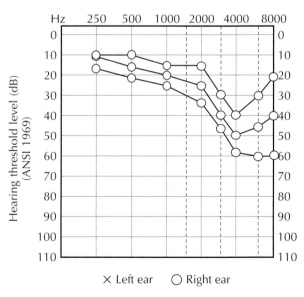

Fig 35.4 Composite audiogram illustrating progression of NIHL and addition of presbyacusis.

Chemical

There has been considerable recent interest in the effect of chemical solvents on hearing. They are widely used in industry; examples include toluene in the printing and tanning industry; carbon disulphide in the manufacture of rayon and the manufacture and use of paint and styrene used to make plastics. Of these, toluene is probably the most widely used. It has been shown in animal experiments and in human epidemiological studies that exposure to these chemicals produces hearing loss not found in control subjects and that the hearing loss is worse when there is also exposure to noise. The effect may be synergistic. Toluene is cochleotoxic, others may also be neurotoxic; the mechanisms are not yet clear.

Presbyacusis

NIHL is often assessed in workers only in their fifties or sixties, by which time presbyacusis also occurs. What is the exact relationship between the two? Are they additive, synergistic or protective? After all, the same OHCs are affected by both. Noise damage is important early in a worker's life; presbyacusis is dominant in later years. Current opinion suggests that at most the two are additive, but in more severe NIHL the affect of presbyacusis is less (Fig 35.4).

CLINICAL EVALUATION

History

NIHL is a clinical diagnosis based upon history, physical examination and audiometric evaluation. The history is important because it will reveal other potential causes of hearing loss in addition to noise exposure. It is important that childhood ear disease, ototoxic drug exposure, vertigo, familial hearing loss, noise exposure that is not work-related, sudden hearing loss and head injury all be looked for. It is surprising how few people actually know their family history. When I was evaluating all claimants for NIHL in the province of Ontario, I found that about 6 per cent had a reason other than noise exposure as their major cause of hearing loss, for example otosclerosis or a sudden hearing loss. A careful history of the noise exposure is also important. Workers will know their loudest employment and they will also remember mechanical failure, which may be blamed for their hearing loss and which is frequently not identified by the employer. They will also usually know whether there has been an asymmetrical noise exposure. In

my experience it is extremely rare to obtain a reasonable quantification of noise exposure. It is not enough to know the sound level at the work place, it is also necessary to know the sound dosage that was received by the worker; how much overtime was worked and whether it included back-to-back shifts. The amount of detail required depends upon the specifics of local compensation practices.

Tinnitus

Tinnitus is a common companion of hearing loss that occurs in about 60 per cent of claimants for compensation for NIHL and is more common in those exposed to impact than steady-state noise. The management is that of any other form of tinnitus.

Examination

It is important to observe the demeanour of the patient. In examinations for pension purposes there is often some exaggeration of hearing loss (EHL) during the audiometry. The frank malingerer can often be spotted in the clinical examination by their exaggerated listening, but they can still hear when the examiner's mouth is covered or when the topic turns to local events rather than the history. Physical examination will identify a conductive hearing loss. As with any hearing loss, the details of examination and investigations are determined by the history and are usually those of any sensorineural hearing loss.

AUDIOLOGY: FORENSIC

The audiometric evaluation for pension purposes is known as 'forensic audiometry' and is not a trivial matter. The test should be conducted in appropriately sound-proofed facilities, using properly calibrated equipment; the patient should have been free from noise for at least 24 and preferably 48 hours unless the assessment is being made after exposure to an explosion or blast from which there may be recovery over a period of several weeks. The minimum test battery is a full pure tone audiogram (PTA) by air and bone conduction, speech reception threshold (SRT) measurement and thereafter whatever clinical tests may be indicated by the findings. If there is an unexplained asymmetrical sensorineural hearing loss, I investigate as I would in non-forensic otology. The occasional acoustic neuroma is discovered this way. There are some warning signs of EHL such as a PTA/SRT discrepancy of 10 dB or more, or a pure tone threshold at 500 Hz of >35 dB, which is caused by either some other condition or inaccurate testing; it is unlikely that noise will cause so much low frequency loss. I place considerable faith in late auditory evoked responses to help quantify the hearing in EHL, unlike the brainstem auditory evoked potentials, they provide frequency-specific thresholds.

AUDIOMETRIC SHAPE

There is considerable audiometric variation in NIHL claimants. The international standard ISO 1999 gives the risk of hearing loss from sound exposure from 85 to 100 dB Leq_8 for the 5th to the 95th percentile, for 1–40 years. The individual variation is large and it does not effectively deal with levels of above Leq_8 100 dBA, which are found in the construction and resource industries. Most industrial noise is broad band and thus fits the pattern of these tables. There may be exceptions: in certain industries noise is predominantly low frequency and the audiometric configuration may show a hearing loss in the lower frequencies; it is suggested that high impact noise levels, as may be found in for example drop forgers, produce a more precipitous hearing loss. Dealing with a population composed mainly of heavy industrial workers and hard rock miners, I am consistently impressed by the number of exceptions

to the standards that I see (Fig 35.5). An audiogram is deemed accurate but atypical and no other cause of hearing loss can be determined. The three main issues are the slope of the audiogram, that is, how flat an audiogram can be before it is no longer attributed to noise exposure; the significance of an asymmetrical hearing loss and, finally, the position or absence of a notch. In general terms, however, a predominantly low frequency hearing loss is not caused by noise exposure and nor is a saucer-shaped loss with its maximum loss at 750, 1000 or 1500 Hz (Fig 35.6).

Asymmetrical hearing loss

It is generally assumed that both ears are equally susceptible to noise exposure. This is a good approximation. However, it cannot be assumed that noise exposure of both ears is identical; for example, concert violinists almost always have an asymmetrical notched hearing loss in the ear closest to the body of the instrument. Similarly it has long been known that the ear nearer the muzzle of a rifle sustains more hearing loss than the other ear protected by the head shadow. There are many similar industrial examples: construction workers using electric drills to pierce concrete may have a 10 dB difference in sound intensity between the two ears;

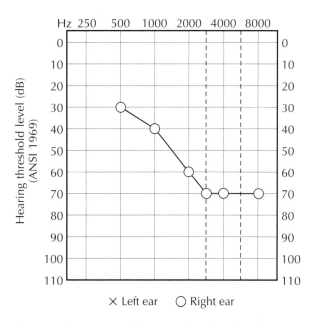

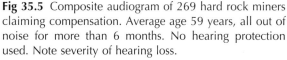

Fig 35.5 Composite audiogram of 269 hard rock miners claiming compensation. Average age 59 years, all out of noise for more than 6 months. No hearing protection used. Note severity of hearing loss.

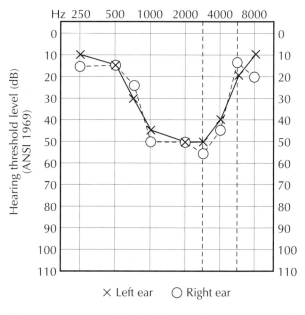

Fig 35.6 Progressive familial hearing loss. Woman aged 51 years, NIHL claim that she believes is due to carpet weaving 20 years earlier. Hearing continues to worsen.

tractor drivers frequently sit with their heads turned protecting one ear and exposing the other to the exhaust pipe; in some industrial processes metal parts fall into a bin beside one ear of an operator with the other ear protected. Until dosimeter studies are undertaken with a microphone at each ear the scale of asymmetrical exposure and hearing loss will not be known.

Progression of hearing loss after cessation of noise exposure

Compensation claims are frequently made only years after noise exposure has ceased and the documented hearing loss may have worsened in the intervening period. Is the further loss due to the prior noise exposure? Conventional wisdom states quite emphatically that it is not; indeed, if anything, hearing may recover a few decibels when noise exposure ceases. Further loss is almost always to do with presbyacusis or other problems.

Multiple pathology

It is certainly possible for more than one cause of hearing loss to affect a cochlea. Presbyacusis and noise have already been mentioned. Someone with a congenital hearing loss may also develop an addi-

tional loss from noise; this may produce an audiogram that at first shows a saucer-shaped loss with recovery to 2000 Hz and a high frequency notch characteristic of noise (Fig 35.7), but that with time loses the recovery at 2000 Hz, leading to a W-shaped loss and finally one that is severe from about 750 Hz upwards (Fig 35.8).

Conductive hearing loss

It is intuitive to think that a conductive hearing loss will protect the ear from further damage by noise, rather like having a built-in earplug. Although this is the conventional wisdom, it is not substantiated by fact. Several studies have shown that neither otosclerosis nor chronic suppurative otitis media protect the ear in any significant way and only one has demonstrated the opposite. There is room for further study.

REHABILITATION

Psychosocial problems

Recently there has been considerable interest in the psychosocial problems of the hearing impaired. It has become evident that even slightly hearing

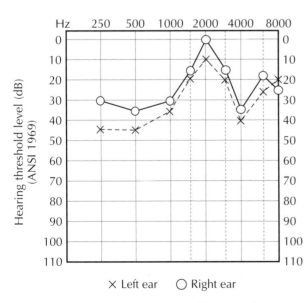

Fig 35.7 Audiogram of a 47-year-old man who was a sheet metal worker for 20 years, with a strong family history of hearing loss. Low frequency loss attributed to familial loss, high frequency notch to noise.

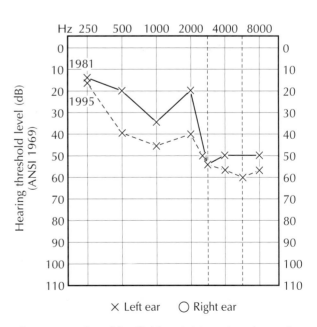

Fig 35.8 Combined familial loss, NIHL and presbyacusis. Spring maker. Composite audiogram: the first was at the age of 44 years, combined familial saucer-shaped loss and noise notch; the second at age 59 years, spread of noise to 2000 Hz, worsening of familial loss and presbyacusis.

impaired workers tend to be reclusive at work because they are subjected to teasing and they may have significant problems at home. Communication with teenage children becomes difficult and father becomes an object of derision or alternatively is identified as disinterested in the family. The relationship between spouses alters, traditional male tasks such as ordering in restaurants and dealing with visitors are delegated to the woman, often causing family friction.

Hearing aids and assistive devices

Much can be done to rehabilitate the injured worker. Current hearing aids are extremely helpful for those with high frequency mild to moderate sensorineural hearing loss; there are many assistive listening devices that are also useful, such as amplifying telephone handsets and personal television amplifiers that allow the television to be used at normal volumes but yet enable the hearing-impaired listener to hear what is being said. Rehabilitation of injured workers is important but has been neglected.

Compensation

Compensation for NIHL has become big business. The underlying philosophy, method and amount of compensation vary between jurisdictions. What is being compensated? Originally workers' compensation was for loss of earnings. It is difficult to demonstrate a loss of earnings from NIHL because few people lose their jobs. Most compensation now contains an element of payment for loss of quality of life. Thus in Ontario, my home, hearing loss compensation has two parts, a lump sum payment for demonstrated loss of quality of life and a pension during the working years if loss of earnings can be demonstrated. In addition, medical aid is provided, that is, hearing aid(s) and assistive devices. Some jurisdictions compensate hearing impairment, defined as any deviation of the audiogram from normal or above a lower limit that may be set at varying levels: 25 dB four-frequency average in the USA; 50 dB three-frequency average in the UK (1, 2 and 3 kHz) and 60 dB in Japan. The pure tone audiogram is used as a surrogate measure (albeit not a good one) for hearing disability because the latter is difficult to measure. Some jurisdictions allow claims to be settled in courts of law, others only in compensation tribunals and yet others allow both. The issues are complex and readers are referred to their own national standards for further details.

Hearing conservation

Hearing conservation programmes exist to prevent hearing loss. They consist of several phases: risk identification, engineering, administrative controls, personal hearing protection and monitoring. A good hearing conservation programme is multidisciplinary, involving the employees, management, engineering, industrial hygiene, audiology (technicians and supervisors), industrial nursing and otolaryngology. The most effective programmes involve the worker from the start. If people are empowered to look after themselves they usually do a better job than if the task is mandated from above.

METHODS

Risk identification

Risk identification is critical. If no hazard is recognized, no steps are taken to deal with it.

Sound level measurement

Sound level measurements determine whether there is risk and if so how much. These are usually made as spot checks at various work stations using a sound level meter calibrated to dBA, an overall scale filtered to resemble the sensitivity of the human ear. If the length of time spent in the workplace is known, the risk can be calculated. However, sound levels often fluctuate throughout the work shift and workers also may move. If this is the case it may be necessary to monitor sound levels at a work site throughout the working day and also to measure individual exposure by fitting the worker with an integrating dosimeter.

Engineering

Although the mainstay of such programmes, engineering controls are outside the scope of this chapter.

Administrative controls

Administrative controls can be used to monitor and limit individual exposure, for example by limiting lengths of work shifts or overtime.

Hearing screening

Hearing testing like much industrial monitoring is contentious and not universally accepted. However, conventional wisdom suggests that it is a valuable monitoring tool. Pre-employment hearing tests will identify the worker with pre-existing hearing loss and perhaps even ear disease. Regular audiometry throughout the period of employment will identify changes in hearing or, better yet, no change. Batch analysis will demonstrate whether the program itself is effective and individual results will show whether each worker is protected. Specialized handbooks should be consulted for details of such programmes.

Education

No hearing conservation programme can be effective without worker commitment and understanding. Time spent educating and empowering the work force is invaluable in ensuring the proper working of such a programme. A hearing protector that is not worn is of no value, but an effective programme saves large sums of money in reduced compensation costs and better productivity.

Hearing protectors

Personal hearing protection is effective but disliked because it is uncomfortable to wear and may appear to interfere with verbal communication and listening to machinery and warning signals. If sound levels are high enough to require its use it is unlikely that oral communication will be possible and warning signals are designed to be heard above the level of the background noise. Hearing protectors do not completely eradicate all sound; they are like wearing sunglasses in bright sunlight, they make the sound more comfortable to hear. However, unlike neutral grey sunglasses, the standard hearing protectors, muffs and plugs, attenuate more at high frequencies, thus they do distort hearing and in the presence of high frequency hearing loss they exaggerate the high frequency loss.

Hearing protectors fall into three major categories: passive protectors, active protectors and communication headsets.

Passive protectors

Passive protectors are either earplugs, semi-insert devices or muffs. Plugs are commonly used; the most widely available effective type is the universal fitting preformed polyurethane foam plug. There are many other types, for example, air-filled and flanged to seal the ear canal. These require sizing to accommodate different shapes of ear canal.

Semi-insert protectors
Semi-insert protectors are plugs on a spring band and are useful if protection is worn intermittently, if high levels of protection are not required and in circumstances in which there is concern about plugs falling into the product as, for example, in the food industry. They are the least commonly used.

Ear muffs
Ear muffs consist of an outer shell lined with a sound absorbent material, a malleable seal that fits closely to the head, enclosing the ear, and a spring band usually made of plastic that holds the cups tightly on the head. In theory the most effective, they suffer from leaks caused by wearing safety glasses and by long hair.

Flat response protectors
In recent years several manufacturers have introduced plugs and muffs with filters built in, which reduce the high frequency attenuation and thus produce a flat attenuation, usually of about 10 dB. As earplugs these are worn by musicians and, in general, workers find them less isolating, the same difference that neutral grey sunglasses make over a tinted colour. Their drawback is that they cost more.

Active hearing protection

For workers in intermittent noise, active hearing protectors are useful. Usually muffs, they have amplifiers built-in that bring ambient sound to the ear up to a predetermined cut-off intensity at which point the amplifier shuts down and they become effective hearing protectors. These are particularly liked by sports hunters, by the military, by miners and by those working in the construction industry. Their drawback is a higher initial cost and higher maintenance fees because of battery costs.

Communication headsets

When communication is important, as for example in fighter pilots, crane operators or heavy equipment drivers, communication headsets that also act as earmuffs should be used. This is much more effective than carrying walkie-talkies and not wearing any protection.

Monitoring

It is important to monitor the effectiveness of these programmes. This is done by routine updating of the sound level measurements, by recording the use of personal protection, by analysing the audiometric data, by various jobs and sections of the plant, by monitoring the individual changes in audiometric records and by monitoring compensation awards. Educational programmes should be evaluated and periodically updated.

NON-ACOUSTIC TRAUMA

Head injury

Head injury may produce hearing loss. This may result from brain injury, from direct trauma to the temporal bone or from a combination of both.

BRAIN INJURY

Trauma to the brain from a closed head injury may produce a flat or sloping bilateral sensorineural hearing loss. This is difficult to diagnose, the cause is surmised from the history and must be differentiated from a feigned hearing loss. The blows are usually on the back or the side of the head; loss of consciousness is not a necessary antecedent. Hearing loss is often overlooked in the management of patients with head injury because of other more serious problems and is frequently coupled with some amnesia of the event so an accurate history is rarely obtained.

Temporal bone fracture

The reader is referred to Chapter 32.

Suggested reading

Axelsson A, Borchgrevink H, Hamernik RP, Hellstrom P-A, Henderson D, Salvi RJ. *Scientific basis of noise-induced hearing loss.* New York: Thieme, 1996.

Clark WW. Noise exposure for leisure activities: a review. *Journal of the Acoustical Society of America* 1991; **90**:175–81.

Dancer AL, Henderson D, Salvi RJ, Hamernik RP. *Noise-induced hearing loss.* St. Louis: Mosby Year Book, 1992.

Dobie RA. *Medical-legal evaluation of hearing loss.* New York: Van Nostrand Reinhold, 1993.

Gao WW, King DL, Zheng XY, Ruan FM, Liu YJ. Comparison in the changes in the stereocilia between temporary and permanent threshold shift. *Hearing Research* 1992; **62**:27–41.

Gasaway DC. *Hearing conservation: a practical guide and manual.* Englewood Cliffs, Prentice–Hall, 1985.

International Organization for Standardization (ISO). *Acoustics: determination of occupational noise exposure for hearing conservation purposes, ISO 1999.* Geneva: International Organization for Standardization, 1990.

King PF, Coles RRA, Lutman E, Robinson DW. *Assessment of hearing disability.* London: Whurr, 1992.

Morata TC, Dunn DE. Occupational hearing loss. In: *Occupational medicine: state of the art reviews, vol 10.* Philadelphia: Hanley and Belfus, 1995.

Robinson DW. *Noise exposure and hearing: a new look at the experimental data. Health and Safety Executive Research Report, 1/1987.* London: HMSO, 1987.

Royster JD, Royster LH. *Hearing conservation programs.* Chelsea, MI: Lewis, 1990.

Vallet M ed. *Noise and Man '93: noise as a public health problem.* Arcueil: INRETS, 1993.

Zajchuck JT, Phillips YY eds. Effects of blast overpressure on the ear. *Annals of Otology, Rhinology and Laryngology* 1989; **98(suppl 140)**.

CHAPTER 36

Acquired sensorineural hearing loss

NICK JONES AND HAROLD LUDMAN

Sensorineural hearing loss is auditory dysfunction caused by a disorder or lesion of the inner ear or of the auditory nervous system. Several classifications for sensorineural hearing loss have been proposed.[1-4] The threshold level at which it is regarded as being material varies from >30 dB at three contiguous frequencies,[5] and 25 dB over 0.5, 1, 2 and 4 kHz,[6] to >20 dB at any one frequency 0.5, 1, 2 and 4 kHz.[7] An air–bone gap is not regarded as significant unless there is an air–bone gap >15 dB in the test ear over the average for 0.5, 1 and 2 kHz.

Population studies of hearing show that age is by far the most important determinant of hearing impairment. Next to this a history of noise exposure is the most influential factor.

Historically, many factors have been implicated as causing hearing loss,[2] but for many of these the link has not been proved scientifically. One problem that has arisen is that the high prevalence of many systemic conditions such as hypertension, atherosclerosis and hyperlipidaemia has led to these frequently being cited as contributing factors, or even causes, when they may be incidental findings. Atherosclerosis and hearing loss, just like white hair, are more prevalent with ageing. This does not mean that one causes the other. Another problem is that when a patient with a rare condition develops a hearing loss, which may or may not be related to their other illness, it will often unquestioningly be attributed to it. The fact that published work is biased in favour of cases or studies with a positive finding may have helped many possible, but unproved, associations to enter the medical literature. The majority of reports studying the possi-

ble factors associated with hearing loss are retrospective, lack adequate controls, may represent incidental findings and not a true causal relationship or, most important of all, fail to account for the known effects of age and noise. Animal work has been sparse, often with inadequate numbers and largely based on herbivores, and is frequently of unsound methodology.

This chapter sets out to present the conditions for which there is good clinical, pathological or experimental evidence to support an association between a disease and sensorineural hearing loss and to qualify conditions for which the proof is poor.

For taxonomic and practical reasons, sensorineural hearing loss can be divided into sudden, progressive or chronic hearing loss.

Sudden sensorineural hearing loss

There is no consistent definition of sudden sensorineural hearing loss in spite of it being an important syndrome. Should the term apply to a loss from a previously normal level, or should rapid deterioration in an ear, already damaged say by Menière's disease, be included? What is sudden? Do we mean overnight, or during the course of a week or a month? How severe must a loss be to merit inclusion? A slight loss developing over a few hours may seem to a patient to be more sudden than a moderate one developing over a few months. As there is no universal agreement on the answers to these and similar questions, readers should be wary when comparing published accounts of the natural history and response to treatment. A practical working definition could be a loss of more than 35 dB in at least three adjacent frequencies over a period of 3 days or less.

There are many possible reasons for the sudden onset of sensorineural hearing loss, but in most instances a reliable diagnosis of cause is impossible, and the condition has to be labelled idiopathic. Fortunately, from whatever cause, the syndrome is usually unilateral. Possible explanations to be considered in every instance include:

- trauma and labyrinthine membrane rupture (see Chapter 32). It occurs occasionally after a neurosurgical procedure, possibly as a result of a reduction in cerebrospinal fluid pressure, which may affect the perilymph
- ototoxic drugs (see Chapter 37)
- bacterial infections – suppurative labyrinthitis (see Chapter 29), syphilis, meningitis
- viral infections – mumps, measles, rubella and varicella-zoster viruses are known possible causes; less certainly, poliovirus, adenovirus III, cytomegalovirus (CMV), coxsackie virus, Epstein–Barr viruses, rubella and herpes simplex have been blamed. A rise in antiviral titre has been shown for mumps, rubella, and influenza B
- acoustic neuroma (see Chapter 39). A small percentage (perhaps 15 per cent) of these tumours manifest with sudden hearing loss. As many as 5 per cent of the victims of sudden sensorineural hearing loss may have an VIIIth nerve tumour – a fact of great practical and medicolegal importance
- vascular lesions. Haemorrhage, arterial occlusion and vasospasm are theoretical causes
- autoimmune diseases such as Wegener's granulomatosis, systemic lupus erythematosus and polyarteritis nodosa. These are discussed elsewhere in this chapter. These may result from immunological reactions to inner ear proteins or as an VIIIth nerve neuritis (mono or poly)
- multiple sclerosis (rare, usually occurs when other areas of the brainstem are affected, but cochlear loss has been reported)
- endolymphatic hydrops
- psychogenic

This list cannot be complete, and it must be obvious that only rarely will a definite cause be established. More often an inference of cause is made from associated findings, but these could be incidental rather than causal. It is better to label the condition 'idiopathic' than to attribute a viral or vascular explanation.

INVESTIGATION

The aim of investigation is first to localize the lesion within the auditory system, and then, when possible, to identify a cause. The investigations of auditory function, to distinguish between sensory and neural lesions, have been described in Chapter 4.

MRI examination is essential to exclude an acoustic neuroma. Serological tests for syphilis must always be arranged, and the appropriate tests for immunological disorders are described later in this chapter.

Other investigations such as chest X-ray and tests for diabetes should be undertaken to establish whether the use of steroids in management will be safe (see below).

PROGNOSIS

As there is no homogeneous group of patients suffering this syndrome, it is not surprising that published accounts of rates of spontaneous recovery vary greatly. Overall, in the majority that is made up of the idiopathic group, about 60 per cent recover spontaneously, and the greater part of that recovery occurs in the first few weeks after onset. These facts alone have polluted comparisons between series and lead to the probably erroneous suggestion that treatment is effective if started early. It must be appreciated that recovery is often not complete, and the criteria for improvement used in different reports vary and need careful scrutiny. Some poor prognostic features have been identified. These include a raised erythrocyte sedimentation rate (ESR), the presence of severe vertigo and old age. Patients presenting late are, of course, self-selected as unfavourable, as they are a group from which those who have enjoyed early spontaneous recovery have been excluded.

MANAGEMENT

In the absence of a diagnosis, the medical treatment of the deafness must be 'empirical'. The main sensible options are systemic steroids and vasodilator drugs and there may be evidence to support this approach.[5,8] Any vascular lesion might theoretically benefit from the use of vasodilators. Although ischaemia of the organ of Corti is rapidly followed by irreversible death of the sensory hair cells, ischaemia of the stria vascularis may cause lowering of the endolymphatic potential, which is reversible. Steroids may help if there are inflammatory neural changes or when immunological processes are at work.

Severe sudden sensorineural deafness is a serious otological emergency, and even if the hearing loss cannot reliably be helped by the doctor, the patient must be treated. Management currently requires:

- admission of the patient to hospital
- investigation to try to establish a diagnosis, and to treat whatever is discovered
- empirical medication, unless specifically contraindicated
- psychological help and rehabilitation (see Chapter 8)

Much of this is recommended by convention rather than on the basis of evidence.

The patient should be nursed in bed, with the head raised in case of labyrinthine membrane rupture (see Chapter 38). Sedation may be needed to alleviate anxiety, and appropriate vestibular sedatives may be used for vertigo. The extent, order and planning of the investigations discussed above will depend on the individual circumstances and clinical judgement of possible cause, but medication should not be started before major contraindications have been excluded. This will be mainly by history-taking and an examination to exclude peptic ulceration, active systemic infection, tuberculosis, diabetes or pregnancy. Prednisolone by mouth is suitable: a 10-day course, 20 mg three times a day, followed by tailing off over a week.

Vasodilatation can include intravenous histamine acid phosphate; each day 2.75 mg in 500 ml normal saline is infused over a 2-hour period. The risk of gastric bleeding can be minimized by the administration of cimetidine, 200 mg three times a day and 400 mg at night time. Some workers also prescribe carbon dioxide inhalations, using a mix of carbon dioxide (90%) and oxygen (10%).

Throughout this time the patient must have what is often loosely described as 'moral support'. In fact, if there is severe hearing loss in both ears, psychiatric support may be vital to help the catastrophic emotional and psychological problems that the illness will entail. In such cases, a hearing aid should be tried as an emergency measure as soon as possible after admission. If bilateral deafness persists, skilled professional rehabilitation will be needed (see Chapter 8) for the patient and their family to adjust and to help them adapt to changed work potential. Ideally this could entail a period of residential care after hospitalization under otological management.

No patient should ever be discharged to a silent outside world and left to fend alone when the otologist has nothing more to offer. The patient should be offered contact with a teacher of the deaf and their general practitioner should be involved.

Progressive hearing loss

Progressive hearing loss is frightening and frustrating for the patient and the doctor. This group might be defined by sequential audiometry showing a progressive hearing loss with three audiometric assessments over a 3-day to 1-year period. The prognosis is worse than for a sudden sensorineural hearing loss, as 68 per cent have no improvement and only 29 per cent make a slight recovery.[9] The differential diagnosis is almost identical to that of sudden sensorineural hearing loss and if the patient feels that their hearing is deteriorating, and this is confirmed by audiometry, then the same urgent investigations and intervention, are indicated. This group also includes patients with cochlear otosclerosis (see Chapter 33), and probably a range of hereditary hearing disorders. The diagnosis of recessive deafness is likely to be conjectural unless there is a large family with a history available over more than one generation.

Chronic hearing loss

The most prevalent cause of chronic hearing loss is termed presbyacusis. This is a term used to describe a common, but not universal, deterioration in hearing with ageing. It is a bilateral hearing loss that initially affects frequencies above 2 kHz; later it also affects lower frequencies, but to a lesser extent. It affects approximately one-third of individuals over the age of 65 years. Some authors have hypothesized that presbyacusis is the cumulative effect of a number of disorders such as atherosclerosis and hyperlipidaemia, or insults such as noise, and is not the result of an innate process 'caused' by old age. Hinchcliffe[10] eloquently put the question '. . .is the deterioration of hearing due to some unavoidable intrinsic degeneration process, or is it merely the result of the individual being exposed to so many surdogens (agents that damage hearing) over the lifespan?'

The concept that vascular disease might be an aetiological factor entered the literature on the basis of a series of poorly controlled trials[11] and an uncritical retrospective analysis of a series of selected patients.[12] This is surprising in view of the good previous pathological work done by Fabinyi,[13] Crowe,[14] and Saxen.[15] Saxen described presbyacusis as

a process of wear, peculiar to old age and comparable with senile atrophy in other structures and tissues of the body. . . as to the degree of hearing loss, this does not depend so much on the changes in the inner ear resulting from atherosclerosis, of decisive importance is the extent to which nerve elements have disappeared.

Saxen concluded that

> Senile atrophy of the spiral ganglion and atherosclerotic degeneration of the inner ear are two diseases of the auditory apparatus peculiar to old age; they are both fairly common and their anatomy and pathogenesis are characteristic. The former is an independent and self-contained disease, the latter but rarely so, being nearly always complicated by the former. Atherosclerotic degeneration of the inner ear alone does not, however, cause any important functional disturbances in the acoustic apparatus. The hearing is well preserved in fairly advanced cases of atherosclerotic degeneration.

The studies that relate to vascular disorders and hearing are inconclusive. This is illustrated by one of the largest and most recent human studies, by Gates *et al.*,[16] which followed 1662 patients from the Framingham Heart Cohort Study. After adjusting for age the only risk factor associated with hearing loss was systolic blood pressure in women and that was a small effect (1 dB low frequency elevation for every 20 mmHg); there was no effect with diastolic pressure.

It is important that a hypothesis that implicates a variable as a cause of a disease has biological credibility. This is particularly important if a multitude of variables are to be examined, otherwise a statistically significant factor may be found by chance. The proposed mechanism by which atherosclerosis might cause a hearing loss varies from author to author, and often several possibilities are suggested in each paper. Blood vessel narrowing, hypercoagulation, sludging of blood, thrombosis with subsequent ischaemia of the end artery or an independent metabolic error have all been suggested.

The cochlea would appear to be vulnerable to ischaemia as the labyrinthine artery has no collateral supply, although the cochlear vein has collaterals to dural veins near the basal coil. The cochlea may have a built-in safety device, because anatomical studies have shown that if one small arteriolar branch is blocked it reduces the flow to the stria vascularis, but does not interfere with the local supply at any particular point.[17] A review of the literature shows that in some studies cochlear function can be altered by relatively minor levels of hypoxia, but that this function returns to normal unless there is such severe anoxia that it affects cerebral function or the cochlear artery is totally occluded with no residual cochlear function. There are no pathological studies showing changes suggesting that a large solitary embolus or small microemboli, even on a background of atherosclerosis, have caused a

hearing loss. Lack of consistency in evidence concerning a particular hypothesis should result in a high degree of caution in any causal interpretation of the findings.

It has been proposed that hyperviscosity can affect hearing by reducing cochlear perfusion through hypoxia.[18] However, this would have only a temporary effect while the blood remained hyperviscous, and the oxygen saturation required to produce a permanent change in hearing threshold experimentally has to be as low as 35 per cent before the cochlea is damaged irreversibly.[19] The inconsistencies between the few existing rheological studies make further research necessary.

One alternative explanation is that presbyacusis is an ageing process that is influenced by the person's genome. Over the last 2 years over 20 autosomal loci for non-syndromic deafness in humans have been identified.[20] These findings raise the possibility that gene expression may play a role in the rate of deterioration of the auditory system.

Schuknecht[1] on the basis of pathological examinations and audiograms, suggested four different sites of cochlear lesions, which give rise to four different forms of presbyacusis: sensory, neural, metabolic and mechanical. He categorized them as follows. In the sensory form there is a loss of outer hair cells and supporting cells, which primarily affects the basilar turn with a high frequency hearing loss. In the neural form he suggested that a loss of speech discrimination with a comparatively well preserved pure tone audiogram coexists with a loss of spiral ganglion cells but with a well preserved organ of Corti. In this form the hypothesis is that the hearing loss is attributable to degeneration of the central auditory pathway. In the strial or metabolic form there is a flat hearing loss with good speech discrimination, said to occur with atrophy of the stria vascularis. In the cochlear form he described a thickening and stiffening of the basilar membrane and cystic degeneration of the stria. These four categories have been quoted in many subsequent texts, but the number of patients for whom there is an adequate history and temporal bone pathology is far too small for this classification to stand unquestioned. A critical appraisal of this work in the light of other studies suggests that the only consistent feature in presbyacusis is a loss of outer hair cells along with a smaller reduction in inner hair cells towards the basal end of the cochlea.[21] In several other studies changes in the stria vascularis have not been found to correlate with hearing loss and some of those noted may have been the result of postmortem changes. A reduction in spiral ganglion cells, along with a loss of hair cells, is usually found with presbyacusis. Conversely, there are reports of well preserved hearing with a marked reduction in the number of spiral ganglion cells. Schuknecht's classification may be an over-interpretation of the pathological changes he found, and more temporal bone studies would be needed to support his concept of neural, strial and cochlear presbyacusis.

The probable causes of chronic hearing loss include:

- presbyacusis. The term presbyacusis means hearing loss associated with ageing in the absence of identifiable causes. Some workers prefer the term age-associated hearing loss[22]
- noise-induced hearing loss (see Chapter 35)
- bacterial infections (see Chapter 29). Tertiary syphilis produces a progressive, often asymmetrical, flat hearing loss and acute vertiginous episodes may occur. There is an osteitis and hydrops. Steroids should be given with benzyl penicillin but the prognosis for hearing is poor
- acoustic neuroma (see Chapter 39) and meningiomas
- endolymphatic hydrops
- autoimmune disease

Organ-specific autoimmune ear disease

Workers have harvested inner ear membranes to produce cochlear antigens.[23] Attempts have been made to see whether these can induce lymphocyte transformation or migration in blood samples taken from patients who are suspected of being affected with organ-specific autoimmune ear disease, but the results are non-specific. The *in vitro* reactions demonstrated may be due to cross-reactivity, particularly as specific antigens have not been identified. Antibody responses have been produced experimentally to type II collagen but this is not specific enough to prove autoimmune cochlear disease. There is no reliable diagnostic test, no definite inner ear antigen and no temporal bone pathology to substantiate organ-specific autoimmune inner ear disease.

Wegener's granulomatosis

Wegener's granulomatosis affects hearing in up to 20 per cent of patients but it is usually because of a middle ear effusion. It affects men twice as frequently as women and it usually starts after 40 years of age. The patient often feels and looks unwell. Other symptoms include a cough and pleuritic pain, a petechial rash, conjunctivitis, iritis or scleritis. It produces a focal necrotizing glomerulonephritis and if unrecognized or untreated is associated with an 80 per cent mortality. Nasal involvement often occurs with crusting, an erythematous granular

lining and later a septal perforation. Sensorineural hearing loss occurs and may respond with treatment of the systemic disease.

Systemic lupus erythematosus

Renowned for the butterfly rash it produces, systematic lupus erythematosus can also cause a polyarteritis, pericarditis, pneumonitis, nephritis and cranial nerve palsies. These patients have antibodies to nuclear components. Immune complexes are found in the basement membranes of renal and other blood vessels. A tiny minority have a sensorineural hearing loss and examination of the rheumatological literature suggests that it is very rare and may possibly be an incidental finding. In one controlled study of 65 patients those affected were asymptomatic and the findings were inconsistent.[24]

Polyarteritis nodosa

There is a polymorphonuclear leucocyte infiltrate of vessels and perivascular tissue with a necrotizing vasculitis of medium-sized and small vessels in polyarteritis nodosa. The associated features include retinal haemorrhages, pericarditis, mucosal ulceration and renal involvement. Patients may be anaemic and neutropenic. Temporal bone studies have shown evidence of ischaemic changes, an arteritis and osteoneogenesis.

Cogan's syndrome

Cogan's syndrome comprises a non-syphilitic interstitial keratitis, vertigo and hearing loss. The ESR reflects disease activity. Temporal bones from affected individuals have varied but have shown hydrops, atrophy of the organ of Corti and an infiltration with lymphocytes and plasma cells.

Relapsing polychondritis

Relapsing polychondritis is an inflammatory disorder of cartilage that can produce a saddle nose and collapse of the trachea or auricle. It is associated with a raised ESR and IgG level, a false-positive VDRL and antibodies to type II and type IV collagen. Sporadic cases of sensorineural hearing loss occur in this rare condition.

Rheumatoid arthritis

The association between chronic hearing loss and rheumatoid arthritis has not been proved and may be incidental or secondary to high doses of salicylates.

Ulcerative colitis

Sporadic cases of ulcerative colitis have been reported.

Behçet's syndrome

Symptoms associated with Behçet's syndrome include orogenital ulceration, vasculitis, iritis, uveitis and arthritis. There is no substantial evidence that this can cause a sensorineural hearing loss.

Assessing response to treatment is difficult as all these diagnoses are rare and patients often have fluctuating episodic symptoms, which make a comparative trial difficult.

Further probable causes of chronic hearing loss include:

• Tumours. The rare occurrence of rhabdomyosarcoma, malignant paraganglionoma, leukaemic deposits and extramedullary plasmacytoma can produce a hearing loss. The latter can occur as an isolated lesion or as part of multiple myeloma.
• Sarcoidosis. This is a multisystem granulomatous disease with histological features of non-caseating epitheliod follicles. Extrapulmonary involvement of the central nervous system can involve the VIIth and VIIIth cranial nerves. Apart from hilar lymphadenopathy there may be an iridocyclitis, keratoconjunctivitis, myalgia, hepatosplenomegaly or hypercalcaemia. The mainstay of treatment is steroids but the response when there is a hearing loss in chronic extrapulmonary disease is often disappointing.
• Multiple sclerosis. This may be either a reversible or progressive high frequency hearing loss, which is said to occur in 4 per cent of patients. It usually occurs when other areas of the brainstem are affected. Brainstem auditory evoked potential (BAEP) studies have shown that there is no consistent site that is affected. MRI has shown that the inferior colliculus can be affected.
• Benign intracranial hypertension. The patient, usually an obese woman, may present with a headache with or without pulsatile tinnitus and blurred vision. Hearing loss has been reported and may be due to brainstem or cochlear nerve compression. If it is severe a cerebrospinal fluid shunt is required.
• Psychogenic. In adolescence the patient usually presents with a history of problems at school but good audiometric thresholds are relatively easily obtained and quickly disperse any concern about hearing. In adults malingering is often part of a claim for compensation after noise exposure.

• Paget's disease. This is an abnormality of bone remodelling and is rare before 40 years of age. It occurs four times more frequently in men and there is typically an enlarged skull with involvement of the pelvis, tibia or femur. The serum alkaline phosphatase is raised. It is said to cause a hearing loss through cochlear nerve compression, but both this and direct involvement of the cochlea probably only occur in advanced cases as the otic capsule is often spared. A study of 1066 patients showed that although many had a hearing loss there was little evidence that any were due to Paget's disease.[25]
• Cortical deafness. This is a rare event and occurs when there is diffuse cortical damage usually due to multiple areas of cerebral infarction; it is just one part of a more serious picture.

Possible causes of chronic hearing loss for which an association has been suggested but the evidence is inadequate include:

• Diabetes mellitus. In the otological literature there are reports that say, without reservation, that diabetes is associated with a sensorineural hearing loss.[2] The main body of evidence is that people with diabetes mellitus as a group have hearing thresholds that do not differ significantly from the normal population. There are several electrophysiological studies that show objective differences between diabetic and normal patients, but it is notable that the diabetic subjects studied in almost all of these have normal pure tone thresholds and no subjective hearing loss. Diabetes and hearing loss have been linked by the identification of the maternally inherited mitochondrial gene tRNA$^{leu(UUR)}$ and the 10.4 kb mitochondrial deletion. The prevalence of these within a diabetic population is under investigation. The association of these with the DIDMOAD syndrome, that is, diabetes mellitus and insipidus, optic atrophy and deafness, is unknown.
• Sickle-cell disease. In view of the prevalence of this condition there are few reports linking it with hearing loss. One suboptimally controlled study examined 83 patients and found a greater than 25 dB loss at one or more frequencies in 4 per cent of the controls and 22 per cent of the sickle-cell group, but only 4 per cent had noticed any hearing loss.[26]
• AIDS. Approximately 8 per cent of AIDS patients suffer from middle ear effusion, although the prevalence is at its highest when the patient's immune mechanism is at a low ebb. Patients with AIDS are not only subject to the effects of ototoxic drugs but they can also suffer lesions of the cochlea and central nervous

system.[27] Cytomegalovirus appears to be the primary culprit and although objective changes have been found at autopsy, the patients studied have been asymptomatic.

- Chronic suppurative otitis media. It has been postulated that bacterial toxins can pass through the round window membrane to produce cochlear damage. There is inadequate evidence to support this.
- Renal dialysis. No consistent pathological changes have been found. There are sporadic reports and it is uncertain if there is an association with either renal failure or dialysis.
- Osteomalacia and vitamin D deficiency. A study of 27 Asian immigrants presenting to the Royal London Hospital showed a high prevalence of hearing loss,[28] but there was no control group and no consistent radiographic evidence of reduced bone density and the data were confounded by several patients having otosclerosis.
- Osteopetrosis. There is a reduction in bone resorption with narrowing of the skull forumina, which may affect hearing.
- Acromegaly and hypothyroidism. There is no material evidence.

We are left with a sizeable group in whom the hearing loss is idiopathic.

HISTORY AND EXAMINATION

After enquiring about the presence of tinnitus, vertigo or hearing asymmetry it is important to clarify the disability that is caused by the hearing loss. A history, otoscopy, tuning fork tests and audiometry (see Chapter 4) are often enough to establish a diagnosis of presbyacusis. A quiet question about the patient's family asked while moving behind them may elicit a response and catch out the malingerer. If a vasculitis or sarcoid is suspected, the nasal mucosa and other relevant systems especially the eyes, joints and skin should be examined.

INVESTIGATION

Audiometry with appropriate masking is done. When there are features in the history or an audiometric pattern uncharacteristic of presbyacusis then the possibility of a remediable condition warrants investigation. As detailed, the search for systemic disease such as diabetes, hypertension or hyperlipidaemia is not justified solely on the basis of a patient's hearing loss. The relevant tests may include a full blood count (anaemia in vasculitis), urinalysis (haematuria in vasculitis), ESR (raised in

Cogan's, vasculitis and sarcoid), autoimmune screen, angiotensin converting enzyme measurement (sarcoid), anti-neutrophil cytoplasmic antibody test (Wegener's), syphilis serology, a plain chest X-ray (sarcoid and vasculitis), MRI (acoustic neuroma or central pathology), cortical auditory evoked potentials if malingering is suspected, and electrocochleography if there is a clinical indication to confirm Menière's disease.

PROGNOSIS AND MANAGEMENT

Prognosis and management are determined by the diagnosis. Although the majority of sensorineural hearing losses are irreversible, it is important to establish a diagnosis as in a few patients further hearing loss may be prevented. In a minority an improvement can be obtained, for example Wegener's granulomatosis and Cogan's syndrome. Once the remediable causes of hearing loss have been excluded, treatment should focus on how the patient can be helped in practical terms, for example an elderly person living on their own may be helped as much by a doorbell and telephone light as by the provision of a hearing aid (see Chapter 8).

References

1. Schuknecht HF. *Pathology of the ear.* Cambridge, MA. Harvard University Press, 1974.
2. Proctor C. Diagnosis, prevention and treatment of hereditary sensorineural hearing loss. *Laryngoscope* 1977; **87(suppl 7)**: 1–60.
3. Ginsberg IA, White TP. Otologic considerations in audiology. In: Katz J ed. *Handbook of clinical audiology, 3rd ed.* London: William and Wilkins, 1985:
4. Nager GT. *Pathology of the ear and temporal bone.* Baltimore: Williams and Wilkins, 1993.
5. Wilson WR, Byl FM, Laird N. The efficacy of steroids in the treatment of idiopathic sudden hearing loss: a double-blind clinical study. *Archives of Otolaryngology* 1980; **106**:772–6.
6. Davis AC. The prevalence of hearing impairment and reported hearing disability among adults in Great Britain. *International Journal of Epidemiology* 1989; **18**:911–7.
7. Moscicki EK, Elkins EF, Baum HM, McNamara PM. Hearing loss in the elderly: an epidemiologic study of the Framingham Heart Study. *Ear and Hearing* 1985; **6**:184–90.
8. Fetterman BL, Saunders JE, Luxford WM. Prognosis and treatment of sudden sensorineural deafness. *American Journal of Otology* 1996; **17**:529–36.
9. Hirayama M, Shitara T, Okamoto M, Sano H. Idiopathic bilateral sensorineural hearing loss: its clinical study in cases with rapidly progressive deafness. *Acta Otolaryngologica (Stockholm)* 1996; **(suppl 524)**:39–42.

10. Hinchcliffe R. The age function of hearing – aspects of the epidemiology. *Acta Otolaryngologica (Stockholm)* 1991; **(suppl 476)**:7–11.
11. Rosen S, Olin P. Hearing loss and coronary heart disease. *Archives of Otolaryngology* 1965; **82**:236–43.
12. Spencer JT. Hyperlipoproteinemia in the etiology of inner ear disease. *Laryngoscope* 1973; **83**:639–78.
13. Fabinyi G. Regarding morphological and functional changes of the inner ear in atherosclerosis. *Laryngoscope* 1931; **41**:663–70.
14. Crowe SJ, Guild SR, Polvogt LM. Observations on the pathology of high tone deafness. *Bulletin of Johns Hopkins Hospital* 1934; **54**:315–79.
15. Saxen H. Inner ear in presbyacusis. *Acta Otolaryngologica (Stockholm)* 1952; **41**:213–27.
16. Gates G, Cobb JL, D'Agostino RB, Wolf PA. The relation of hearing in the elderly to the presence of cardiovascular disease and cardiovascular risk factors. *Archives of Otolaryngology – Head and Neck Surgery* 1993; **119**:156–61.
17. Smith CA. Vascular patterns of the membranous labyrinth. In: Darin de Lorenzo AJ ed. *Vascular disorders and hearing defects*. Baltimore: University Park Press, 1972:1–21.
18. Gatehouse S, Lowe GDO. Whole blood viscosity and red cell filterability as factors in sensorineural hearing impairment in the elderly. *Acta Otolaryngologica (Stockholm)* 1991; **(suppl 476)**:37–43.
19. Gulick WL. The effects of hypoxaemia upon the electrical response of the cochlea. *Annals of Otology, Rhinology and Laryngology* 1958; **67**:148–69.
20. Steel K, Brown SDM. Genetics and deafness. *Current Opinion in Neurobiology* 1996; **6**:520–5.
21. Wright A, Davis A, Bredberg G, Ulehlova L, Spencer H. Hair cell distribution in the normal human cochlea. *Acta Otolaryngologica* 1987; **(suppl 444)**:1–48.
22. King PF, Coles RRA, Lutman ME, Robinson DW. *Assessment of hearing disability*. London: Whurr, 1993.
23. Harris JP. Autoimmune diseases affecting the inner ear. In: Myers EN, Bluestone CD, Brackmann DE, Krause CJ eds. *Advances in Otolaryngology – Head and Neck Surgery*. St.Louis: Mosby, 1993:59–77.
24. Andonopopoulos S, Naxakis S, Goumas P, Lygatsikas C. Sensorineural hearing disorders in systemic lupus erythematosus. A controlled study. *Clinical and Experimental Rheumatology* 1995; **13**:137–41.
25. Harner SG, Rose DE, Facer GW. Paget's disease and hearing loss. *Otorhinolaryngology* 1978; **86**:869–74.
26. Todd GB, Sergeant GR, Larson MR. Sensorineural hearing loss in Jamaicans with SS disease. *Acta Otolaryngology* 1973; **76**:268–72.
27. Soucek S, Michaels L. The ear in the acquired immunodeficiency syndrome: II. Clinical and audiometric investigation. *American Journal of Otology* 1996; **17**:35–9.
28. Brookes GB. Vitamin D deficiency and deafness: 1984 update. *American Journal of Otology* 1985; **6**:102–7.

CHAPTER 37

Ototoxicity

TONY WRIGHT

Introduction

Many agents, including noise, direct trauma, infections and drugs, can damage the inner ear. Ototoxicity is generally considered to be that damage caused by medications and has been defined by Joe Hawkins[1] as

> the tendency of certain therapeutic agents and other chemical substances to cause functional impairment and cellular degeneration of the tissues of the inner ear and especially of the end organs and neurons of the cochlear and vestibular divisions of the VIIIth cranial nerve.

In the same publication Hawkins also gives a historical review, which is complemented by that of Stephens.[2]

One of the problems with evaluating the presence or the severity of the ototoxicity of specific drugs is the possible contribution made by the disease process for which the drug was given. For example, in former times could it have been tuberculous meningitis or the treatment that caused the vertigo and deafness that frequently arose during the course of the disease when it was being treated with streptomycin? More recently the question has arisen as to whether a middle ear and mastoid infection with a purulent discharge can cause a sensorineural hearing loss as the bacterial toxins enter the inner ear or whether it is prolonged treatment with aminoglycoside-containing eardrops that causes the damage. This latter subject will be discussed in depth further on in this chapter.

Generalized illness can alter the hearing for a variety of reasons. In a well planned study by Davey et al.[3] it was found that in a group of similarly ill people who were admitted to hospital and who had their hearing tested at the beginning of their illness and at a 3-month follow-up those who were treated with aminoglycosides had less long-term hearing loss than the control group. This suggested to the authors that had the control group been treated with aminoglycosides then the hearing loss that this group sustained could easily have been labelled as having been caused by the drug. An alternative interpretation is that the aminoglycosides protected against the damaging effects of infection. Thus any study to evaluate the incidence of hearing loss that could be drug-related needs pretreatment audiometry, follow-up and, importantly, a proper control group for the study to be valid. The authors also questioned the value of bedside audiometry in providing reliable evaluation of changes in threshold of less than 20 dB sound pressure level (SPL).

Nevertheless, it is quite clear that several classes of drugs regularly damage the inner ear, whereas some occasionally do and others might. These different groups are shown in Table 37.1.

Table 37.1 Classes of ototoxic agents

Drugs that are certainly ototoxic
    Aminoglycoside antibiotics
    Cis-platinum
    Salicylates
    Quinine
    Loop diuretics e.g. furosemide, bumetanide
Drugs that certainly cause a hearing loss
    Macrolide antibiotics e.g. erythromycin
Drugs that may alter hearing and balance
    Glycopeptide antibiotics e.g. vancomycin
Centrally acting agents
    Imipramine
    5-Hydroxytryptamine
    Carbamazepine

The clinical features of ototoxicity

Whatever drug is the cause of suspected ototoxicity, the clinical features are much the same, differing only in the severity of the symptom, the timing of onset and the duration of effect. The cardinal symptoms are tinnitus, hearing loss and balance disturbances, with a feeling of pressure in the ears being a frequently added complaint.

TINNITUS

Tinnitus is very often the first warning that something is affecting the inner ear or its innervation. The site of 'production' of the abnormal neural output that is recognized by the higher auditory centres as 'tinnitus' is unknown, but probably varies between the different classes of ototoxic drugs. The aminoglycosides may generate tinnitus by altering hair cell function whereas the salicylates may involve the afferent or efferent neural pathways directly. The loop diuretics, by altering the activity of the stria vascularis, change not only the endocochlear potential but also the endolymphatic ion concentrations, thereby causing many changes in the transduction process. Any drug that alters the hearing is likely to alter central 'awareness' so that more attention is paid by the brain to the ear, which in turn enhances appreciation of the background internal 'noise' of the cochlea. Whatever the origin of the tinnitus, it is frequently high-pitched and continuous when it starts and, at least with the aminoglycosides, is often a relatively pure tone. The loop diuretics frequently cause a more severe crashing noise after rapid intravenous administration. If damage progresses the noises change and additional sounds often add themselves to the background tinnitus, the pitch of which may drop in tone as the damage extends. This tinnitus can be unilateral or bilateral or be heard centrally.

HEARING LOSS

Different patterns of hearing loss can be found with different ototoxic agents and these will be described in more detail in the following sections. There is frequently some question as to whether a particular drug did cause a hearing loss in an individual. The pattern of the loss, the proximity of the loss to the treatment and the lack of other possible causes of such a loss make it more likely than not that the treatment itself did cause the damage in the absence of any other contributory factors that are known to be associated with a similar pattern of loss. There is often a delay in the onset of hearing loss when the aminoglycosides are the culprit and indeed the hearing losses may not be blamed on the drug as they can be insidious. The use of dihydrostreptomycin, which is powerfully cochleotoxic, prompted this response from an eminent group of American otologists in 1959

> Cases of irreversible hearing loss attributable to dihydrostreptomycin are continuing to occur, usually without the knowledge of the prescribing physician because of the latent period from several weeks to as long as six months between administration of the drug and the onset of the hearing loss.[4]

Dihydrostreptomycin was subsequently withdrawn from the market in the USA and UK.

BALANCE DISTURBANCES

The severe, acute vertigo that arises from damage to one labyrinth is not a common feature of vestibulotoxic damage from systemic administration, although it can arise from the topical administration of an aminoglycoside to one ear if the damage occurs rapidly. More commonly the patients are severely unsteady, even bed-bound in the worse cases, as there are altered labyrinthine responses to head movement. There may be strange sensations of unreal movement (which is the classic description of vertigo), although this is usually in response to head movement rather than being spontaneous. Patients with bilateral labyrinthine disturbances are extremely unsteady and need to hold on to solid objects for stability. All the symptoms are worse in the dark, as the individual can only rely on their proprioceptive input and their impaired labyrinthine information for stability and these together are not adequate for functionally normal balance. Once the damage has stabilized and if there is some labyrinthine function left, then central compensation can occur and with practice and exercise balance can return, if not to normality then at least to a useful state. In general, the younger the patient the quicker the return to normal. In the elderly, normal balance may never be restored and they may continue to be unsteady for the rest of their lives.

If there has been total loss of labyrinthine balance responses as measured by absent cold caloric tests or the loss of the vestibulo-ocular reflex on rotating chair testing, then the symptom of 'oscillopsia' can arise. The rapid labyrinthine responses to head movement are missing and visual fixation is difficult to maintain when the head is moved quickly. Objects seen by the patient appear to continue to move as eye movement lags behind head movement. Thus in a car on a bumpy road the surroundings seem to bob up and down thereby giving the condition the name of 'bobbing oscillopsia'.

Bilateral severe labyrinthine failure is extremely difficult to manage successfully and is a serious handicap that is better avoided.

THE HISTORY

There are important features in the history that need to be obtained if the diagnosis of ototoxicity is to be made. The details of the onset of the tinnitus, the hearing loss or the balance disturbance need to be fully explained by the patient or their carer. The use of sprays in the treatment of scalds or burns in children is a classic example of a treatment that was often not thought worthy of mention by the parents to the doctor investigating a progressive sensorineural hearing loss in their child. Neomycin was a common additive to antibiotic sprays and was extremely effective in controlling superficial infection of raw areas. Unfortunately the aminoglycosides are completely water soluble and are absorbed down their concentration gradient across these 'open' tissues. These losses in children were often labelled as 'autosomal recessive hearing losses', which is an easy term for doctors to use rather like the notion of an acute viral hearing loss, and means that the real cause is probably not understood. There is no reason why parents should associate a successfully treated burn or scald with a subsequent and possibly disastrous hearing loss.

The same constraints apply to the use of aminoglycosides to sterilize the gut before abdominal surgery. If the lining of the small and large intestine is inflamed then the usual resistance to the passage of the aminoglycosides into the lymphatics is lost and ototoxicity can and has occurred.

Absorption also occurs with the use of aminoglycosides in nebulizers used in the treatment of chest infections. Large doses of the drug can be absorbed across the alveolar membranes and in due course damage the ear. To a lay person, and even to some doctors, the association is obscure.

The description of the pattern of onset of any balance disturbance, the troubles the patient experiences and the circumstances surrounding the development of the problem are very important because of the close interaction between the psyche and the symptoms as far as balance is concerned. This has been discussed in detail in Chapter 14.

The classes of drugs

Table 37.1 lists the drugs most commonly involved in ototoxicity and these will be described in some detail below. Most attention will be paid to the aminoglycosides as this class of drug has been extensively studied and forms a model for the assessment of the other ototoxic agents.

THE AMINOGLYCOSIDES

The first of a family of antimicrobial agents derived from soil organisms and discovered by Waksman[5] in 1944 was soon put into clinical use against tuberculosis. This drug was streptomycin and the very first report of its use in humans mentions the

STREPTOMYCIN

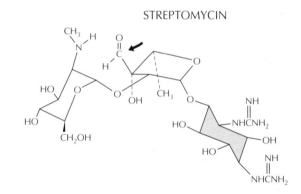

NEOMYCIN B

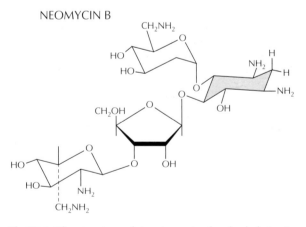

Fig 37.1 The structure of streptomycin: the shaded ring is the terminal aminocyclitol called streptidine. The heavy arrow indicates the site of reduction of the side chain –CHO to CH₂OH during the formation of dihydrostreptomycin. (b) The structure of Neomycin B: the shaded ring is the aminocyclitol 2-deoxystreptamine and is in a central position as it is for all the newer aminoglycosides.

Table 37.2 Relative toxicity of the aminoglycosides

	Vestibular	Methylamine Total	Methylamine Glycosidic	Cochlear	Amino Total	Amino Glycosidic
Streptomycin	+++	1	1	+	2	0
DHSM	+	1	1	++	2	0
Netilmicin	?+	1	1	?(+)	3	2
Sisomycin	?++	1	1	?+	4	2
Gentamicin						
C_{1a}	+	1	1	+	4	2
C_1	++	1	1	+	3	1
Amikacin	+	0	0	++	3	2
Kanamycin A	+	0	0	+++	4	2
Tobramycin	+	1	1	++++	5	3
Neomycin	+	0	0	+++++	6	4

DHSM, dihydrostreptomycin.

unexpected finding that of the 34 patients treated, one developed a transient deafness and three had disturbances of balance. Whether these changes were due to the drug or the disease will never be known, but all of the aminoglycosides that have subsequently been developed have some effect on hearing or balance or both. The reason for the propensity of the drug to damage the cochlear or vestibular sensory cells preferentially is unknown, but might be related to biochemical features such as the number of amino groupings present on the surface of the aminoglycoside molecule (Fig 37.1 and Table 37.2).

Whatever the precise mechanism, these drugs are ototoxic and nephrotoxic and need to be prescribed with caution, although they are very effective agents to use against a wide range of serious Gram-negative bacteria such as *Pseudomonas, Klebsiella* and *Proteus* species which are often resistant to other antibiotic treatments.

Incidence and assessment

The definition of what comprises cochlear ototoxicity is not uniform. Using pure tone data a bilateral change in the hearing level of 10 dB at one or more frequencies is commonly taken to be indicative of some change. To be this accurate requires pure tone audiometry to be carried out in high-class sound-proofed booths. This is rarely possible in sick patients and so perhaps the more realistic level of a persisting bilateral change in the threshold of 20 dB or more should be adopted. Despite this reservation, the reported rates of aminoglycoside toxicity are around 5–10 per cent for gentam-

icin, tobramycin and amikacin, whereas netilmicin has had consistently less cochlear toxicity attributed to it.

There are papers reporting recovery from cochlear toxicity in 50 per cent, or more, of patients who have sustained a hearing loss during their illness and treatment with an aminoglycoside. This claim should be treated with some scepticism as there are no studies in adult mammalian species that have ever indicated any recovery of cochlear hair cells, although there may be reversible structural changes in the afferent innervation arising from the cochlea. The aminoglycosides are neurotoxic to a small degree and any recovery may have been a result of this reversible action, which has been shown as an acute change in the cochlear action potentials after intravenous administration. Alternatively the effect could easily have been caused by the intercurrent illness that prompted the administration of the drug in the first place.

The use of transient evoked otoacoustic emissions (TEOAEs) to detect changes in the function of the outer hair cells, which as we will see are the prime site of action of the cochleotoxic aminoglycosides, will undoubtedly alter the degree of true detection of the problem and revise our definitions. The tests do not need to be performed in sound-proofed rooms and do not even require much patient compliance, although permission to perform the test should always be sought when appropriate. There are no contemporary papers on the widespread use of this technique.

As far as the objective assessment of vestibular function is concerned there are even more problems. There is an extremely wide spread of the variables for any standard test in the 'normal' population. However, rotational tests that attempt to measure the threshold of an individual detecting a change in the angular velocity of a rotating chair do seem to be the most specific and sensitive of the available tests, although not only is the equipment that is needed to perform this assessment properly not widely available, but the test still only evaluates the lateral semicircular canals effectively. The use of dynamic posturography (e.g. the Equitest balance platform) may be helpful, although once again the equipment is expensive and patients may be too unwell to use it. See Chapter 5 for an appraisal of vestibular testing.

The basis of aminoglycoside toxicity

The aminoglycosides damage sensory hair cells. In the cochlea they damage the outer hair cells (OHCs) of the basal turn preferentially. This damage extends apically and when all the outer hair cells in any particular section of the cochlea are gone, then the inner hair cells (IHCs) start to die. This IHC loss may well be due to damage to the supporting cells.

In the vestibular system, hair cell loss first occurs on the crest of the cristae and in the striolar regions of the maculae, spreading outwards as damage progresses.

Aminoglycosides enter the perilymph fairly slowly (peak concentrations 4 hours after a single dose) and the endolymph even more slowly. Once in the endolymph, the aminoglycosides are extremely slow to leave and may be present for days. They may also be sequestered within lysosomal-like bodies within the hair cells and persist for up to a year, which may account for the ability of a subtoxic dose of an aminoglycoside to predispose the cochlea to subsequent damage by a further noxious stimulus be it more aminoglycoside, a different drug or noise.

Although the aminoglycosides can cause changes in the cell membrane of the endolymphatic surface of the hair cell and its stereocilia (Fig 37.2), this does not seem to be the cause of cell degeneration and death.

It seems more likely that irreversible interactions occur with various membrane phospholipids – specifically phosphatidylinositol-4-5-biphosphate (PhIP$_2$) – which are important second messengers in essential intracellular enzyme cascades. Damage to these pathways results in eventual cell death.[6] It is of interest that PhIP$_2$, although found in all tissues, is in high concentrations in neural tissues, including the ear and in the kidney.

Interactions

The aminoglycosides are only excreted by the kidneys, so that any form of renal impairment can lead to an increase in the blood levels of the aminoglycosides and this, in turn can result in toxic levels in the perilymph and endolymph. However, renal failure itself is often associated with hearing loss, not only because of the possibly altered ionic environment in the cochlea, but also because the stria vascularis and dark cell regions of the inner ear, which maintain the homeostasis of the endolymphatic ion composition and the endocochlear potential, show many of the characteristics of the cells of the loop of Henle in the kidney. These characteristics are not only structural, but functional by way of shared antigens and shared responses to some drugs, that is, the loop diuretics. There are several cochleo-renal syndromes with altered hearing and renal failure.

From what has just been written, it is also clear that the loop diuretics are likely to interact with the ototoxic effect of the aminoglycosides. This was first shown in 1969 when the then unexpected synergistic interaction between the aminoglycosides and loop diuretics was reported. A synergistic interaction occurs when the effect of two drugs (or any agent) is more than that which would be expected from the addition of the effects of each drug if they were used separately. In other words the use of 'safe' doses of the loop diuretics along with 'safe' doses of the aminoglycosides can result in damage. The situation would be worse in the presence of renal failure.

As mentioned above, there are suggestions that previous exposure to a subtoxic dose of the aminoglycosides predisposes ears to subsequent damage when there is further exposure to, again, subtoxic doses of aminoglycosides or industrial or occupational noise or other ototoxic agents.

Routes of administration and 'safe' levels

Although aminoglycosides are completely water-soluble, they are positively charged molecules and do not cross normal skin or intact bowel epithelium. Thus they need to be given by systemic (intravenous or intramuscular) administration to reach effective blood levels capable of overcoming pathogenic bacteria. To minimize the ototoxic and nephrotoxic damage that could be caused by their use, divided daily doses have been advised. The serum levels of the aminoglycosides can be determined by bioassay and fairly complicated and expensive schemes of administration based on peak or trough serum levels have been derived.

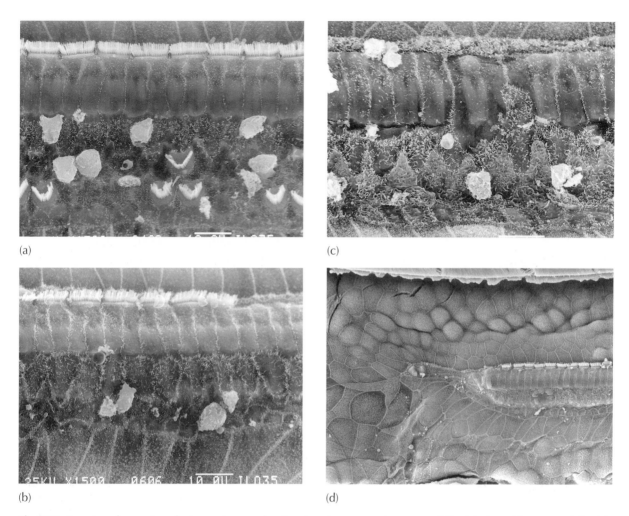

(a)

(c)

(b)

(d)

Fig 37.2 A series of scanning electron micrographs showing damage to the organ of Corti induced by gentamicin. (a), (b) and (c) There is progressive damage to the hair cells in order of their sensitivity. First the first row of inner hair cells is lost followed by the middle and then outer rows. If damage is severe enough to have destroyed these, then the inner hair cells are vulnerable and eventually die. After loss of all the hair cell population in one region of the organ of Corti then there can be collapse of the supporting cells and disappearance of all the normal features, as seen in (d), which is taken at a lower magnification. (Reproduced with permission of Dr Andrew Forge.)

However, a major meta-analysis from Barza *et al.*[7] has shown that a single daily dose is just as efficient (based on otologic or renal toxicity outcomes), and is easy to administer. The study did not recommend the dosage per kilogram and the reduction that would be necessary in the presence of renal failure, but suggested that there was no indication for measuring the peak serum values. From a medicolegal point of view it would, however, seem wiser to ensure that serum levels are assessed, especially in patients with renal impairment. A confounding feature to the value of bioassay of blood levels is the frequent idiosyncratic nature of aminoglycoside toxicity. Patients with well maintained 'safe' levels

sometimes lose their hearing whereas others, who have very high levels, escape damage. This has never been satisfactorily explained.

The drug data sheets that come with the loop diuretics indicate that the aminoglycosides should only be given concomitantly with great caution. However, it is probably wiser never to give these two classes of drugs together as there are always alternatives. By similar argument, there is almost certainly no reason to give an aminoglycoside in the presence of renal failure, despite the cost benefit, if there is an alternative choice.

Having said this, the aminoglycosides are very effective agents for some patients with serious, life-

Table 37.3 Approximate cost in pounds sterling of 5 days of treatment for commonly used intravenous doses at the lower end of recommended range (for 70 kg patient)

meropenem (500 mg three times daily)	£225
imipenem/cilastatin (imipenem 500 mg three times daily)	£225
cefotaxime (1 g three times daily)	£73
ceftazidime (1 g three times daily)	£149
ceftriaxone (1 g/day)	£57
clindamycin (0.6 g/day)	£51
metronidazole (500 mg three times daily)	£54
gentamicin (2 mg/kg/day)	£14
ciprofloxacin (200 mg twice daily)	£199
tobramycin (3 mg/kg/day)	£32
amikacin (15 mg/kg/day)	£106

threatening infections and in balancing the risks of their use with their non-use, ototoxicity may be a small price to pay for survival.

Table 37.3 is derived from a recent publication of the British Drugs and Therapeutics Bulletin published by the Consumers Association and gives the relative costs of various antibiotics effective when bacterial drug resistance is a problem.

Topical administration

Because many cases of otitis externa or chronic suppurative otitis media have a purulent discharge containing *Pseudomonas, Klebsiella* or *Proteus* species, antibiotic ear drops containing aminoglycosides are marketed in preference to other antibiotic preparations, despite the theoretical risk of damage to the inner ear.

This theoretical risk arises from the possibility of the drugs entering the inner ear from the middle ear directly by way of the round window membrane and the annular ligament of the oval window. The round window membrane, by virtue of its far greater surface area, would be the more likely candidate as a route of access, although in humans the membrane itself is far thicker than in the commonly used experimental animals.

The manufacturers of antibiotic ear drops recognize this potential and indicate caution in their product information sheets. However, there has not been good evidence that aminoglycosides instilled into the middle ears of humans with chronic suppurative otitis media cause sensorineural hearing loss. Professor Browning, in one of his studies on the whole problem of deafness in discharging ears and the effects and risks of treatments, states:

> the risk of inner ear damage occurring following topical Gentamicin therapy in active chronic otitis media must be low. However, it is unlikely that the actual risk will ever be known because of the size of the study that would be required to assess it. It is estimated from this study that, if the incidence of damage of greater than 15 dB to the inner ear with gentamicin were to be 1%, it would require 300–500 individuals in both the therapy and placebo control groups to demonstrate it.[8]

Because of this lack of ototoxic effect in clinical practice, the British Association of Otolaryngologists has recommended to the British National Formulary that the suggested restriction on the use of aminoglycosides in situations in which there is a perforation of the eardrum should be lifted and be replaced by the suggestion that ear drops should not be used for long periods. However, it is a practice for many otolaryngologists to use aminoglycoside-containing ear drops in situations in which the middle ear is open and infected for several weeks or even for 2–3 months in order to try to clear the infection. Indeed, the study by Professor Browning[8] quoted above was a trial of treatment with gentamicin-containing ear drops used over a period of 4–6 weeks.

Potentially ototoxic agents are used to treat suppurating ears because 'prolonged chronic suppurative otitis media may eventually, without evidence of direct spread of the infection into the labyrinth, lead to sensorineural hearing loss'. However, much of the evidence for this statement is anecdotal or relates to individual patients who may well have had other causes for these losses. Another report, again from Professor Browning, of a very large prospective study concluded: 'There was no difference in bone conduction thresholds in 395 patients with chronic otitis media compared with those in 920 control ears.'[9] Despite this it is quite clear that gentamicin instilled into normal human middle ears can cause sensorineural hearing loss.

In Menière's disease one current form of therapy is to instil gentamicin solution into the middle ear so that it is absorbed into and damages the inner ear thereby reducing the vertigo, which is usually the most serious symptom as far as the patient is concerned. The mechanism of action is direct damage to the sensory cells subserving balance, but in addition the cochlear sensory cells can also be destroyed as an unwanted side effect of the treatment. Bagger-Sjoback *et al.*[10] described patients treated with gentamicin in whom the balance failed to get better, although the hearing was completely lost. The authors were able to collect specimens from the inner ear at a subsequent labyrinthectomy.

The vestibular epithelium was severely damaged with signs of marked degeneration but the hair cells in the cochlea were completely missing.

Thus, loss of hearing is an unfortunate complication of this form of treatment for Menière's disease and it has been well documented. Odkvist[11] has collected the results of treatment of Menière's disease by gentamicin infusion into the middle ear from the literature and has been able to correlate the hearing loss against the days of treatment. He states: 'it is obvious from the figures that the greatest risk to the hearing arises when treatment is prolonged for more than six days.' The concentration of gentamicin used in this so-called therapeutic procedure was 40 mg/ml (that is, 4% w/v, approximately). In another study by Parnes and Riddell[12] a lower concentration of gentamicin – 3% w/v – was used and the authors stated: 'Despite our patients having a higher incidence of hearing loss compared to the reported rates, our results of this treatment are encouraging'!

An even lower exposure of two injections on 2 consecutive days was enough to damage the labyrinth although 'hearing levels were about the same compared to before treatment'.[13]

A different approach was taken by a German group, who used continuous treatment by irrigation with a low dose of 3 ml gentamicin solution (0.3% w/v) per day for several days. Patients were compared with other groups who had discontinuous treatment, again with gentamicin in standard doses. In the discontinuous treatment group, 3 out of 40 had total deafness and in the continuous treatment group 2 out of 42 patients had losses of up to 60 dB.[14] The discontinuous therapy group received on average 95 mg gentamicin whereas the other group received 325 mg.

Thus it is quite clear that gentamicin in solution is capable of passing through the round window membrane and of being severely ototoxic to the inner ear in very short courses at high concentration or in longer courses if a lesser concentration is used and when the middle ear mucosa is normal.

The concentration of gentamicin in Gentisone HC ear drops (which is one of a group of commonly used aminoglycoside-containing ear drops) is 0.3% and one bottle contains 10 ml, which is equivalent to 30 mg gentamicin. Three bottles would thus be required to provide a dose of 90 mg, which is a dose that can cause a profound sensorineural hearing loss. If neomycin were the drug used in the antibiotic ear drops then, because it is so cochleotoxic, it can only be assumed that a lesser dose would be needed to cause some hearing loss.

These results have all been derived from the installation of aminoglycoside-containing ear drops into otherwise normal middle ears. The situation is obviously different in infected, congested middle ears but, nevertheless, when the surface mucosa is altered, aminoglycosides can quite quickly be absorbed down their concentration gradient as described earlier in the chapter. It would thus seem very sensible to limit the dosage of aminoglycosides to the middle ear from an open perforation. If after two or three courses of appropriate antibiotic treatment the ear fails to settle then it is more likely than not that a surgical procedure to treat the infected middle ear mucosa and mend the perforated eardrum is indicated.

CISPLATIN

Cisplatin has been in use since the 1970s and can produce not only renal damage and neurotoxicity, but a permanent mainly high-frequency sensorineural hearing loss, the mechanism of which is not really understood although the pattern of hair cell loss in experimental animals is similar to that found with aminoglycosides. As well as damage to the hair cells, atrophy of the stria vascularis can occur, as also happens with long-term aminoglycoside treatment. Once again, the mechanism is not known.

Various chemoprotective agents, which have been called rescue or blocking agents, have been used in an attempt to reduce the various toxicities of this otherwise useful chemotherapeutic agent. These blocking agents include

- diuresis by salt and fluid loading
- carbonic anhydrase inhibitors – acetazolamide
- sulphur nucleophiles – which block the interaction of cisplatin with the sulphydryl groups of various enzymes
- free radical oxygen scavengers
- phosphonic acid antibiotics

It seems, as might be expected, that anything that reduces the otoneuronephrotoxic effects of this class of drugs also reduces the effectiveness of these drugs as antineoplastic agents.

SALICYLATES

Aspirin use is probably the most common cause of drug-induced auditory symptoms. In the UK an analysis of the adverse reaction register database of the two decades 1964–1984, has shown that the most commonly reported cochleotoxic effect was secondary to the salicylates. Fortunately, however, most of this is reversible, although the occasional permanent hearing loss has been reported.

The main features that develop are a high-frequency, usually pure tone tinnitus rather than a crashing broad band tinnitus, and this precedes the hearing loss. This loss is often reported as affecting the whole range of frequencies so that an audiometric 'flat' loss develops. These two symptoms nearly always recover within a few days of aspirin withdrawal. The dose required to cause these symptoms is variable, but at serum levels of 35 mg/dl (100 ml) most individuals have some symptoms.

The precise site of action of the salicylates is not known, but they may well exert a direct effect on the OHCs, although a change in the blood supply may also play a part. There is no decrease in the endocholear potential which indicates that the stria vascularis is not affected; however, the electrical and acoustic responses of the OHCs do change, suggesting that the membrane permeability of the OHC is altered and this might damage its mechanical function within the cochlear amplifier.

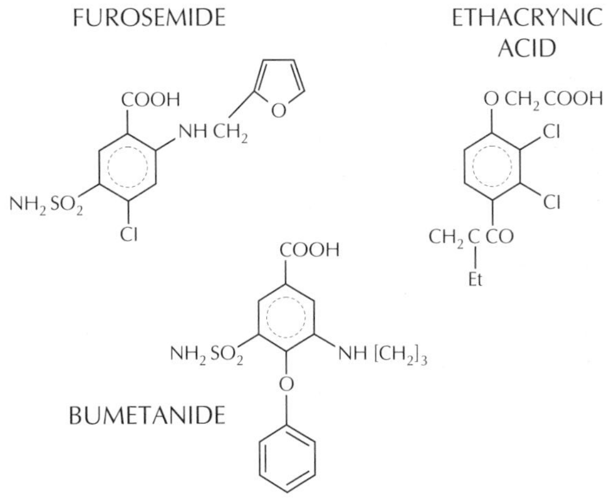

Fig 37.3 The structures of furosemide, bumetanide and ethacrynic acid. The major structural dissimilarities between the three molecules are apparent so that the uniformity of their actions, both diuretic and ototoxic, becomes more remarkable.

QUININE

Quinine is, in some ways, similar to aspirin in that it produces a hearing loss and an associated tinnitus that is usually reversible and that occurs at consistent blood plasma levels.[15]

Its mode of action is probably different to that of the salicylates. Quinine seems to affect the membrane of the OHCs directly, especially the region of the lateral cisternae, and alter the ionic properties and thereby the mechanical responses of this essential part of the cochlear amplifier (see Chapter 2).

Some years ago in the UK the formulation of generic quinine was changed from a 30 mg to a 300 mg tablet. This brought forth a small epidemic of tinnitus among the elderly who continued to take one or two tablets each night to counteract nocturnal cramps.

LOOP DIURETICS

The loop diuretics are an important group of powerful diuretics that have a widely different chemical structure (Fig 37.3) despite a similarity of their mechanism of action. The members of this group of drugs include furosemide (frusemide), ethacrynic acid, bumetanide and piretanide. The reversible toxic effect was first reported in 1965 by Maher and Schreiner[16] after intravenous administration of ethacrynic acid.

The site of the ototoxic action of the loop diuretics is the stria vascularis, which, as discussed in Chapter 1, has a marked similarity to the active cellular regions of the loop of Henle in the kidney. It is clear that the loop diuretics interfere with ion transport, and if suitable doses are given there results a precipitous fall in the endocochlear potential. There is then a slow recovery over many hours after a single dose. The decline in the endocochlear potential occurs at the same time as intercellular oedema develops in the stria vascularis (Fig 37.4), though the precise mechanism of action is not understood.

It is certainly not the strial Na/K ATPase or adenyl cyclase that is the prime target and a Na/K/Cl cotransport mechanism may be involved.

Nevertheless, after intravenous administration individuals develop a crashing tinnitus that is extremely unpleasant and they can only be reassured that it will nearly always settle over the day. Vast quantities of loop diuretics are prescribed for the elderly who are in mild congestive cardiac failure. The effects of these agents on cochlear and vestibular function is not known and has not, apparently, been researched. It is my concern that these drugs may well have a small effect on the stria vascularis and consequently upon auditory discrimination, as well as balance, in a group that are already subject to the effects of presbyacusis and presbyastasia. I suggest that an alternative diuretic be prescribed if patients have auditory or vestibular problems.

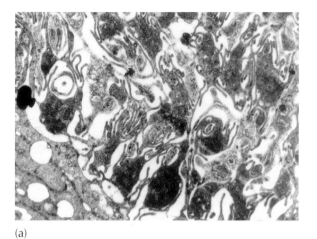

(a)

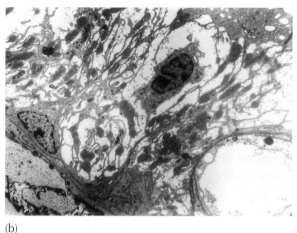

(b)

Fig 37.4 (a) Transmission electron micrograph of sections of the human stria vascularis from a patient in renal failure given large doses of intravenous loop diuretics (furosemide). There are large, oedematous intercellular spaces and the intermediate cells of the stria have shrunk down. This section should be compared with (b), which is a similar section from a guinea pig that had received intraperitoneal furosemide. The similarity of change is striking and almost certainly allows the use of this species as a model for assessing the damage that can happen in humans. (Reproduced with permission of Dr Andrew Forge.)

ERYTHROMYCIN

The macrolide antibiotics, of which erythromycin is one, have on rare occasions been associated with hearing loss. Some 15 years elapsed between the introduction of the drug and the first mention of a possible ototoxic action.[17] In most subsequent patients the hearing loss was thought to be reversible, although in one 73-year-old patient treated with erythromycin lactobionate, 500 mg 6 hourly, a right-sided hearing loss developed that failed to recover after stopping the drug.

As mentioned, the vast majority of losses are reversible, but the precise cause of the loss is unknown. It may well be that erythromycin acts more centrally, as there are many reports of disorders occurring during treatment and that are associated with the brainstem or the higher centres, such as hallucinations, behavioural disturbances, diplopia and slurred speech.

It seems poor hepatic and renal function increases the likelihood of problems with erythromycin.

THE GLYCOPEPTIDES – VANCOMYCIN

The clinical and scientific basis upon which the purported ototoxicity of this powerful antibiotic is founded is not particularly robust. Nearly all the patients in whom otoxocity has been reported have

been severely ill with overwhelming infections and have often been prescribed other ototoxic agents and have had renal failure. Indeed, animal studies in guinea pigs and gerbils have not shown any change in the cochlear hair cells when vancomycin has been used alone, although it does appear to augment the ototoxicity of gentamicin in guinea pigs.[18] It may well be that vancomycin has received an unjustified label, partly because its name suggests that it is an aminoglycoside. It does, however, appear to potentiate the ototoxic actions of the aminoglycosides and must, therefore, be used with extreme care.

Centrally acting agents

Apart from the huge range of drugs that depress consciousness and generally dull awareness, a few individual drugs seem to effect the central auditory pathways and delay brainstem auditory potentials or alter central auditory function. Chronic treatment with imipramine significantly delays the large negative wave of the middle latency responses at 17 ms (N17). 5-Hydoxytryptamine (5HT), which also causes an increase in N17 latency, enhances the effect of imipramine.

Carbamazepine seems to dampen central responses to sound by delaying the N1 response on cortical auditory evoked potential testing.

Hair cell regeneration

The specialized sensory cells in the inner ear of mammals have long been thought to be incapable of regeneration after damage, although there have been some reports of improvement in vestibular function after hair cell loss.

In fish the production of vestibular sensory cells continues throughout life so that in, for example, a baby shark there may be only 2000 vestibular hair cells whereas in old age the shark may have at least 200 000 or more hair cells.

In birds there is not the continuous production of hair cells seen in fish, but a process of regeneration of auditory and vestibular cells after damage does exist. This has been well documented following on from the earlier, pioneering work by Cotanche.[19] After structural recovery, functional recovery as measured by an improvement in the audiogram almost inevitably follows.

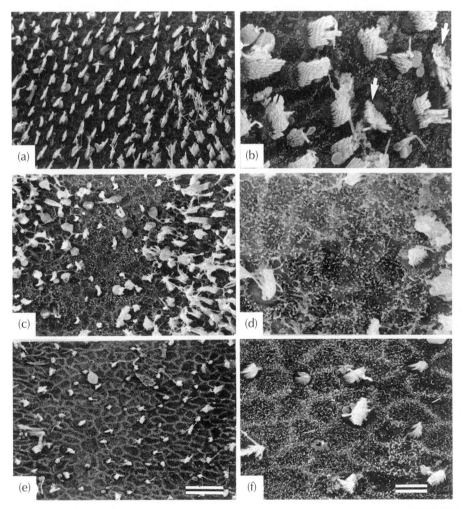

Fig 37.5 Scanning electron micrographs of the striolar region of the normal guinea pig utricular macula. (a) and (b) are controls, (c) and (d) are at 4 days and (e) and (f) are at 4 weeks after treatment with gentamicin. The normal utricle is evenly covered with hair cells. Each hair cell bundle consists of stereocilia, which increase in height in one direction towards the the single kinocilium marked. In the striolar region, hair cell orientation changes by 180°. In (b) the white arrowheads point to two hair cell bundles in opposite orientation to the rest. By 4 days after treatment hair cells within the striola are lost (c) and have been replaced by expansion of neighbouring supporting cells (d). By 4 weeks immature hair cell bundles are appearing within the region where hair cell bundle loss was earlier most pronounced. Scale bars (a), (c) and (e), 20 μm; (b), (d) and (e), 5 μm. (Reproduced with permission of Dr Andrew Forge.)

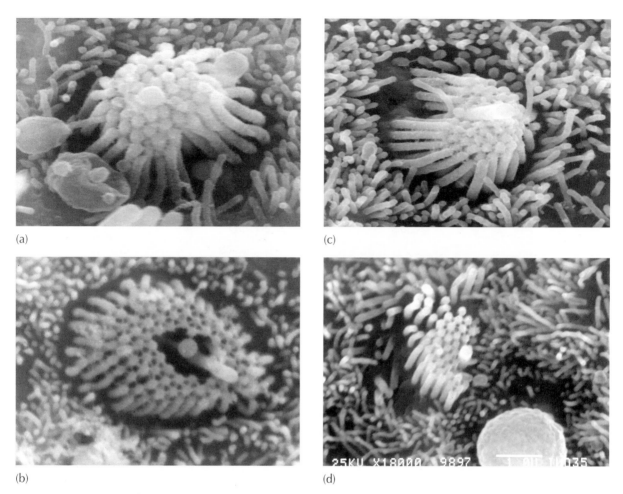

(a)

(c)

(b)

(d)

Fig 37.6 Scanning electron micrographs showing immature hair cell bundles in the guinea pig utricle 4 weeks after gentamicin administration. The bundles consist of immature stereocilia and a thicker, single kinocilium. The stereocilia are approximately of equal height and the cross link can be easily seen. The illustrations (a)–(d) show what appears to be successive stages in the development and orientation of the bundle. (Reproduced with permission of Dr Andrew Forge.)

In 1993 Forge *et al.*[20] were the first to show in mammals that after controlled chronic treatment with gentamicin there was a major loss of vestibular sensory cells, as predicted, but that with time immature hair cell bundles could be seen to have developed from the remaining mass of cells (Figs 37.5 and 37.6). These immature cells subsequently matured and, indeed, in transmission electron microscopy could be seen to have nerve terminals developing and proliferating near their lower poles.

It appears that the supporting cells in the vestibular sensory areas change in the presence of sensory cell damage and in some way become destined to differentiate into vestibular sensory cells. By the end of 1996 there was no conclusive evidence that the new hair cells had arisen through simulation of renewed cell division, although this is the intuitive route for regeneration. It is unclear whether the new sensory cells could arise from the 'reprogramming' of the supporting cells or whether some other mechanism was in process. It does seem clear, however, that once a sensory cell is set on the process of apoptosis (programmed cell death) then recovery from this state is not possible.

The other salient feature of hair cell regeneration was that by the end of 1997 no group had been able to induce regeneration in the mature organ of Corti, although this can be achieved in the developing, immature auditory system. The difference between the two systems is that the adult outer hair cell is surrounded by fluid and that the Deiter's cells are reduced to thin finger-like processes between the outer hair cell bodies. In the immature auditory system the organ of Corti is a solid mass, rather like the vestibular sensory cell region. The highly specialized arrangement of the organ of Corti in the adult is closely related to the mechanism of the cochlear amplifier, which gives the mammalian cochlea its remarkable sensitivity and frequency specificity. The price to pay for this might just be a loss of the ability to self-repair after damage. The next 20 years promises exciting discoveries that will surely lead to the ability to induce repair in the vestibular system and the possibility of some augmentation of cochlear hair cells or their associated innervation as an aid to cochlear implantation.

References

1. Hawkins JE. Drug ototoxicity. In: Kiedel WD, Neff WD eds. *Handbook of sensory physiology, vol 5.* Berlin: Springer–Verlag, 1976:707–48.
2. Stephens SDG. Some historical aspects of ototoxicity. *British Journal of Audiology* 1982; **16**:76–80.
3. Davey PG, Jabeen FJ, Harpur ES, Shenoi PM, Geddes AM. A controlled study of the reliability of pure tone audiometry for the detection of gentamicin auditory toxicity. *Journal of Laryngology and Otology* 1983; **97**:27–36.
4. Shambaugh GE, Derlacki EL, Harrison WH, *et al.* Dihydrostreptomycin deafness. *Journal of the American Medical Association* 1959; **170**:1657–60.
5. Waksman SA, Bugie E, Schatz A. Isolation of antibiotic substances from soil microorganisms with special reference to streptothricin and streptomycin. *Proceedings of the Staff Meetings of the Mayo Clinic* 1944; **19**:537–48.
6. Schacht J. Molecular mechanisms of drug induced hearing loss. *Hearing Research* 1986; **22**:297–304.
7. Barza M, Ioanniais JPA, Cappelleri JC, Lau J. Single or multiple daily doses of aminoglycosides: a meta-analysis *British Medical Journal* 1996; **312**:338–45.
8. Browning GG, Gatehouse S, Calder IT. Medical management of active chronic otitis media: a controlled study. *Journal of Laryngology and Otology* 1988; **102**:491–5.
9. Browning GG, Gatehouse S. Hearing in chronic suppurative otitis media. *Annals of Otology, Rhinology and Laryngology* 1989; **98**:245–50.
10. Bagger-Sjoback D, Bergenius J, Lundberg AM. Inner ear effects of topical gentamicin treatment in patients with Menière disease. *American Journal of Otology* 1990; **11**:406–10.
11. Odkvist LM. Middle ear ototoxic treatment for inner ear disease. *Acta Otolaryngologica* 1989; **(suppl 457)**:83–6.
12. Parnes LS, Riddell D. Irritative spontaneous nystagmus following intratympanic gentamicin for Menière's disease. *Laryngoscope* 1993; **103**:745–9.
13. Magnusson M, Padoan A, Karlberg M, Johansson R. Delayed onset of ototoxic effects of gentamicin in patients with Menière's disease. *Acta Otolaryngologica* 1991; **(suppl 485)**:120–2.
14. Küppers P, Ahrens H, Blessing R. Continuous intratympanic gentamicin infusion in Menière's disease [in German]. *HNO* 1994; **42**:429–33.
15. Alvan G, Karlsson KK, Hellgren U, Villen T. Hearing impairment related to plasma quinine levels in healthy volunteers. *British Journal of Clinical Pharmacology* 1991; **31**:409–12.
16. Maher JF, Schreiner GE. Studies on ethacrynic acid in patients with refractory edema. *Annals of Internal Medicine* 1965; **62**:15–29.
17. Mintz U, Amir J, Pinkhas J, DeVries A. Transient perceptive deafness due to erythromycin lactobionate. *Journal of the American Medical Association* 1973; **225**:1122–3.
18. Brummett RE, Fox KE, Jacobs F, Kempton JB, Stokes Z, Richmond AB. Augmented gentamicin toxicity induced by vancomycin in the guinea pig. *Archives of Otolaryngology – Head and Neck Surgery* 1990; **116**:61–4.
19. Cotanche DA. Regeneration of hair cell stereociliary bundles in the chick cochlea following severe acoustic trauma. *Hearing Research* 1987; **30**:181–95.
20. Forge A, Li L, Corwin JT, Nevill G. Ultrastructural evidence for hair cell regeneration in the mammalian inner ear. *Science* 1993; **259**:1616–9.

CHAPTER 38

Vestibular disorders

HAROLD LUDMAN

Vertigo is defined as an illusion or hallucination of movement. The majority of the causes of vertigo lie in the peripheral vestibular system, by which is meant the labyrinthine receptors and their first order neuronal supply, together with the vestibular neurons in the brainstem. The assessment and investigation of this symptom is extensively explored in Chapters 5 and 14.

Vestibular disorders may be classified as extrinsic, peripheral or central.

Extrinsic vestibular disorders

Extrinsic vestibular disorders are those in which the vestibular apparatus is affected either peripherally or centrally by some disturbance not arising in the system itself. They include the toxic effect of drugs and any systemic disorder that prevents the normal provision of metabolic requirements to the labyrinth or the brain – disorders such as anaemia, hypoglycaemia and hypotension. These are discussed in Chapter 14. Many of the causes of sudden sensorineural deafness, discussed in Chapter 36, can also affect the vestibular system, with the sudden onset of the characteristic vertigo of vestibular failure. Also in this group of extrinsic causes is erosion of the labyrinth and the spread of infection from the adjacent middle ear cleft. This is discussed with the complications of middle ear disease (see Chapter 29). Sudden vestibular failure from injury to the labyrinth, in skull fracture, has also been described (see Chapter 32).

Also classified as extrinsic vestibular disorders are the syndromes of pressured-induced vertigo. This term can describe a group of 'extrinsic' labyrinthine disorders provoked by pressure changes. Included among them are perilymph fistulae and vertigo provoked by sound (Tullio); external air pressure changes (Hennebert) and Valsalva's manoeuvre. Appreciation of their clinical features is easier after studying the intrinsic peripheral labyrinthine disorders, so their description is relegated to a later part of the chapter.

Intrinsic vestibular disorders – peripheral vestibular disorders

Under this heading we are concerned with the main topic of this chapter – a small group of disorders intrinsic to the peripheral vestibular system in that the immediate cause of the vertigo is a lesion arising within that system and peculiar to it. The principle conditions to be considered are Menière's disease; sudden vestibular failure and benign paroxysmal positional vertigo.

Menière's disease

This condition derives its name from the Paris physician Prosper Menière, who first described it. In 1861, the last year of his life, Menière drew attention to the syndrome characterized by paroxysmal attacks of vertigo associated with vomiting, tinnitus and deafness. Menière also showed, from a postmortem study (but not actually of the disease bearing his name), that symptoms, which we now readily associate with vestibular disease, do arise from damage to the labyrinth. Indeed this was the first time that such violent systemic symptoms had been connected with derangement of the tiny structures of the inner ear. Menière wrote 'la lesion reside dans les canaux demicirculaires'.

For pathological reasons, discussed below, the term 'endolymphatic hydrops' may be used to describe the disorder. If the condition is secondary to known diseases of the otic capsule, it may be called Menière's *disorder* or *syndrome*. The term Menière's *disease* is reserved for idiopathic endolymphatic hydrops.

AETIOLOGY AND PATHOLOGY

The pathological features yet to be described may be secondary to a number of diseases of the otic capsule. These include syphilis, trauma, infection – viral or bacterial – chronic suppurative otitis media and otosclerosis. These account for possibly 25 per cent of cases of endolymphatic hydrops. The remaining 75 per cent are idiopathic and hence Menière's disease by definition. The incidence is not known for certain, but is thought to be about 15 per 100 000 of population per year, with a prevalence of about 200 per 100 000 in Europe and the USA. The disease may occur at any age, but the first attack usually strikes between the ages of 30 and 60 years. It is rare but not unknown in childhood, and it does not often arise for the first time after the age of 60 years. The disease is equally common in the two sexes. There is a family history in around 10 per cent of patients.

The condition is usually unilateral, but several long-term studies indicate that it is bilateral more often than was formerly believed. After 2 years the disease is bilateral in only 15 per cent of patients, but after 20 years at least 40 per cent show disease in both ears. Some authors have suggested that the incidence of bilateral affection may be even higher. The uncertainty about the frequency of bilaterality can be partly attributed to different criteria used by different workers for recognizing involvement of the second ear. Some accounts depend on pure tone audiometric evidence of hearing impairment, whereas in others the second ear has been deemed abnormal, despite good hearing, if there have been radiological changes considered typical of the condition – similar to those of the diseased ear – or if there have been electrocochleographic abnormalities. Rehydration of the cochlea by the drug acetazolamide may unmask 'latent' hydrops in up to 5 per cent of apparently normal opposite ears.

The principal morphological change in Menière's disease is an increase in volume of part of the endolymphatic space – hence the name 'endolymphatic hydrops'. This was recognized for the first time in 1938 from two temporal bone studies by Hallpike and Cairns. Whether the distension is associated with raised endolymphatic pressure or with lowered perilymphatic pressure, and precisely how the distension is related to the symptoms is still unknown. The endolymphatic distension first affects the scala media of the cochlea and the saccule, which together constitute the *pars inferior* of the membranous labyrinth. The *pars superior*, composed of the utricle and semicircular canals, is less affected, perhaps because its walls are thicker. The dilatation may be so extreme that the scala vestibuli is completely filled by the cochlear duct into which Reissner's membrane bulges, and the saccule may fill the vestibule and abut against the inner surface of the stapes footplate. Reissner's membrane sometimes herniates through the helicotrema into the scala tympani, and the distended saccule may bulge into, and obstruct, the lateral semicircular canal. In places there may be dilatations, or outpouchings, of the membranous labyrinth. Their significance is uncertain as they are also found in some ears not affected by Menière's disease. Ruptures of the membranous labyrinth are probably an important finding, and these are seen most commonly in Reissner's membrane. In long-standing disease there is atrophy of sensory structures.

Menière's disease is probably the result of some disorder of endolymph homeostasis and one current view is that it may arise from a defect in normal endolymph absorption by the endolymphatic system. Experimental destruction of the sac or obstruction of its duct has produced hydrops in guinea pigs, cats and rabbits, after a time that is species dependent. However, perversely, neither vestibular symptoms nor audiometric changes develop despite the soft-tissue changes.

Endolymph is maintained by the stria vascularis of the cochlea and the dark cell regions of the vestibular labyrinth. There is no flow of endolymph per se, although ions may move by diffusion through it. Furthermore, communication between the cochlear endolymph and that in the saccule and the rest of the vestibular labyrinth is very restricted as the ductus reuniens, which links the two systems, is extremely narrow and rather long. Alterations in the function of the stria vascularis and the dark cell regions of the vestibular labyrinth result in alterations of the ionic environment of the endolymph with probable alterations in the endocochlear potential (reflected by changes in the summating potential on the electrocochleogram) and osmotic changes between endolymph and perilymph, which consequently cause the feature of endolymphatic hydrops, which is a non-specific histological change seen in many end-stage chronic ear diseases.

Radiological examination of the temporal bones of patients with Menière's disease show certain features that are present more often than in normal controls. These changes include hypocellularity of the mastoid, anterior displacement of the sigmoid sinus and a shorter and straighter vestibular aqueduct than is normal. CT scanning has shown narrowing, even ablation, of the vestibular aqueduct in a statistically significant number of patients. It may well be that the disposition to Menière's disease is associated with such changes in a mastoid, which are not causal. There is also an association with otosclerosis. This may be coincidental but it could possibly be due, in some cases, to the massive otosclerotic deposits (see Chapter 33) that are found in these cases. Many factors influence the maintenance of the endolymph.

Immune complex disorders have been implicated by the finding of raised complement levels, and immune complexes, in the serum of patients with the disease, and immunological implications have increasing importance in most workers' ideas. There may be hormonal factors – the disease is more common in myxoedematous patients than in the euthyroid population. Recent work suggests that the familial form of the disease (from 2.5 to 12 per cent) might be due to a genetic abnormality on chromosome 6. For many years there have been theories about an aetiology based on changes in, or failure to control, labyrinthine blood flow. Some ideas have been based on the effects of ischaemia of the stria vascularis. It has been argued that this could result in the accumulation of metabolites of small molecular size emanating from a relatively anoxic cochlea, and that the increased osmotic potential created by these ionic particles in the endolymph would suck fluid from the perilymphatic compartment. It has also been suggested that changes in the microcirculation could cause engorgement and hence obstruction to venous return from the paravestibular canalicular vein. Clearly, there could be many ways to explain deviations from normal in the microcirculation, and especially in the venous drainage, of the labyrinth.

The cause of the symptoms that characterize the attacks is uncertain. One theory that is difficult to sustain is that ruptures of the membranous labyrinth allow contamination of perilymph with potassium-rich endolymph. It seems more likely that some alteration to the blood supply or to the delivery of nutrients to, or removal of byproducts from, the stria vascularis or dark cell regions of the vestibular labyrinth, or both, results in the subsequent alteration in the constituents of the endolymph, which brings about the attacks of hearing loss, tinnitus, vertigo and the feelings of pressure in the affected ear. It is also quite clear that the variations in this disturbance to the blood supply to the cochlear or the vestibular side of the labyrinth can be the cause

of the wide variation in symptoms that are found in any large group of patients and that are discussed further on in this chapter. A problem that any otolaryngologist has with understanding the process of Menière's disease is that the sensory cells of hearing and balance are remarkably sensitive and the amount of distortion required to produce a symptom is disproportionately small compared with the central perception of a change in hearing, tinnitus or vertigo. It will be recalled from the chapters on the anatomy and physiology that minute changes in endolymphatic pressure or distortion of the sensory hair cells is enough to cause loss of the frequency tuning curves in the cochlea or to stimulate vestibular sensory cells in the vestibular labyrinth. It has been shown, from the assessment of the personality traits of patients with Menière's disease, that this group comprises patients who tend to have a highly structured and particularly tidy way of life, with predetermined levels of achievement, a neat and tidy approach to their environment and a feeling of frustration when their particular life patterns are disrupted. This is similar (but not the same) personality profile to those who suffer from migraine and, indeed, there is a strong family cross-correlation between the disorders.

The morphological changes seen in the histology of end-stage disease might represent an attempt by the membranous labyrinth to overcome the minor osmotic differences between normal perilymph and ionically altered endolymph, which result from failure of homeostasis.

CLINICAL FEATURES

Menière's disease is characterized by attacks of paroxysmal vertigo associated with deafness and tinnitus. The attacks occur at any time, often without warning, although premonitory symptoms in the form of a sensation of pressure in the ear and in the side of the head and neck are common. A single episode of vertigo may be followed by a long period of freedom; but often a 'cluster' of attacks occurs over a period of weeks or months to be followed by a long period of remission before the next cluster. This tendency to long remission has always made it difficult to assess the value of treatment. The vertigo of each attack is violent and prostrating, and is usually associated with nausea and vomiting. The sensation is most often one of rotation, but linear movement or side to side swaying may be described. Very rarely, brief sudden falling attacks occur. In these so called *utricular crises* the patient feels as if pole-axed. It is unusual for the typical vertiginous episode to last for less than half an hour, and rare for it to persist for longer than 12 hours.

Occasionally, frequently recurring episodes may suggest to the patient an impression of much longer lasting vertigo. During an attack the victim is grossly ataxic and cannot stand, but when the vertigo ceases normal balance is rapidly regained. Loss of consciousness is very rare indeed in Menière's disease and should always suggest the possibility of epilepsy.

The deafness is a fluctuating sensorineural loss associated with distortion and intolerance of loud noises. Episodes of impaired hearing may precede the first attack of vertigo, but the symptoms often occur together, although the vertigo is so all-consuming and distressing an experience that its effects may prevent recollection of the lesser symptom of impaired hearing. After and between attacks, the hearing loss, which is at first for low tones, improves – even to a normal level. During remission this improvement is maintained, but when the disease is active the hearing again deteriorates, with more marked deafness just before and during each episode of vertigo. This fluctuation in hearing level is characteristic, as is the discomfort produced in the ear by clattering crockery and violin music, for example. Music may be unbearably discordant, with a higher pitch in the affected ear (disharmonic diplacusis). If the disease progresses, the hearing inexorably deteriorates over years, with less and less recovery between the clusters of attacks. Eventually hearing becomes impaired at all frequencies, with a flat audiometric pattern. The tinnitus is low pitched, rumbling or roaring, and is associated in severity with the degree of hearing loss, changing in intensity and sometimes in pitch before an attack of vertigo. These typical attacks have been designated by the American Academy of Ophthalmology and Otology (AAOO), as *definitive* attacks of vertigo. The AAOO also recognizes so-called *adjunctive* vertiginous symptoms. These consist of long-lasting feelings of unsteadiness, often with a sensation of tilting or floating. They are believed to arise from permanent irreversible damage to the vestibular sensory structures and they can be considered as symptoms of vestibular deficit – a state that can be expected, especially in bilateral Menière's disease, after many years. It is very important to recognize the gradual change of emphasis in the vestibular symptoms of long-standing disease from one of erratic overactivity to one of sensory deficit. Without that recognition, treatment decisions and prognostic expectations will be irrational (see Chapter 15).

INVESTIGATION

A careful detailed history is the most important guide to correct diagnosis, although full neuro-oto-logical assessment is necessary for confirmation and exclusion of other possible causes.

General examination

General examination between attacks will reveal normal stance and gait, without spontaneous nystagmus or central nervous system abnormalities. *Positional testing* rarely provokes either vertigo or nystagmus. *Otoscopy* nearly always reveals normal tympanic membranes, although the disorder can arise secondarily after fenestration or stapedectomy operations. The tuning fork tests show a sensorineural hearing loss.

Tests of auditory function

Pure tone audiometry (see Chapter 4) shows that the sensorineural hearing loss is predominantly low tone in the early stages. The fluctuation in level can usually be observed by serial audiometry over weeks or months, and improvement in the audiometric threshold is a useful diagnostic feature. Other tests confirm that the hearing loss is sensory rather than neural. Recruitment is almost always full, adaptation slight and speech discrimination relatively good.

Electrocochleography

Electrocochleography (see Chapter 4) shows changes that are characteristic of, and probably diagnostic of, endolymphatic hydrops. There is broadening of the summating potential (SP)/action potential (AP) wave form due to a relative enhancement of the summating potential (SP) (see Chapter 3). The normal SP/AP ratio is around 20 per cent. In an ear with hydrops, the ratio is often as high as 30 per cent (Fig 38.1). If the cochlear microphonic is separated from the trace, it is found to be small and distorted. These abnormalities may be reversed towards normal by dehydration of the cochlea after the administration of oral glycerol. This glycerol dehydration test is performed by administering glycerol, flavoured with orange juice, by mouth in a dose of 1–5 ml/kg. A pure tone audiogram and electrocochleography are carried out before ingestion of the dose, and again 1.5–2 hours later. Plasma osmolality should also be measured as there can be no effect on the cochlea unless that rises by more than 10 mOsm/kg. A variant of this test involves overhydrating the cochlea by the administration of acetazolamide. This drug lowers plasma osmolatity and, in patients with Menière's disease, causes an increase in pure tone audiometric threshold and enlargement of the SP on the electrocochleogram. It must be noted that electro-

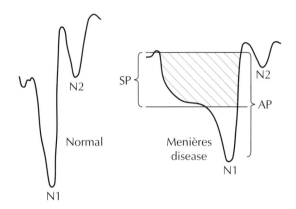

Fig 38.1 Electrocochleogram in Menière's disease.

cochleographic changes are found only in the presence of an abnormal audiogram. The normal responses found in remission do not exclude the presence of Menière's disease.

Caloric responses

Caloric responses are abnormal in about three-quarters of patients. The commonest pattern is a canal paresis (see Chapter 5), but a directional preponderance towards the normal ear or a combination of reduced canal sensitivity and directional preponderance may be found.

Differential diagnosis

Menière's disease must be separated from all the other causes of vertigo listed at the start of this chapter. In particular it must be distinguished from central causes of vertigo and from other peripheral labyrinthine diseases – infection spreading from the middle ear cleft, benign paroxysmal positional vertigo and sudden vestibular failure. Of special importance is the distinction from acoustic neuroma, a possibility to consider whenever unilateral sensorineural deafness is under discussion.

Central causes of vertigo do not generally produce such clear-cut paroxysmal attacks as those of Menière's disease, and they are often associated with persisting imbalance, which is never found in Menière's disease. Examination may expose spontaneous nystagmus, which is not to be expected between attacks of Menière's disease, and this may well have central characteristics (see Chapter 3). Often, other neurological abnormalities will be found. Unconsciousness suggests epilepsy.

Infective erosion of the labyrinth should be recognized by the otoscopic evidence of middle ear disease. If there is any suspicion of cholesteatoma, provoked, say, by the appearance of an attic crust, that should be the presumed cause until it can definitely be excluded by an exploratory operation. This principle should apply to vertigo when middle ear disease is suspected.

Positional vertigo of the benign paroxysmal type (see below) is distinguished by the very brief duration of each attack – seconds only – and the absence of auditory symptoms.

Vestibular failure (see below) can be recognized by the story of much longer lasting vertigo, worst at onset, with gradual steady recovery over more than a week. Indeed, the duration of continuous vertigo is an important aspect in distinguishing these two disorders from Menière's disease.

Acoustic neuroma must be seriously considered and excluded in every instance of supposed Menière's disease. A small proportion, about 5 per cent, of acoustic neuromas masquerade as Menière's disease. The diagnostic features of acoustic neuroma are discussed in Chapter 39. As a counsel of perfection, any patient thought to have Menière's disease ought to have radiological examination of the internal auditory meatuses, preferably by MRI. Features in the history that are not typical, such as periods of imbalance, and any neuro-otological findings that are not expected, such as audiological evidence in favour of a neural lesion (absent recruitment, pathological adaptation or poor speech discrimination), are compelling reasons for insisting on MRI examination, with injection of gadolinium, even if the internal auditory canals appear radiologically normal on conventional X-ray imaging.

Menière's disease may be confused with other disorders such as migraine affecting the inner ear blood supply, and other forms of hydrops affecting only the vestibular labyrinth or just the cochlea (see below). In other words Menière's disease as an idiopathic condition should not be diagnosed until hydrops secondary to other causes has been excluded.

OTHER FORMS OF HYDROPS

Lermoyez syndrome

Lermoyez syndrome is a rare variation of Menière's disease in which the symptoms arise in the reverse order. Progressive deterioration of hearing is followed by episodic vertigo, at which time the hearing recovers. Patients with Lermoyez syndrome often give a history of migraine. The course of the condition resembles that of Menière's disease proper.

Cochlear hydrops

Cochlear hydrops is a relatively common disorder that is characterized by the sudden development of unilateral hearing loss and tinnitus. It may be due to obstruction to the ductus reuniens, causing hydrops confined to the cochlear duct, or to an isolated disorder of the stria vascularis. The impairment of hearing is found to be due to a low tone, recruiting sensorineural deafness. The level of the hearing fluctuates and, indeed, the symptoms are those of endolymphatic hydrops affecting only the cochlea. Most patients probably recover spontaneously, although a number later experience episodic vertigo and develop typical Menière's disease as the dark cell regions of the vestibular labyrinth become involved.

Vestibular hydrops

It is believed, but not known with certainty, that, in a similar way, hydrops may affect only the vestibular system, perhaps if the utriculo-endolymphatic valve is deficient, with a clinical pattern of intermittent episodic vertigo identical to that of Menière's disease. Auditory function is found to be normal, whereas vestibular testing shows the abnormalities expected in Menière's disease. Some patients with this pattern of episodic vertigo can probably be found among members of the category described as vestibular neuronitis.

TREATMENT

Any discussion about the success of treatment in Menière's disease must be prefaced by the warning that the natural history of a disease with a spontaneous remission rate of 60–80 per cent for vertigo, and a tendency for remission as a placebo effect following attentive care by the physician bedevils attempts at assessment and trials of treatment. At the time of writing, no form of medication has been shown, in a way that has satisfied later statistical criticisms, to influence the long-term course of the disease, although many drugs may be helpful in symptomatic control of vertigo.

Medical treatment

The drugs used in the treatment of Menière's disease are chosen to control the vestibular symptoms – vestibular sedatives – or are selected for a possible effect on a particular mechanism thought to cause endolymphatic hydrops. Most drugs have several actions, and in most instances it is not known which effect is beneficial.

Vestibular sedatives

Drugs with antihistamine properties, including phenothiazines and especially those active against H3-histamine receptors in the brainstem, are strong vestibular suppressants. Prochlorperazine is a frequently prescribed example. Antihistamines such as promethazine theoclate (Avomine) and promethazine hydrochloride (Phenergan) are also useful as vestibular sedatives. Diazepam may usefully relieve some of the attendant anxiety and is also a gamma-aminobutyric acid (GABA) receptor inhibitor, decreasing activity in the vestibular nuclei. Its relative clonazepam has similar actions. Cinnarizine is a valuable vestibular suppressant with several actions. It is a calcium antagonist and an antihistamine, thereby reducing the responses of histamine receptors in the vestibular nuclei. In addition it blocks 5-hydroxytryptamine (5HT) receptors and reduces blood viscosity. Flunarizine works in similar ways. Any of these drugs may suppress symptoms sufficiently during an active phase, but must be withdrawn during periods of remission.

Drugs and regimes used on a theoretically aetiological basis are aimed at the following possible causes.

- **Vascular**. Numerous vasodilator drugs are available. Betahistine hydrochloride releases histamine in the body, when taken by mouth, and has been shown to increase cochlear blood flow. It causes vasodilatation in the stria vascularis and lowers endolymph pressure. This drug also has vestibular sedative capabilities as a powerful H3-antagonist (although to complicate the issue still further, it is a weak H1-receptor stimulator and H2-agonist). Carbon dioxide inhalations also induce strong cerebral vasodilatation. Many other vasodilator drugs such as nicotinic acid are in common use. Lipoflavonoid capsules have advocates. The active constituent is eriodictyol glycoside (lemon bioflavonoid complex), a histidine decarboxylase blocking agent and hence an antidote to the liberation of toxic amounts of histamine from the capillary bed. As with all other forms of medication, there is no evidence of results better than the natural history of the disease.
- **Electrolyte water balance**. Fluid and salt restricted diets have long been recommended and adherence to a salt-limited diet may be of value. This regime can be accompanied by the use of diuretic drugs such as hydrochlorthiazide. In theory the loop diuretics should not be prescribed, as they themselves affect the stria vascularis and dark cell regions of the vestibular labyrinth. Theoretical support for such a regime

can be found in the known fact that dehydration with osmotic diuretics such as glycerol is often followed, within hours, by audiometrically confirmable hearing improvement, albeit temporary. Oral urea in a dose of 25 g per day is an effective osmotic diuretic used by some otologists, especially for those female patients who suffer more during the premenstrual phase.

- **Immunological**. Rational medication directed at possible immune complex causes includes the prescription of systemic steroids and injections of dexamethasone through the tympanic membrane into the middle ear cavity. Plasmapheresis to remove circulating immune complexes from the bloodstream has support in desperate instances of rapidly deteriorating hearing loss. These are often instances in which the true diagnosis of classic idiopathic hydrops is not secure, and may be a subgroup of patients suffering from other immunological disorders.

Surgical treatment

Relief from vertigo can be achieved most certainly by total ablation of the erratically active labyrinth; but that entails total loss of hearing in the affected ear. This may be acceptable in those patients with severe deafness and distortion, whose hearing is no more than a painful shred, but in many others the hearing is too valuable to sacrifice. This is particularly so when there is any doubt about the integrity of the other ear. As has been indicated, it is impossible to be sure that an apparently normal opposite ear is not the seat of latent disease, which will become manifest many years in the future. Some patients, particularly those over the age of 60 years, do not compensate fully for the loss of one labyrinth. Others, who may have lost a labyrinth earlier in life, suffer imbalance from progressive loss of compensation as they grow older (see Chapter 15). For all these reasons, the role of radical surgical treatment by labyrinthectomy is limited.

CONSERVATIVE SURGICAL TREATMENT

Much attention has been given to the development of so-called 'conservative' operative procedures that are aimed at relieving vertigo while attempting to preserve auditory function. These operations are in two main groups: those addressing a presumed cause of hydrops and those eliminating or reducing vestibular nuclear excitation by the labyrinth, without damaging the cochlea.

Some of these procedures are obsolete. After enjoying a few years of vogue attention, they are now of only historical interest. Others are of dubious

rationality. They are mentioned or described here (bracketed in lists below) so that the reader will appreciate the extent to which ideas have changed, to provide an historical perspective against which to view current practice and to testify to the difficulty of assessing the results of any procedure. It is axiomatic in surgical practice that profusion of surgical solutions is evidence of the efficacy of none.

Operations in the first group include

- endolymphatic sac decompression
- [cochleostomy (cochlear endolymphatic shunt)]
- [cochlear dialysis]
- [sacculotomy]
- grommet insertion
- [cervical sympathectomy]

The second group of 'conservative' procedures includes

- vestibular nerve division
- [ultrasonic destruction of the vestibular labyrinth]
- intratympanic injection of ototoxic drugs

At the time of writing, the most favoured procedure in the first group is decompression or drainage of the endolymphatic sac, and in the second group vestibular nerve section.

Saccus decompression operations

Operations on the saccus endolymphaticus were first described in the 1920s, but their use lapsed until the renaissance of saccus surgery began over 25 years ago. Since then they have become the most commonly applied techniques of conservative treatment for Menière's disease. It is hoped that by dealing fundamentally with the main functional defect of the disorder the natural history of the disease may be altered, with preservation of hearing otherwise doomed to inexorable deterioration – this in addition to eliminating or diminishing the attacks of vertigo and reducing tinnitus.

The technique by which the operation is performed involves exposing the endolymphatic sac through a cortical mastoidectomy, in front of the sigmoid sinus and just below the posterior semicircular canal (Fig 38.2). The endolymphatic sac can usually be found without difficulty by following the posterior fossa dura, deep to Trautmann's triangle, forwards and medially, using a diamond paste burr to avoid damage to the dura. If a bulging sinus prevents easy access to the posterior fossa dura, it may be compressed by developing a trapdoor of thin bone on its surface, on which to press medially with a blunt dissector (Fig 38.3). The saccus can be recognized by its thick texture and whitish colour, which contrasts with the thin bluish dura above and

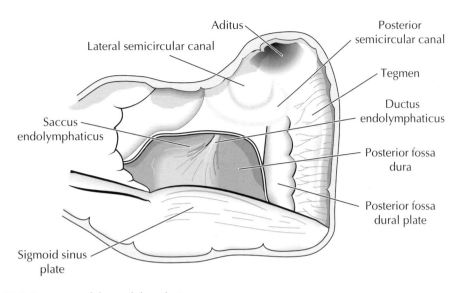

Fig 38.2 Exposure of the endolymphatic sac.

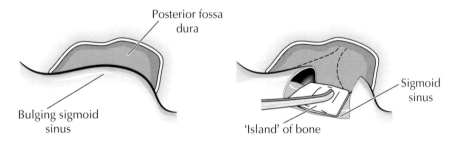

Fig 38.3 Saccus decompression – displacement of a bulging sigmoid sinus.

below its extent. It can be defined positively by following it medially and identifying the ductus, which is the only structure in this region passing from the dural surface into the posterior surface of the petrous temporal bone (Fig 38.4). When exposed the saccus can be left untouched, or it may be opened with a sharp knife into the mastoidectomy cavity. In the earlier days of this procedure, it was usual to place a shunt tube between the lumen of the saccus and the subarachnoid space in the posterior cranial fossa, even though it has been known from earlier structural studies that any lumen in the sac is multiloculated and of minute dimensions. If the saccus is opened, a tube or a sheet of silastic may be placed from the mastoid cavity into its lumen. It has also been suggested that it is possible to cannulate the ductus and to place within its lumen a valved tube designed to open in a controlled way as endolymphatic pressure rises, despite the refuting histological evidence. It is by no means certain that different ways of handling the saccus affect the outcome of the operation. Perhaps this is

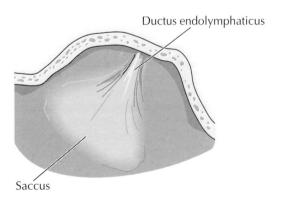

Fig 38.4 Saccus decompression – demonstration of ductus passing into posterior surface of temporal bone.

not surprising, as the effect of saccus decompression surgery in helping to cure the disease is not well understood and sham operations seem to be just as good at preventing the vertigo.

The main risk of operation is to the hearing. Cochlear function may be destroyed if, accidentally, the posterior semicircular canal is breached during exposure of the saccus. This can best be avoided by a detailed understanding of the anatomy and by working close to the dura with very small burrs. It is undesirable to identify the canal by 'blue lining'.

The results of saccus surgery reveal that overall about 80 per cent of patients should be relieved from attacks of vertigo. It is only fair to comment that belief in the value of this operation is not universal, as a similar number of patients seem to benefit from most procedures offered for this disease – even so-called 'placebo' operations. The benefits are likely to be greater early in the disease, while the hearing is fluctuating. Fifty per cent of patients at this stage gain useful improvement in hearing, but only 25 per cent report improvement in tinnitus. In an attempt to standardize the reporting of results, the AAOO has defined significant vestibular improvement as relief from attacks for at least 10 times the average interval between those attacks before treatment. Four categories of result are defined:

- relief from vertigo, as defined above, with improved hearing
- relief from vertigo with no change in hearing
- relief from vertigo with poorer hearing
- failure to control vertigo

Predictive tests for the results of saccus surgery include electrocochleography and its response to the glycerol dehydration test, described earlier. The greater the enhancement of the SP before operation, the less chance there is of benefit from operation. The improvements of pure tone hearing threshold and the response of the SP seem to give an indication of the possible benefits of saccus decompression, but if there is no improvement with dehydration, it is possible that the plasma osmolality has not been increased sufficiently (by at least 10 mOsm/kg) to affect the endolymph. No sensible prediction can be made from a negative response to dehydration, unless plasma osmolality is measured at the same time as the post-ingestion audiometric measurements are made.

Grommet insertion

Placing a grommet into the tympanic membrane through a myringotomy incision has had advocates for many years. This rather unlikely procedure derives from a theory that hydrops might follow intermittent obstruction of the auditory tube – causing a pull on the round window – in patients with abnormally narrow cochlear aqueducts. Although the benefits may stem from the 'placebo' effect of interference, the procedure has the merit of safety and simplicity.

Vestibular nerve section

Division of the vestibular nerve, to prevent abnormal and erratic sensory labyrinthine stimuli from reaching the vestibular neurons, can be performed through a number of different routes: posterior fossa, middle fossa, retrolabyrinthine and retrosigmoid.

Posterior fossa
A standard neurosurgical approach to the posterior cranial fossa by the neurosurgeon allows division of vestibular fibres, with attempted preservation of the cochlear nerve.

Middle fossa
The extradural approach to the middle cranial fossa allows access to the internal acoustic meatus through its roof. The vestibular nerve and Scarpa's ganglion can be excised. The procedure has some risks, especially of damage to the facial nerve and to hearing. The skull is opened above the root of the zygoma by removing a large rectangle of squamous temporal bone. The middle fossa dura is then elevated from the anterior surface of the petrous bone and retracted with the temporal lobe above it. The elevation must not extend forwards and medially too far lest the middle meningeal artery be damaged. The superior petrosal sinus comes into view and guides the dissection over the bulge of the arcuate eminence, overlying the dome of the superior semicircular canal. The roof of the internal meatus lies anteromedially to this structure, and drilling downwards in this position will open the meatus by removal of bone with diamond paste burrs.

Retrolabyrinthine
The posterior fossa dura is exposed, as it is for saccus decompression, and an extradural dissection medial to the labyrinth leads to the porus of the internal acoustic meatus, where the vestibular portion of the VIIIth nerve is identified and divided. The problem with this approach, as with the neurosurgical suboccipital approach, is that the inferior vestibular nerve and the cochlear nerve are not always easily separable. Cochlear nerve damage is then a risk, and there is also a chance that vestibular section may be incomplete.

Retrosigmoid
This route entails a neurosurgical exposure of the porus of the internal meatus, by a suboccipital route, just behind the sigmoid sinus. The bony posterior wall of the internal acoustic meatus is then removed with a drill as far laterally as the fovea for the endolymphatic sac, on the posterior surface of the temporal bone. This exposes the contents of the

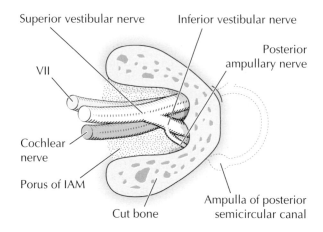

Fig 38.5 Contents of internal auditory meatus (IAM) after drilling away its posterior wall.

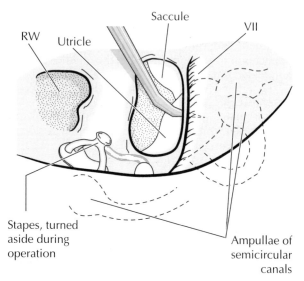

Fig 38.6 Transtympanic labyrinthectomy.

meatus as far laterally as the origin of the singular nerve from the inferior vestibular nerve before it enters the singular canal on its way to the ampulla of the posterior semicircular canal (Fig 38.5). The superior vestibular nerve is divided. The singular nerve is divided as is the inferior vestibular nerve.

RADICAL SURGICAL TREATMENT

Total destruction of the membranous labyrinth offers the most certain guarantee of relief from the attacks of vertigo of Menière's disease. This may be achieved by virtually any operation that transgresses the membranous labyrinth. There will be almost inevitable total loss of cochlear and vestibular function.

Transtympanic access through a tympanotomy operation allows removal of the stapes from the oval window, after dividing the stapediovestibular ligament. A specially shaped 'double-angled' hook is introduced into the vestibule, and the utricle and saccule are impaled and removed (Fig 38.6). The end of the hook is then introduced upwards and anteriorly into the ampullae of the lateral and the superior semicircular canals, and then downwards and backwards into the ampulla of the posterior canal. Instillation of alcohol into the vestibule has been advocated, but that is potentially dangerous and is not necessary as gentamicin can be used in the same way without the risks. Some workers advise drilling between the oval window and round window as the first intratympanic manoeuvre. Before replacing the tympanomeatal flap the oval window can be sealed by replacing the undamaged stapes.

Transmastoid access through a postaural incision allows exposure of the lateral semicircular canal. The canal is opened and its membranous contents

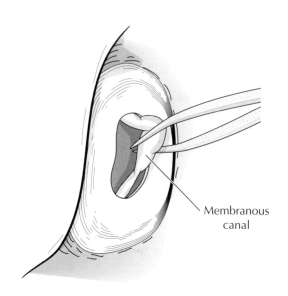

Fig 38.7 Transmastoid labyrinthectomy – through lateral semicircular canal.

removed with watchmaker's forceps (Fig 38.7). No further damage is needed, but, if desired, the posterior and the superior canals can be opened and their contents extirpated. Subsequently the vestibule may be opened to allow removal of its contents. A full vestibular labyrinthectomy should leave no potentially active vestibular neurons.

Medical labyrinthectomy: medical destruction of the vestibular labyrinth was in earlier days achieved by systemic intramuscular streptomycin, 2 g daily, to destroy selectively the dark cells in the ampullary cristae and maculae of the saccule and utricle. Deafness frequently occurred. In a revival of this form of treatment, labyrinthectomy is achieved by the local application of gentamicin within the middle ear. The aminoglycoside is absorbed through the round and oval windows. Various regimens exist, but the commonest is the filling of the middle ear with a solution of 30 mg/ml gentamicin on a daily basis for a variable period.

Choice of treatment

It is traditionally and generally accepted that after medical treatment 80 per cent of patients can live with their symptoms and confidently follow their normal employment. Of course, activities in which balance is important, such as climbing scaffolding or working at heights, must be avoided. There is also a view that if operations such as those on the saccus endolymphaticus do modify the natural history of the disease, they should be offered early, in place of medical treatment, before the hearing is much affected, even though evidence that hearing can be protected is lacking. Conventionally, however, surgical treatment will be considered when a medical regime has failed to control symptoms – that is when the vertigo is disabling and the distortion of hearing is intolerable. No promises of hearing improvement should be offered.

Trial of medical treatment

In the average patient the initial attack of acute vertigo is treated with bedrest. If vomiting allows, a vestibular sedative is given orally, for example, dimenhydrinate tablets, 50 mg 4-hourly. If vomiting prevents oral administration, the drug can be given intramuscularly or intravenously or can be taken as suppositories. A low-salt diet and fluid restriction may be helpful. Once the acute phase is over and the patient is ambulant, cinnarizine in a dose of 45–90 mg per day or prochlorperazine 30 mg per day can be used orally for a short time only, as the sedatives prevent central compensation. The patient must be warned against the side effects of drowsiness. An alternative initial regime after recovery from the acute attack is by the oral administration of betahistine, 8–16 mg three times a day. This drug must not be prescribed if there is a history of gastric ulceration or asthma and, theoretically, it should not be administered concurrently with an antihistamine, as the latter would tend to negate the pharmacological action of betahistine. Failure to control with either of these regimes is an indication for a trial of salt restriction and the administration of bendrofluazide as a diuretic, 5 mg daily. A potassium supplement should also be used if long-term treatment

with a thiazide is contemplated. Medication is generally discontinued when the condition becomes quiescent. At the first instance of impending recurrence, suggested by increase in tinnitus or deafness, the drug of choice is again taken in full dosage.

In every patient psychological support is of great value, diazepam may be useful for sedation and its other effects. Many patients fear serious intracranial disease or impending cerebral catastrophe, and reassurance, with an explanation of the nature of the disorder, works wonders. If vertigo is uncontrollable *surgical treatment* must be considered. For *unilateral* disease, if the hearing is *unserviceable*, the treatment of choice is labyrinthectomy. If the hearing is *serviceable* the choice lies between saccus decompression and vestibular nerve section. The difficulties entailed in assuring that disease is strictly unilateral have been discussed earlier.

Patients with *bilateral disease* and medically uncontrollable vertigo are very difficult to manage. Often the deafness is a greater problem than the vertigo. Furthermore, vertigo and imbalance sometimes result from the vestibular deficit caused by damage to the labyrinth rather than overactivity in one diseased ear. Even when the vertigo is due to the activity of the disease, it is not always easy to identify the active side. A change in tinnitus often gives an indication. If one ear is very deaf and thought to be active, labyrinthectomy is worth considering. If the better hearing ear is believed to be the active one, saccus decompression on that side should be considered. Purely on the grounds of its safety, insertion of a grommet through anterior myringotomy might be tried before either of the more major procedures, but the honest surgeon will accept that this, like saccus surgery, is a placebo operation. The concept that a procedure has a strong placebo effect should not deter its use, but it should discourage the doctor from believing the mechanism rather than appreciating the effect.

If both ears are moderately or severely deaf and if the deafness is the main problem, saccus decompression may be appropriate and might even be considered for each ear. When vertigo and imbalance are the principal complaints, the part played by vestibular deficit should be recognized. Vestibular rehabilitation exercises will often help (see Chapter 15), whereas vestibular sedatives may exacerbate the imbalance by preventing central compensation.

Sudden vestibular failure

Sudden vestibular failure is the name applied to the clinical syndrome that arises when vestibular function on one side is suddenly lost. It is no more a diagnostic label than is sudden sensorineural deafness. There are many possible causes, not always identifiable, and it is a useful description of a not uncommon disorder.

AETIOLOGY

The cause of sudden vestibular failure may be as obvious as skull fracture, or as doubtful as some viral infections. The syndrome can follow sudden occlusion of the anterior vestibular artery, and it is also one feature of a more extensive neurological disturbance when the posterior inferior cerebellar or vertebral arteries are occluded. Other possible causes include multiple sclerosis, varicella-zoster infection, brainstem encephalitis and diabetic neuropathy. Usually no cause can be established. Many patients with idiopathic vestibular failure are included in the group of disorders described as vestibular neuronitis, or vestibular neuritis, on the basis of a supposed anatomical localization between the labyrinth and the vestibular neurons. Some confusion affects the use of all these terms. As a clinical description the name 'acute vestibular failure' has much to commend it. Difficulties of nomenclature are further compounded by the terms 'epidemic labyrinthitis' and 'viral labyrinthitis', which are in common but unfortunate use. It seems possible that sudden vestibular failure sometimes occurs in small groups of the population, perhaps when caused by viral infection, and for that reason acquires the epidemic epithet.

CLINICAL FEATURES

The illness starts with the sudden onset of violent rotatory vertigo, nausea and vomiting, followed by slow but gradual recovery of balance over a period of 10 days to 3 weeks – a time scale and pattern quite different from that of Menière's disease, in which the vertigo lasts for hours, or benign paroxysmal positional vertigo, which lasts for only seconds. Auditory symptoms are conspicuously absent. Shortly after onset the patient is found to have a large amplitude first, second and third degree jerk nystagmus to the unaffected side, a so-called paralytic nystagmus (see Chapter 14). Gradually, as the symptoms subside, the nystagmus diminishes, becoming first and second and then first degree in magnitude until it is no longer visible in the presence of visual fixation. For a long time afterwards nystagmus will reappear when the eyes are examined without fixation, in the dark or with Frenzel's glasses. Caloric tests at first show no response to any stimulus, but later the tendency to a nystagmus, which had previously been overt, appears as a directional preponderance on caloric stimulation of the unaffected ear (see Chapter 5). Balance is recovered by a process of compensation (see Chapter 15). If, as occasionally happens, vestibular function actually recovers, then restoration of activity to the previously inactive side recreates tonic imbalance and may cause a further period of vertigo and disequilibrium. Compensation develops more slowly and is less complete in the elderly, and it may break down long after it has been acquired as the result of ill health, fatigue or a failing central nervous system. Here is another explanation for a recurrence of imbalance and even vertigo.

DIAGNOSIS

As with Menière's disease the history is of paramount diagnostic importance, with particular attention to the time course of the vertigo. The story of sudden vestibular failure is usually clear cut. The absence of auditory abnormalities and the typical caloric findings provide confirmation. Brainstem disorders causing vestibular failure are usually accompanied by other neurological features, but an episode of demyelination may be overlooked unless there are other reasons to suspect multiple sclerosis.

TREATMENT

Treatment of an episode of sudden vestibular failure requires bedrest and vestibular sedation, exactly as is advocated for the treatment of an acute attack of Menière's disease. Normally recovery is gradual and complete, but in an elderly patient or when compensation is slow vestibular head exercises help (see Chapter 15).

Vestibular neuronitis

Vestibular neuronitis is an unsatisfactory diagnostic label sometimes applied to patients with one or more episodes of vertigo without auditory or central nervous system involvement. It used to be thought, from these negative features, that any causative lesion must lie central to the labyrinth but no more so than the vestibular neurons in the brainstem. To widen the possible anatomical involvement, vestibular neuritis is sometimes used as an alternative term. Two distinct groups of patients tend to be classified under this heading, and would be better separated. First are those patients with the syndrome of 'sudden vestibular failure' described above. The second comprises those patients who have repeated episodes of vertigo similar in timing and character to those of Menière's disease but without any cochlear symptoms. It is quite likely that this group includes patients suffering from several different entities that tend to be diagnosed by inference and guess. These include vestibular hydrops, repeated slight inflammatory damage to the vestibular nerve or neurons (never severe enough to cause total vestibular failure) and migrainous disturbances of the vestibular system.

The caloric responses of patients with a diagnosis of vestibular neuronitis are often, if not always, abnormal, with reduced or absent responses from one or both sides. Unilateral loss of activity is of course expected in those who have suffered sudden vestibular failure. Bilateral loss of caloric response may indicate either a reduction in sensitivity of both labyrinths, or an enhanced ability to suppress caloric-induced nystagmus by optic fixation – so-called habituation.

Benign paroxysmal positional vertigo

Benign paroxysmal positional vertigo is characterized by brief but violent attacks of paroxysmal vertigo provoked by certain positions of the head. There are no auditory symptoms. It is without doubt the commonest cause of peripheral aural vertigo and is further described in Chapter 15. The attacks cease after a variable period. This is usually about 3 weeks, but quite often may be several months or even years. Recurrence even after intervals as long as several years is common

AETIOLOGY

It has long been known that the provoking lesion lies in the labyrinth, probably in the utricle, of the ear that is undermost when the vertigo is provoked, and recent evidence suggested that the mechanism is one that Schuknecht has called 'cupulolithiasis'. In this explanation calcium carbonate from otoconia of the otolith organs becomes deposited on the cupula of the posterior semicircular canal. Changing the head position from erect to the provoking supine position displaces the cupula away from the utricle under the gravitational force of the attached deposit.

There are certain objections to this explanation. In the first place the neurological connections of the posterior semicircular canal crista are to external ocular muscles causing vertical depression of the eyes, and so a stimulus to that crista alone should cause a vertically beating nystagmus with no rotatory component. Second, the cupulolithiasis theory does not adequately explain the way in which the provoked nystagmus ceases after 20 seconds or so. It ought to continue for as long as the cupula remains deflected, and that deflection should continue as long as the head remains down, as the lightly damped cupula would not be able to return to its neutral position against the force of a distorting load of otoconial deposits.

A more acceptable explanation of the role of displaced otoconia in this syndrome is provided by the concept of 'canalolithiasis', described in Chapter 15. The wadge of particulate material from the otoconia is believed to become lodged in the membranous posterior canal, and to move endolymph by a piston-like action when the head is moved, so bending the posterior canal stereocilia.

Either theory accords with the observation that denervation of the sensory nerve supply to the posterior canal crista relieves the symptoms of the disorder. The syndrome of benign paroxysmal positional vertigo frequently arises with no apparent antecedent cause, in adults of all ages. It is the most common vestibular disturbance after closed-head injury, and may develop with degenerative changes in the labyrinth of the aged. The disorder is sometimes encountered after stapes surgery and it may also be caused by vestibular artery occlusion.

CLINICAL FEATURES

The history of violent vertigo provoked by turning over to a particular position in bed, or reaching upwards in a particular direction, say to remove a book from a shelf, is typical. The patient often wakes after turning over in sleep, a diagnostic feature to be sought in any history. Sometimes the symptoms are so severe and so often repeated that the patient describes continuous vertigo lasting for hours or even days, while lying in bed. Careful analysis of the story, minute by minute, may be needed to reveal the intermittent paroxysmal nature of the vertigo that distinguishes the condition from vestibular failure.

DIAGNOSIS

The syndrome can be suspected from the typical history, and is diagnosed by provoking the typical nystagmus in the positional tests (see Chapter 15). When the head is turned 30° towards the examiner and taken backwards into the provoking position 30° below the horizontal the nystagmus observed has the following characteristics:

- there is a latent period of several seconds, after the assumption of the provoking posture, before the nystagmus appears and before the patient complains of vertigo
- the nystagmus is rotatory, beating towards the underlying ear
- the nystagmus abates and disappears after a period of 20–40 seconds, while the head is retained in the provoking posture
- the nystagmus is fatiguable, in that repetition of the test produces smaller and smaller responses
- the nystagmus does not change direction, either on repeated testing, or with changes of head position
- the accompanying vertigo is so violent that the patient may cry out and try to sit up

These features together support the suspicion of benign paroxysmal positional vertigo and are necessary and sufficient for its diagnosis. Deviation from any one of these characteristics should suggest that the positional vertigo could be central in origin, arising from the vestibular centres or the cerebellum, and a full neurological assessment is then necessary. Rare positional nystagmus of the central variety should be considered not as a syndrome, but as a physical sign of central nervous system disease.

Clearly, then, the diagnosis depends on the correct assessment of the results of positional testing. Central positional nystagmus is often accompanied by little or no vertigo, and the direction of the beat is frequently vertical or to the uppermost ear. Rarely, benign paroxysmal positional nystagmus, arising peripherally and typical of the syndrome of benign paroxysmal positional vertigo, can be provoked by putting the head down to the left and down to the right. In this form of bilateral benign paroxysmal positional vertigo, the nystagmus, which is preceded by a latent period and is fatiguable, beats clockwise when the head is down to the left and anticlockwise with the head down to the right. The inference is that there is disease in the utricles of both labyrinths.

TREATMENT

Reassurance about the innocent nature of the complaint, and that the natural course is usually for self-resolution, is very important. Although the symptom can be relieved by labyrinthine destruction, this is rarely advisable. Severely afflicted patients, in whom the condition has lasted for more

than a few weeks, may be helped by so-called Brandt–Daroff vestibular head exercises. The deliberate provocation of attacks by head movement can help central adaptation to the abnormal stimulus. Alternatively, particle repositioning manoeuvres may be used. Epley's technique for persuading the detached particulate otoconia to move from the posterior canal into the utricle is described in detail in Chapter 15. If a severely affected patient, who has had the symptoms for many months or years, cannot be helped in any other way, relief may be provided by one of two possible operations: posterior ampullary (singular nerve) section or posterior canal obliteration.

Posterior ampullary (singular nerve) nerve section

The posterior ampullary nerve carries the sensory fibres of the posterior canal crista to the inferior vestibular nerve. After leaving the internal acoustic meatus, it travels backwards to the posterior semicircular canal ampulla, in a channel that takes it just below the lower border of attachment of the round window membrane. It can be reached through a permeatal tympanotomy approach (Fig 38.8). The bony overhang of the round window niche is drilled away with fine diamond paste burrs until the round window membrane is exposed. Drilling further bone below and medially to its inferior edge will expose the singular nerve, so that it can be avulsed. Accessibility of the nerve depends on its relationship to the round window – if too far superomedial, it may not become visible without damage to the cochlea. This procedure offers relief from the symptoms of benign paroxysmal positional vertigo, but carries a high risk of severe sensorineural hearing loss, so should not be advocated lightly.

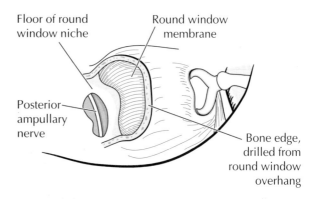

Fig 38.8 Posterior ampullary nerve section.

Posterior canal obliteration

Compression of the membranous posterior semi-circular canal can prevent movement of material within it. The bony canal is exposed through a cortical mastoidectomy approach (see Chapter 29). Diamond paste burrs are used to 'blue line' the canal, which is gently opened. It is important to avoid damage to the membranous labyrinth within. Bone wax or bone pate is then used to fill the peri-lymph space to squash the membranous tube within and prevent movement of the endolymph it contains.

Vascular lesions

Many vascular disorders affect labyrinthine function. Mention has already been made of the effects of anterior vestibular artery occlusion, which produces the symptoms of vestibular failure and benign paroxysmal positional vertigo.

MIGRAINE

Migraine can cause vertigo, which is episodic in nature, and it is often associated with Menière's disease – an association noticed by Menière himself. Some migrainous patients have an aura of vertigo presaging an attack of headache. In others, the headaches are replaced by attacks of vertigo – a so-called migraine equivalent. Finally, there are patients who, having suffered from typical migraine, develop Menière's disease and then are no longer afflicted with migraine. When the vertigo is thought to be a migraine equivalent, even though it is accompanied by deafness and tinnitus, no neuro-otological abormalities will be demonstrable after the attack. Antimigrainous preparations are often effective.

Perilymph fistula or labyrinthine membrane rupture

Perilymph fistula or labyrinthine membrane rupture is a condition of controversial interest that has exercised otologists for the past 20 years or so. Under certain conditions, the inner ear membranes may be ruptured and then the oval window or round window may leak perilymph into the middle ear. The external pressure trauma needed to produce this damage may be severe, as in concussive head injuries and diving barotrauma, or perhaps trivial, as with pressure changes caused by sneezing, straining at a stool, light head blows or sexual intercourse. That perilymph leakages can be caused by the more severe insults is generally accepted, but there is a great deal of argument still about the less violent causes and whether so-called 'spontaneous' peri-lymph fistulae exist at all.

The name perilymph fistula is in a way misleading, as the damage arising in the inner ear is attributable to tearing of intralabyrinthine membranes, disruption of sensory structures and biochemical harm from mixing inner ear fluids. The perilymph leak itself is simply the final evidence, found at operation, of this damage, and it cannot rationally be suggested that the closure of a fistula, which is just the injury at the most lateral extent of the insult, will repair irreversibly disrupted inner ear structures.

The clinical result of labyrinthine membrane ruptures has never been consistently agreed, which is hardly surprising when the very existence of 'spontaneous' perilymph leaks is uncertain. Suspicion should be directed, it is argued, at all patients who develop sudden sensorineural hearing loss after trauma of the kinds mentioned, and when there are attacks of Menière-like vertigo, with atypical features such as persisting imbalance between attacks of proper vertigo. Patients with untypical features of otherwise characteristic benign paroxysmal positional vertigo should also be suspected. There are no useful diagnostic predictable clues, beyond the clinician's suspicion. A great deal has been written about the status of a positive fistula sign (see Chapter 3), but in fact no series of presumed peri-lymph fistulae has shown the presence of a fistula sign to be more than a useful pointer, and its absence is of no value at all.

Diagnostic proof can be sought only by observation during a tympanotomy operation. Even this is subjective and not reliable; false-positive leaks have been described by the observation of fluid accumulating in the round window niche, which actually has come from tissue exudate or preoperative infiltration of the ear canal, whereas false-negative reports may arise from the lowering of perilymph pressure. There have been descriptions of 'shredding' of the round window membrane later shown to be mucosal strands across the round window niche, which normally hides the actual membrane from view. Enthusiasts encourage watching the windows for several minutes, with the head lowered on the operating table to raise cerebrospinal fluid pressure, before the absence of a leak is declared. Absence of leak discovery is sometimes ascribed to spontaneous healing, which is an argument in the enthusiast's armamentarium very difficult to gainsay. To see the round window membrane clearly it is usually necessary to drill away bone overhanging it, but this actually risks causing a leak.

If a leak is found, or suspected, it can easily be patched operatively with a piece of connective tissue or fat from the ear lobe. There have certainly been reliable anecdotal accounts of immediate relief from ataxia and imbalance after this procedure in some instances. There are few reliable accounts of any improvement in the patient's hearing. The rational otologist should keep an open mind on the existence of this syndrome. Any patient developing vertigo or sensorineural hearing loss after diving or definite head injury should be a legitimate suspect for the diagnosis, and ought to be nursed sitting up, as, if healing can occur, it will do so more readily with low cerebrospinal fluid pressure. After a week or so with no improvement it is reasonable to explore the middle ear surgically.

Pressure-induced vertigo syndrome

There are three rare interesting disorders that arise, for reasons that are not fully understood, in which vertigo is caused by pressure changes. Patients may exhibit any singly, or two or three of the group in inexplicable combinations, and for this reason the disorders are grouped here as instances of one syndrome – the pressure-induced vertigo syndrome (PIVS). In each, rises in pressure in the external air or in internal fluids – cerebrospinal fluid and perilymph – cause vertigo, instability and abnormal eye movements. Oscillopsia is often the presenting symptom. A curious feature is that the syndrome may develop spontaneously, with no apparent provocation, in adult life. The components of the syndrome are

- Tullio phenomenon
- Hennebert's sign (or phenomenon)
- Valsalva-induced vertigo

Unresolved mysteries are the identity of the labyrinthine receptors causing the vertigo, and the route of transmission of the pressure changes exciting them.

The Tullio phenomenon is the excitation of vertigo and imbalance by loud sound. The stimulus is usually specific in frequency and intensity for any one patient. Usually it is unilateral. One well known variety of this is associated with a fistula into the lateral semicircular canal, and has been recognized for many years. This is known to be a feature of any ear with two mobile windows on the same side of

the basilar membrane (a fistula into the lateral semicircular canal and the stapes), and is thought to be associated with excitation, by sound pressure change, of the lateral semicircular canal crista. This is not what concerns us here, when noise causes the symptoms in otherwise normal ears with no suspicion of a fistula. There is evidence to believe that it may arise by stimulation of sound receptors in the saccule. The mechanism of pressure transfer is probably directly through the ossicular chain to the stapes, but some writers have blamed a displaced stapes footplate moved by an abnormally vigorous stapedius or tensor tympani reflex. (This is an explanation that does not stand up to critical examination.)

Hennebert's is a fistula sign (see Chapter 3) induced with a pneumatic speculum when there is no fistula. When first described in the nineteenth century it was though to be due to syphilitic softening of the stapediovestibular attachment – a suggestion that can no longer be sustained. Here pressure is being transmitted to the middle ear, by tympanic membrane movement, but what happens more medially is a mystery. It may have something in common, as a very low frequency stimulus, with the Tullio phenomenon, but there are differences, as the Tullio phenomenon may also be provoked by loud sound generated internally travelling from the nasopharynx through the Eustachian tube.

Valsalva's manoeuvre induced vertigo is the most difficult of all three to analyse for several reasons. First there are variations in its performance. The glottis may be closed, in which case the only effect is to raise cerebrospinal fluid pressure. The glottis may be open, in which case there will be a change in pharyngeal air pressure. This may be passed directly to the middle ear space, but only if the Eustachian tube and the nasopharynx open and the tube is patent. Raised cerebrospinal fluid pressure may be partly transmitted to the inner ear fluids through connections at the lateral end of the internal auditory meatus or through the aqueduct of the cochlea. Unfortunately aqueductal patency in the normal adult is uncertain. Anatomical studies suggest that the aqueduct is usually partly obstructed in adult life by a kind of spongy connective tissue material, which would not allow rapid fluid pressure transfers; however, studies based on changes in middle ear impedance have suggested that it is usually able to transmit such pressure changes. So the perilymph fluid pressure might rise, but the effect of that would be partly counteracted or even overcome by a rise in middle ear air pressure transmitted through the Eustachian tube.

These pressure relationships of Valsalva may be further confused by the possible acoustic events in a patient who also has the Tullio phenomenon, from the exterior, and separately through the Eustachian tube. Clearly it is difficult to analyse the mechanics when a wind instrument player, whose technique may or may not require a closed raised palate, commits Valsalva by blowing an instrument, excites the Tullio phenomenon and develops oscillopsia.

Central vestibular disorders

Vertigo may be a feature of any disease process affecting the vestibular pathways and their connections with the cerebellum and the temporal lobe cortex (see Chapter 14). A central cause should be suspected

- whenever the history includes other neurological symptoms, such as disturbance of vision, dysphasia, numbness, diplopia or limb weakness
- when the story does not clearly fit the pattern of any recognized peripheral disorder. Vertigo from central derangements is often much less sharply defined than in peripheral disease, less clearly associated with nausea and vomiting and often overshadowed by persisting or increasing imbalance
- when other neurological abnormalities can be demonstrated
- when spontaneous nystagmus shows central characteristics (see Chapter 3). Spontaneous nystagmus of central origin may last for many weeks. Nystagmus beating vertically upwards is caused by high brainstem lesions, whereas downbeat nystagmus suggests a lesion in the medulla. Nystagmus that changes direction, either with time or with direction of gaze, is nearly always central in origin. Disjunctive nystagmus, with a difference in beating in the two eyes – often being absent from the adducting one – implies a lesion in the medial longitudinal bundle
- when positional nystagmus of central type can be provoked (see above). That is, indeed, whenever a positionally provoked nystagmus does not show all the features expected in the peripheral variety. This suggests a lesion in the vestibular centres of the brainstem and cerebellum
- when caloric testing produces responses that are only slightly prolonged by the removal of optic fixation with Frenzel's glasses or in the dark
- when electronystagmography shows that spontaneous nystagmus is abolished by eye closure

No list of suspicious features can hope to be comprehensive. The recognition of a central cause demands detailed knowledge and experience of the patterns of central nervous system disease. Here only brief comments can be made about some disorders of the central nervous system, of which vertigo is a common feature.

TUMOURS

Intracranial tumours may cause vertigo either by direct destruction of vestibular structures, or, when cerebrospinal fluid pressure is raised, by interference with arterial blood supply to vestibular neurons. Common in the adult are gliomas, meningiomas and secondary tumour deposits, particularly from bronchus and breast. These may occur with no physical signs other than the central variety of positional nystagmus. In children, medulloblastomas must be considered. Cystic space-occupying lesions of the fourth ventricle may cause episodic vertigo with nausea and vomiting (Brun's syndrome).

MULTIPLE SCLEROSIS

Demyelinating plaques may be found anywhere in the central VIIIth-nerve system. The part played by multiple sclerosis as a possible cause of sudden vestibular failure has already been described. The clinician's suspicion of this cause is likely to be aroused by any mention in the history of other symptoms such as transient numbness or visual disturbance. Disjunctive nystagmus, already mentioned, due to a lesion in the medial longitudinal bundle, is caused by this disease more often than by any other.

EPILEPSY

Vertigo may be the aura of an epileptic attack arising in the temporal lobe cortex, and indeed may be the only symptom. Unconsciousness should raise suspicion, but does not always occur, nor is the EEG always abnormal. A story of amnesia or mental dullness after the attack is suggestive.

POSTERIOR INFERIOR CEREBELLAR ARTERY OCCLUSION (LATERAL MEDULLARY INFARCTION, WALLENBERG'S SYNDROME)

Wallenberg's syndrome is associated with infarction of a wedge-shaped area of the lateral aspect of the medulla and the inferior surface of the cerebellum. Traditionally attributed to obstruction of the posterior inferior cerebellar artery, it is probably more often due to thrombosis of one vertebral artery.

The syndrome has otological interest in that the onset is very much that of sudden vestibular failure, with severe vertigo and vomiting. The additional neurological symptoms of headache, dysphagia, sensory disturbance and sometimes diplopia point to the central nature of the cause. Examination shows a spontaneous nystagmus to the unaffected side. Involvement of the spinal tract of the Vth nerve causes numbness of the face on the side of the lesion, and involvement of the crossed spinothalamic fibres shows as a dissociated sensory loss, for pain and temperature sensation only, on the opposite side of the trunk and extremities. Destruction of the nucleus ambiguus causes ipsilateral paralysis of the palate and larynx, and sensory impairment of the oropharyanx. Ipsilateral Horner's syndrome is the result of damage to sympathetic fibres descending in the brainstem from the hypothalamus. Variably, there may be involvement of the facial nucleus – with facial palsy – and the VIth nerve nucleus – with lateral rectus palsy. The central structures of the medulla, including the hypoglossal nucleus, are spared. The hearing is normal, and caloric studies have shown a directional preponderance to the undamaged side associated, at postmortem, with destruction of vestibular nuclei receiving afferents from the utricle – the descending vestibular nucleus and the caudal part of the medial vestibular nucleus.

BASILAR MIGRAINE

Attacks of this syndrome are initiated by visual phenomena that differ a little from those common in migraine in that they consist of dimming or loss of vision in the whole of both visual fields with flashes or blobs of light, rather than of typical fortification spectra. These arise from spasm of the posterior cerebral artery and ischaemia of its territory of supply in the occipital cortex. This stage is rapidly followed by vertigo, unsteadiness of gait and sometimes tinnitus, also by disturbance of speech (dysarthria), and by tingling of the hands and feet on both sides and sometimes tingling around both sides of the mouth. The symptoms last 10–30 seconds and are followed by severe, usually occipital, headache, or in some instances, by unconsciousness. The diagnosis cannot be sustained in the absence of these additional central nervous system symptoms. Basilar migraine tends to occur in adolescent girls. There is a strong menstrual relationship and a clear family history of migraine, often against a background of other easily recognizable migrainous episodes. As with migraine equivalents mentioned earlier in this chapter, vestibular investigation fails to reveal any abnormality, and treatment is the province of a neurologist.

VERTEBROBASILAR ISCHAEMIA

Ischaemia within the territory of supply of the two vertebral arteries and their basilar union may arise from intermittent compression of the vessels when the neck is hyperextended or excessively rotated, in the presence of osteophytes and degenerative cervical arthritic disease. More persistent ischaemia with intermittent exacerbations, provoked by head movement and posture, is found in patients with atherosclerotic narrowing of these vessels. More rare is the subclavian steal syndrome, in which obstruction of the subclavian or innominate artery proximal to the vertebral artery results in supply of blood to the arm at the expense of the vertebral territory, with blood flowing downwards through the neck.

The history is of intermittent vertigo, particularly associated with change in posture on lateral rotation or extension of the head on the neck. The repeated attacks of vertigo are associated with other symptoms, of which transient dysphasia and hemiparesis are common. Blurred vision and hemianopia may also accompany the attacks.

Persistent ischaemia sometimes produces chronic instability with vertigo on rising in the morning. As the sufferers are usually elderly, high tone bilateral hearing loss is often found, but vestibular investigations rarely indicate localizing abnormalities.

A diagnosis of cervical spine disease is made radiologically and treated orthopaedically. A radiological abnormality is so common in the elderly that it is only rarely related to the cause of vertigo, and it is improper to blame the cervical spine simply on radiological evidence. In the absence of other symptoms, X-ray of the cervical spine in the elderly never helps with the diagnosis or management of vertigo. All too often the results mislead doctor and patient. Arteriography is hardly ever justified to demonstrate the impaired blood flow because its risks are usually too great, but occasionally there may be justification for a neurologist to advise Doppler or other non-invasive studies of arterial blood flow.

PSYCHOGENIC VERTIGO

Feelings of instability or disorientation may be present in anxiety states and agoraphobia, whereas depersonalization, which can be confused with vertigo, features in hysteric illnesses and schizophrenia (see also Chapter 14).

Suggested reading

Alford B.R. Committee on hearing and equilibrium, Report of Subcommittee on Equilibrium and its Measurement. Meniere's Disease: Criteria for Diagnosis and Evaluation of Therapy for Reporting. *Transactions of the American Academy of Ophthalmology and Otolaryngology* 1972; **76**:1462–4.

Aso S, Watanabe Y, Mizukoshi K. A clinical study of electrocochleography in Meniere's disease. *Acta Otolaryngologica* 1991; **111**:44–52.

Balkany T, Sires B, Arenberg IK. Bilateral aspects of Meniere's disease: an underestimated entity. *Otolaryngology Clinics of North America* 1980; **13**:603–9.

Brookes G. The pharmacological treatment of Meniere's disease. *Clinical Otolaryngology* 1996; **21**:3–11.

Cawthorne TE. Perilabyrinthitis. *Laryngoscope* 1957; **67**:1233–6.

Clemis JD, Valvassori GE. Radiographic and clinical observations on the vestibular aqueduct. *Otolaryngology Clinics of North America* 1968; **1**:339–46.

Colebatch J, Rothwell J, Bronstein A, Ludman H. Click-evoked vestibular activation in the Tullio Phenomenon. *Journal of Neurology, Neurosurgery and Psychiatry* 1994; **57**:1538–40.

Davis LE. Viruses and vestibular neuritis: review of human and animal studies [Review]. *Acta Otolaryngologica* 1993; **(suppl 503)**:70–3.

Derebery MJ, Valenzuela S. Meniere's syndrome and allergy. *Otolaryngology Clinics of North America* 1992; **25**:213–24.

Dingle AF, Hawthorne MR, Kumar BU. Fenestration and occlusion of the posterior semicircular canal for benign positional vertigo. *Clinical Otolaryngology* 1992; **17**:300–2.

Dornhoffer JL, Arenberg IK. Diagnosis of vestibular Meniere's disease with electrocochleography [Review]. *American Journal of Otology* 1993; **14**:161–4.

Gacek R. Singular neurectomy update. II Review of 102 cases. *Laryngoscope* 1992; **101**:855–62.

Gibson WP. The use of electrocochleography in the diagnosis of Meniere's disease. *Acta Otolaryngologica* 1991; **(suppl 485)**:46–52.

Gibson WP. The use of intraoperative electrocochleography in Meniere's disease. *Acta Otolaryngologica* 1991; **(suppl 485)**:65–73.

Graham MD, Goldsmith MM. Labyrinthectomy. Indications and surgical technique. *Otolaryngology Clinics of North America* 1994; **27**:325–35.

Hallpike CS, Cairns H. Pathology of Meniere's Syndrome. *Journal of Laryngology and Otology* 1938; **53**:625–55.

Horner KC. Auditory and vestibular function in experimental hydrops [Review]. *Otolaryngology – Head and Neck Surgery* 1995; **112**:84–9.

Kohut RI. Perilymph fistula – clinical criteria. *Archives of Otolaryngology – Head and Neck Surgery* 1992; **118**:687–92.

Ludman H. Meniere's disease (editorial). *British Medical Journal* 1990; **301**:1232–3.

Moffat DA. Endolymphatic sac surgery: analysis of 100 operations. *Clinical Otolaryngology* 1994; **19**:261–6.

Morrison AW, Mowbray JF, Williamson R, Sheeka S, Sodha N, Koskinen N. On genetic and environmental factors in Meniere's disease. *American Journal of Otology* 1994; **15**:35–9.

Nakagawa H, Watanabe Y, Mizukoshi K, Ohi H. Plain radiological findings in Meniere's disease. *Auris, Nasus, Larynx* 1994; **21**:137–42.

Pearson BW, Brackmann DE. Committee on Hearing and Equilibrium Guidelines for Reporting Treatment Results in Meniere's Disease. *Otolaryngology – Head and Neck Surgery* 1985; **93**:579–81.

Schmidt JT, Huizing EH. The clinical drug trial in Meniere's disease – with emphasis on the effect of betahistine SR. *Acta Otolaryngologica* 1992; **(suppl 497)**:1–89.

Schuknecht HF. Myths in neurology [see comments] [Review]. *American Journal of Otology* 1992; **13**:124–6.

Shea JJ. Classification of Meniere's disease [Review]. *American Journal of Otology* 1993; **14**:224–9.

Silverstein H, Norrell H, Haberkamp T. A comparison of retrosigmoid EAV, retrolabyrinthine, and middle fossa vestibular neurectomy for treatment of vertigo. *Laryngoscope* 1987; **97**:165–73.

Smith WC, Pillsbury HC. Surgical treatment of Meniere's disease since Thomsen. *American Journal of Otology* 1988; **9**:39–43.

CHAPTER 39

Tumours of the auditory–vestibular nerve

DERALD E BRACKMANN AND CHARLES A SYMS III*

The purpose of this chapter is to provide a brief overview of the diagnosis and management of acoustic neuromas (vestibular schwannomas). Although the chapter is titled tumours of the auditory–vestibular nerve, acoustic tumours represent the most common lesion encountered in this region and are the subject of this discussion.

History

The first recorded case, according to Cushing,[1] of an acoustic tumour with an adequate case history was probably by Sandifort. In the years before Cushing's famous monograph in 1917, the primary advances were not in the treatment of these tumours, but rather in the identification of the symptoms caused by their relentless growth. In addition to the increased accuracy of diagnosis from clinical symptomatology, advances in anaesthesia and asepsis were necessary before surgical treatment could be effective.[2] Without the important contributions of Morton and Cushing to anaesthesia and Semmelweis, Pasteur and Lister to asepsis, modern surgical procedures would not be possible. The first successful removal of an acoustic tumour was probably performed by Annandale in 1895.[3] Most reviews credit this achievement to Balance in

1892; however, the record reflects that this tumour had a broad base of attachment to dura[3] and Cushing felt it was a meningioma.[1]

The first real advance in the treatment of acoustic tumours was through Cushing's work at the Johns Hopkins Hospital, Baltimore, USA. Cushing trained under Halstead and further developed his interest in brain tumours at this institution. Patients were diagnosed when their tumours reached a far advanced state. 'Their suffering was intense, including headache, blindness, vomiting, dizziness, and ataxia.'[2] Against this background, it is easy to see why Cushing's work centred on bilateral suboccipital decompression of the posterior fossa and eventually a subcapsular, subtotal removal. Cushing's meticulous documentation of the progression of the symptoms of patients with acoustic tumours enabled the diagnosis to be made earlier in their clinical course.

One of Cushing's residents was Walter Dandy, a technically brilliant neurosurgeon. Dandy treated several patients with acoustic neuromas with a decompression and intracapsular dissection with less than satisfactory results. He advocated total extirpation via a unilateral suboccipital approach. This became the standard neurosurgical operation for the next 50 years or more. Dandy also contributed to the earlier diagnosis of acoustic tumours by introducing pneumoencephalography. At this stage in the development of acoustic tumour surgery, complete removal of the tumour was the goal, and permanent facial paralysis was the inevitable result. The operative mortality still remained unacceptably high. It was not until Atkinson[3] identified the

* The opinions expressed in this chapter are those of the authors and do not necessarily reflect the official policy of the United States Department of Defense or the United States Air Force.

importance of preserving the anteroinferior cerebellar artery that any substantial reduction in perioperative mortality was obtained. Even after this advance, the operative mortality remained greater than 10 per cent when William House began to attack the problem.

The next revolution in acoustic tumour surgery came in the early 1960s. William House collaborated with William Hitselberger, and they assembled a team of associates and colleagues to tackle the problem of acoustic neuromas. There was formidable opposition to the concepts that they espoused, but thankfully they persevered. William House introduced microsurgical technique to neurosurgery in first the middle fossa and later the translabyrinthine approaches. The successful removal of cerebellopontine angle tumours was now possible with acceptable morbidity and perioperative mortality. The concept of a neurotological examination and work-up for patients with unilateral audiological symptoms and disequilibrium was introduced. The accuracy of the evaluation of patients was progressively increased by Pantopaque polytomography,[4] audiometric brainstem response,[5] computer cranial tomography[6] enhanced with gas cisternography, and magnetic resonance imaging (MRI),[7] eventually with gadolinium.[8] Although delay in diagnosis is still encountered, it is not because of a lack of adequate tools developed during this exciting time. The contemporary issues are not much different from what they were 30 years ago. Deciding when and on whom to operate are still the difficult issues, albeit for entirely different reasons.

Classification

There is no formal classification scheme for acoustic neuromas. We sort these tumours on the basis of size. Intracanalicular tumours are those confined to the internal auditory canal. Small tumours include intracanalicular tumours and tumours with less than 1 cm extension into the cerebellopontine angle cistern. These tumours are less than 2 cm in overall size. The patient usually has only auditory symptoms, although there may be balance problems also. Medium-sized tumours are from 2 to 4 cm and there may be brainstem compression. There is progressive worsening of the auditory symptoms and there may be a decreased corneal reflex. When tumours are 4 cm or larger, they can progress through the 'syndrome of the cerebellopontine angle' as described by Cushing. There can be progressive headache, Vth cranial nerve signs, ataxia and, after obstruction of the

fourth ventricle, papilloedema and eventually blindness. With improved diagnostic testing and a heightened awareness, the percentage of tumours manifesting while small, even intracanalicular, is steadily increasing.[9]

Epidemiology

Acoustic tumours account for 8–10 per cent of all intracranial tumours, but in the House Ear Clinics' population over 90 per cent of all cerebellopontine angle neoplasms.[10] Acoustic neuromas occur in two distinct clinical forms. The less common, hereditary form is neurofibromatosis type-2, which occurs as an autosomal dominant disorder and accounts for approximately 5 per cent of acoustic tumours. The gene was mapped to chromosome 22[11] some time ago and it has recently been identified.[12,13] The gene protein product, 'merlin' or 'schwannomin', is thought to be a tumour suppressor. Neurofibromatosis type-2 has an incidence of one in 100 000.[14] In addition to the acoustic tumours occur that bilaterally, there are associated posterior subcapsular cataracts, meningiomas, facial nerve neuromas, gliomas, neurofibromas and spinal lesions such as ependymomas. These patients generally present at a younger age than the patients with sporadic tumours.

The more common condition of sporadic acoustic neuromas accounts for approximately 95 per cent of all acoustic neuroma operations. The reported annual incidence of acoustic tumours is between 1 in 50 000[15] to 1 in 100 000.[16] Recently it has been suggested that sporadic acoustic tumours are the result of mutations of the same gene through a 'two-hit' mutation.[17,18] This tumour usually manifests in mid-life, around 50 years of age.[19]

Clinical manifestations

SYMPTOMS

The most common symptom is a unilateral or asymmetric hearing loss. The loss is usually slowly progressive, but approximately 10 per cent of patients with an acoustic neuroma will present with sudden hearing loss.[20] Among patients with sudden hearing loss, however, only about 3 per cent will have an acoustic tumour.[21]

Tinnitus, although present, is not usually the manifesting symptom. Unexplained unilateral tinnitus, however, should be investigated thoroughly. There is no characteristic pattern to the tinnitus.

Vertigo is an uncommon complaint among patients with acoustic tumours. Patients much more commonly relate disequilibrium, imbalance or inco-ordination.

Once the tumour reaches a medium to large size, there can be numbness in the distribution of the trigeminal nerve. Advanced tumours manifest the characteristics of increased intracranial pressure and brainstem compression outlined previously.

Facial nerve weakness and spasm are exceedingly rare. Numerous other diagnoses should be entertained before an acoustic neuroma in the presence of facial nerve symptoms.

CLINICAL SIGNS

In the majority of patients the clinical examination will be normal. An early finding may be the presence of a positive Hitselberger sign. Whereas the motor portion of the facial nerve is relatively resistant to the effects of an expanding tumour, the same cannot be said about the sensory division, nervus intermedius (of Wrisberg). Hypaesthesia of the posterior external ear canal on the side with the hearing loss should raise the index of suspicion of the presence of a tumour.[22] A recent report re-examining the sensitivity and specificity of the Hitselberger sign has confirmed its accuracy.[23,24]

In larger tumours loss of first the corneal reflex and later sensation in the trigeminal distribution can be seen. Papilloedema, a positive Romberg or tandem Romberg, ataxia and dysdiadochokinesis can all be seen in advanced tumours.

Audiometric testing usually reveals a unilateral hearing impairment. Fewer than 5 per cent of patients operated on for acoustic neuroma will have normal hearing. Brainstem auditory evoked potential (BAEP) testing is usually abnormal, with an interaural latency of wave V being the most sensitive measure, although this appears to be size-related. Now that tumours are being discovered at earlier stages, the sensitivity of BAEPs has dropped from 93–98 per cent to 83 per cent, when tumours are less than 1.0 cm.[25] Concern over 'missed' tumours and the increasing ability of imaging to detect even the smallest tumours, at lower cost, has led to imaging protocols replacing BAEP screening.[26,27] In the past, over 90 per cent of patients had abnormal electronystagmography testing, but that percentage is decreasing as the percentage of intra-canalicular tumours increases. If the caloric response is normal, the classic teaching is that there is a higher probability of the tumour originating from the inferior vestibular nerve. Although this is often the case, this is not a universal finding.

The definitive diagnosis of an acoustic tumour is made with MRI, with gadolinium, examination of the cerebellopontine angle and internal auditory canal (IAC). This test is extremely sensitive and very specific, although other lesions can masquerade as an acoustic neuroma (Tables 39.1 and 39.2, Fig 39.1; see Chapter 6).

Table 39.1 Cerebellopontine angle lesions

Primary tumours of the cerebellopontine angle
    Acoustic schwannoma
    Meningioma
    Epidermoid
    Arachnoid cyst
    Schwannoma of cranial nerves V, VII, IX, X and XI
    Primary melanoma
    Haemangioma
    Lipoma
    Dermoid
    Teratoma
Secondary tumours of the cerebellopontine angle
    Paraganglioma
    Ceruminoma
    Chondroma/chondrosarcoma
    Chordoma
    Extension of cerebellar and temporal bone tumours
    Metastasis
Vascular lesions
    Aneurysms
    Arteriovenous malformations
    Vertebrobasilar dolichoectasia

Table 39.2 Intracanalicular lesions

Neoplastic
    Vestibular schwannoma
    Facial schwannoma
    Haemangioma
    Meningioma
    Lipoma
    Metastasis
    Lymphoma
    Melanoma
    Glioma
    Osteoma
Non-neoplastic
    AICA (anterior inferior cerebellar artery) loop
    AICA aneurysm
    Meningitis
    Neuritis
    Hamartoma

From Lo[28] with permission.

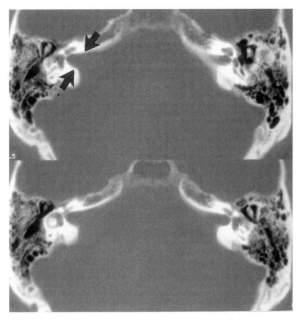

(a)

Fig 39.1 (a) Axial CT scans showing widening of the left internal auditory meatus, but no indication of an 'iso-dense' tumour, even with enhancement. (b) Gadolinium-enhanced MRI scan of the same patient showing the small acoustic neruoma. (c) T2-weighted fast spin echo MRI showing normal structures on the left side, and a small right-sided acoustic neuroma.

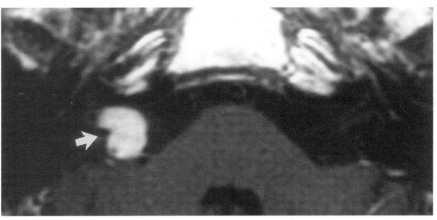

(b)

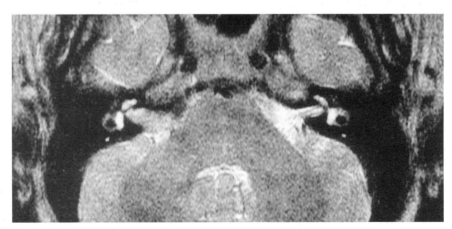

(c)

Management goals

The aim in the management of patients with an acoustic neuroma is to enable the individual to live life with as little disability as possible, while removing the threat of the devastating effects of a cerebellopontine tumour that robs the patient of expected years. This usually entails treating these tumours as soon as they are found, and finding them as early as possible. If the patient's overall life expectancy is limited because of coexisting disease, then no intervention may be the best course of action. Most individuals, however, should have these lesions treated, as prediction of future medical outcomes is difficult.

Preservation of binaural hearing is the ideal goal, when possible. Patients with small tumours and normal or near normal hearing can have their hearing preserved at or near their preoperative level about two-thirds of the time.[29] However, 22–56 per cent[30,31] of patients will have a significant decline in their long-term hearing. Preservation of hearing in patients with tumours larger than 2 cm is so infrequent that hearing should not be an issue when discussing options. The overwhelming majority of individuals will have a unilateral profound hearing impairment as a result of either the tumour or the treatment.

Major advances have been made in the preservation of facial nerve function in acoustic tumour surgery. Ninety per cent of patients undergoing acoustic neuroma resection will eventually have normal or near normal facial nerve function.[32] Larger tumours have poorer facial nerve results, which has implications for a 'watchful waiting' strategy.

Recommended approaches

SURGERY

When seeing a patient with an acoustic neuroma in consultation, we recommend surgery in most cases. In patients with small tumours who desire to have a hearing preservation operation, we usually recommend removal by the middle cranial fossa approach. For patients with a small to medium-sized tumour primarily based in the cerebellopontine angle cistern, with little extension out into the IAC, we recommend removal by the retrosigmoid approach. In the majority of patients, however, our recommendation is removal by the translabyrinthine approach.

All of our neurotological procedures are performed with the patient in the supine position, without head fixation devices or muscle paralysis, and with VIIth cranial nerve and, if appropriate, VIIIth cranial nerve monitoring. We use prophylactic antibiotics in all craniotomies, as a recent meta-analysis demonstrated their efficacy.[33] Furosemide, mannitol, dexamethasone and hyperventilation are used as necessary for brain relaxation and to prevent oedema.

MIDDLE FOSSA APPROACH

The patient is placed on the operating table with the head turned so that the affected ear is uppermost. The surgeon is seated at the head of the table (Fig 39.2). Our current incision forms an open question mark (Fig 39.3), rather than the previously used vertical incision. The incision extends to the plane of the temporalis muscle, and once this plane is encountered, the incision is extended by blunt dissection. The temporalis muscle is then incised posteriorly, elevated from the squamous portion of the temporal bone with a periosteal elevator and retracted anteriorly and inferiorly.

A 5.5 cm (anteroposterior) × 5.0 cm (superoinferior) craniotomy is then made with its centre located two-thirds anterior and one-third posterior to the external auditory canal. The inferior aspect of the craniotomy should be flush with the floor of the middle cranial fossa.

The dura is elevated from posterior to anterior and a House–Urban self-retaining middle fossa retractor is placed. Posterior to anterior elevation is important to avoid elevation of the greater superficial petrosal nerve and injury of the geniculate ganglion. Identification of the landmarks of the middle fossa approach is important at this point. The greater superficial petrosal nerve, the middle meningeal artery and the arcuate eminence are viewed. We now commence our dissection in the technique described by Garcia-Ibàñez and Garcia-Ibàñez[34] (Fig 39.4). Drilling starts at the most medial aspect of the temporal bone in an area identified by the bisection of an angle formed by the greater superficial petrosal nerve and the arcuate eminence. All bone dissection is done with diamond burrs. The dura of the IAC is identified and bone is removed from 270° around the medial aspect of the IAC. Dissection then proceeds in a medial to lateral direction. Only 90° of the IAC can be exposed at the fundus because of the proximity of the superior semicircular canal posteriorly and the cochlea anteriorly.

After all bone removal is completed, the dura is incised posteriorly and reflected anteriorly to

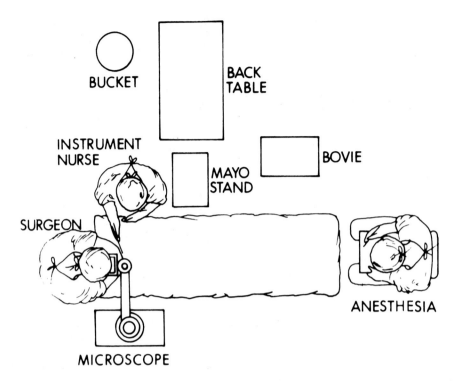

Fig 39.2 The operating room set-up. The surgeon is seated at the head of the table. (Reproduced with permission of House Ear Institute.)

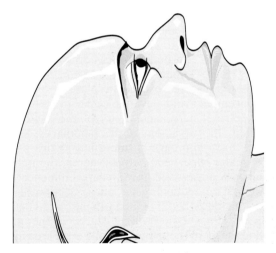

Fig 39.3 Our current incision utilizes a longer, curved incision, rather than a vertical incision. (Reproduced with permission of House Ear Institute.)

expose the tumour and the facial nerve (Fig 39.5). Bill's bar (vertical crest) is identified and the tumour is separated from the facial nerve. Care is taken to stay in the plane of the tumour so that the cochlear nerve or the blood supply of the cochlea are not disturbed. The blood supply to the cochlea

runs between the facial and cochlear nerves. The dissection is continued in a medial to lateral direction as much as possible in order to avoid avulsing the cochlear nerve. Continuous facial nerve monitoring has greatly facilitated the dissection of the tumour from the facial nerve. Direct cochlear nerve and near-field BAEP recordings have aided in the dissection, but our experience with these techniques has yet to prove a definitive improvement in hearing preservation.

After all the tumour is removed, the wound is copiously irrigated and haemostasis obtained. Abdominal fat is used to close the defect in the roof of the IAC. The retractor is removed, the bone flap replaced and the wound closed in layers over a Penrose drain.

SUBOCCIPITAL APPROACH

The patient is placed on the operating table facing away from the surgeon. A lazy S-shaped postauricular incision is made (Fig 39.6) and the subcutaneous tissues divided and moved out of the way with a self-retaining retractor. The mastoid periosteum is elevated and the external auditory canal identified. A complete mastoidectomy is performed from the posterior semicircular canal to the sigmoid

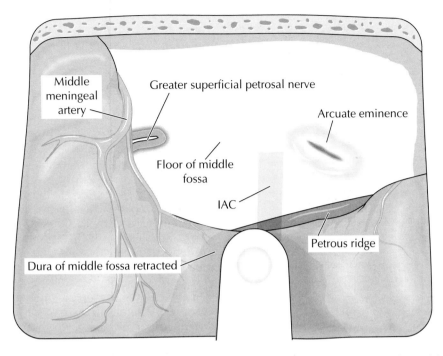

Fig 39.4 The IAC is visualized using the technique of Garcia-Ibàñez. The angle formed by the greater superficial petrosal nerve and the arcuate eminence is bisected to identify the IAC at its medial aspect. Drilling is started in this safe area. (Reproduced with permission of House Ear Institute.)

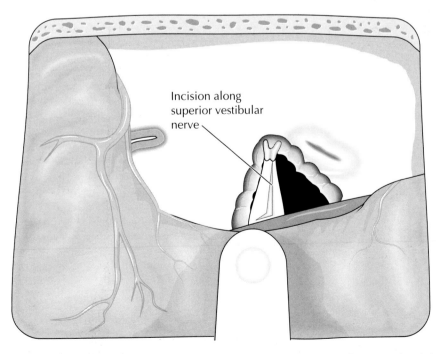

Fig 39.5 The exposure at the porus acusticus is 270°. Once the bone work is completed the dura is incised posteriorly and reflected anteriorly. (Reproduced with permission of House Ear Institute.)

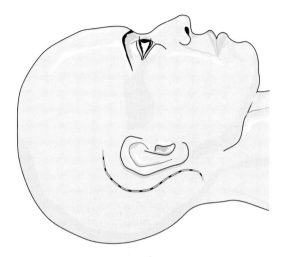

Fig 39.6 A lazy S-shaped postauricular incision. (Reproduced with permission of House Ear Institute.)

sinus. A 5×5 cm suboccipital bone flap is then developed just posterior to the sigmoid sinus and inferior to the lateral sinus (Fig 39.7). The mastoid emissary vein is bipolar, coagulated and divided. The posterior fossa dura is then incised just posterior to the sigmoid sinus, and stay sutures are used to retract the sinus anteriorly (Fig 39.8).

The cerebellum is protected with neurosurgical gauze patties and the cisternas lateralis is decompressed. All bone on the posterior aspect of the IAC is removed to expose the intracanalicular aspect of the tumour. The lateral aspect of the tumour should be seen. Inadvertent labyrinthine injury can be avoided by removing bone only medial to the vestibular aqueduct.

The posterior aspect of the tumour is inspected visually and with the facial nerve monitor, to identify the facial nerve. Usually the facial nerve is on the anterior or superior aspect of the tumour, in which case it is identified at the medial aspect of the tumour. Once the facial nerve has been identified, the tumour is debulked with cup forceps and the Urban dissector, or with ultrasonic dissection apparatus. After debulking, the tumour is removed from the facial nerve by sharp dissection. Tumour dissection once again proceeds in a medial to lateral direction (traction on the nerves in a lateral to medial direction places traction on the facial and cochlear nerves, which are fixed in the IAC). The remaining tumour is then removed from the IAC.

After tumour removal, the wound is irrigated copiously and haemostasis secured with bipolar electrocautery. Bone wax is used to seal any exposed air-cell tracts around the IAC, and muscle is used to fill the defect. The dura is closed with silk sutures and the mastoid defect obliterated with

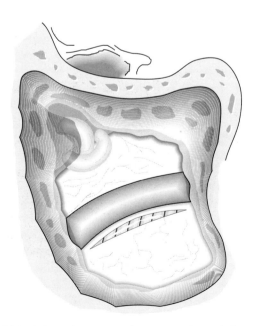

Fig 39.7 A complete mastoidectomy with total decompression of the sigmoid sinus. The dural incision is made just posterior to the sigmoid sinus. (Reproduced with permission of House Ear Institute.)

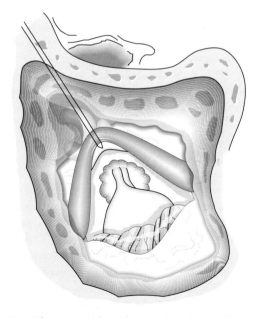

Fig 39.8 The sigmoid and posterior fossa dura are retracted with stay sutures. (Reproduced with permission of House Ear Institute.)

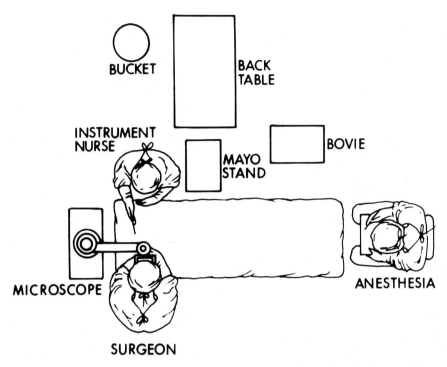

Fig 39.9 The operating room set-up for the translabyrinthine and retrosigmoid approaches. (Reproduced with permission of House Ear Institute.)

abdominal fat. The bone flap is replaced and the wound is closed in layers.

Recently, an additional procedure, the enhanced retrosigmoid exposure with posterior semicircular canal resection, has been described.[35] The extradural dissection is identical to the routine retrosigmoid dissection; however, the posterior semicircular canal is carefully occluded and the surrounding bone removed. In this procedure hearing preservation is possible and the majority of the IAC can be directly exposed. In addition, no intradural drilling is necessary. Further experience with this technique is necessary before it joins the routine neurotological armamentarium.

TRANSLABYRINTHINE APPROACH

There is no tumour that is too large to be removed by the translabyrinthine approach. The positioning is identical to the retrosigmoid approach (Fig 39.9). A postauricular incision is made 2 cm behind the postauricular crease and the periosteum elevated and moved away with self-retaining retractors.

A complete mastoidectomy is performed (Fig 39.10). The sigmoid sinus, posterior and middle

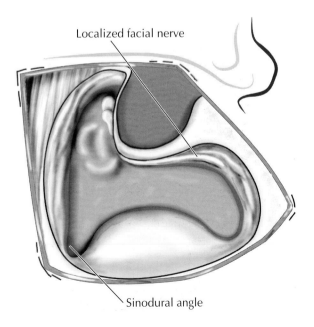

Localized facial nerve

Sinodural angle

Fig 39.10 A complete mastoidectomy with skeletonization of the sigmoid, middle and posterior fossa dura and the facial nerve. (Reproduced with permission of House Ear Institute.)

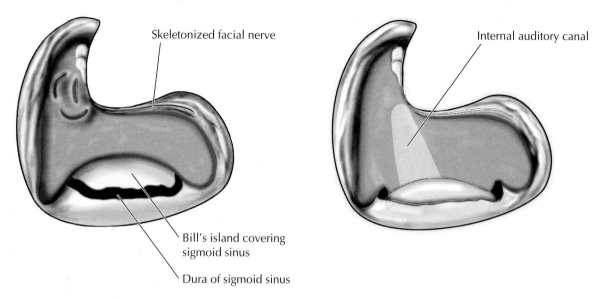

Fig 39.11 A labyrinthectomy is performed. (Reprinted with permission of House Ear Institute.)

Fig 39.12 The internal auditory canal is skeletonized. (Reproduced with permission of House Ear Institute.)

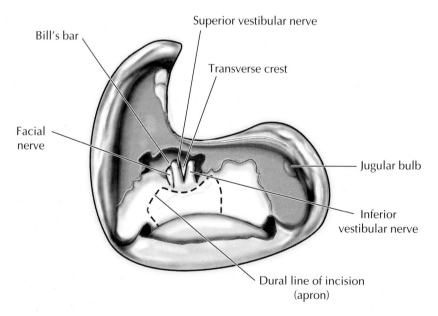

Fig 39.13 Bill's bar is clearly identified and the dural incision made. (Reproduced with permission of House Ear Institute.)

fossa dura and facial nerve are skeletonized. When the tumour is large, additional bone behind the sigmoid is removed. A labyrinthectomy is then accomplished (Fig 39.11). The jugular bulb and cochlear aqueduct are identified inferiorly. Dissection continues superior to the aqueduct to avoid inadvertent injury to the IXth and Xth cranial nerves. Bone removal is then continued until 270° around the entire length of the IAC is exposed (Fig 39.12). Bone removal is continued laterally until Bill's bar is clearly identified, separating the facial and superior vestibular nerves (Fig 39.13).

The posterior fossa dura is then incised and the cerebellum protected with patties. Vessels on the surface of the tumour are also protected with patties. The tumour is first debulked with cup forceps and the Urban dissector, or with ultrasonic dissector. The dissection is then started at Bill's bar, separating the tumour from the facial nerve as far as safely possible. The tumour is often extremely adherent to the facial nerve in the area of the porus acusticus. Identifying the facial nerve at the brainstem is very helpful for dissecting in a medial to lateral direction. After the tumour is freed from the facial nerve, its attachment to the VIIIth cranial nerve is divided and the tumour remnant removed. Haemostasis is secured and the wound copiously irrigated. The incus is removed and the Eustachian tube packed with Surgicel. The middle ear is packed with muscle. The defect is then filled with abdominal fat and the wound closed in layers.

Management alternatives

OBSERVATION

We recommend 'watchful waiting' only to those patients whose medical problems create a situation in which their life expectancy is shorter than the time it would take for them to get in trouble from their acoustic neuroma. There are no absolute guidelines and each case must be individualized. A patient with an extremely small tumour and very advanced age can probably be observed, but occasionally even these patients will have problems. If observation is elected by the patient, then frequent scanning is necessary to monitor growth. We recommend scanning every 6 months for 18 months and then scanning every year[36] or at least every other year.

IRRADIATION

We are unsure why stereotactic irradiation has enjoyed such popularity recently. Its ascendancy has come just when improved surgical techniques have made hearing preservation for small tumours a consistent reality. If a similar benign tumour was located in almost any other area of the body, irradiation would be considered ludicrous. Irradiation of adenoids, tonsils, thymus and acne was also accepted treatment at one time, but when followed for extended periods, unacceptable complications were noted.

Surgery after irradiation is more difficult and the facial nerve is in greater jeopardy.[37] We do not recommend stereotactic irradiation for the management of acoustic neuromas.

Complications

Complications occur no matter what approach is used. Fortunately, complications are infrequent and more bothersome than life-threatening.

Postoperative haemorrhage and haematoma is the most serious complication. This is a clinical diagnosis, and most frequently there is not time for scanning. In a patient with deteriorating levels of consciousness and other signs of increased intracranial pressure, the wound should be opened in the intensive care unit. The patient can then be taken back to the operating theatre for formal wound exploration, control of bleeding and wound closure.

Hearing loss occurs in all patients with a translabyrinthine approach and many patients in whom a hearing conservation operation is attempted. If the loss is unaidable then a CROS (contralateral routing of signal) hearing aid can be tried. This is well accepted in individuals whose occupations require frequent meetings or for whom sound perception from all directions is important.

Meningitis is fortunately an infrequent occurrence. Bacitracin in the irrigating solution and prophylactic antibiotics have greatly reduced the infection rate. When a patient has a postoperative temperature, the threshold for a spinal tap is low. Waiting until overt signs of meningitis develop can be a lethal approach. If the spinal tap is suggestive of an infectious process, then the appropriate antibiotics are started. This usually prolongs the hospital stay, but it is seldom a critical situation if diagnosed and treated early.

As previously mentioned, the preponderance of patients will have a normal or near normal facial nerve result in the long term. Many patients, however, will have weakness or paralysis that may last for weeks or months. In the interim, eye protection must be instituted to prevent corneal ulceration and vision loss. Moisture chambers, lubricating eye drops and ointment, contact lenses and, if necessary, palpebral springs or gold weights are used. If the nerve is disrupted during the procedure, it is repaired at the time. If the nerve is intact at the end of the procedure, and yet no function returns after 1 year, a hypoglossal – facial anastomosis is offered.

Conclusion

In recent years, the diagnosis, treatment and basic understanding of acoustic tumours have experienced remarkable growth. Patients are no longer

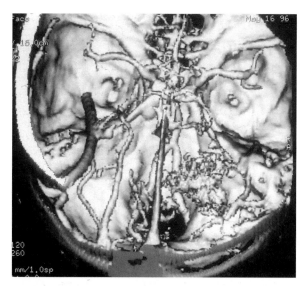

Fig 39.14 Three-dimensional reconstruction, from CT scans, of a large right-sided acoustic neuroma. This is not cited in the text, but is reproduced to end this chapter – and this book – with a demonstration of advanced technological techniques in the service of otology, as we approach the end of this twentieth century. *[Eds.]*

suffering the mortality, from the tumour or the surgery, that they did in years past. Death is an infrequent, if not rare, occurrence after microsurgical removal. Cranial nerve monitoring techniques have facilitated the dissection and will continue to enhance hearing and facial nerve preservation. The basic pathogenesis, on a molecular level, is rapidly being defined. Eventually this may open the avenue to molecular genetic treatment of this problem. The future is exciting, but for the clinician today we have the tools and skills necessary to treat this once lethal disease.

References

1. Cushing H. *Tumors of the nervus acousticus and the syndrome of the cerebellopontine angle, 2nd ed.* New York: Hafner, 1917.
2. House WF. A history of acoustic tumour surgery, 1800-1900, early history. In: House WF, Luetje CM eds. *Acoustic tumours, volume 1: diagnosis.* Los Angeles: House Ear Institute, 1985:3–8.
3. Atkinson WJ. Anterior-inferior cerebellar artery. *Journal of Neurology, Neurosurgery and Psychiatry* 1949; **12**:137–51.
4. Glasscock ME, Overfield RE, Miller GW. Polytomography in an otologic practice. *Southern Medical Journal* 1976; **69**:1433–7.
5. Selters WA, Brackmann DE. Acoustic tumour detection with brain stem electric response audiometry. *Archives of Otolaryngology* 1977; **103**:181–7.
6. Bergeron RT, Cohen NL, Pinto RS. Role of computerized tomography in the diagnosis of acoustic neuromas. *Archives of Otolaryngology* 1977; **103**:314–7.
7. House JW, Waluch V, Jackler RK. Magnetic resonance imaging in acoustic neuroma diagnosis. *Annals of Otology, Rhinology and Laryngology* 1986; **95**:16–20.
8. Jackler RK, Shapiro MS, Dillon WP, Pitts L, Lanser MJ. Gadolinium-DTPA enhanced magnetic resonance imaging in acoustic neuroma diagnosis and management. *Otolaryngology – Head and Neck Surgery* 1990; **102**:670–7.
9. Angeli SI, Jackson C. Neurotologic evaluation. In: House WF, Luetje CM, Doyle KJ eds. *Acoustic tumors: diagnosis and management, 2nd ed.* San Diego, California: Singular, 1997:85–91.
10. Brackmann DE, Arriaga MA. Differential diagnosis of neoplasms of the posterior fossa. In: Cummings CW ed. *Otolaryngology – Head and Neck Surgery.* St. Louis: Mosby-Yearbook, 1993:3271–91.
11. Seizinger BR, Martuza RL, Gusella JF. Loss of genes on chromosome 22 in tumourigenesis of human acoustic neuroma. *Nature* 1986; **322**:644–7.
12. Rouleau GA, Merel P, Lutchman M, Sanson M, Zucman J, Marineau C, et al. Alteration in a new gene encoding a putative membrane-organizing protein causes neuro-fibromatosis type 2. *Nature* 1993; **363**:515–21.
13. Trofatter JA, MacCollin MM, Rutler JL, Murrell JR, Duyao MR, Parry DM, et al. A novel moesin-, ezrin-, radixin-like gene is a candidate for the neurofibromatosis 2 tumour suppressor. *Cell* 1993; **72**:791–800.
14. Evans DG, Huson SM, Donnai D, Neary W, Blair V, Teare D, et al. A genetic study of type 2 neurofibromatosis in the United Kingdom. 1. Prevalence, mutation rate, fitness, and confirmation of maternal transmission effect on severity. *Journal of Medical Genetics* 1992; **25**:841–6.
15. Moffat DA, Hardy DG, Irving RM, Viani L, Beynon GJ, Baguley DM. Referral patterns in vestibular schwannoma. *Clinical Otolaryngology* 1995; **20**:80–3.
16. Tos M, Thomsen J. Epidemiology of acoustic neuromas. *Journal of Laryngology and Otology* 1984; **98**:685–92.
17. Lanser MJ, Sussman SA, Frazer K. Epidemiology, pathogenesis, and genetics of acoustic tumours. *Otolaryngology Clinics of North America* 1992; **25**:499–520.
18. Moffat DA, Irving RM. The molecular genetics of vestibular schwannoma. *Journal of Laryngology and Otology* 1995; **109**:381–4.
19. Selesnick SH, Jackler RK, Pitts LW. The changing clinical presentation of acoustic tumours in the MRI era. *Laryngoscope* 1993. **103**:431–6.
20. Moffat DA, Baguley DM, von Blumenthal H, Irving RM, Hardy DG. Sudden deafness in vestibular schwannoma. *Journal of Laryngology and Otology* 1994; **108**:116–9.

21. Saunders JE, Luxford WM, Devgan KK, Fetterman BL. Sudden hearing loss in acoustic neuroma patients. *Otolaryngology – Head and Neck Surgery* 1995; **113**:23–31.

22. Hitselberger WE, House WF. Acoustic neuroma diagnosis. External auditory canal hypesthesia as an early sign. *Archives of Otolaryngology* 1966; **83**:218–21.

23. Ballagh RH, Moffat DA, Harada T, Baguley DM. The Hitselberger sign and acoustic neuroma diagnosis [Abstract]. *Journal of Laryngology and Otology* 1994; **108**:909.

24. Ballagh RH, Moffat DA, Harada T, Baguley DM. The Hitselberger sign and acoustic neuroma diagnosis [Abstract]. *Otolaryngology – Head and Neck Surgery* 1994; **111**:P108.

25. Chandrasekhar SS, Brackmann DE, Devgan KK. Utility of auditory brainstem response audiometry in diagnosis of acoustic neuromas. *American Journal of Otology* 1995; **16**:63–7.

26. Phelps PD. Fast spin echo MRI in otology. *Journal of Laryngology and Otology* 1994; **108**:383–94.

27. Carrier DA, Arriaga MA. Cost-effective internal auditory canal evaluation with screening, enhanced magnetic resonance imaging. [Abstract]. *Otolaryngology – Head and Neck Surgery* 1995; **113**:P60-1.

28. Lo WWM. Tumours of the cerebellopontine angle. In: Som P, Bergeron RT eds. *Head and neck imaging, 2nd ed.* St Louis: Mosby-Yearbook, 1991:

29. Brackmann DE, House JR III, Hitselberger WE. Technical modifications to the middle fossa craniotomy approach in removal of acoustic neuromas. *American Journal of Otology* 1994; **15**:614–9.

30. McKenna MJ, Halpin C, Ojemann RG, Nadol JB Jr, Montgomery WW, Levine RA, Carlisle E, *et al.* Long-term hearing results in patients after surgical removal of acoustic tumours with hearing preservation. *American Journal of Otology* 1992; **13**:134–6.

31. Shelton C, Hitselberger WE, House WF, Brackmann DE. Long-term results of hearing preservation after acoustic tumour removal. In: Tos M, Thomsen J eds. *Acoustic neuroma. Proceedings of the First International Conference on Acoustic Neuroma 1991.* Amsterdam: Kugler, 1992:661–4.

32. Arriaga MA, Luxford WM, Atkins JS Jr, Kwartler JA. Predicting long-term facial nerve outcome after acoustic neuroma surgery. *Otolaryngology – Head and Neck Surgery* 1993; **108**:220–4.

33. Barker FG II. Efficacy of prophylactic antibiotics for craniotomy. *Neurosurgery* 1994; **35**:484–92.

34. Garcia-Ibàñez E, Garcia-Ibàñez JL. Middle fossa vestibular neurectomy: a report of 373 cases. *Otolaryngology – Head and Neck Surgery* 1980; **88**:486–90.

35. Arriaga M, Gorum M. Enhanced retrosigmoid exposure with posterior semicircular canal resection. *Otolaryngology – Head and Neck Surgery* 1996; **115**:46–8.

36. Bederson JB, von Ammon K, Wichmann WW, Yasargil MG. Conservative treatment of patients with acoustic tumours. *Neurosurgery* 1991; **28**:646–51.

37. Slattery WH, Brackmann DE. Results of surgery following stereotactic irradiation for acoustic neuromas. *American Journal of Otology* 1995; **16**:315–9.

Index

Figures and tables occurring away from their text are indicated in **bold** and *italic* respectively